# Psychiatry: Essential Aspects

# Psychiatry: Essential Aspects

Edited by Fernando Hogan

hayle
medical

New York

Hayle Medical,
750 Third Avenue, 9th Floor,
New York, NY 10017, USA


Visit us on the World Wide Web at:
www.haylemedical.com

ISBN: 978-1-63241-739-8

**Cataloging-in-Publication Data**

Psychiatry : essential aspects / edited by Fernando Hogan.
    p. cm.
Includes bibliographical references and index.
ISBN 978-1-63241-739-8
1. Psychiatry. 2. Psychology, Pathological. 3. Mental health.
4. Medicine and psychology. I. Hogan, Fernando.
RC454 .P79 2019
616.89--dc23

# Table of Contents

**Permissions**

**List of Contributors**

**Index**

# Preface

Psychiatry is a field of science and medicine that deals with mental disorders. It involves the study of several maladaptations related to perception, behavior and mood. Mental disorders and personality disorders are two of the main types of disorders treated under psychiatry. A mental disorder is a behavioral or mental pattern which causes impairment of personal functioning. Disorders related to the maladaptive patterns of behavior, cognition, inner experience and the act of deviating from the generally acceptable behavior patterns are classified as personality disorder. Psychotherapy and psychiatric medication are two of the most common ways to treat psychiatric disorders. This book studies, analyzes and upholds the pillars of psychiatry and its utmost significance in modern times. It strives to provide a fair idea about this discipline and to help develop a better understanding of the latest advances within this field. The book is appropriate for students seeking detailed information in this area as well as for experts.

This book is a result of research of several months to collate the most relevant data in the field.

When I was approached with the idea of this book and the proposal to edit it, I was overwhelmed. It gave me an opportunity to reach out to all those who share a common interest with me in this field. I had 3 main parameters for editing this text:

1. Accuracy – The data and information provided in this book should be up-to-date and valuable to the readers.

2. Structure – The data must be presented in a structured format for easy understanding and better grasping of the readers.

3. Universal Approach – This book not only targets students but also experts and innovators in the field, thus my aim was to present topics which are of use to all.

Thus, it took me a couple of months to finish the editing of this book.

I would like to make a special mention of my publisher who considered me worthy of this opportunity and also supported me throughout the editing process. I would also like to thank the editing team at the back-end who extended their help whenever required.

**Editor**

# Personality functioning in anxiety disorders

Stephan Doering[1]* [iD], Victor Blüml[1], Karoline Parth[1,2], Karin Feichtinger[1], Maria Gruber[3], Martin Aigner[4], Hemma Rössler-Schülein[5], Marion Freidl[3] and Antonia Wininger[1]

## Abstract

**Background:** The Alternative DSM-5 Model for Personality Disorders as well as the upcoming IDC-11 have established a new focus on diagnosing personality disorders (PD): personality functioning. An impairment of self and interpersonal functioning in these models represents a general diagnostic criterion for a personality disorder. Little is known so far about the impairment of personality functioning in patients with other mental disorders than PD. This study aims to assess personality functioning in patients with anxiety disorders.

**Methods:** Ninety-seven patients with the diagnosis of generalized anxiety disorder, panic disorder, or phobia, and 16 healthy control persons were diagnosed using the Structured Clinical Interview for DSM-IV (SCID-I and -II) and were assessed by means of the Structured Interview for Personality Organization (STIPO) to determine the level of personality functioning.

**Results:** While all three patient groups showed significant impairment in personality functioning compared to the control group, no significant differences were observed between the different patient groups. In all three groups of anxiety disorders patients with comorbid PD showed significantly worse personality functioning than patients without. Patients without comorbid PD also yielded a significant impairment in their personality functioning when compared to the control group.

**Conclusions:** Anxiety disorders are associated with a significant impairment in personality functioning, which is significantly increased by comorbid PD. There are no differences in terms of personality functioning between patients with different anxiety disorders.

**Keywords:** Personality functioning, Generalized anxiety disorder, Panic disorder, Phobia, Personality disorder

## Background

Personality functioning has been introduced into the diagnosis of personality disorders (PD) by the two new classifications of mental disorders. Section III of the fifth edition of the Diagnostic and Statistical Manual of Mental Disorders (DSM-5) [1] contains an Alternative Model for Personality Disorders (AMPD; p. 761). In this model the general criterion A for PD is a "moderate or greater impairment in personality (self/interpersonal) functioning" (p. 761). This impairment is assessed by means of the DSM-5 Levels of Personality Functioning Scale (p.775) that comprises four dimensions: (1) self: identity, (2) self: self-direction, (3) interpersonal: empathy, and (4) interpersonal: intimacy. The so called beta draft of the upcoming International Classification of Diseases

(ICD-11) contains a very similar description of "problems in functioning" as a general diagnostic criterion for PD, consisting of impaired functioning of "aspects of the self (e.g., identity, self-worth, accuracy of self-view, self-direction), and/or interpersonal dysfunction (e.g., ability to develop and maintain close and mutually satisfying relationships, ability to understand others' perspectives and to manage conflict in relationships)" [2, 3].

Mental health and, as a consequence, psychosocial functioning are not only determined by the presence or absence of psychopathological symptoms, but also by basic functions of personality. In psychoanalytic theory, these functions are subsumed under the heading of psychic structure. Synonyms like personality structure, personality organization, or personality function are used frequently. Historically, Sigmund Freud was the first one who conceptualized psychic structure within his topographical model of conscious, preconscious, and unconscious psychic realms [4]. Later he developed his

---

* Correspondence: stephan.doering@meduniwien.ac.at
[1]Department of Psychoanalysis and Psychotherapy, Medical University of Vienna, Währinger Gürtel 18-20, A-1090 Wien, Austria
Full list of author information is available at the end of the article

structural model by separating the ego, the id, and the super-ego as psychic structures [5]. Hartmann emphasized the relevance of ego functions for psychosocial adaptation as opposed to neurotic conflicts in the aetiology of mental disorders [6]. In his conceptual work Kernberg [7, 8] elaborated the impact of early experiences in relationships on the maturation of psychic structure or – in his words – personality organization. He was the first to define different levels of personality functioning and developed the *Structural Interview* as a clinical instrument for the assessment of personality organization [9]. The Structural Interview focuses key dimensions of personality function, i.e., identity integration, quality of object relations, defence mechanisms, superego integration (moral values), aggression, and reality testing. According to Kernberg, individuals with good (normal/ neurotic) personality functioning show a consolidated identity, good quality of object relations, mature defence mechanisms, solid moral values and behaviour, secure reality testing, and are able to control their aggressive impulses. Patients with impaired personality function (Kernberg coined the term "borderline personality organization" for this group) suffer from identity diffusion, i.e., their internal images of the self and significant others are contradictory, superficial, and not integrated. Moreover, they are not able to maintain stable interpersonal relationships, are vulnerable to stress (employ primitive defence mechanisms), suffer from impaired impulse control, especially in terms of self-directed and other-directed aggression, and tend to have less stable moral values and behaviour. The most severely disturbed patients function on a psychotic level. In addition to an even worse personality functioning in all of the described domains they suffer from an impaired reality testing.

Since the Structural Interview is a clinical tool that does not allow for a reliable quantification of personality functioning, Kernberg and colleagues developed the Structured Interview for Personality organization (STIPO) [10] for research purposes. This 100-item interview addresses the domains mentioned above and results in a profile of personality functioning on seven dimensions and a total score on a six-point scale. The interview has been validated in its English original version and the German translation [11, 12]. The STIPO contains seven dimensions (see Methods section), the first two of which – identity and object relations – correspond to the two dimensions of the AMPD of DSM-5 and the personality functioning domains of the ICD-11 draft [1, 2].

During the last decade, a growing number of studies have been published that focus on personality functioning. It was demonstrated that patients with PD, especially borderline, show a worse personality functioning compared to patients with previously so called axis I disorders [11, 13], and that a higher symptom severity in borderline patients goes along with worse personality functioning [14]. However, very few studies have yet assessed personality functioning in disorders other than PD, e.g. in substance use disorders [15, 16].

The investigation of personality functioning in anxiety disorders seems of particular interest, since theoretical assumptions postulate different levels of functioning in different anxiety disorders. Eckhardt-Henn et al. (p.91) published a model that assigned the lowest level of personality functioning to patients with generalized anxiety disorder, a higher one to agoraphobic and panic disorder patients, and the highest one to individuals with specific phobias [17].

This study was undertaken to test the hypothesis that patients with different anxiety disorders reveal different levels of personality functioning, by assessing mental disorders including PD (formerly axis I and II disorders) according to DSM-IV [18] as well as personality functioning.

## Methods

### Study design

This study was approved by the ethics committee of the Medical University of Vienna, Austria on March 27, 2012 (IRB No. 1037/2012). After receiving detailed information about the study all subjects gave written informed consent. Patients and control subjects were diagnosed according to DSM-IV [18] by means of SCID-I and -II [19, 20] and underwent the Structured Interview for Personality Organization (STIPO) [10].

The patients were recruited between 2012 and 2017 at (1) the outpatient unit of the Department of Psychoanalysis and Psychotherapy, (2) the inpatient and outpatient units of the Department of Psychiatry and Psychotherapy, Division of Social Psychiatry of the Medical University of Vienna, (3) the Department of Psychiatry of the University Hospital Tulln, and (4) the outpatient clinic of the Vienna Psychoanalytic Society. In addition, a healthy control group from the community was recruited. In these individuals a screening with the Brief Symptom Inventory (BSI) [21] took place before the interviews (results are not reported here). All patients and control subjects received a compensation of € 50 for the participation in the study.

### Subjects

Inclusion criteria for all subjects were: (1) age ≥ 18 years and (2) sufficient knowledge of the German language. An additional inclusion criterion for patients was: (3) diagnosis of generalized anxiety disorder or panic disorder or specific phobia.

Exclusion criteria for all patients were: (1) organic brain disease, (2) mental disease with cognitive impairment (dementia, acute psychosis, severe depression), (3) substance dependence with acute intoxication, (4) comorbidity of two or all of the above mentioned anxiety disorders. Exclusion criteria for control subjects were:

(5) a GSI (Global Severity Index) > 0.26 in the BSI screening and (6) any DSM-IV diagnosis according to SCID-I and -II.

## Instruments
### Demographic data
The following demographic data were collected by means of a questionnaire: name, age, gender, marital status, educational status, and occupational status.

### Structured clinical interview for DSM-IV (SCID-I and -II)
The SCID represents the American Psychiatric Association's official instrument for the diagnosis of mental disorders according to DSM-IV. The structured interview contains questions addressing every single diagnostic criterion of the mental disorders of DSM-IV. The interview consists of two parts: SCID-I [20] for the assessment of all mental disorders except PD, which are evaluated by the SCID-II [19].

### Structured interview for personality organization (STIPO)
The STIPO [10] was developed by Otto F. Kernberg and colleagues at the Cornell University New York. It represents the structured version of the Structural Interview that was developed by Kernberg in the 1980s [8, 9]. The interview contains 100 items that are addressed by one or more specific questions. The single-item rating is made by the interviewer on a three point scale with operationalized descriptions for each level: 0 = pathology absent, 1 = minor impairment, 2 = significant to severe impairment. The interview covers seven domains: (1) identity, (2) object relations, (3) primitive defences, (4) coping/rigidity, (5) aggression, (6) moral values, and (7) reality testing and perceptual distortions. Two different scoring systems can be used: (a) Guided by operationalized anchors each domain and subdomain is rated on a five-point scale with "1" standing for the absence of pathology to "5" indicating most severe impairment of personality functioning, an overall rating is generated from the ratings of the seven dimensions; (b) the arithmetic mean values are calculated for all dimensions and sub-dimensions from the single item scores (range: 0–2). Based on scoring system (a) six different levels of personality organization (i.e., personality functioning) are provided for the overall rating: (1) normal, (2) neurotic 1, (3) neurotic 2, (4) borderline 1, (5) borderline 2, and (6) borderline 3. Satisfactory reliability and validity of the English as well as of the German version of the instrument have been demonstrated [10, 11].

Both interviews were conducted by four well-trained postgraduate psychologists or medical doctors (A.F., K.F., K. P., M.G.) with proven reliability for the STIPO (ICC with expert ratings ≥0.7). One interviewer conducted both interviews in one and the same patient.

## Statistics
T-tests and one-way ANOVA were used for group comparisons of the level of personality functioning. Due to multiple testing in the group comparisons of the STIPO dimensions Bonferroni correction was employed and a level of significance of $p < 0.006$ was defined. Linear regression analyses were calculated for the evaluation of the effects of the type of anxiety disorder and comorbidity with personality disorder(s). IBM SPSS Statistics 24 (IBM Corporation, Armonk, New York, USA) was employed.

## Results
### Sample characteristics
In total, 97 patients and 16 healthy control subjects were included into the study. In the patient group, 22 were suffering from generalized anxiety disorder, 47 had panic disorder (with or without agoraphobia), and 22 phobias. Demographic data and diagnoses according to DSM-IV (American Psychiatric Association 1994) are given in Table 1. Regarding disorders other than PD (including the anxiety disorder) 26 (26.8%) had one diagnosis, 37 (38.1%) had two, 22 (22.7%) had three, 9 (9.3%) four, and 3 (3.1%) five or more diagnoses. Sixty-three (64.9%) were suffering from a comorbid personality disorder. Twenty-two (22.7%) had one personality disorder, 23 (23.7%) had two, 14 (14.4%) three, 2 (2.1%) four, and 2 (2.1%) five or more. There were no significant differences regarding comorbidity between the three groups of patients with anxiety disorders.

### Tests for normality of homogeneity of variance
Before using t-tests and ANOVA, tests for normality and homogeneity of variance were conducted. Neither the presence of PD nor the STIPO overall scores were normally distributed in the three subgroups of anxiety disorders. Shapiro-Wilk statistics for presence of PD in the three groups ranged from W = .508 to .628 with $p < .001$ and for the STIPO overall score W = .865 to .896 with $p < .001$, except for GAD with $p = .011$.

However, no significant inhomogeneity of variances occurred in the above mentioned subgroups. For this reason, it was decided to use the parametric tests the results of which are reported below.

### Level of personality functioning in the groups of anxiety disorders
There were no significant differences between the different groups of patients with anxiety disorders regarding their level of personality functioning (see Table 2). The total mean score of the STIPO differed almost not at all. The mean values of 3.55 to 3.68 depict a moderate impairment of general personality functioning, or in terms of the STIPO model an organization between lower neurotic and higher borderline functioning. Compared to the healthy control group with a mean STIPO score of 1.50, all three patient

**Table 1** Sample characteristics ($n = 113$)

| | Phobias ($n = 28$) | Panic disorder ($n = 47$) | GAD ($n = 22$) | Controls ($n = 16$) |
|---|---|---|---|---|
| | Mean (s.d.) | Mean (s.d.) | Mean (s.d.) | Mean (s.d.) |
| Age (years) | 30.96 (14.72) range: 18–73 | 35.26 (13.48) range: 19–74 | 36.55 (13.89) range: 19–70 | 31.88 (14.49) range: 20–60 |
| | n (%) | n (%) | n (%) | n (%) |
| Gender | | | | |
| Female | 17 (60.7) | 32 (68.1) | 18 (81.8) | 12 (75.0) |
| Male | 11 (39.3) | 15 (31.9) | 4 (18.2) | 4 (25.0) |
| Education | | | | |
| No compulsory school | 0 (0.0) | 0 (0.0) | 0 (0.0) | 0 (0.0) |
| Compulsory school | 5 (17.9) | 11 (23.4) | 5 (22.7) | 0 (0.0) |
| Apprenticeship/ vocational school | 9 (32.1) | 11 (23.4) | 6 (27.3) | 3 (18.8) |
| High school | 13 (46.4) | 17 (36.2) | 8 (36.4) | 10 (62.5) |
| Academic | 0 (0.0) | 4 (8.5) | 3 (13.6) | 3 (18.8) |
| Other | 1 (3.6) | 3 (6.4) | 0 (0.0) | 0 (0.0) |
| Missing | 0 (0.0) | 1 (2.1) | 0 (0.0) | 0 (0.0) |
| Employment | | | | |
| In occupational training | 6 (21.4) | 6 (12.8) | 4 (18.2) | 7 (43.8) |
| Unemployed | 10 (35.7) | 12 (25.5) | 8 (36.4) | 0 (0.0) |
| Part-time | 1 (3.6) | 8 (17.0) | 4 (18.2) | 5 (31.3) |
| Full-time | 4 (14.3) | 11 (23.4) | 1 (4.5) | 3 (18.8) |
| Homemaker | 1 (3.6) | 2 (4.3) | 1 (4.5) | 0 (0.0) |
| Retired | 4 (14.3) | 7 (14.9) | 4 (18.2) | 1 (6.3) |
| Missing | 2 (7.1) | 1 (2.1) | 0 (0.0) | 0 (0.0) |
| Family status | | | | |
| Single | 16 (57.1) | 20 (42.6) | 8 (36.4) | 3 (18.8) |
| Unmarried with partner | 9 (32.1) | 12 (25.5) | 5 (22.7) | 9 (56.3) |
| Married | 2 (7.1) | 11 (23.4) | 6 (27.3) | 3 (18.8) |
| Divorced/ separated | 1 (3.6) | 2 (4.3) | 3 (13.6) | 1 (6.3) |
| Widowed | 0 (0.0) | 1 (2.1) | 0 (0.0) | 0 (0.0) |
| Missing values | 0 (0.0) | 1 (2.1) | 0 (0.0) | 0 (0.0) |
| DSM-IV diagnoses other than PD (anxiety disorders excluded)[a] | | | n | |
| Substance abuse disorders | 4 | 15 | 2 | 0 |
| Mood disorders | 20 | 32 | 14 | 0 |
| Brief psychotic disorder | 1 | 2 | 0 | 0 |
| Posttraumatic stress disorder | 2 | 3 | 1 | 0 |
| Obsessive-compulsive disorder | 7 | 5 | 0 | 0 |
| Somatoform disorders | 3 | 2 | 0 | 0 |
| Eating disorders | 2 | 3 | 2 | 0 |
| Adjustment disorders | 1 | 0 | 0 | 0 |
| DSM-IV PD Diagnoses[a] | | | n | |
| Paranoid | 5 | 7 | 1 | 0 |
| Schizoid | 0 | 0 | 0 | 0 |
| Schizotypal | 0 | 0 | 0 | 0 |
| Obsessive-compulsive | 6 | 1 | 0 | 0 |

5

**Table 1** Sample characteristics (*n* = 113) *(Continued)*

| | Phobias (*n* = 28) Mean (s.d.) | Panic disorder (*n* = 47) Mean (s.d.) | GAD (*n* = 22) Mean (s.d.) | Controls (*n* = 16) Mean (s.d.) |
|---|---|---|---|---|
| Histrionic | 0 | 2 | 0 | 0 |
| Dependent | 4 | 2 | 2 | 0 |
| Antisocial | 1 | 0 | 0 | 0 |
| Narcissistic | 0 | 1 | 1 | 0 |
| Avoidant | 14 | 15 | 7 | 0 |
| Borderline | 10 | 9 | 4 | 0 |
| Depressive | 11 | 12 | 6 | 0 |
| Passive-aggressive | 0 | 2 | 1 | 0 |

*PD* personality disorder, *GAD* generalized anxiety disorder
[a]More than one diagnosis per patient included

groups showed significant impairment. The distribution of the level of personality organization in the four groups is depicted in Table 3. Post-hoc comparisons (least significant difference; Bonferroni corrected level of significance *p* < .004) revealed highly significant differences between controls and all three groups of anxiety disorders (*p* < .001) and non-significant results between the groups of anxiety disorders (*p* = .625 to .838).

In correspondence to the overall score, the seven dimensions of the STIPO did not show relevant differences between the groups of anxiety disorders. Within all groups the best personality functioning occurred in the domain of moral values, which indicates a low level of antisocial tendencies. Also the aggression and reality testing domains yielded slightly higher levels of personality functioning than the remaining scales.

### Comorbid personality disorders and level of personality functioning

In view of the high number of comorbid personality disorder diagnoses in the sample it was tested, whether a PD is of more relevance for personality functioning than the type of anxiety disorder.

A linear regression analysis was conducted to further explore the influence of anxiety disorders as well as comorbid PD on personality functioning. It turned out that only the presence of a PD was significantly associated to with personality functioning, but not any of the three anxiety disorders - a comorbid PD impaired personality functioning ($T = 8.121$, $p < .001$).

However, an ANOVA excluding all patients with PD still yielded a significantly worse personality functioning in patients compared to controls (F = 14.020, df = 3, $p < .001$). Patients without comorbid PD showed a moderate impairment of personality function with a mean STIPO score of around 3, which indicates a lower neurotic level, whereas patients with comorbid PD revealed a mean STIPO score around 4, which stands for a higher borderline organization (see Table 4).

Finally, when all 113 subjects were included in a correlation analysis of number of PDs diagnosed and the

**Table 2** Personality organization in the different groups of anxiety disorders (*n* = 113)

| | Phobias (*n* = 28) Mean (s.d.) | Panic disorder (*n* = 47) Mean (s.d.) | GAD (*n* = 22) Mean (s.d.) | Controls (*n* = 16) Mean (s.d.) | ANOVA (including controls) F | df | $p^a$ | ANOVA (without controls) F | df | $p^a$ |
|---|---|---|---|---|---|---|---|---|---|---|
| STIPO dimensions | | | | | | | | | | |
| Identity | 2.79 (±0.83) | 2.62 (±0.85) | 2.64 (±0.95) | 1.25 (±0.45) | 13.88 | 3 | <.001 | 0.35 | 3 | .70 |
| Object relations | 2.68 (±0.86) | 2.51 (±0.98) | 2.45 (±0.91) | 1.44 (±0.63) | 7.34 | 3 | <.001 | 0.43 | 3 | .66 |
| Primitve defenses | 2.86 (±0.85) | 2.70 (±0.98) | 2.77 (±0.92) | 1.19 (±0.40) | 15.01 | 3 | <.001 | 0.27 | 3 | .78 |
| Coping/ rigidity | 3.43 (±0.69) | 3.04 (±0.81) | 3.36 (±0.79) | 1.56 (±0.51) | 25.03 | 3 | <.001 | 2.65 | 3 | .08 |
| Aggression | 1.89 (±0.88) | 2.09 (±0.91) | 2.05 (±1.09) | 1.00 (±0.00) | 6.53 | 3 | <.001 | 0.38 | 3 | .69 |
| Moral values | 1.61 (±0.69) | 1.60 (±0.71) | 1.68 (±0.95) | 1.19 (±0.54) | 1.64 | 3 | .19 | 0.10 | 3 | .91 |
| Reality testing and perceptual distortions | 2.04 (±1.04) | 2.26 (±1.01) | 1.86(±1.04) | 1.13 (±0.34) | 5.66 | 3 | .001 | 1.18 | 3 | .31 |
| Total score | 3.68 (±0.95) | 3.60 (±1.04) | 3.55 (0.96) | 1.50 (±0.63) | 22.52 | 3 | <.001 | 0.12 | 3 | .89 |

*GAD* generalized anxiety disorder, *ANOVA* analysis of variance, *STIPO* Structured Interview for Personality Organization
[a]Bonferroni corrected, level of significance *p* < 0.006

**Table 3** Personality organization in the different groups of anxiety disorders (*n* = 113)

|  | Phobias (*n* = 28) | Panic disorder (*n* = 47) | GAD (*n* = 22) | Controls (*n* = 16) |
|---|---|---|---|---|
|  | n (%) | n (%) | n (%) | n (%) |
| STIPO level of personality organization |  |  |  |  |
| 1 – normal | 0 (0.0) | 0 (0.0) | 0 (0.0) | 9 (56.3) |
| 2 – neurotic 1 | 2 (7.1) | 7 (14.9) | 2 (9.1) | 6 (37.5) |
| 3 – neurotic 2 | 11 (39.3) | 17 (36.2) | 10 (45.5) | 1 (6.3) |
| 4 – borderline 1 | 10 (35.7) | 11 (23.4) | 7 (31.8) | 0 (0.0) |
| 5 – borderline 2 | 4 (14.3) | 12 (25.5) | 2 (9.1) | 0 (0.0) |
| 6 – borderline 3 | 1 (3.6) | 0 (0.0) | 1 (4.5) | 0 (0.0) |

*GAD* generalized anxiety disorder, *STIPO* Structured Interview for Personality Organization

STIPO overall score a highly significant correlation emerged ($r$ = 0.596, $p$ < .01).

## Discussion

Our data demonstrate that anxiety disorders are associated with an impaired personality functioning, which is moderate when no comorbid personality disorder is present and more severe in case of comorbid PD. There are no differences in personality functioning between phobias, GAD, and panic disorder, either with or without comorbid PD.

The hypothesis derived from psychoanalytic theory that GAD patients are characterized by a worse personality functioning followed by panic disorder patients and phobia patients with the best functioning could therefore not be confirmed. In contrast, it seems that anxiety disorders can occur on all levels of personality organization from mild impairment ("high neurotic level") to the lowest level ("low borderline level") (see Table 3). It is possible that in first level care settings patients with anxiety disorders with higher personality function can be found

compared to patients in our study of secondary and tertiary care settings. In a Swedish study by Sundquist et al. about half of the patients with PD were only present in the primary care setting and never showed up in secondary or tertiary care settings [22].

The pattern of personality functioning within the seven domains of the STIPO seems to reflect the comparably high ratio of avoidant and depressive PD and the lower prevalence of Cluster A and B PD in the sample (see Table 1). One might assume that Cluster C PD show a higher impairment in the realms of relational functioning as well as coping with and defending against stress. However, the validity study of the German version of the STIPO [10] revealed a similar pattern in a sample with a much higher ratio of Cluster A and B PD. Thus, personality functioning appears to be rather independent from the symptoms and characteristics of specific PDs.

A very high comorbidity between anxiety disorders and PDs has previously been shown. Grant et al. [23] reported from the National epidemiologic survey on alcohol and related conditions (NESARC) that in 41.8% of patients with any anxiety disorder a comorbid personality disorder is present. In treatment seeking patients with anxiety disorders this number rises to 59.6%. Thus, our finding of 64.9% of comorbid PDs in a population from psychiatric in- and outpatient units is in line with this earlier finding. It can be assumed that a study recruiting subjects with anxiety disorders outside the mental health care system would have found somewhat lower rates of comorbid PDs and, thus, a slightly better personality functioning.

Our study adds to these previous findings the result that even in absence of a personality disorder patients with an anxiety disorder show significant impairment in their personality functioning. As a consequence, the treatment of patients with anxiety disorders should take into consideration the presence of personality problems.

**Table 4** Personality organization (STIPO overall scores) in the different groups of anxiety disorders with and without comorbid personality disorders (*n* = 97)

|  | STIPO level of personality organization | ANOVA | | |
|---|---|---|---|---|
|  | Mean (s.d.) | F | df | p |
| Anxiety disorder |  |  |  |  |
| Phobias without PD (*n* = 6) | 2.83 (±0.75) |  |  |  |
| Phobias with PD (*n* = 22) | 3.91 (±0.87) | −2.76 | 26 | .011 |
| Panic disorder without PD (*n* = 19) | 2.84 (±0.83) |  |  |  |
| Panic disorder with PD (*n* = 28) | 4.11 (±0.83) | −5.11 | 45 | <.001 |
| GAD without PD (*n* = 9) | 3.11 (±0.60) |  |  |  |
| GAD with PD (*n* = 13) | 3.85 (±1.07) | −1.86 | 20 | .077 |
| All patients without PD (*n* = 34) | 2.91 (±0.75) |  |  |  |
| All patients with PD (*n* = 63) | 3.98 (±0.89) | −5.97 | 95 | <.001 |

*PD* comorbid personality disorder, *GAD* generalized anxiety disorder, *ANOVA* Analysis of Variance, *STIPO* Structured Interview for Personality Organization

On the one hand, a diagnosis of personality functioning as well as PD should be mandatory in every patient. The newly developed instruments for the assessment of the levels of personality functioning according to DSM-5 serve this purpose, e.g., the self-report form of the DSM-5 Level of Personality Functioning Scale [24, 25]. Moreover, well-established questionnaires and interviews exist that can be employed. For example, the Inventory of Personality Organization (IPO) [26, 27], the Structured Interview for Personality Organization (STIPO) [10, 11], and the Operationalized Psychodynamic Diagnosis (OPD-2) [28]. It has recently been shown that the DSM-5 levels of personality functioning can be reliably assessed by untrained raters from audio-recorded STIPO interviews [29] as well as OPD-2 interviews [30]. For a general assessment of personality function and screening purposes, the DSM-5 LPFS or questionnaires can be used, while the multidimensional and more extensive interviews like the STIPO or OPD-2 yield a much more comprehensive assessment of the different domains of personality functioning, which is highly valuable for clinical treatment planning as well as for detailed research questions.

On the other hand many treatment failures in patients with anxiety disorders might be attributable to impaired personality functioning and comorbid PD [31–33]. This is of high clinical relevance, since it is known, that treatment response rates are low, e.g. 48% in generalized anxiety disorder as reported by Hunot et al. [34] in their Cochrane review. If one assumes, that most of the randomized-controlled treatment studies exclude patients with comorbid PD, the relevance of sub-threshold/ mild impairment of personality functioning might be of even greater importance for treatment outcome. Personality functioning can be improved by psychotherapy, which has been shown by Doering et al. [35], but it will need specialized treatment approaches that focus not only on symptoms of the anxiety disorder, but also on specific domains of the patient's personality [36]. If we follow the presumption that personality pathology complicates the treatment of anxiety disorders and has to be addressed before sustainable symptom remission can occur, specific treatments should be offered to patients with both, anxiety disorder and impaired personality functioning. Treatments that have demonstrated their efficacy in improving personality functioning are Transference-focused Psychotherapy (TFP) [35, 37–39] and - with some limitations due to the lack of specific outcome criteria in the conducted RCTs - Schema-focused Psychotherapy (SFT) [40, 41], Mentalization-based Treatment (MBT) [42–44], and Dialectical Behavior Therapy (DBT) [45, 46].

Limitations of this study can be found in the relatively low sample size in two of the three groups of patients with anxiety disorders, and in the recruitment at psychiatric hospital units. This reduces the generalizability of the absolute numbers regarding personality functioning in anxiety disorders, which probably is somewhat better in the general population than in the treatment seeking sub-population. However, the result that all anxiety disorders occur on almost all levels of personality functioning can be regarded as mainly independent from the recruitment bias. In future studies with larger sample sizes it will be interesting to evaluate the specific influence of cluster B vs. cluster A or C PDs, or even of specific PDs like borderline.

## Conclusions

An impairment of personality functioning is highly frequent in all anxiety disorders and has to be taken into consideration for diagnosis and treatment of patients with anxiety disorders. There are no differences between the anxiety disorders with regard to their personality functioning, and comorbid PD further impair personality functioning.

**Abbreviations**
AMPD: Alternative Model for Personality Disorders; ANOVA: Analysis of Variance; BSI: Brief Symptom Inventory; DBT: Dialectical Behavior Therapy; DSM-5: Diagnostic and Statistical Manual of Mental Disorders – Fifth Edition; DSM-IV: Diagnostic and Statistical Manual of Mental Disorders – Fourth Edition; GAD: Generalized Anxiety Disorder; GSI: Global Severity Index; ICC: Intraclass Correlation; ICD-11: International Classification of Mental and Behavioral Disorders, 11th Revision; IPO: Inventory of Personality Organization; LPFS: Levels of Personality Functioning Scale; MBT: Mentalization-based Treatment; NESARC: National Epidemiologic Survey on Alcohol and Related Conditions; OPD-2: Operationalized Psychodynamic Diagnosis, Second Edition; PD: Personality Disorder; SCID-I: Structured Clinical Interview for DSM-IV, Axis I; SCID-II: Structured Clinical Interview for DSM-IV, Axis II; SFT: Schema-focused Psychotherapy; STIPO: Structured Interview of Personality Organization; TFP: Transference-focused Psychotherapy

**Funding**
This study was funded by the Jubilaeumsfonds of the Austrian National Bank, project # 15078. The funding body did not take any influence on the design of the study and collection, analysis, and interpretation of the data and on writing the manuscript.

**Authors' contributions**
SD developed the study design, carried out the statistical analyses, and drafted the manuscript, AW, KP, KF, MG recruited the patients, have been responsible for data acquisition, VB, MF, HRS, MA contributed substantially to data analyses and interpretation of data. All authors contributed substantially to a number of revisions of the manuscript and gave final approval for its submission.

**Consent for publication**
Not applicable.

## Competing interests

None of the authors reports any competing interests. Stephan Doering and Victor Blueml are currently acting as Associate Editors for BMC Psychiatry.

## Author details

[1]Department of Psychoanalysis and Psychotherapy, Medical University of Vienna, Währinger Gürtel 18-20, A-1090 Wien, Austria. [2]Department of Psychology, Webster Vienna Private University, Wien, Austria. [3]Department of Social Psychiatry, Medical University of Vienna, Wien, Austria. [4]Department of Psychiatry, University Hospital Tulln, Tulln, Austria. [5]Vienna Psychoanalytic Society, Wien, Austria.

## References

1. American Psychiatric Association. Diagnostic and Statistical Manual. 5th ed. Washington, DC: American Psychiatric Publishing; 2013.
2. Reed GM. Progress in developing a classification of personality disorders for ICD-11. World Psychiatry. 2018;17(2):227–9.
3. World Health Organization. ICD-11 for Mortality and Morbidity Statistics (ICD-11 MMS) 2018 version. 6D10 Personality disorder. https://icd.who.int/browse11/l-m/en#/http%3a%2f%2fid.who.int%2ficd%2fentity%2f941859884 (2018). Accessed 9 August 2018.
4. Freud S. Die Traumdeutung. Gesammelte Werke Bd. II/III. Frankfurt am Main: Fischer Taschenbuchverlag; 1900/1999.
5. Freud S. Das ich und das Es. Gesammelte Werke Bd. XIII. Frankfurt am Main: Fischer Taschenbuchverlag; 1923/1999. p. 235–89.
6. Hartmann H. Ich-Psychologie und Anpassungsproblem. Int Z Psychoanal Imago. 1939;24:62–135.
7. Kernberg OF. Borderline conditions and pathological narcissism. New York: Jason Aronson; 1975.
8. Kernberg OF. Severe personality disorders. New Haven: Yale University Press; 1984.
9. Kernberg OF. The structural interviewing. Psychiatr Clin North Am. 1981;4: 169–95.
10. Clarkin JF, Caligor E, Stern B, Kernberg OF. Structured interview of personality organization (STIPO). New York: Weill Medical College of Cornell University; 2003.
11. Stern BL, Caligor E, Clarkin JF, Critchfield KL, Hörz S, Maccornack V, Lenzenweger MF, Kernberg OF. Structured interview of personality organization (STIPO): preliminary psychometrics in a clinical sample. J Pers Assess. 2010;92:35–44.
12. Doering S, Burgmer M, Heuft G, Menke D, Bäumer B, Lübking M, Feldmann M, Hörz S, Schneider G. Reliability and validity of the German version of the structured interview of personality organization (STIPO). BMC Psychiatry. 2013;13:210.
13. Huber D, Klug G, Wallerstein RS. Skalen psychischer Kompetenzen (SPK). Ein Messinstrument für therapeutische Veränderung in der psychischen Struktur. Incl. Manual und Interviewleitfaden. Stuttgart: Kohlhammer; 2006.
14. Hörz S, Rentrop M, Fischer-Kern M, Schuster P, Kapusta N, Buchheim P, Doering S. Strukturniveau und klinischer Schweregrad der Borderline-Persönlichkeitsstörung. Z Psychosom Med Psychother. 2010;56(2):136–49.
15. Rentrop M, Zilker T, Lederle A, Birkhofer A, Hörz S. Psychiatric comorbidity and personality structure in patients with polyvalent addiction. Psychopathology. 2014;47(2):133–40.
16. Di Pierro R, Preti E, Vurro N, Mededdu F. Dimensions of personality structure among patients with substance use disorders and co-occuring personality disorders: a comparison with psychiatric outpatients and healthy controls. Compr Psychiatry. 2014;55(6):1398–404.
17. Eckhardt-Henn A, Heuft G, Hochapfel G, Hoffmann SO. Neurotische Störungen und Psychosomatische Medizin. 8. Auflage ed. Stuttgart: Schattauer; 2009.
18. American Psychiatric Association. Diagnostic and Statistical Manual. 4th ed. Washington, DC: American Psychiatric Publishing; 1994.
19. Fydrich T, Renneberg B, Schmitz B, Wittchen HU. Strukturiertes Klinisches Interview für DSM-IV Achse II: Persönlichkeitsstörungen. Göttingen: Hogrefe; 1997.
20. Wittchen HU, Zaudig M, SKID-I FT. Strukturiertes Klinisches Interview für DSM-IV, Achse I. Göttingen: Hogrefe; 1997.
21. Franke RB. BSI: brief symptom inventory von Derogatis - deutsche version. Göttingen: Beltz; 2000.
22. Sundquist J, Ohlsson H, Sundquist K, Kendler KS. Common adult psychiatric disorders in Swedish primary care where most mental health patients are treated. BMC Psychiatry. 2017;17:235.
23. Grant BF, Hasin DS, Stinson FS, Dawson DA, Chou SP, Ruan WJ, Huang B. Co-occurence of 12-month mood and anxiety disorders and personality disorders in the US: results from the national epidemiologic survey on alcohol and related conditions. J Psychiatr Res. 2005;39:1–9.
24. Morey LC. Development and initial evaluation of a self-report form of the DSM-5 Level of Personality Functioning Scale. Psychol Assess. 2017; 29(10):1302–8.
25. Hopwood CJ, Good EW, Morey LC. Validity of the DSM-5 levels of personality functioning scale-self report. J Pers Assess. 2018; https://doi.org/10.1080/00223891.2017.1420660.
26. Clarkin JF, Foelsch PA, Kernberg OF. The inventory of personality organization (IPO). Unpublished manuscript. New York: Weill Medical College of Cornell University; 1995.
27. Lenzenweger MF, Clarkin JF, Kernberg OF, Foelsch PA. The inventory of personality organization: psychometric properties, factorial composition, and criterion relations with affect, aggressive dyscontrol, psychosis proneness, and self-domains in a nonclinical sample. Psychol Assess. 2001;13:577–91.
28. OPD Task Force. Operationalized Psychodynamic Diagnosis – OPD-2. Manual of diagnosis and treatment planning. Cambridge, MA: Hogrefe & Huber Publishers; 2008.
29. Preti E, Di Pierro R, Costantini G, Benzi IMA, De Panfilis C, Madeddu F. Using the structured interview of personality organization for DSM-5 level of personality functioning rating performed by inexperienced raters. J Pers Assess. 2018; https://doi.org/10.1080/00223891.2018.1448985.
30. Zimmermann J, Benecke C, Bender DS, Skodol AE, Schauenburg H, Cierpka M, Leising D. Assessing DSM-5 level of personality functioning from videotaped clinical interviews: a pilot study with untrained and clinically inexperienced students. J Pers Assess. 2014;96(4):397–409.
31. Ansell EB, Pinto A, Edelen MO, Markowitz JC, Sanislow CA, Yen S, Zanarini M, Skodol AE, Shea MT, Morey LC, Gunderson JG, McGlashan TH, Grilo CM. The association of personality disorders with the prospective 7-year course of anxiety disorders. Psychol Med. 2011;41(5):1019–28.
32. Crawford TN, Cohen P, First MB, Skodol AE, Johnson JG, Kasen S. Comorbid Axis I and Axis II disorders in early adolescence: outcomes 20 years later. Arch Gen Psychiatry. 2008;65(6):641–8.
33. Skodol AE, Geier T, Grant BF, Hasin DS. Personality disorders and the persistence of anxiety disorders in a nationally representative sample. Depress Anxiety. 2014;31(9):721–8.
34. Hunot V, Churchill R, Teixera V, Silva de Lima M. Psychological therapies for generalised anxiety disorder (Review). Cochrane Database Syst Rev. 2007;(1): CD001848.
35. Doering S, Hörz S, Rentrop M, Fischer-Kern M, Schuster P, Benecke C, Buchheim A, Martius P, Buchheim P. Transference-focused psychotherapy v. Treatment by experienced community psychotherapists for borderline personality disorder: randomized controlled trial. Br J Psychiatry. 2010;196(5):389–95.
36. Benecke C, Huber D, Staats H, Zimmermann J, Henkel M, Deserno H, Wiegand-Grefe S, Schauenburg H. A comparison of psychoanalytic therapy and cognitive behavioral therapy for anxiety (panic/agoraphobia) and personality disorders (APD study): presentation of the RCT study design. Z Psychosom Med Psychother. 2016;62(3):252–69.
37. Yeomans F, Clarkin J, Kernberg O. Transference-focused psychotherapy for borderline personality disorder: a clinical guide. Washington DC: American Psychiatric Publishing; 2015.
38. Levy KN, Meehan KB, Kelly KM, Reynoso JS, Weber M, Clarkin JF, Kernberg OF. Change in attachment patterns and reflective function in a randomized control trial of transference-focused psychotherapy for borderline personality disorder. J Consult Clin Psychol. 2006;74:1027–40.
39. Tmej A, Fischer-Kern M, Doering S, Buchheim A. Psychotherapy and changes from insecurity to security in borderline patients – a detailed descriptive study of AAI subcategories. Z Psychosom Med Psychother. 2018; 64:222–36.

40. Arntz A, van Genderen H. Schema therapy for borderline personality disorder. Chichester: Wiley-Blackwell; 2009.

41. Giesen-Bloo J, van Dyck R, Spinhoven P, van Tilburg W, Dirksen C, van Asselt T, Kremers I, Nadort M, Arntz A. Outpatient psychotherapy for borderline personality disorder. Randomized trial of Schema-focused therapy vs transference-focused psychotherapy. Arch Gen Psychiatry. 2006;63:649–58.

42. Bateman A, Fonagy A. Psychotherapy for borderline personality disorder. Mentalization-based treatment. Oxford: Oxford University Press; 2004.

43. Bateman A, Fonagy P. Effectiveness of partial hospitalization in the treatment of borderline personality disorder: a randomized controlled trial. Am J Psychiatry. 1999;156:1563–9.

44. Bateman A, Fonagy P. 8-year follow-up of patients treated for borderline personality disorder: mentalization-based treatment versus treatment as usual. Am J Psychiatry. 2008;165(5):631–8.

45. Linehan MM. Cognitive-behavioral treatment of borderline personality disorder. New York: Guilford Press; 1993.

46. Linehan MM, Comtois KA, Murray AM, Brown MZ, Gallop RJ, Heard HL, Korslund KE, Tutek DA, Reynolds SK, Lindenboim N. Two-year randomized controlled trial and follow-up of dialectical behavior therapy vs therapy by experts for suicidal behaviors and borderline personality disorder. Arch Gen Psychiatry. 2006;63(7):757–66.

# 2

# A qualitative study on the stigma experienced by people with mental health problems and epilepsy in the Philippines

Chika Tanaka[1*] ⓘ, Maria Teresa Reyes Tuliao[2], Eizaburo Tanaka[3], Tadashi Yamashita[4] and Hiroya Matsuo[1]

## Abstract

**Background:** Stigma towards people with mental health problems (PMHP) is known to have substantial negative impacts on their lives. More in-depth exploration of the stigma and discrimination experienced by PMHP in low- and middle-income countries is needed. Previous research suggests that negative attitudes towards PMHP are widespread among the Filipino general public. However, no study has investigated PMHP's own experiences of being stigmatised in the Philippines.

**Methods:** A qualitative study was conducted on the stigma experienced by PMHP (including people with epilepsy) and its related factors in the Philippines, employing the constructivist grounded theory approach. We analysed data on 39 PMHP collected through interviews with PMHP, their carers, and community health volunteers who know them well.

**Results:** The findings highlight the culturally and socio-economically specific contexts, consequences, and impact modifiers of experiences of stigma. Participants emphasised that PMHP face stigma because of the cultural traits such as the perception of mental health problem as a disease of the family and the tendency to be overly optimistic about the severity of the mental health problem and its impact on their life. Further, stigma was experienced under conditions where mental health care was not readily available and people in the local community could not resolve the PMHP's mental health crisis. Stigma experiences reduced social networks and opportunities for PMHP, threatened the economic survival of their entire family, and exacerbated their mental health problems. An individual's reaction to negative experiences can be fatalistic in nature (e.g. believing in it is God's will). This fatalism can help PMHP to remain hopeful. In addition, traditional communal unity alleviated some of the social exclusion associated with stigma.

**Conclusions:** The study indicates that existing stigma-reduction strategies might have limitations in their effectiveness across cultural settings. Therefore, we propose context-specific practical implications (e.g. emphasis on environmental factors as a cause of mental health problems, messages to increase understanding not only of the possibility of recovery but also of challenges PMHP face) for the Philippines.

**Keywords:** Stigma, Discrimination, Mental illness, The Philippines, Qualitative

## Background

Stigma and discrimination against people with mental health problems (PMHP) are a global public health issue [1–3] and can have substantial negative impacts on all aspects of a person's life, from employment and housing to social and family life [4–7]. Public stigma, the general public's reaction towards a stigmatised group, can be conceptualised as having three distinct elements [8]. First, a negative belief about a stigmatised group is seen as stereotype. Second, an emotional reaction to the stereotype is seen as prejudice. Third, a behavioural manifestation of the prejudice is discrimination. Historically, research on stigma related to mental health has been conducted mainly on stereotypes, prejudices, and intentions to discriminate that are held by the general public with regard to PMHP. Such research revealed that the general public frequently label PMHP as dangerous, blameworthy, incompetent and weak, which is often accompanied with emotions of fear and anger and can lead to

* Correspondence: chika128@gmail.com
[1]Graduate School of Health Sciences, Kobe University, 701, 2-6-2, Yamamoto-dori, Chuo-ku, Kobe, Hyogo 650-0003, Japan
Full list of author information is available at the end of the article

behavioural intention of avoidance, punishment, and coercion [9–12]. Further, the literature shows that internalisation of public stigma or self-stigma is also frequent among PMHP, which reduces self-esteem, causes social isolation, and inhibits help-seeking behaviour [6, 13–15].

Recent research has more often investigated levels of discrimination using direct reports from PMHP. The results of such research suggest that discrimination against PMHP is a universal phenomenon around the world [2, 3, 16]; however, PMHP's experiences of discrimination and its related factors might differ in high-income countries (HICs) versus low- and middle- income countries (LMICs). Some studies suggest that PMHP experience a lower level of stigma in LMICs [17], such as India [18], China [19], and Nigeria [20], compared with HICs. The reasons for the more positive acceptance of PMHP in those settings have been considered to be a more supportive environment with social cohesion as well as more social role options that PMHP are able to fulfil [21, 22]. At the same time, there is also accumulating evidence revealing that in LMICs, experiences of stigma, discrimination and human rights abuses related to mental health problems are common and severe [23–27]. The stigmatisation in LMICs has been attributed to the combined effects of socioeconomic and ethno-cultural characteristics of the setting [28]. For example, the economic situation of widespread poverty may contribute to further marginalisation of PMHP who are not able to financially contribute to society [29]. Moreover, the cultural value of collectivism may results in discrimination towards PMHP especially with regarding to marriage and childrearing, since a person's mental health problem is often seen as the family's mental health problem [30]. Overall, practices and outcomes of stigma differ across cultures and socioeconomic backgrounds [29, 31, 32], and meaningful comparison across cultural settings may not be achievable with cross-cultural measures [33]. In consideration of this, researchers have called for an in-depth qualitative exploration of the experiences of stigma among PMHP in LMICs settings, where about 85% of the world's population live [21].

PMHP in the Philippines, a lower-middle income country in Asia, might experience a significant level of stigma and discrimination. Filipino immigrants believed that personal characteristics (i.e. self-centeredness and "soul weakness") resulted in mental health problems [34, 35], which have been shown to be related to blaming PMHP and discriminatory behaviour in other settings [36]. Also, a multi-country survey revealed that, among 16 countries surveyed, the Philippines had the second highest proportion of citizens who agreed that PMHP should not be hired for a job even if they are qualified [37]. Further, some studies that involved interviews with Filipino immigrants living in Australia and the United States and that sampled from the general population revealed that a fear of being labelled as 'crazy' and spoiling their family's reputation made Filipinos hesitate to seek help from mental health professionals [35, 38, 39]. Although these previous studies provide some knowledge regarding public stigma in the Filipino context, all of them looked at stereotypes, prejudices and intentions to discriminate held by the general public towards PMHP. To our knowledge, there is no study investigating PMHP's own experiences of being stigmatised and discriminated against and the related factors in the Philippines.

To fill the gaps in the literature, we conducted a qualitative study on the factors related to experiences of stigma as well as the experiences itself of PMHP in the Philippines, using interviews with PMHP and people who know them well. Revealing the existence, types, and sources of stigma experienced by PMHP in the Philippines can contribute to the stigma research in Asian LMIC settings. Further, exploring the experiences of stigma and its related factors can provide fundamental knowledge for the design of an effective stigma reduction program in the Filipino setting.

## Methods

The current research utilised the principles of constructivist grounded theory, which is deemed suitable for revealing the social phenomenon of PMHP's experiences of stigma [40] in the Filipino context. The constructivist grounded theory assumes a relativist ontology (accepting that multiple realities exist) and a subjectivist epistemology (involving a co-construction of meaning through interaction between the researcher and participant) [41]. It provides a means of studying power, inequality, and marginality [42].

### Setting

Our study was conducted in Muntinlupa, the southernmost city in the Philippines' National Capital Region. The city has a population of 481,461 as of 2016. The majority comprises Tagalog ethnic groups and professes Christian, primarily Roman Catholic, faith. Households below the food threshold, the minimum income required to meet basic food needs, account for 21.5% of the total in the city [43]. The majority of citizens cannot afford private medical services, which cost five times more than the public medical services [44]. With respect to public psychiatric service, the city has one outpatient and no in-patient facility. The nearest public in-patient psychiatric facility is located about 23 km away.

### Main data collection
#### Participants
We collected data on PMHP from three different sources of information: PMHP themselves, their carers, and community health volunteers who knew them well. The eligibility criteria for PMHP were 1) having a mental

health problem, listed in the Diagnostic and Statistical Manual of Mental Disorders 5 (DSM-5), or epilepsy, and 2) currently not using residential care. Epilepsy was included for several reasons. First, people with epilepsy are known to suffer stigma and discrimination [45, 46]. Second, the condition has a long history of being classified as a psychiatric problem [47]. Third, even with the present-day efforts promoting mental health in LMICs, epilepsy is often treated together with mental health issues [48]. Last, pilot interviews revealed that local lay people do not clearly differentiate epilepsy from mental health problems.

For the recruitment, we approached 42 PMHP in person; one of them declined to participate owing to time constraints. Thus, we obtained informed consent from 41 PMHP. Among them, two PMHP were excluded because they were confirmed to have only physical health problems and no mental health problems as listed in DSM-5. Consequently, we used data of 39 PMHP for our analysis. The profiles of the final sample are shown in Table 1. In 20 of the PMHP, we interviewed the PMHP and their main carer, usually a parent or sibling. In the remaining 19 PMHP, only a main carer was interviewed, as the 19 PMHP had communication difficulties that hindered them from answering interview questions. Additionally, in 11 PMHP, we conducted interviews with a community health volunteer who was in charge of the district in which the PMHP lived.

### Recruitment

We aimed to include a wide variation in the characteristics of the PMHP, namely, gender, age, marital status, educational attainment, employment status, religion, type of mental health problem, and history of using health and welfare services. To achieve this, the participants were recruited by purposive sampling in cooperation with two different collaborating stakeholders. First, as stigma was considered to inhibit Filipino people from seeking professional help for their mental condition [35, 49], we recruited the majority of PMHP ($n = 36$) in cooperation with community health volunteers, which enabled us to recruit PMHP regardless of their history of receiving health care. The community health volunteers had good knowledge of the profiles of the residents of the district under their charge and covered all the areas of the city. Second, we recruited a small number of PMHP ($n = 3$) with common mental health problems (e.g. anxiety and depressive problems) from the outpatient clinical practice of a psychiatrist, as the community health volunteers did not identify any people with these types of problems.

To check the eligibility of those who had never been diagnosed by a specialist as having a mental health problem, a research member, ET, carefully reviewed the data

**Table 1** Profiles of people with mental health problems

|  | n | N = 39 (%) |
|---|---|---|
| Sex |  |  |
| Male | 26 | (66.7) |
| Female | 13 | (33.3) |
| Age range |  |  |
| 0–19 years | 11 | (28.2) |
| 20–39 years | 18 | (46.2) |
| 40–59 years | 8 | (20.5) |
| 60–69 years | 2 | (5.1) |
| Highest educational attainment |  |  |
| No formal education | 4 | (10.3) |
| Primary school or lower | 16 | (41.0) |
| High school or higher | 17 | (43.6) |
| Still in full-time education | 2 | (5.1) |
| Employment status |  |  |
| Out of work[a] | 34 | (87.2) |
| Employed for wages | 4 | (10.3) |
| Self-employed | 1 | (2.6) |
| Marital status |  |  |
| Single[b] | 32 | (82.1) |
| Married/ Domestic partnership | 5 | (12.8) |
| Widowed/ Separated | 2 | (5.1) |
| Religion |  |  |
| Roman Catholic | 28 | (71.8) |
| Iglesia ni Cristo | 3 | (7.7) |
| Protestant | 3 | (7.7) |
| Islam | 1 | (2.6) |
| Other Christian | 4 | (10.3) |
| Classification of mental health problems |  |  |
| Neurodevelopmental | 13 | (33.3) |
| Schizophrenia Spectrum and Other Psychotic | 10 | (25.6) |
| Substance-related and Addictive | 8 | (20.5) |
| Epilepsy | 2 | (5.1) |
| Anxiety | 2 | (5.1) |
| Trauma and Stressor-related | 1 | (2.6) |
| Depressive | 1 | (2.6) |
| Sleep -Wake | 1 | (2.6) |
| Data deficient | 1 | (2.6) |
| Lifetime mental health or welfare service use |  |  |
| Yes | 26 | (66.7) |
| No | 13 | (33.3) |
| Current mental health or welfare service use |  |  |
| Yes | 12 | (30.8) |
| No | 27 | (69.2) |

[a]Children under 15 years old, the legal working age, ($n = 3$) are included
[b]Children under 18 years old, the legal marriage age, ($n = 8$) are included

of the individual participants, including interview recordings, transcriptions, and field notes, and then provided informed presumption if the participants had a mental health problem or not. ET also assessed which chapter, the broadest classification in DSM-5, the participant most fitted. ET has clinical experience as a psychiatrist in Japan for over 15 years.

### Interview procedures

Data on the PMHP were collected through semi-structured in-depth interviews. Prior to the beginning of data collection, an interview guide was developed, referring to previous research [18, 50], and then modified based on six pilot interviews in the setting. The interview guide had a series of open questions on three major topics: onset of mental health problems and coping behaviours, experiences of being treated negatively owing to the problem and its consequences, and activities PMHP gave up because of how others might respond to their health problem. The interview guides for interviews with PMHP and for interviews with carers and community health volunteers can be accessed in Additional files 1 and 2, respectively. Consistent with the grounded theory methods, we used the interview guide as a flexible tool that could be revised as the analysis progressed. The carers and community health volunteers were not asked about their own experiences of stigma as a carer or person working in mental health. Instead, we asked them about the PMHP's experiences regarding the same topics, based on their observations. Demographic data of the PMHP were also obtained at the beginning of the interview.

The first author, CT (female, a Japanese public health nurse), conducted all of the data collection between January and March 2017. During the interview, Tagalog or English was used as preferred by the participants. When Tagalog was chosen, the interviews were interpreted by one of two health workers who had lived in the city for more than 30 years and were fluent in both Tagalog and English. After explaining the study and gaining informed consent, the interviews were conducted in their home, a health centre, or the city hospital, depending on the participants' preference. Wherever possible, we conducted interviews in a space where there was no one but the interviewee, interviewer, and interpreter around. However, five PMHP were not willing to be interviewed alone. In which case, a family member was in the same place and assisted the interview. All the interviews were digitally recorded with interviewees' permission and lasted between 19 and 53 min; the median length was 29 min. The participants received 100 Philippine pesos (1.9 US dollars) as acknowledgement for their participation.

### Supplementary data collection

We included data of interviews with seven health workers into our analysis to gain a wider perspective on the stigma experienced by PMHP. CT conducted the interviews during her one-month participant observation at health services provided by the city government. During the observation, CT discussed the role of stigma and its impact on PMHP with more than 85 health and welfare workers. We analysed seven interviews with those who shared episodes on PMHP with whom they were in direct contact as a part of their duty at work. The interviewees were three community health volunteers, two nurses, one doctor, and one rehabilitation program officer. Notes were taken during the interviews and six out of seven interviews were audiotaped with their permission.

### Analyses

All of the recordings were transcribed verbatim by two trained transcribers. Tagalog recordings were simultaneously translated into English by the transcribers fluent in English and Tagalog. An independent research assistant randomly selected 10% of the English transcripts and checked their accuracy by matching them with the Tagalog and English recordings. During this checking process, no significant errors were found thus the transcripts were quality assured.

Data analysis started as soon as the initial data were collected. We set aside theoretical ideas from the existing literature; instead, we remained open to exploring the theoretical possibilities we could discern from the data. After reading each of the transcripts at least twice, CT and ET independently conducted the initial coding. Simple codes were created to describe the phenomenon in each segment of data, using the qualitative data analysis software, Nvivo Version 11.4.1 (QSR International, 2016). The initial codes with identical meanings were merged through discussion, whereas those with different meanings were left unchanged to increase the variety in the interpretation of the data. We used data from interviews with cares, health volunteers, health and welfare workers to increase variety of data on stigma experienced by PMHP and gain comprehensive understanding of its context. Thus, when accounts showed some discrepancy between a person with mental health problem and his/her carer or a person who knew him/her well, we used the data from both accounts for our analysis.

The authors gradually moved on to the focus coding, in which the initial codes were concentrated on or collapsed into categories that make analytical sense, and then tested these against extensive data. The interpersonal interaction between people with and without mental health problems was treated as the central phenomenon of our interest. To explore comprehensively PMHP's experiences of stigma, we decided to treat any "uncomfortable treatments from others" reported as stigma experience, regardless of the actors' motivation. We constantly compared data on similarities and differences within a participant as well as across participants to examine the categories and develop links among them. CT led the preliminary focus coding. Subsequently, discussions were held between CT, ET, and HM, in which we reviewed the developed categories and links to determine if they were grounded in data and sufficiently explained the phenomenon.

After analysing the data of the 35 PMHP, a tentative model that explains the relations between categories was developed. We then collected and analysed data on four additional PMHP. Through discussion, the full research team determined that the categories and themes were sufficiently relevant and that the model held true for these additional PMHP. We then concluded that the model was theoretically saturated.

## Results

Analyses revealed four interrelated themes surrounding stigma experienced by PMHP: (1) the context affecting stigma experience, (2) stigma experience, (3) impact modifier of the stigma experience, and (4) consequence of the stigma experience. Figure 1 shows the relationship among the themes.

### Context affecting stigma experience

We identified two contextual categories that changed how others treated PMHP in a negative way.

#### Public belief about mental health problems

Public beliefs surrounding mental health issues are a contextual category of stigma experienced by PMHP in the Philippines. It consists of three themes: familial problems, unrealistic pessimism and optimism about severity, and oversimplified chronic course.

#### Familial problems

Community health volunteers and health workers observed that families of PMHP and people in the local community do not provide appropriate support for PMHP because they perceive mental affliction as a family problem and indicative of so-called "bad blood". The belief that mental health problems can

be transmitted among relatives pushed families of PMHP to deny the existence of mental health issues and people in the community to distance themselves from PMHP. A nurse shared an episode of a male patient with depression:

*His family could not accept the idea that one of their relatives is actually depressed. (...) It's because in our culture, when it comes to mental illness, it tends to be a family affair. People think if one of you has a history of mental illness, there is a chance that almost all of you already have that as well. We care about how others think about our family more than anything else. And other people feel that it is not their place to intervene in some family matters. (Interview 48, Nurse, Female)*

In particular, marrying age PMHP faced stigma because of the belief in heredity. People in the community often believe that PMHP have mental health problems in their family's blood and are afraid of developing those problems in their kinship via marriage.

*I had one neighbour that I reported to the barangay [district government] because she mocked me. She was saying that I had mental illness in our blood and no one dare marry me and get in trouble. (Interview 51, PMHP, Male)*

#### Unrealistic pessimism and optimism about severity

PMHP experienced stigma when others were overly pessimistic about the severity of a mental health problem. Participants often criticised those who believe that mental health problems generally cause severe functional impairments. This belief has resulted in unfair treatment towards PMHP in the Philippines.

*[Researcher: What is the biggest challenge for the [social inclusion] program?] Finding a job. It's very difficult. The community people don't believe they*

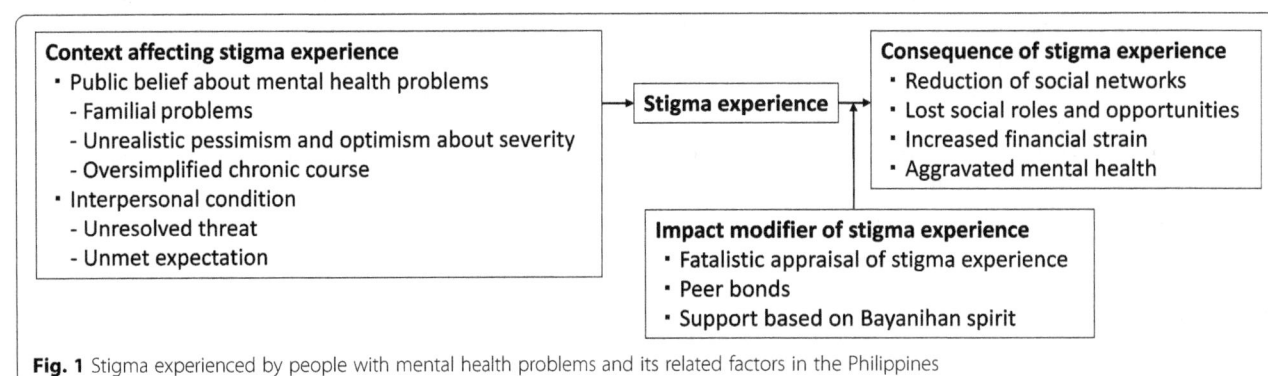

**Context affecting stigma experience**
- Public belief about mental health problems
  - Familial problems
  - Unrealistic pessimism and optimism about severity
  - Oversimplified chronic course
- Interpersonal condition
  - Unresolved threat
  - Unmet expectation

**Stigma experience**

**Consequence of stigma experience**
- Reduction of social networks
- Lost social roles and opportunities
- Increased financial strain
- Aggravated mental health

**Impact modifier of stigma experience**
- Fatalistic appraisal of stigma experience
- Peer bonds
- Support based on Bayanihan spirit

**Fig. 1** Stigma experienced by people with mental health problems and its related factors in the Philippines

*[PMHP] are functional and don't hire them. (...) So now some barangays [district governments] have started to hire them. We hope people see them working hard and start to trust them. (Interview 27, Rehabilitation program officer, Male)*

Meanwhile, unrealistic optimism about its severity also caused stigma. The commonly held belief is that individuals are able to overcome any psychological suffering by themselves, and as a result, it will not become a serious problem. It was common for PMHP to be doubted or withheld empathy in such a culture that emphasises resilience and humour under stressful situations.

*Filipinos are proud of being resilient. We find something funny in any difficult situation. But when you have this illness, that kind of thinking gives you a huge pressure. (...) One day, I opened up about my mental illness to my friends, but they all had the same reaction. They laughed at me and didn't take it seriously. (Interview 71, PMHP, Female)*

### Oversimplified chronic course
The *oversimplified chronic course* of mental health problems emerged as one of the causes of stigma. People without any experience of a mental health problem often misunderstand the repetitive relapse and remission in the course of a mental health problem. They tend to apply an acute illness model and expect a complete cure in the short term. However, as the symptoms are prolonged, they begin to mistrust the PMHP's account.

*After one month of no work, I was able to work and sleep. But in February, it came back. I couldn't sleep for several days. (...) My supervisors were thinking that I should be working a night shift duty, but I told them that I would have to take sick leave. But because it was the same reason for my previous absent, they are already thinking that I am making up stories. (Interview 30, PMHP, Male)*

### Interpersonal condition
*Interpersonal condition* was identified as a direct trigger of stigma experience. It consists of two themes: unresolved threat and unmet expectation.

### Unresolved threat
*Unresolved threat* is a condition where PMHP are at risk of hurting themselves or others owing to their mental health problems, with the people in contact with the PMHP failing to manage such risks. Under such conditions, PMHP often experience physical violence, being

avoided, and being restricted by others. Although the PMHP, their families, and community health volunteers attributed the threats to PMHP's personal factors, such as personality and outwardly noticeable symptoms, they also emphasised the culpability of people in the local community for their lack of understanding and skills in interacting with PMHP. When others became familiar with PMHP, they successfully managed those threats and prevented PMHP from experiencing stigma. The mother of a boy with a neurodevelopmental problem told us:

*My son easily becomes violent. For example, when someone takes and plays with his toy. The neighbours don't understand why he is angry and they bully him. But there are also some playmates who fully understand him. When they know that my son is about to be angry, they immediately keep distance from him. And after a while, my son calms down and they start playing around together. (Interview 4, Mother of a boy with a mental health problem)*

### Unmet expectation
*Unmet expectation* was another context of stigma. In this context, there is a gap between PMHP's abilities and other people's expectations of them. Some PMHP reported suffering from stigma when others' expectations were too high for their situation. People in this cultural setting tend to value strong bonds and reciprocity among families and neighbours. PMHP sometimes were unable to perform in accordance with this value owing to their mental health conditions. Violation of this value was judged as morally wrong.

*They [the neighbours] say I should help my mum by doing washing, cleaning, and taking care of my brother, even when I say I feel weak or don't know how to. (Interview 5, PMHP, Female)*

*She is big but still doesn't help her mother. That's why the neighbours don't like her. They say she is not a good daughter. (Interview 18, Community health volunteer, Female)*

Meanwhile, some other PMHP experienced stigma when others underestimated PMHP's abilities. Families often criticised other people that looked only at PMHP's disabilities but not at their abilities.

*When someone in our neighbourhood was trying to talk to my sister and she did not respond back, they started bullying her and calling her crazy. [Researcher: How do you think we can change such situation?] I think proper communication towards her would be the best since she's really a good listener. The problem is that other people don't know she actually understands things really well. (Interview 8, Sister of a woman with a mental health problem)*

## Stigma experience

Although we frequently found that PMHP were positively treated by others because of their mental health problems, we also discovered that almost all the PMHP participants were faced with negative treatment from others. PMHP experienced *psychological abuse* (e.g. being verbally insulted, laughed at, stared at, gossiped about, doubted), *physical violence* (e.g. being hit, stones being thrown at them), being *restricted* (e.g. being told not to go outside alone, tied with a rope to a pillar), not being *supported* (e.g. lack of understanding and sympathy), being *taken advantage of* (e.g. being cheated out of money and belongings), being *neglected* (e.g. privacy not being protected, medical care not being provided), and being *rejected* (e.g. not being associated with, not being hired). Families were an important source of stigma in terms of prominence as stigma from families was often repetitive (e.g. frequently being slapped) and prolonged (e.g. being locked up in a room for several months). PMHP also experienced stigma frequently from their neighbours, and sometimes from school friends, co-workers and employers. People who were involved with PMHP as a part of their duty at work (i.e. health workers and public safety officers) were a source of stigma as well. For complete information on the stigma experience by source, please see Table 2.

## Impact modifier of stigma experience

Even if the nature of stigma experiences were similar, the extent and degree of its influence on PMHP's life varied depending on *impact modifier of stigma experience*. PMHP had three impact modifiers consisting of internal (i.e. fatalistic appraisal) and external (i.e. peer bonds, community unity) factors.

### Fatalistic appraisal of stigma experience

*Fatalistic appraisal of stigma experience* offered PMHP and their families a strategy to cope with the emotional pain caused by stigma experience. People in the setting generally believed that God predetermined life events in the past, present and future. Some PMHP and their family accepted unfair treatments from others as "fate." They were able to remain hopeful because they believed that God would help them if they had faith in God.

*Sometimes people say he is crazy. [Researcher: What do you do in response to that?] Nothing. People say*

**Table 2** Stigma experience by type and source and its examples[a]

| | |
|---|---|
| **Psychological abuse** | |
| Family | My other siblings say that she's crazy. (Interview 70, Sister of PMHP) |
| Friends | Her classmates were bullying her (Interview 21, Mother of PMHP) |
| Neighbours | They [neighbours] say bad things to me like "abnoy" ["abnormal" in Tagalog]. (Interview 55, PMHP) |
| Coworkers, Employers | I don't like them [coworkers] gossiping about me. (Interview 32, PMHP) |
| Health care providers | They told me that I was lazy. (Interview 42, PMHP) |
| Strangers on the street | When a vehicle stopped and the driver stared at her I got mad. (Interview 38, Father of PMHP) |
| **Physical violence** | |
| Family | He [Father] sometimes slaps him. (Interview 15, Mother of PMHP) |
| Friends | My high school friends started throwing stones at me and saying I'm crazy (Interview 6, PMHP) |
| Neighbours | When my neighbour hit him I needed to bring him to the hospital (Interview 1, Mother of PMHP) |
| Public safety officers | They [public safety officers] hit me and I was very scared. (Interview 58, PMHP) |
| **Restricted** | |
| Family | We tied him down with a rope because he would always wander around. (Interview 43, Mother of PMHP) |
| **Not supported** | |
| Family | Her brothers don't understand her. (Interview 8, Sister of PMHP) |
| Friends | No one really understands me, even my friends. (Interview 60, PMHP) |
| Coworkers, Employers | They [coworkers] usually laugh because they don't know it's hard having this problem. (Interview 12, PMHP) |
| **Taken advantage of** | |
| Neighbours | He usually rents a bike in our neighbour for five pesos, but sometimes he'll pay with twenty pesos and they won't give him the change. (Interview 7, Mother of PMHP) |
| **Neglected** | |
| Family | We had to let him live with us because his parents abandoned him when he was little. (Interview 44, Aunt of PMHP) |
| Health care providers | When we visited the hospital, we saw that she was naked and she was already held with other mental patients in the room. There were no assessments done for her [for urinary tract infection]. (Interview 38, Father of PMHP) |
| **Rejected** | |
| Family | My brother says to "keep her out of the home." (Interview 63, Sister of PMHP) |
| Friends | [Researcher: Did he have many friends?] Yes, before. But now, they avoid him. (Interview 65, Mother of PMHP) |
| Coworkers, Employers | I kept failing to find a job. That's why I need to hide it [mental health problem]. (Interview 16, PMHP) |

[a]A listed source with an example of a particular type of stigma experience indicates that at least one incidence of that type was reported by the participant

*what they want to say. We just say "God is good." As long as we believe in Him, it will be alright. (Interview 23, Sister of a man with a mental health problem)*

### Peer bonds

*Peer bonds*, the emotional bonds with other people with similar mental health problems, empowered PMHP to change their stigmatised situation in a positive way. Stigma experience could marginalise them in the community, but when they were together with peers who understood not only their health condition but also their lowered social status, they were empowered and motivated to change the situation for themselves and their peers.

> *[Researcher: What are the barriers to your recovery?] The different perceptions of people towards us [she and other people with mental health problems]. It is so discouraging for us. And we are the only ones who can understand each other very well. We are like brothers and sisters already. Nevertheless, we make sure that the reason we join the [rehabilitation] program is not only for ourselves but to show them that we can change ourselves for the better. If we will be given a chance to work again, we will make 100 percent effort to get things done accordingly. (Interview 34, PMHP, Female)*

### Support based on Bayanihan spirit

*Support based on Bayanihan spirit*, a traditional concept of community unity, relieved the negative impacts of stigma on PMHP. It was not rare that community people gave food or rented a house free to PMHP and their family who had little income. Helping one another in a time of need was inherent in their lives, called Bayanihan in Tagalog. For example, a homeless woman with schizophrenia told us that she had felt hopeless because she had been bullied at school and was in a materially deprived circumstance. However, she was now enjoying her life and managing to make a living because some of her neighbours treated her as a valued community member (e.g. regularly invited her to a local dancing event) and occasionally gave her food. A community health volunteer explained why she had good relationships with the community as follows:

> *That is natural here. When your family member is sick, neighbours and friends are there to pay for medicines, bring food, help with housework, and take care of small kids. We call it Bayanihan. (Interview 3, Community health volunteer, Female)*

### Consequence of stigma experience

Stigma experience was found to bring about a substantial negative impact on PMHP's social networks, roles, opportunities, and mental health.

### Reduction of social networks

Stigma experience reduced PMHP's social networks, which led to them spending their days isolated at home without any interaction with people outside of their immediate family. This was due not only to the direct influence of experiences of stigma (i.e. being *physically restrained*, being *avoided by others*) but also the indirect influence of changes in three aspects: PMHP's behaviour, restriction by families, and relationships with others. First, after being negatively treated, PMHP tended to "close off to everybody" and distanced themselves from others.

> *Going out is sometimes like an obstacle. (...) After that [hearing my friends gossiping about me], I have been afraid of people's judgments. (Interview 62, PMHP, Female)*

Second, families started to restrict PMHP's behaviour to protect them from further stigma experiences.

> *We do not allow him to go out. We are afraid that something like that [neighbours calling him crazy] might happen to him again or someone might abduct him. (Interview 9, Sister of a man with a mental health problem)*

Third, stigma experiences provoked conflicts, from a quarrel to a physical fight, and worsened the relationship between PMHP and others. The conflicting relationships produced a further stigmatising attitude towards PMHP.

> *He got into a fight with his playmates because they said bad words to him. (...) Many of our neighbours told me that he should be in a cell. They told me that they knew a policeman who could put him in jail. (Interview 1, Mother of a man with metal health problem)*

### Lost social roles and opportunities

As a result of stigma experience, PMHP *lost social roles and opportunities*, such as being employed, going to school, having a romantic partner, getting married, parenting, helping with household chores and the family business, taking care of younger siblings and joining religious activities.

> *She was a member of the choir in church. She likes singing and has a good voice. And plenty of friends visited her in the past and they went to church together. But no more. Nobody visits her, and she quit attending it. (Interview 10, Mother of a woman with a mental health problem)*

### Increased financial strain

Lost social roles and opportunities increased financial strain, which negatively affected the families as well as PMHP themselves. In this setting, PMHP and their families lived in communities where many people find it difficult to make a living. The cost of transportation to medical facilities and treatment fees put them in a further difficult situation economically. In such conditions, entire families often suffered from the financial strain that was due to stigma to the degree that they could not afford basic items including food and clothing.

> If only I could find a good job like when I was well. Even though we do not have enough money to buy things, my family really makes an effort to find ways that we can buy those medicines. (Interview 20, PMHP, Male)

### Aggravated mental health

The participants reported that the stigma experiences *aggravated mental health* in PMHP. The memory of negative treatment from others often stuck in their mind and its influence lasted for a long time. A 32-year-old woman with anxiety problem explained how the experience of being bullied when she was a teenager influenced her current condition:

> It triggers my anxiety. When I remember their facial expressions, even now, I feel overwhelmed and breathless (Interview 39, PMHP, Female).

The experience of stigma also affected the mental health condition of PMHP by preventing them from seeking help. Some PMHP and their families choose to keep their mental health status a secret. However, families have limited capacities to take care of a person with a mental health problem, especially in the case of someone with severe symptoms. In the worst case in terms of the influence of stigma on PMHP's mental health, a community health volunteer reported that the parents of a daughter with a mental health problem locked her up in her room and took care of her without seeking professional help. However, her condition kept deteriorating and eventually she committed suicide inside her room.

## Discussion

To our knowledge, this is the first study to document the stigma experienced by PMHP in the Philippines. This study adds to the understanding of discrimination in LMIC settings and its related contextual factors in the Philippines.

First, our results showed that PMHP in the Philippines experienced stigma, which brought about negative impacts on PMHP's social networks, roles and opportunities, financial burden, and mental health. Although stigma types, sources, and areas of impact were generally consistent with the existing literature in this field [4, 6, 51], we found that experiences of stigma threatened the economic survival of the entire family of PMHP and increased the mental health crisis in the LMIC context, given the minimal welfare and mental health care provisions. Several studies with participants recruited from clinical settings have shown that PMHP in LMICs suffered less from stigma [2, 18–20]. In this study, we involved PMHP without psychiatric service use, which prevented us from overlooking the stigma experienced by the poorest and most marginalised PMHP. Our findings might better reflect the reality in LMIC settings, where it is estimated that more than 70% of PMHP receive no treatment for their mental health conditions [52].

Second, we found that pessimistic and over-optimistic reactions to a mental health problem are among the important contexts of experiences of stigma in the Philippines. Historically, stigma research has mainly focused on the pessimistic view on the prognosis and its negative effects [10, 53–56]. Meanwhile, when the over-optimistic view on the outcome of mental health problems has been documented among Filipino immigrants, it was only recognised as a barrier to help-seeking [35, 39]. Our qualitative exploration's original finding is that the over-optimistic belief among the community regarding the severity of mental health problems results in PMHP's receiving inappropriate or negative treatment. This is an important finding for the Philippines, because resilience and optimism under difficult situations are among the well-known cultural traits of Filipinos [57, 58]. Stigma resulting from optimism might be prevalent in the Philippines; a prior study showed that among the 16 countries, the Philippines posted the highest proportion of respondents who agreed that mental illness would improve on its own [59].

Third, the results indicated that mental health problems were perceived as problems of the family and discouraged people from accepting mental health problems. The finding is consistent with psychiatrists' clinical experiences with Filipino patients [60, 61]. We also found that a belief in transmissibility among relatives led to PMHP experiencing reduced marriage opportunities. Previous studies conducted on Chinese descent groups [62–64] showed that the threat of genetic contamination was related to endorsement of reproductive restriction. We propose that it might hold true in the Filipino context, meaning that the threat to family lineage through genetic contamination via marriage accounts for some of the discrimination experienced by PMHP.

Fourth, we revealed a context-specific impact modifier of stigma experiences, namely, *fatalistic appraisal of stigma experience*. Existing studies have discussed that Filipinos typically attribute illness to "the will of God" [39, 49, 65]. A new finding of this study is that negative treatments from others were also attributed to fate. Globally, it is known that fatalistic appraisal of negative events inhibits active coping and worsens health [66, 67]. However, we found that fatalism offered a spiritual coping strategy and shielded PMHP from the adverse effects of stigma in the Catholic dominant setting of the Philippines. These findings are consistent with the literature that have showed that fatalism facilitates adjustment to negative life events [49, 68, 69]. Moreover, *support based on Bayanihan spirit* was another culturally relevant impact modifier. The origin of the Bayanihan spirit is traced back to the country's tradition wherein towns' people cooperate to carry a family's entire house on their shoulders to a new location. It is considered a core essence of the Filipino culture. Our finding supports the arguments by Lasalvia [21] and Mascayano et al. [29] that communal network, which tends to be better maintained in LMICs, is among the existing strengths to reduce the negative effects of stigma.

Lastly, the research method of obtaining perspectives from multiple participants who witnessed and experienced stigma allowed us to reveal that the interpersonal conditions (i.e. *unresolved threat* and *unmet expectations*) preceded stigma experiences. Consistent with previous research from India [24] and Indonesia [70], in the setting where mental health care is not readily available at a local level, people in the community needed to cope with the possible danger of PMHP to self or others and can violate PMHP's human rights. Similar to the results of prior qualitative analyses of interviews with PMHP and their families [18, 71], the expectations of others in contrast to PMHP's actual capabilities caused negative reactions from others. Those interpersonal conditions might be a more important determinant of stigma experiences than PMHP's personal factors, considering the previous studies showing individual variables (e.g. employment status, symptom, and treatment experiences) accounted for only less than 30% of total variance of experienced stigma [2, 3].

### Practical implications

Our results suggest that mental health care must have the objective of the reduction of stigma towards PMHP. The Department of Health and Local Government Units are required by the Mental Health Act [72], established in 2018 as the first law of its kind in the Philippines, to initiate and sustain nationwide campaigns to raise the level of awareness on the protection and promotion of mental health and rights. In conducting stigma reduction campaigns, they should: 1) target families of PMHP, community people, health workers, and public safety officers; 2) avoid genetic explanations for mental health problems and emphasise the role of environmental and social factors as its cause; 3) increase public understanding of not only the possibility of

recovery but also the challenges that PMHP face; and 4) improve families' and community members' skills in assessing and coping with possible danger posed by PMHP to self or others [73–76]. These interventions might be more effective when they utilise the existing communal network and increase social contact between PMHP and others [77, 78] We also propose that mental health and welfare services for PMHP should: 1) be community-based and support PMHP in meeting expectations that are meaningful for themselves and others; 2) provide opportunities for PMHP to share their experiences with peers to empower them [79–81]; and 3) prevent PMHP from internalising experiences of stigma with acknowledgement of fatalistic appraisal of them as a coping strategy. Lastly, to mitigate the adverse influences of stigma, it is necessary to change the structure of health care and welfare service provision for PMHP (e.g. inclusive education, welfare benefits, and job schemes). It is also essential to provide effective and accessible mental health care.

### Study limitations

We were unable to recruit people with common mental health problems who were not using psychiatric services. In fact, community health volunteers do not recognise any people having common mental health problems. This may reflect stigma-related situations where local people do not recognise the manifestation of symptoms of those problems as a health issue, or where people with those problems hide their conditions. Additionally, cultural and language barriers may have played a part in data collection and interpretation. However, we also encountered a number of situations where the interviewee provided the data collector, who was from another cultural background, with further explanations, especially on their culture. Further, some interviews were too short to be considered an in-depth interview. Also, we needed to rely in part on data from narratives of people who know PMHP well, instead of from PMHP themselves. These were because the interviewer had difficulty encouraging some participants, especially PMHP, to talk about sensitive topics. Thus, there might be experiences and related themes that we could not explore. Lastly, we conducted the study in one city; thus, the results may not be generalisable to another part of the Philippines (e.g. rural and Muslim-dominant areas).

### Conclusions

Our findings highlight that PMHP in the Philippines experience substantial discrimination and its adverse effects are severe to the degree that it threatens the financial survival of the entire family. Culture-bound beliefs and social structure (e.g. perceiving mental health problems as a familial problems, traditional communal unity) played important roles in shaping and modifying stigma experiences. More research is needed to develop stigma reduction interventions utilising these findings and to evaluate their effectiveness.

## Additional files

**Additional file 1:** Interview guide for interviews with people with mental health problems. A set of questions we referred while interviewing PMHP. (DOCX 88 kb)

**Additional file 2:** Interview guide for interviews with carers and community health volunteers. A set of questions we referred while interviewing carers and community health volunteers. (DOCX 90 kb)

## Abbreviations

DSM: The Diagnostic and Statistical Manual of Mental Disorders; HICs: High-income countries; LMICs: Low- and middle-income countries; PMHP: People with mental health problems

## Acknowledgments

We are grateful to the interviewees for their participation. We would like to thank Dr. Magdalena C. Meana, Dr. Ma. Luisa Babaran-Echavez, and barangay health workers for their assistance with data collection.

## Availability of data and materials

The transcripts from the interviews are confidential and will not be shared.

## Authors' contributions

CT had a major role in the conception of the study, undertook the data collection, carried out the data analysis, and had a major role in writing the manuscript. MT contributed to the design of the study, assisted the data collection and interpretation, and supervised writing the manuscript. ET assisted data collection, conducted data analysis, and revised the manuscript. YT assisted data collection and revised the manuscript. HM supervised the design of the study, had a role in data analysis, and revised the manuscript. All authors read and approved the final manuscript.

## Consent for publication

Participants were informed that the information they shared in the interviews would be published in anonymised form. Written informed consent for publication was obtained.

## Competing interests

The authors declare that they have no competing interest.

## Author details

[1]Graduate School of Health Sciences, Kobe University, 701, 2-6-2, Yamamoto-dori, Chuo-ku, Kobe, Hyogo 650-0003, Japan. [2]City Health Office, City Government of Muntinlupa, Muntinlupa, Philippines. [3]Hyogo Institute for Traumatic Stress, Kobe, Japan. [4]Kobe City College of Nursing, Kobe, Japan.

## References

1. Seeman N, Tang S, Brown AD, Ing A. World survey of mental illness stigma. J Affect Disord. 2016;190:115–121. Available from: https://doi.org/10.1016/j.jad.2015.10.011 Elsevier.
2. Lasalvia A, Zoppei S, Van Bortel T, Bonetto C, Cristofalo D, Wahlbeck K, et al. Global pattern of experienced and anticipated discrimination reported by people with major depressive disorder: a cross-sectional survey. Lancet. 2013;381:55–62. Available from: https://doi.org/10.1016/S0140-6736(12)61379-8 Elsevier Ltd
3. Thornicroft G, Brohan E, Rose D, Sartorius N, Leese M. Global pattern of experienced and anticipated discrimination against people with schizophrenia: a cross-sectional survey. Lancet; 2009;373:408–415. Available from: https://doi.org/10.1016/S0140-6736(08)61817-6. Elsevier Ltd
4. Sharac J, McCrone P, Clement S, Thornicroft G. The economic impact of mental health stigma and discrimination: a systematic review. Epidemiol Psichiatr Soc. 2010;19:223. Available from: https://www.ncbi.nlm.nih.gov/pubmed/21261218.
5. Clement S, Schauman O, Graham T, Maggioni F, Evans-Lacko S, Bezborodovs N, et al. What is the impact of mental health-related stigma on help-seeking? A systematic review of quantitative and qualitative studies. Psychol Med. 2015;45:11–27 Available from: http://www.ncbi.nlm.nih.gov/pubmed/24569086.
6. Livingston JD, Boyd JE. Correlates and consequences of internalized stigma for people living with mental illness: a systematic review and meta-analysis. Soc Sci Med. 2010;71:2150–2161. Available from: https://doi.org/10.1016/j.socscimed.2010.09.030 Elsevier Ltd
7. Link BG, Phelan JC. Conceptualising stigma. Annu Rev Sociol. 2001 [cited 2018 Jul 3];27:363–385. Available from: https://www.annualreviews.org/doi/pdf/10.1146/annurev.soc.27.1.363
8. Corrigan PW. Mental health stigma as social attribution: implications for research methods and attitude change. Clin Psychol Sci Pract. 2006;7:48–67 Available from: http://doi.wiley.com/10.1093/clipsy.7.1.48.
9. Mannarini S, Boffo M. Anxiety, bulimia, drug and alcohol addiction, depression, and schizophrenia: what do you think about their aetiology, dangerousness, social distance, and treatment? A latent class analysis approach. Soc Psychiatry Psychiatr Epidemiol. 2015;50:27–37.
10. McGinty EE, Goldman HH, Pescosolido B, Barry CL. Portraying mental illness and drug addiction as treatable health conditions: effects of a randomized experiment on stigma and discrimination. Soc Sci Med; 2015;126:73–85. Available from: https://doi.org/10.1016/j.socscimed.2014.12.010. Elsevier Ltd
11. Angermeyer MC, Dietrich S. Public beliefs about and attitudes towards people with mental illness: a review of population studies. Acta Psychiatr Scand. 2006;113:163–79.
12. Corrigan PW, Markowitz FE, Watson A, Rowan D, Kubiak MA. An attribution model of public discrimination towards persons with mental illness. J Health Soc Behav. 2003;44:162–79.
13. Corrigan P, Watson A. The paradox of self-stigma and mental illness. Clin Psychol Sci Pract. 2002;9:35–53 Available from: https://onlinelibrary.wiley.com/doi/10.1093/clipsy.9.1.35.
14. Evans-Lacko S, Brohan E, Mojtabai R, Thornicroft G. Association between public views of mental illness and self-stigma among individuals with mental illness in 14 European countries. Psychol Med. 2012;42:1741–52.
15. Mccann TV, Renzaho A, Mugavin J, Lubman DI. Stigma of mental illness and substance misuse in sub-Saharan African migrants: a qualitative study. Int J Ment Health Nurs. 2017;27:956–65.
16. Camden Schizoph E, Corker EA, Beldie A, Brain C, Jakovljevic M, Jarema M, et al. Experience of stigma and discrimination reported by people experiencing the first episode of schizophrenia and those with a first episode of depression: The FEDORA project Anamaria Vasilache 2 , Margda Waern 3,4 , Norman Sartorius 10 , Graham Thornicroft 1 and the FEDORA study group. Int J Soc Psychiatry. 2015 [cited 2018 Jul 3];61:438–445. Available from: http://journals.sagepub.com/doi/pdf/10.1177/0020764014551941
17. Lasalvia A, Van Bortel T, Bonetto C, Jayaram G, Van Weeghel J, Zoppei S, et al. Cross-national variations in reported discrimination among people treated for major depression worldwide : the ASPEN / INDIGO international study. Br J Psychiatry. 2015;207:507–14.
18. Koschorke M, Padmavati R, Kumar S, Cohen A, Weiss HA, Chatterjee S, et al. Experiences of stigma and discrimination of people with schizophrenia in

India. Soc Sci Med; 2014;123:149–159. Available from: https://doi.org/10.1016/j.socscimed.2014.10.035. Elsevier Ltd

19. Lv Y, Wolf A, Wang X. Experienced stigma and self-stigma in Chinese patients with schizophrenia. Gen Hosp Psychiatry. 2013;35:83–8. Available from: https://doi.org/10.1016/j.genhosppsych.2012.07.007 Elsevier Inc.

20. Oshodi YO, Abdulmalik J, Ola B, James BO, Bonetto C, Cristofalo D, et al. Pattern of experienced and anticipated discrimination among people with depression in Nigeria: a cross-sectional study. Soc Psychiatry Psychiatr Epidemiol. 2014;49:259–66.

21. Lasalvia A. Tackling the mental illness stigma in low- and middle-income countries: lessons learned from high-income countries and mistakes to avoid. Epidemiol Psychiatr Sci. 2015;24:395–8 Available from: https://www.cambridge.org/core/journals/epidemiology-and-psychiatric-sciences/article/tackling-the-mental-illness-stigma-in-low-and-middleincome-countries-lessonslearned-from-highincome-countries-and-mistakes-to-avoid/83D63EA7FD15A3A3F2F9085E7E1700A2.

22. Rosen A. Destigmatizing day-to-day practices: what developed countries can learn from developing countries. World Psychiatry. 2006;5:21–24. https://www.ncbi.nlm.nih.gov/pmc/articles/PMC1472257/.

23. Alonso J, Buron A, Bruffaerts R, He Y, Posada-Villa J, Lepine JP, et al. Association of perceived stigma and mood and anxiety disorders: results from the world mental health surveys. Acta Psychiatr Scand. 2008;118:305–14.

24. Mathias K, Kermode M, San Sebastian M, Koschorke M, Goicolea I. Under the banyan tree--exclusion and inclusion of people with mental disorders in rural North India. BMC Public Health. 2015;15:-446 Available from: https://bmcpublichealth.biomedcentral.com/articles/10.1186/s12889-015-1778-2.

25. Maramis A, Van Tuan N, Minas H. Mental health in Southeast Asia. Lancet. 2011;377:700–2.

26. Minas H, Diatri H. Pasung: Physical restraint and confinement of the mentally ill in the community. Int J Ment Health Syst. 2008;2 Available from: https://www.ncbi.nlm.nih.gov/pmc/articles/PMC2442049/.

27. Tawiah PE, Adongo PB, Aikins M. Mental Health-Related Stigma and Discrimination in Ghana: Experience of Patients and Their Caregivers. Ghana Med J. 2015 [cited 2018 Jul 3];49:30–6. Available from: http://www.ncbi.nlm.nih.gov/pubmed/26339082.

28. Lauber C, Rössler W. Stigma towards people with mental illness in developing countries in Asia. Int Rev Psychiatry [Internet]. 2007;19:157–78 Available from: https://www.ncbi.nlm.nih.gov/pubmed/17464793.

29. Mascayano F, Armijo JE, Yang LH. Addressing stigma relating to mental illness in low- and middle-income countries. Front Psychiatry. 2015;6:1–4.

30. Abdullah T, Brown TL. Mental illness stigma and ethnocultural beliefs, values, and norms. Clin Psychol Rev. 2011;31:934–48.

31. Semrau M, Evans-Lacko S, Koschorke M, Ashenafi L, Thornicroft G. stugma and discrimination related to mental illness in low- and middle-income countries. Epidemiol. Psychiatr. Sci. [Internet]. 2015;24:382–94. Available from: https://www.ncbi.nlm.nih.gov/pubmed/25937022.

32. Yang LH, Kleinman A, Link BG, Phelan JC, Lee S, Good B. Culture and stigma: adding moral experience to stigma theory. Soc Sci Med. 2007;64:1524–35.

33. Yang LH, Thornicroft G, Alvarado R, Vega E, Link BG. Recent advances in cross-cultural measurement in psychiatric epidemiology: utilizing "what matters most" to identify culture-specific aspects of stigma. Int. J. Epidemiol. [internet]. 2014;43:494–510. Available from. https://www.ncbi.nlm.nih.gov/pubmed/24639447.

34. Edman JL, Johnson RC. Filipino American and Caucasian American beliefs about the causes and treatment of mental problems. Cultur Divers Ethnic Minor Psychol. 1999;5:380–6.

35. Thompson S, Hartel G, Manderson L, Woelz-Stirling N, Kelaher M. The mental health status of Filipinas in Queensland. Aust N Z J Psychiatry. 2002;36:674–80.

36. Corrigan PW, Rowan D, Green A, Lundin R, River P, Uphoff-Wasowski K, et al. Challenging two mental illness Stigmas : personal responsibility and dangerousness. Schizophr Bull. 2002;28:293–310.

37. Pescosolido BA, Medina TR, Martin JK, Long JS. The "Backbone" of Stigma: Identifying the Global Core of Public Prejudice Associated With Mental Illness. Am. J. Public Health [Internet]. 2013;103:853–60. Available from: https://www.ncbi.nlm.nih.gov/pubmed/23488508.

38. Gong F, Gage SJL, Tacata LA. Helpseeking behavior among Filipino Americans: a cultural analysis of face and language. J Community Psychol. 2003;31:469–88.

39. Javier JR, Supan J, Lansang A, Beyer W, Kubicek K, Palinkas LA. Preventing Filipino mental health disparities: perspectives from adolescents, caregivers,

providers, and advocates. Asian Am J Psychol [Internet]. 2014;5:316–24 Available from: https://www.ncbi.nlm.nih.gov/pmc/articles/PMC4319658/.

40. Charmaz K. Constructing Grounded Theory. 2nd ed. SAGE Publications Ltd; 2014.

41. Charmaz K. Grounded theory methods in social justice research. In: Denzin NK, Lincoln YS, editors. SAGE Handb. Qual. Res. SAGE; 2011. p. 359–380.

42. Charmaz K. The Power of Constructivist Grounded Theory for Critical Inquiry. Qual. Inq. [Internet]. 2017;23:34–45. Available from: http://journals.sagepub.com/doi/10.1177/1077800416657105

43. City Government of Muntinlupa. POVERTY AND EMPLOYMENT STATISTICS [Internet]. 2017 [cited 2017 Jun 30].

44. Philippine Statistics Authority. Philippines National Demographic and Health Survey 2013. 2013 [cited 2017 Jun 30]. Available from: https://dhsprogram.com/pubs/pdf/FR294/FR294.pdf.

45. Boling W, Means M, Fletcher A. Quality of Life and Stigma in Epilepsy, Perspectives from Selected Regions of Asia and Sub-Saharan Africa. Brain Sci. [Internet]. Multidisciplinary Digital Publishing Institute (MDPI); 2018 [cited 2018 Jun 27];8. Available from: http://www.ncbi.nlm.nih.gov/pubmed/29614761.

46. Herrmann LK, Welter E, Berg AT, Perzynski AT, Van Doren JR, Sajatovic M. Epilepsy misconceptions and stigma reduction: Current status in Western countries. Epilepsy Behav. [Internet]. 2016 [cited 2018 Jun 27];60:165–73. Available from: http://www.ncbi.nlm.nih.gov/pubmed/27208826.

47. Koch-Stoecker S. Neuropsychiatric issues in epilepsy. In: Matsuura M, Inoue Y, editors. Neuropsychiatr. issues epilepsy [Internet]. John Libbey Eurotext; 2010 [cited 2018 Jun 27]. p. 233. Available from: https://books.google.co.jp/books?id=FQXhAAAAQBAJ&pg=PA174&lpg=PA174&dq=epilepsy+Emil+Kraepelin&source=bl&ots=r35Oh0rwjA&sig=IZa-67-5hrTVkzSl4HEloGkaobQ&hl=en&sa=X&ved=0ahUKEwjd26SwkvPbAhWEnZQKHUvrDZsQ6AEIsAEwEw#v=onepage&q=epilepsyAQ28EmilKraepelin&f=false.

48. World Health Organization. mhGAP Training Manuals - for the mhGAP Intervention Guide for mental, neurological and substance use disorders in non-specialized health settings, version 2.0 [Internet]. WHO. World Health Organization; 2017 [cited 2018 Jun 27]. Available from: http://www.who.int/mental_health/mhgap/training_manuals/en/

49. Tuliao AP. Mental health help seeking among Filipinos: a review of the literature. Asia Pacific J Couns Psychother [Internet]. 2014;5:124–36 Available from: http://www.tandfonline.com/doi/abs/10.1080/21507686.2014.913641.

50. Yang LH, Valencia E, Alvarado R, Link B, Huynh N, Nguyen K, et al. A theoretical and empirical framework for constructing culture-specific stigma instruments for Chile. Cad. saude coletiva [Internet]. 2013;21:71–9. Available from: /pmc/articles/PMC3753780/?report=abstract.

51. Hamilton S, Pinfold V, Cotney J, Couperthwaite L, Matthews J, Barret K, et al. Qualitative analysis of mental health service users' reported experiences of discrimination. Acta Psychiatr Scand. 2016;134:14–22.

52. Demyttenaere K, Bruffaerts R, Posada-Villa J, Gasquet I, Kovess V, Lepine JP, et al. Prevalence, severity, and unmet need for treatment of mental disorders in the World Health Organization world mental health surveys. JAMA [internet]. 2004;291:2581–90. Available from. http://www.ncbi.nlm.nih.gov/pubmed/15173149.

53. Wig NN, Suleiman MA, Routledge R, Murthy RS, Ladrido-Ignacio L, Ibrahim HH, et al. Community reactions to mental disorders. A key informant study in three developing countries. Acta Psychiatr. Scand. [Internet]. 1980;61:111–26. Available from: https://www.ncbi.nlm.nih.gov/pubmed/7361584.

54. Ando S, Yamaguchi S, Aoki Y, Thornicroft G. Review of mental-health-related stigma in Japan. Psychiatry Clin Neurosci. 2013;67:471–82.

55. van Boekel LC, Brouwers EP, van Weeghel J, Garretsen HF. Comparing stigmatising attitudes towards people with substance use disorders between the general public, GPs, mental health and addiction specialists and clients. Int J Soc Psychiatry [Internet]. 2014;61:539–49 Available from: http://isp.sagepub.com/cgi/doi/10.1177/0020764014562051.

56. Clement S, Jarrett M, Henderson C, Thornicroft G. Messages to use in population-level campaigns to reduce mental health-related stigma: consensus development study. Epidemiol Psichiatr Soc. 2010;19:72–9.

57. Dy MB. Values in Philippine culture and education. Washington, DC: CRVP; 1994.

58. Social Weather Stations. Social Weather Station Survey. [Internet]. 2017 [cited 2017 Nov 9]. Available from: https://www.sws.org.ph/swsmain/artcldisppage/?artcsyscode=ART-20170816103037

59. Pescosolido BA, Martin JK, Olafsdottir S, Long JS, Medina TR, Martin JK. The theory of industrial society and cultural schemata: does the "cultural myth of stigma" underlie the WHO schizophrenia paradox? Am J Sociol. 2015;121:783–825.

60. Araneta EG. Psychiatric Care of Pilipino Americans. In: Gaw AC, editor. Cult. Ethn. Ment. Illn. Washington, DC: American Psychiatric Press; 1993. p. 377–412.

61. Sanchez F, Gaw A. Mental health Care of Filipino Americans. Psychiatr Serv [Internet] 2007;58:810–815. Available from: https://www.ncbi.nlm.nih.gov/pubmed/17535941

62. Wonpat-Borja AJ, Yang LH, Link BG, Phelan JC. Eugenics, genetics, and mental illness stigma in Chinese Americans. Soc Psychiatry Psychiatr Epidemiol. 2012;47:145–56.

63. Yang LH, Purdie-Vaughns V, Kotabe H, Link BG, Saw A, Wong G, et al. Culture, threat, and mental illness stigma: identifying culture-specific threat among Chinese-American groups. Soc. Sci. Med. [internet]. Elsevier Ltd. 2013;88:56–67 Available from: https://doi.org/10.1016/j.socscimed.2013.03.036.

64. Yang LH, Kleinman A. "Face" and the embodiment of stigma in China: the cases of schizophrenia and AIDS. Soc Sci Med. 2008;67:398–408.

65. Abad PJB, Tan ML, Baluyot MMP, Villa AQ, Talapian GL, Reyes ME, et al. Cultural beliefs on disease causation in the Philippines: challenge and implications in genetic counseling. J Community Genet. 2014;5:399–407.

66. De Los Monteros KE, Gallo LC. The relevance of fatalism in the study of Latinas' cancer screening behavior: a systematic review of the literature. Int J Behav Med. 2011;18:310–8.

67. Roberts RE, Roberts CR, Chen IG. Fatalism and risk of adolescent depression. Psychiatry [internet]. 2000;63:239–52. Available from. http://www.ncbi.nlm.nih.gov/pubmed/11125670.

68. Cheng H, Sit JWH, Twinn SF, Cheng KKF, Thorne S. Coping with breast Cancer survivorship in Chinese women the role of fatalism or fatalistic voluntarism. Cancer Nurs. 2013;36:236–44.

69. Gonzalez P, Nuñez A, Wang-Letzkus M, Lim J-W, Flores KF, Nápoles AM. Coping with breast cancer: reflections from Chinese American, Korean American, and Mexican American women. Heal Psychol [Internet] 2016;35: 19–28. Available from: https://www.ncbi.nlm.nih.gov/pubmed/26389720.

70. Nurjannah I ,Mills J PT& UK. Human rights of the mentally ill in Indonesia. Int Nurs Rev. 2015;62:153–61.

71. Habtamu K, Alem A, Hanlon C. Conceptualizing and contextualizing functioning in people with severe mental disorders in rural Ethiopia: a qualitative study. BMC psychiatry [internet]. 2015;15:34. Available from: https://bmcpsychiatry.biomedcentral.com/articles/10.1186/s12888-015-0418-9.

72. An act establishing a national mental health policy for the purpose of enhancing the delivery of integrated mental health services, promoting and protecting the rights of persons utilizing psychiatric, neurologic and psychosocial health services, APPROPRI [Internet]. Republic of the Philippines; 2018. Available from: http://www.officialgazette.gov.ph/2018/06/20/republic-act-no-11036/

73. Kitchener B, Jorm A. Mental health first aid training for the public: evaluation of effects on knowledge, attitudes and helping behavior. BMC Psychiatry [Internet]. 2002;2:10. Available from: http://www.biomedcentral.com/1471-244X/2/10

74. Morgan AJ, Ross A, Reavley NJ. Systematic review and meta-analysis of Mental Health First Aid training: Effects on knowledge, stigma, and helping behaviour. Doran CM, editor. PLoS One [Internet]. 2018 [cited 2018 Jun 28];13:e0197102. Available from: https://journals.plos.org/plosone/article?id=10.1371/journal.pone.0197102.

75. Bond KS, Jorm AF, Kitchener BA, Reavley NJ. Mental health first aid training for Australian medical and nursing students: an evaluation study. BMC Psychol. [Internet]. 2015 [cited 2018 Jun 28];3:11. Available from: http://www.ncbi.nlm.nih.gov/pubmed/25914827.

76. Jorm AF, Kitchener BA, Fischer J-A, Cvetkovski S. Mental Health First Aid Training by e-Learning: A Randomized Controlled Trial. Aust. New Zeal. J. Psychiatry [Internet]. 2010 [cited 2018 Jun 28];44:1072–81. Available from: http://www.ncbi.nlm.nih.gov/pubmed/21070103.

77. Corrigan PW, Morris SB, Michaels PJ, Rafacz JDRN. Challenging the public stigma of mental illness: a meta-analysis of outcome studies. Psychiatr. Serv. [Internet]. 2012;63:963–73 Available from: https://www.ncbi.nlm.nih.gov/pubmed/23032675.

78. Corrigan PW, Michaels PJ, Vega E, Gause M, Larson J, Krzyzanowski R, et al. Key ingredients to contact-based stigma change: A cross-validation. Psychiatr. Rehabil. J. [Internet]. 2014 [cited 2018 Jun 28];37:62–4. Available from: http://www.ncbi.nlm.nih.gov/pubmed/24417232.

79. Corrigan PW, Larson JE, Michaels PJ, Buchholz BA, Del Rossi R, Fontecchio MJ, et al. Diminishing the self-stigma of mental illness by coming out proud. Psychiatry Res. 2015;229:148–54.

80. Rüsch N, Abbruzzese E, Hagedorn E, Hartenhauer D, Kaufmann I, Curschellas J, et al. Efficacy of Coming Out Proud to reduce stigma's impact among people with mental illness: pilot randomised controlled trial. Br. J. Psychiatry [Internet]. 2014 [cited 2018 Jun 28];204:391–7. Available from: http://www.ncbi.nlm.nih.gov/pubmed/24434073.

81. Corrigan PW, Rüsch N, Scior K. Adapting disclosure programs to reduce the stigma of mental illness. Psychiatr. Serv. [internet]. 2018 [cited 2018 Jun 28];appi. Ps.2017004. Available from: http://www.ncbi.nlm.nih.gov/pubmed/29606076.

# 3

# Factors associated with treatment intensification in child and adolescent psychiatry: a cross-sectional study

Richard Vijverberg[1,2,3]*[iD], Robert Ferdinand[1], Aartjan Beekman[2,3] and Berno van Meijel[2,3,4,5,6]

## Abstract

**Background:** More knowledge about characteristics of children and adolescents who need intensive levels of psychiatric treatment is important to improve treatment approaches. These characteristics were investigated in those who need youth Assertive Community Treatment (youth-ACT).

**Method:** A cross-sectional study among children/adolescents and their parents treated in either a regular outpatient clinic or a youth-ACT setting in a specialized mental health treatment center in the Netherlands.

**Results:** Child, parent and family/social context factors were associated with treatment intensification from regular outpatient care to youth-ACT. The combination of the child, parent, and family/social context factors adds substantially to the predictive power of the model (Nagelkerke $R^2$ increasing from 36 to 45% for the three domains separately, to 61% when all domains are combined). The strongest predictors are the severity of psychiatric disorders of the child, parental stress, and domestic violence.

**Conclusions:** Using a wide variety of variables that are potentially associated with treatment intensification from regular outpatient clinic to youth-ACT, we constructed a regression model illustrating a relatively strong relation between the predictor variables and the outcome (Nagelkerke $R^2 = 0.61$), with three strong predictors, i.e. severity of psychiatric disorders of the child, parental stress, and domestic violence. This emphasizes the importance of a system-oriented approach with primary attention for problem solving and stress reduction within the system, in addition to the psychiatric treatment of the child, and possibly also the parents.

**Keywords:** Child and adolescent psychiatry, Assertive community treatment, Assertive outreach, Predictors, Risk factors

## Background

Ten to 20 % of the children and adolescents in the general population suffer from a psychiatric disorder [1–3]. With the general practitioner as the gate keeper, most of the Dutch children and adolescents with psychiatric disorders are referred to outpatient clinics [4, 5]. If more intensive mental health care is necessary, children or adolescents can be referred by the general practitioner or via the outpatient clinic to youth Assertive Community Treatment (youth-ACT). This is an intensive home-based treatment that is provided by a multidisciplinary team of

mental health care professionals who have small caseloads (size< 15).

Existing studies (only four) mainly studied child factors (and not: variables pertaining to parents) [6, 7], only pertained to children (and not to adolescents) [7], used small samples [8], or only studied children with autism spectrum disorder [9]. Two of the four studies were conducted more than 20 years ago [6, 7]. To increase scientific knowledge regarding the intensification of outpatient psychiatric treatment in children and adolescents we (1) studied a larger sample, and (2) examined child, parent, and family/social context factors that might predict intensification of outpatient treatment, in (3) both children and adolescents.

More knowledge about factors associated with intensifying treatment from regular outpatient care into youth-ACT is important from the perspective of prevention because it

* Correspondence: r.vijverberg@ggz-delfland.nl
[1]Department of Child and Adolescent Psychiatry, GGZ Delfland, PO-box 5016, 2600, GA, Delft, The Netherlands
[2]Amsterdam UMC, location VUmc and GGZ inGeest, Department of psychiatry, Amsterdam, The Netherlands
Full list of author information is available at the end of the article

offers opportunities to determine which factors should be targeted with treatment to prevent increase in psychopathology and deterioration of functioning, ultimately leading to referral to a more intensive form of mental health care [6–9]. By identifying factors associated with intensifying treatment, mental health care professionals are encouraged to determine at an early stage whether regular outpatient care can be expected to be effective or if they should consider treatment intensification [9]. More precision in the allocation of care for those who need intensive treatment may help avoid exposure of patients to treatments that will prove to be ineffective, and lead to unnecessary delay in recovery [10, 11]. Conversely, in the vast majority of children and adolescents a more intensive form of treatment than outpatient care is not necessary, so referral to a setting such as youth-ACT would be inefficient for most patients [12–17].

The aim of this study was to investigate factors that are associated with treatment intensification from regular outpatient care into youth-ACT. We aimed to include variables on the child, parent and family/social context levels which are known from the literature to be associated with mental health of children [6–9, 18].

Our a priori hypotheses were that children and adolescents in whom outpatient treatment is intensified into youth-ACT have significantly more severe psychiatric disorders, more care needs, lower quality of life, and an older age [6–9]. Further, we expected that parents of children and adolescents in whom outpatient treatment is intensified into youth-ACT have higher levels of parental psychiatric disorders, more care needs, lower quality of life, higher levels of parental stress, and a poorer parental ability to deal adequately with the psychiatric problems of the child. Studies that link functioning of parents with the utilization of inpatient care of children and adolescents support these hypotheses [7–9]. At the family/social context level, we expected that treatment intensification from regular outpatient care into youth-ACT is associated with a parent being single parent, a larger number of children in the family, more domestic violence, more financial problems, less social support, and low family socioeconomic status (SES) [7–9].

## Method
### Design
We conducted a cross-sectional study with children/adolescents and their parents who were treated in either a regular outpatient clinic or a youth-ACT setting.

### Setting
The study was carried out between September 2014 and July 2016 in a specialized treatment center for psychiatric disorders in the Netherlands, GGZ Delfland. Two

outpatient clinics and one youth-ACT team, who served patients in the same geographical area, were included. The two outpatient clinics carry out diagnostic assessments and treatment of children/adolescents using a multidisciplinary team. Each team consists of one child psychiatrist, six psychologists, and one nurse practitioner.

The youth-ACT team provides treatment based on the following elements and principles: (a) home-based multidisciplinary treatment, (b) intensity of treatment is scaled up or down according to the severity of current psychiatric symptoms and level of functioning of the patient, (c) small caseloads (size< 15), (d) focused on patients who are difficult to reach, (e) case management, (f) early intervention, (g) family support, (h) reintegration/vocational and educational therapy, (i) medication when appropriate. The youth-ACT team consists of one child psychiatrist, five psychologists, three nurse practitioners and two psychiatric nurses.

### Participants
Figure 1 presents the flowchart of the inclusion process. To be included, participants in both treatment settings had to meet the following inclusion criteria: (a) children/adolescents aged between 4 and 18 years; (b) with a DSM-IV diagnosis; and (c) had a parent who fulfilled the role of primary caregiver. Because the involvement of parents in raising a child can vary widely [19], especially when it concerns single parent families [20], only the parent who fulfilled the role of primary caregiver was included in this study. Only children who were referred from an outpatient clinic, were included in the youth-ACT sample.

Included outpatients who were later referred to youth-ACT were excluded from the outpatient sample and included in the youth-ACT sample. Also, children were excluded when a sibling or other child living in the same household already participated in the study.

### Ethical approval
The study was approved by the Medical Ethics Committee on Research Involving Human Subjects of the VU University Medical Centre, Amsterdam (protocol no. 2015.245). Participants received written and oral information, separately for children and parents, about the study and were included after giving informed consent.

### Measurement instruments
#### Child factors
For the assessment of psychiatric diagnoses, we used the Neuropsychiatric Interview for Children and Adolescent (MINI-KID), supplemented with clinical diagnoses that were not included in the MINI-KID [21].

The Health of the Nation Outcomes Scales Child and Adolescents Mental Health (HoNOSCA) was used to

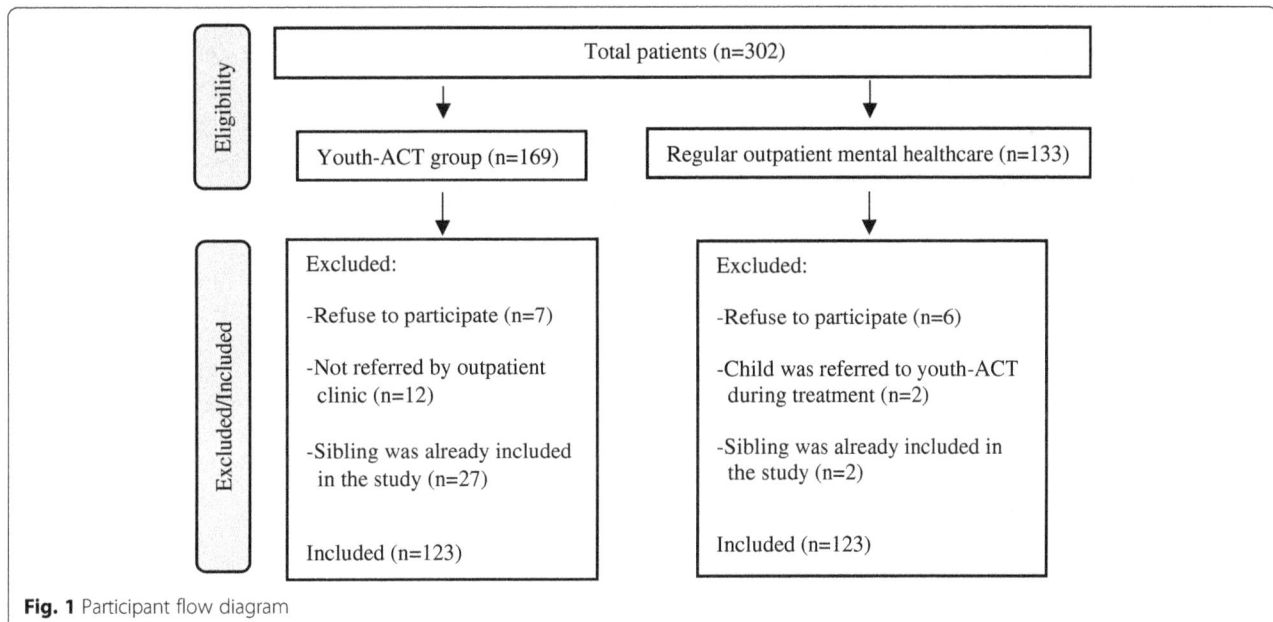

**Fig. 1** Participant flow diagram

assess the severity of psychiatric disorders [22]. The HoNOSCA covers 15 items to be scored on a 5-point severity scale ranging from `no problems' (0) to `severe problems' (4). To calculate HoNOSCA-sum score, we used the items 1 to 13, since items 14 and 15 do not provide information about the mental health situation of the child.

The Camberwell Assessment of Need Short Appraisal Schedule (CANSAS) was used to assess the care needs of the child [23]. The CANSAS covers 25 care need items which are scored on a nominal 3-point scale 'no need' (1), `met need' (2), and 'unmet need' (3). To calculate the CANSAS-sum score, the sum of met and unmet needs of the 25 items was computed.

The Kidscreen-27 was used to assess the health-related quality of life of children [24]. The Kidscreen is a self-report questionnaire that consists of 27 items to be scored on a 5-point scale ranging from 'never' (0) to 'always' (4). The Kidscreen sum score was calculated by adding up the scores of the 27 items.

A designated client-based standardized questionnaire (DEMOG) was used to measure the following demographic characteristics of the child: (a) age, (b) gender, and (c) country of birth [25]. This is a standardized client-based questionnaire to measure demographic characteristics.

### Parental factors

The Health of the Nation Outcomes Scales (HoNOS) was used to assess the severity of psychiatric disorders of the parent [26–28]. The HoNOS covers 12 items to be scored on a 5-point severity scale ranging from `no problems' (0)

to `severe problems' (4). The HoNOS sum score was calculated by adding up the scores of the 12 items.

Item 14 of the HoNOSCA was used to assess the parental knowledge about the difficulties of the child from the perception of the parent.

As with the children, the CANSAS was used by parents as a self-report scale to assess their care needs.

Parenting stress was measured using a Parenting Stress Scale. The primary caregivers rated their level of parenting stress on a scale ranging from 1 to 10.

The Manchester Short Assessment of quality of life (MANSA-16) was used to assess the health-related quality of life of the parent [29, 30]. The MANSA consists of 16 items to be scored on a 7-point scale ranging from `could not be worse' (1) to `could not be better' (7). The MANSA-16 sum score was calculated by adding up the scores of the 16 items.

DEMOG-adult was used to measure the following demographic characteristics of the parent: (a) age, (b) gender, and (c) country of birth [25].

### Family/social context factors

The DEMOG-Adult was also used to assess living situation, family composition, and socio-economic status (SES; expressed in educational achievements and ethnic background).

Domestic violence was registered by a self-developed form to be scored 'yes' or 'no'. It was assessed whether the client, parents, and siblings had used violence against other family members in the present.

Items 3 and 6 of the MANSA were used separately to assess social support and financial problems of the family, respectively.

### Data-analysis

Analyses were performed using SPSS 24.0. The descriptive statistics of the outpatient sample and youth-ACT sample were calculated on item or scale level. Next, we conducted three series of univariable logistic regression analyses, with treatment setting as dependent variable, to identify candidate predictors for the multivariable regression models. The first series concerned candidate predictors at the level of the child: severity of psychiatric disorders, care needs, quality of life, and age. The second series concerned candidate predictors at the level of the parent: severity of psychiatric disorders of the parent, care needs, quality of life, parental stress, and (lack of) knowledge pertaining to difficulties of the child. The third series concerned candidate predictors at the level of family/social context: living situation, the number of children, financial problems, educational achievements and ethnic background of the primary caregiver, domestic violence, social support and financial problems.

By using this step-by-step approach, we created multivariable regression models that did not violate the statistical rule of 10 events per 1 variable and ensured the validity of the analysis [31, 32]. First, for each level (child, parent, and family/social context) we conducted three separate multivariable analyses in which we entered the predictors that were (borderline)-significant ($P < 0.10$) in the univariable analyses. Finally, we conducted a stepwise multivariable analyses investigating the three levels (child, parent, and family/social context) together.

The assumptions of the logistic regression analyses (multicollinearity) were tested for indications of multicollinearity by examining the variance inflation factor (VIF) and tolerance values. No violations of limits were found (VIF range 1.00–2.00; tolerance between 0.45 and 1.00), indicating that there was no indication of multicollinearity [33]. Further, the assumptions of linearity and homoscedasticity were tested by creating a scatter plot of the standardized residuals. The distribution of the residuals was reasonably rectangular, and most of the scores were in the centre. Thus, the assumption of linearity and homoscedasticity were met in this study [33, 34]. The Hosmer and Lemeshow goodness-of-fit test was used to measure the predictive value of the model [33]. To obtain an overall indication of how well the models performed, we used the Omnibus test [33]. The Nagelkerke $R^2$ was used to provide an indication of the strength of the relation between the predictor variables and the outcome variable [33]. The discrimination accuracy of the model was examined by using the area under the curve (AUC) of the receiver operating characteristic

curve (ROC curve) and were categorized as fail (0.50–0.60); poor (0.60–0.70); fair (0.70–0.80); good (0.80–0.90); or excellent (0.90–1.00) [35].

### Results
#### Characteristics of the sample

Characteristics of the study sample ($n = 246$) are presented in Tables 1 and 2. The outpatient sample ($n = 123$) comprised 56 girls (45.5%) and 67 boys (54.5%) with an average age of 11.8 years. The most frequent clinical diagnoses were attention deficit hyperactivity disorder (43.1%), anxiety disorder (31.7%), behavioral disorder (12.0%), or mood disorder (6.5%). In the outpatient sample, most primary care givers ($n = 123$) were mothers (99.2%) with an average age of 41.0 years. The majority of mothers (66.6%) had a

**Table 1** Sample characteristics of the child or adolescent who received treatment

|  | Outpatient | Youth-ACT |
|---|---|---|
|  | Child ($n^1$=123) | Child ($n = 123$) |
| Age (sd[2]) | Total mean 11.8 (3.2) | Total mean 13.0 (3.2) |
|  | range 6–17 | range 4–18 |
|  | Girls mean 13.0 (3.4) | Girls mean 13.7 (3.0) |
|  | range 6–17 | range 4–18 |
|  | Boys mean 11.1 (2.9) | Boys mean 12.5 (3.3) |
|  | range 6–17 | range 6–17 |
| Gender | Girls 45.5% | Girls 42.3% |
|  | Boys 54.5% | Boys 57.7% |
| Country of birth | Holland 96.7% | Holland 95.1% |
|  | Other 3.3% | Other 4.9% |
| Clinical diagnoses | Mood 6.5% | Mood 37.4% |
|  | Anxiety 31.7% | Anxiety 41.5% |
|  | Behavior 12.0% | Behavior 30.0% |
|  | Psychotic 0.0% | Psychotic 4.0% |
|  | ASD[3] 11.4% | ASD 40.7% |
|  | ADHD[4] 43.1% | ADHD 42.3% |
|  | Somatoform 0.8% | Somatoform 13.8% |
|  | Drugs/alcohol 0.0% | Drugs/alcohol 3.2% |
|  | Mental retard 3.2% | Mental retard 8.1% |
|  | Personality 0.0% | Personality 5.7% |
|  | Other 0.8% | Other 3.2% |
| GAF[5]-score (sd) | Mean 55.0 (5.4) | Mean 45.7 (8.1) |
|  | Range 45–75 | Range 15–60 |
| Living situation | Single parent 26.2% | Single parent 42.1% |
|  | Two parent 73.8% | Two parent 57.9% |

[1]$n$ number of included patients
[2]$sd$ standard deviation
[3]$ASD$ Autism spectrum disorder
[4]$ADHD$ Attention deficit hyperactivity disorder
[5]$GAF$ General assessment of functioning

**Table 2** Sample characteristics of the parent who fulfilled the role of primary caregiver

|  | Outpatient Parent[1] (n[2]=123) | Youth-ACT Parent (n = 123) |
|---|---|---|
| Age (sd[3]) | Total mean 41.0 (6.2) | Total mean 43.7 (7.3) |
|  | range 27–55 | range 24–70 |
| Status | Mother 99.2% | Mother 98.4% |
|  | Father 0.8% | Father 1.6% |
| Country of birth | Holland 78.0% | Holland 88.6% |
|  | Other 22.0% | Other 11.4% |
| Education status | Basic 15.4% | Basic 25.3% |
|  | Intermediate 22.0% | Intermediate 29.2% |
|  | High 62.6% | High 45.5% |
| Employment status | Paid job 66.6% | Paid job 35.8% |
|  | No paid job 33.4% | No paid job 64.2% |

[1]Parent primary care giver
[2]n number of included patients
[3]sd standard deviation

paid job and 73.8% of these mothers raised their children in a two-parent household.

The youth-ACT sample (n = 123) comprised 52 girls (42.3%) and boys 71 (57.7%) with an average age of 13.0 years. The most frequent clinical diagnoses were attention deficit hyperactivity disorder (42.3%), anxiety disorder (41.5%), behavioral disorder (30.0%), and mood disorder (37.0%). In the youth-ACT sample 98.4% of the primary caregivers (n = 123) were mothers with an average age of 43.7 years. The majority of mothers (64.2%) did not have a paid job and 57.9% of these mothers raised their children in a two-parent household.

### Predictors youth-ACT
#### Univariable analyses
As presented in Table 3, the univariable analyses shows that treatment intensification from outpatient care into youth-ACT was predicted by all variables, with the exception of educational status of the primary caregiver (P = 0.210, P = 0.312), social support (P = 0.118), and number of children in the household (P = 0.965).

At the child level, the referral to youth-ACT was predicted by the severity of the psychiatric disorders, assessed with the HoNOSCA (OR = 1.29, 95% CI 1.21–1.38, P < 0.001), the child's care needs (OR = 1.06, 95% CI 1.00–1.12, P = 0.034), quality of life (OR = 0.94, 95% CI 0.92–0.97, P < 0.001), and age (OR = 2.24, 95% CI 1.32–3.80, P = 0.003).

At the parent level, the severity of psychiatric disorders of the parent predicted the referral to youth-ACT (OR = 1.22, 95% CI 1.15–1.30, P < 0.001), as did the parents' care needs (OR = 1.12, 95% CI 1.07–112, P < 0.001), and the parents' quality of life (OR = 0.93, 95% CI 0.91–0.96, P < 0.001). Also, the parental knowledge about the

difficulties of the child and the perceived parental stress were significant predictors (respectively OR = 1.53 (95% CI 1.34–1.76, P < 0.001) and OR = 1.66 (95% CI 1.30–2.13, P < 0.001)).

At the family/social context level, being a single parent (OR = 2.05, 95% CI 1.19–3.42, P = 0.009), the presence of domestic violence (OR = 12.05, 95% CI 6.20–23.42, P < 0.001), having financial problems (OR = 1.32, 95% CI 1.11–1.56, P = 0.015), and ethnic background of the primary caregiver (OR = 0.46, 95% CI 0.23–0.92, P = 0.029) were significant predictors.

#### Multivariable analyses for each level separately
Table 3 shows that at the child level, quality of life (P = 0.213), and age of the child (P = 0.322) did not remain significant in the multivariable analysis. The child model showed a good fit of the data (Hosmer-Lemeshow, P = 0.681) and illustrated a relatively strong relation between the predictor variables and the outcome (Nagelkerke $R^2$ = 0.43). The AUC under the ROC curve suggested that the model has a good classification ability to discriminate the referral to regular outpatient care with youth-ACT (AUC = 0.84, 95% CI 0.78–0.89, P < 0.001).

At the parent level, the care needs (P = 0.802) and quality of life (P = 0.568) did not remain significant. The model showed a good fit of the data (Hosmer-Lemeshow, P = 0.912) and illustrated a relatively strong relation between the predictor variables and the outcome (Nagelkerke $R^2$ = 0.45). The model has a good classification ability to discriminate the referral to regular outpatient care with youth-ACT (AUC = 0.85, 95% CI 0.80–0.89, P < 0.001).

At the family/social context level, being a single parent (P = 0.437) and having financial problems (P = 0.593) did not remain significant in the multivariable analysis. The model fitted the data (Hosmer-Lemeshow, P = 0.576) and illustrated a relatively strong relation between predictor variables and the outcome (Nagelkerke $R^2$ = 0.36). The model has a fair classification ability to discriminate the referral to regular outpatient care with youth-ACT (AUC = 0.78, 95% CI 0.72–0.84, P < 0.001).

#### Multivariable analyses for all levels simultaneously
First, in the final logistic model, the severity of the psychiatric disorder of the child (OR = 1.31, 95% CI 1.22–1.41, P < 0.001) remained a significant predictor regarding referral to youth-ACT (see Table 4). However, the child's care needs did not remain significant (P = 0.186). Second, the significant child and parent predictors together showed that all predictors remained significant: the severity of the psychiatric disorder of the child (OR = 1.21, 95% CI 1.12–1.30, P < 0.001) and parent (OR = 1.13, 95% CI 1.05–1.21, P < 0.001), parental stress (OR = 1.36, 95% CI 1.15–1.60, P < 0.001) and parental knowledge about the difficulties of the child (OR = 1.39, 95% CI 1.00–

**Table 3** Predictors of youth-ACT

| Level of predictors | Univariable model[1] | | | Multivariable model[2] | | |
|---|---|---|---|---|---|---|
| | n[3] | OR[4] (95% CI[5]) | P-value | n | OR (95% CI) | P-value[6] |
| Child[8] | | | | 225 | | |
| HoNOSCA[7] | 246 | 1.29 (1.21–1.38) | <.001 | | 1.27 (1.18–1.37) | <.001 |
| CANSAS[7] | 243 | 1.06 (1.00–1.12) | 0.034 | | 0.93 (0.87–1.01) | 0.051 |
| Kidscreen[7] | 228 | 0.94 (0.92–0.97) | <.001 | | 0.97 (0.95–1.00) | 0.213 |
| Age | 246 | | | | | |
| 4–11 years old | 93 | | | | | |
| 12–18 years old | 153 | 2.24 (1.32–3.80) | 0.003 | | 1.41 (0.71–2.81) | 0.322 |
| Parent[9] | | | | 238 | | |
| HoNOS[7] | 244 | 1.22 (1.15–1.30) | <.001 | | 1.22 (1.10–1.35) | <.001 |
| CANSAS[7] | 246 | 1.12 (1.07–1.12) | <.001 | | 0.99 (0.92–1.06) | 0.802 |
| MANSA[7] | 240 | 0.93 (0.91–0.96) | <.001 | | 1.01 (0.97–1.06) | 0.568 |
| Parental stress | 245 | 1.53 (1.34–1.76) | <.001 | | 1.42 (1.21–1.67) | 0.002 |
| Lack of knowledge pertaining to difficulties | 246 | 1.66 (1.30–2.13) | <.001 | | 1.60 (1.19–2.15) | 0.003 |
| Family and social context[10] | | | | 243 | | |
| Living situation | 243 | | | | | |
| Two parents | 160 | | | | | |
| Single parent | 83 | 2.05 (1.19–3.42) | 0.009 | | 1.30 (0.67–2.55) | 0.437 |
| Domestic violence | 245 | 12.05 (6.20–23.42) | <.001 | | 11.27 (5.56–22.86) | <.001 |
| Financial problems | 243 | 1.32 (1.11–1.56) | 0.015 | | 1.06 (0.86–1.31) | 0.593 |
| Ethnic background primary caregiver | 246 | | | | | |
| Dutch | 236 | | | | | |
| Other | 10 | 0.46 (0.23–0.92) | 0.029 | | 0.40 (0.18–0.91) | 0.028 |
| Social support | 243 | 0.52 (0.23–1.18) | 0.118 | | | |
| Educational status | 246 | | | | | |
| Basic | 39 | | | | | |
| Intermediate | 74 | 1.65 (0.75–3.63) | 0.210 | | | |
| High | 133 | 0.69 (0.34–1.41) | 0.312 | | | |
| Number of children | 245 | 0.99 (0.76–1.30) | 0.965 | | | |

[1]Univariable: binary logistic analyses of each candidate predictor preformed separately
[2]Multivariable: binary logistic regression analysis of the predictors that were significant in the univariable analysis, performed simultaneously
[3]n number of patients
[4]OR Odds Ratio
[5]CI Confidence interval
[6]P-value< 0.10 is considered statistically significant
[7]Sum-score
[8]Child-level: Omnibus test, Step $P = 0.00$, Model $P = < 0.00$, Hosmer-Lemeshow, $P = 0.68$, Nagelkerke $R^2=0.43$, AUC = 0.84, 95% CI 0.78–0.89, $P < 0.001$
[9]Parent-level: Omnibus test, Step $P = 0.00$, Model $P = < 0.00$, Hosmer-Lemeshow, $P = 0.91$, Nagelkerke $R^2=0.45$, AUC = 0.85, 95% CI 0.80–0.89, $P < 0.001$
[10]Family-social context-level: Omnibus test, Step $P = 0.00$, Model $P = < 0.00$, Hosmer-Lemeshow, $P = 0.58$, Nagelkerke $R^2 = 0.36$, AUC = 0.78, 95% CI 0.72–0.84, $P < 0.001$

1.92, $P = 0.049$). Third, when the family/social context predictors were added, the severity of the psychiatric disorder of the child (OR = 1.19, 95% CI 1.11–1.29, $P < 0.001$), parental stress (OR = 1.35, 95% CI 1.13–1.62, $P = 0.001$), and domestic violence (OR = 5.19, 95% CI 2.20–12.26, $P < 0.001$) remained significant predictors. The severity of the psychiatric disorder of the parent ($P = 0.085$), parental knowledge about the difficulties of the child ($P = 0.081$) and ethnic background of the primary caregiver ($P = 0.104$) were no longer significantly associated with the dependent variable.

The model of the child, parent and family/social context predictors together showed a good fit of the data (Hosmer-Lemeshow, $P = 0.511$), and illustrated a relatively strong relation between the predictor variables and the outcome (Nagelkerke $R^2 = 0.61$). The AUC under the ROC curve suggested that the model has an excellent classification ability to discriminate the referral to regular outpatient care

**Table 4** Predictors of youth-ACT

| Level of predictors | Child[1] | | Child and parent[2] | | Child, parent and family/social context[3] | |
|---|---|---|---|---|---|---|
| | Multivariable model[4] | | Multivariable model | | Multivariable model | |
| | OR[5](95% CI[6]) | P[7] | OR (95% CI) | P | OR (95% CI) | P |
| Child | | | | | | |
| HoNOSCA[8] | 1.31 (1.22–1.41) | <.001 | 1.21 (1.12–1.30) | <.001 | 1.19 (1.11–1.29) | <.001 |
| CANSAS[8] | 0.96 (0.90–1.02) | 0.186 | | | | |
| Parent[9] | | | | | | |
| HoNOS[8] | | | 1.13 (1.05–1.21) | <.001 | 1.07 (0.99–1.15) | 0.085 |
| Parental stress | | | 1.36 (1.15–1.60) | <.001 | 1.35 (1.13–1.62) | 0.001 |
| Lack of knowledge pertaining to difficulties | | | 1.39 (1.00–1.92) | 0.049 | 1.34 (0.96–1.87) | 0.081 |
| Family/social context | | | | | | |
| Domestic violence | | | | | 5.19 (2.20–12.26) | <.001 |
| Ethnic background primary caregiver | | | | | | |
| Dutch | | | | | | |
| Other | | | | | 0.40 (0.13–1.21) | 0.104 |

[1]Child-level: Omnibus test, Step $P = 0.00$, Model $P = < 0.00$, Hosmer-Lemeshow, $P = 0.26$, Nagelkerke $R^2 = 0.43$, AUC = 0.84, 95% CI 0.78–0.89, $P < 0.001$
[2]Child-parent-level: Omnibus test, Step $P = 0.00$, Model $P = < 0.00$, Hosmer-Lemeshow, $P = 0.17$, Nagelkerke $R^2 = 0.56$, AUC = 0.89, 95% CI 0.85–0.93, $P < 0.001$
[3]Child-parent-family/social context-level: Omnibus test, Step $P = 0.00$, Model $P = < 0.00$, Hosmer-Lemeshow, $P = 0.51$, Nagelkerke $R^2 = 0.61$, AUC = 0.91, 95% CI 0.87–0.95, $P < 0.001$
[4]Multivariable: binary logistic regression analysis of all predictors entered simultaneously
[5]OR Odds Ratio
[6]CI Confidence interval
[7]P-value< 0.10 is considered statistically significant
[8]Sum-score
[9]Parent: primary caregiver

with youth-ACT (AUC = 0.91, 95% CI 0.87–0.95, $P < 0.001$).

## Discussion

This cross-sectional study examined the patient, family and contextual variables that are associated with treatment intensification from regular outpatient care to a more intensive form of treatment: youth-ACT. To our knowledge, this is the first study that provides a much more detailed insight into the variables that are associated with intensifying outpatient treatment towards more intensive treatment. Through the step-by-step logical regression, a view is obtained on the hierarchy of these variables. By applying the step-by-step logistic regressions, we determined which variables are the strongest predictors of intensification of treatment. As hypothesized, we found many univariable associations between candidate predictors and intensification of treatment (see Table 3). However, not all variables that were entered as possible predictors of intensification of treatment were significant (see Table 3). In contrast to our expectations, significant effects of level of social support and educational status of parents on treatment intensification were not found. Number of children in the family did not predict treatment intensification as well.

Our findings indicate that children in whom outpatient care is intensified are likely to have parents with more

psychiatric problems (see Table 3). A cross-sectional relation like this can be explained in three different ways: X caused Y, Y caused X or there is a third variable causing X and Y [36]. Hence, a possible explanation is that severe psychiatric problems of the child negatively affect a parent's mental health [37]. Conversely, severe psychiatric problems in parents may also negatively affect a child's mental health [37, 38]. Finally, third variables, for instance, similar genes, or living in a similar adverse environment, may influence mental health in parents and their children.

We also found that parents of children in whom outpatient care is intensified display high levels of parental distress. This association may indicate that serious psychiatric symptoms in the child, that require more intense treatment, cause a high level of distress in parents, or vice versa. But, a variable influencing both psychiatric symptoms in a child, as well as parental distress, may be present as well.

A relation was also found between treatment intensification and lower quality of life and more care needs in parents (see Table 3). Regardless of the direction or exact nature of associations between, on one hand, treatment intensification, and on the other hand, parental mental health, parental distress, parental quality of life, and parental care needs, it is clear that all associations found possibly indicate a diminished ability of the parent to support children who are at risk for treatment intensification. In other words, several parental characteristics that were found may negatively influence treatment effects in their children [39–42].

Existing guidelines for intensive forms of treatment suggest that children who are living in families where children and parents experience many problems need a system-oriented approach [43, 44]. However, a classical system-oriented approach does not seem to be sufficient, because this approach does not specifically focus on the psychiatric problems of parents, and on their care needs and quality of life. Our findings suggest that this may be necessary, in addition to the classic system-oriented approach.

When conducting multivariable analyses including all levels, three variables - severity of psychiatric disorder of the child, parental stress and domestic violence - remained significant. The logistic regression model that included these three predictors showed a strong relation between the predictor variables and the outcome illustrated by the Nagelkerke $R^2$ of 0.61 and has an excellent ability to discriminate (AUC = 0.91, 95% CI 0.87–0.95, $P < 0.001$), indicating a high predictive value. We may conclude that children with severe psychiatric disorders, who live in a context where parents experience high levels of parental stress and where domestic violence takes place, are most likely to be referred from outpatient care to a more intensive form of treatment. A possible explanation is that there are negative reciprocal interactions patterns between domestic violence, parental stress and the severe psychiatric disorders in children [45]. When health care providers, together with patient and family members, are not able to break through these negative reciprocal interaction patterns when offering regular outpatient care, referral to more intensive treatment (such as youth ACT) is needed.

The effect sizes found in relation to domestic violence and parental stress are remarkable when we consider that existing guidelines for children and adolescents do not contain recommendations regarding stopping domestic violence and reducing parental stress [46–49]. Our results show that it is important to encourage guidelines to include recommendations regarding these issues.

For clinical practice, our findings indicate that health care professionals should pay extra attention to children with severe psychiatric disorders, parents who are stressed, and families characterized by domestic violence. A first step would be to assess (all of these) problems systematically. In case of high HoNOSCA-scores, it is especially important to assess parental stress and domestic violence as well. If problems exist in these areas, it may be important to focus treatment not only on reducing psychiatric problems, but also on parental stress and domestic violence. Another, important finding (see Table 4), is the prediction of treatment intensification by parental stress, and not by HONOS-scores of the parent in the final analysis. Our finding, parental stress scores being very important, is of clinical significance,

because it shows that, instead of screening parents for a broad range of psychiatric disorders, which is time consuming, one single question (parental stress was assessed on a visual analogue scale in our study) regarding parental stress is sufficient to screen for children/adolescents with a poor prognosis.

To our knowledge, regular outpatient treatment and youth-ACT programs do often not incorporate specific modules targeted at parental stress and at domestic violence [43]. The present study shows that, by adding such modules to outpatient treatment and youth-ACT programs might decrease the need for ACT. This is not to say that in the daily practice of an outpatient clinic or youth-ACT team, mental healthcare providers do not pay attention to reducing parental stress and domestic violence, but it is different to focus treatment specifically on these problems.

### Strengths and limitations

This study has several strengths. First, to our knowledge, this is the first study that examined the patient, family and contextual variables that are associated with referral to regular outpatient care or youth-ACT together. Second, a methodological strength of this study is that the youth-ACT sample consisted of patients that were referred directly from outpatient clinics in the same geographical catchment area, which assured a fair comparison of both groups. Third, the data was collected from a relatively large sample ($n$ = 246) and had limited missing values (3%). The power of the analyses was sufficient to draw relatively firm conclusions about the associations between characteristics of patients, their families and living context on the one hand, and treatment intensity on the other hand. Fourth, in order to prevent bias, the data in both samples were collected during the intake-phase of both types of treatment. A clear limitation of the study is that data were collected in one youth-ACT team and two outpatient clinics from the same mental health organization. Therefore, the results of this study cannot be generalized without reservations [36]. However, it is worthwhile to note that this study is not about a specific treatment modality, but about the phenomenon of intensification of outpatient treatment. This intensification may occur in various forms, but always involves the intensification of treatment compared to regular outpatient care. Although the Dutch situation and/or treatment facilities are specific, they are also very similar to the international guideline-based care for children and adolescents. Therefore, generalisability of our findings seems not only limited to Dutch situation, despite the variation in practice across various countries.

### Recommendations

Domestic violence and parental stress are strong predictors of treatment intensification. Therefore, research is needed to determine whether the addition of special modules targeted at domestic violence and parental stress can actually prevent intensification of treatment, but also to improve effects of intensive treatment.

To date, studies examining youth-ACT mainly focussed on child-related factors, such as severity of psychiatric symptoms, general functioning, and duration and frequency of psychiatric hospital admissions [50]. In line with our research, it is important that future research regarding treatment intensification to youth-ACT includes variables at child, parent and family/social context level. The results of this study emphasize the importance of a system-oriented approach with primary attention for problem solving and stress reduction within the system, in addition to the psychiatric treatment of the child, and possibly also the parents.

## Conclusion

To summarize, child, parent and family-social context factors predict treatment intensification from outpatient care to youth-ACT. Although each domain has a unique and important contribution to make, and although variables across domains are correlated, the combination of the three domains adds substantially to the predictive power of the model (increasing from Nagelkerke $R^2$ 0.36–0.45 in the three domains separately, to 0.61 when all domains were combined). Nagelkerke $R^2$ of 0.61 for treatment allocation is a high predictive power.

The strongest predictors regarding treatment intensification from outpatient care to youth-ACT are the severity of psychiatric disorders of the child, parental stress and domestic violence. From the perspective of prevention and effectiveness it is important to examine whether influencing parent and family-social context factors affects the mental health situation of the child and its need for youth-ACT.

## Abbreviations
ACT: Assertive Community Treatment; ADHD: Attention Deficit Hyperactivity Disorder; ASD: Autism Spectrum Disorder; AUC: Area under the curve; CANSAS: Camberwell Assessment of Need Short Appraisal Schedule; CI: Confidence Interval; Fig.: Figure; GAF: Global Assessment of Functioning; HoNOS: Health of the Nation Outcome Scales; HoNOSCA: Health of the Nation Outcome Scales Child and Adolescents Mental Health; MANSA: Manchester Short Assessment of quality of life; MINI-KID: MINI International Neuropsychiatric Interview for Children and Adolescents; OR: Odds Ratio; SD: Standard Deviation; SPSS: Statistical Package for the Social Sciences

## Acknowledgements
The authors gratefully acknowledge the families and mental health care providers who participated, and research assistant Amanda Noorman who helped conducting the study. We thank Marlene Stewart and Adriaan Hoogendoorn for their valuable comments on this paper. We would like to thank Daphne van de Draai for her assistance with building the SPSS-files.

## Funding
This research was funded by GGZ Delfland. The funding body did not have any role in the design of the study or collection, analysis or interpretation of data or in writing the manuscript.

## Authors' contributions
RV, RF, AB and BM designed this study. RV and RF performed the analysis and interpreted the data. RV and RF wrote the manuscript. BM and AB critically revised it. All authors read and approved the final manuscript.

## Consent for publication
Not applicable.

## Competing interests
The authors declare that they have no competing interests.

## Author details
[1]Department of Child and Adolescent Psychiatry, GGZ Delfland, PO-box 5016, 2600, GA, Delft, The Netherlands. [2]Amsterdam UMC, location VUmc and GGZ inGeest, Department of psychiatry, Amsterdam, The Netherlands. [3]Amsterdam Public Health Research Institute, Amsterdam, The Netherlands. [4]Inholland University of Applied Sciences, Amsterdam, The Netherlands. [5]GGZ-VS, Academy for Masters in Advanced Nursing Practice, Utrecht, The Netherlands. [6]Parnassia Psychiatric Institute, The Hague, The Netherlands.

## References
1. Kieling C, Baker-Henningham H, Belfer M, Conti G, Ertem I, Omigbodun O, et al. Child and adolescent mental health worldwide: evidence for action. Lancet. 2011;378(9801):1515–25. https://doi.org/10.1016/s0140-6736(11)60827-1.
2. Costello E, Egger H, Angold A. 10-year research update review: the epidemiology of child and adolescent psychiatric disorders: I. Methods and public health burden. J Am Acad Child Adolesc Psychiatry. 2005;44(10):972–86. https://doi.org/10.1097/01/chi.0000172552.41596.6f.
3. Belfer ML. Child and adolescent mental disorders: the magnitude of the problem across the globe. J Child Psychol Psychiatry. 2008;49(3):226–36. https://doi.org/10.1111/j.1469-7610.2007.01855.x.
4. Nederlands Jeugdinstituut (NJI). Gemeente-is-vaker-verwijzer-naar-verwijzer-naar-jeugdhulp. In: NJI; 2016. http://www.nji.nl/nl/Actueel/Nieuws-over-de-jeugdsector/2016/Gemeente-is-vaker-verwijzer-naar-jeugdhulp.
5. Nederlandse overheid. Overheid.nl. In: Nederlandse overheid; 2017. http://wetten.overheid.nl/BWBR0018450/2016-08-01.
6. Pottick K, Hansell S, Gutterman E, Raskin White H. Factors associated with inpatient and outpatient treatment for children and adolescents with serious mental illness. J Am Acad Child Adolesc Psychiatry. 1995;34(4):425–33.
7. Pfeffer C.R., Plutchik R., Mizruchi M.S. A comparison of psychopathology in child psychiatric inpatients, outpatients, and nonpatients. 1986;179(9): 529–535.
8. Golubchik P, Sever J, Finzi-Dottan R, Kosov I, Weizman A. The factors influencing decision making on children's pychiatric hospitalization: a retrospective chart review. Community Ment Health J. 2013;49(1):73–8. https://doi.org/10.1007/s10597-012-9487-00650.
9. Righi G, Benevides J, Mazefsky C, Siegel M, Sheinkopf SJ, Morrow EM. Predictors of inpatient psychiatric hospitalization for children and adolescents with autism spectrum disorder. J Autism Dev Disord 2017. dio: https://doi.org/10.1007/s10803-017-3154-9

10. Davidson GC. Stepped care: doing more with less? J Consult Clin Psychol. 2000;68:580–5.

11. Goldberg D, Huxley P. Mental illness in the community: the pathway to psychiatric care. London: Tavistock; 1980.

12. Prabhu A, Pandit L, Vardhan GV. Pathways to tertiary care adopted by individuals with psychiatric illness. Asian J Psychiatr. 2015;16:32–5. https://doi.org/10.1016/j.ajp.2015.06.005.

13. Dvir Y, Wenz-Gross M, Jeffers-Terry M, Peter-Metz W. An assessment of satisfaction with ambulatory child psychiatric consultation services to primary care providers by parents of children with emotional and behavioral needs. Front Psychiatry. 2012;3:1–7. https://doi.org/10.3389/fpsyt.2012.00007.

14. Hickie IB, Scott EM, Hermens DF. Applying clinical staging to young people who present for mental health care. Early Interv Psychiatry. 2013;7(1):31–43. https://doi.org/10.1111/j.1751-7893.2012.00366.x.

15. Hetrick S, Parker A, Hickie I, Purcell R, Yung A, McGorry P. Early identification and intervention in depressive disorders: towards a clinical staging model. Psychother Psychosom. 2008;77(5):263–70. https://doi.org/10.1159/000140085.

16. Scott E, Hermens D, Glozier N, Naismith S, Guastella A, Hickie I. Targeted primary case-based mental health services for young Australians. Med J Aust. 2012;196(10):136–40.

17. Cross S, Hermens D, Scott E, Ottavio A, McGorry P, Hickie I. A clinical staging model for early intervention youth mental health services. Psych serv. 2014; 65(7):939–43. https://doi.org/10.1176/appi.ps.201300221.

18. Bronfenbrenner U. Readings on the development of children. In: Ecological models of human development. Freeman; 1993.

19. McBride B, Schoppe S, Rane T. Child characteristics, parenting stress, and parental involvement: fathers versus mothers. J Marriage Fam. 2002;64(4):998–1011. https://doi.org/10.1111/j.1741-3737.2002.00998.x.

20. Halme N, Astedt-Kurki P, Tarkka M. Fathers' involvement with their preschool-age children. Child Youth Care Forum. 2009;38(3):103–19. https://doi.org/10.1007/s10566-009-9069-7.

21. Sheehan D, Sheehan K, Shytle R, Janavs J, Bannon Y, Rogers J. Reliability and validity of the Mini international neuropsychiatric interview for children and adolescents. J Clin Psychiatry. 2010;71(3):313–26. https://doi.org/10.4088/JCP.09m05305whi.

22. Gowers S, Harrington R, Whitton A, Beevor A, Lellitiot P, Wing J. Brief scale for measuring the outcomes of emotional and behavioural disorders in children. Health of the nation outcomes scales of children and adolescents (HoNOSCA). Br J Psychiatry. 1999;174(5):413–6. https://doi.org/10.1192/bjp.174.5.413.

23. Phelan M, Slade M, Thornicroft G, Dunn G, Holloway F, Wykes T. The Camberwell assessment of need: the validity and reliability of an instrument to assess the needs of people with severe mental illness. Br J Psychiatry. 1995;167(5):589–95. https://doi.org/10.1192/bjp.167.5.589.

24. Ravens-Sieberer U, Herdman M, Devine J, Otto C, Bullinger M, Rose M, et al. The european kidscreen approach to measure quality of life measure for and well being of children: development, current application, and future advances. Qual Life Res. 2014;23(3):791–803. https://doi.org/10.1007/s11136-013-0428-3.

25. Reflectum. Bibliotheek vragenlijsten NVPP/LVE. Deventer: Reflectum.

26. Wing J, Beevor A, Curtis R, Park S, Hadden S, Burns A. Health of the nation outcome scales (HONOS): research and development. Br J Psychiatry. 1998; 172(1):11–8. https://doi.org/10.1192/bjp.172.1.11.

27. Mulder C, Staring A, Loos J, Kuijpers D, Sytema S, Wierdsma A. Health of the nation outcome scales (HoNOS). Tijdschrift voor de psychiatrie. 2004;46(5):273–85.

28. Adams M, Palmer A, Crook W. Health of the nation outcome scales for psychiatry: are they valid? J Ment Health. 2000;9(2):193–201. https://doi.org/10.1080/09638230050009186.

29. Björkman T, Svensson B. Quality of life in people with severe mental illness. Reliability and validity of the Manchester short assessment of quality of life (MANSA). Nord J Psychiatry. 2005;59(4):302–6. https://doi.org/10.1080/08039480500213733.

30. Priebe S, Huxley P, Knight S, Evans S. Application of the Manchester short assessment of quality of life (MANSA). Int J Soc Psychiatry. 1999;45(1):7–12. https://doi.org/10.1177/002076409904500102.

31. Belle van G. Statistical rules of tumb, 2 red. In: John Wiley and sons Ldt; 2008.

32. Vittinghoff E, McCulloch C. Relaxing the rule of ten events per variable in logistic and cox regression. Am J Epidemiol 2006;165(6):710–718. dio: https://doi.org/10.1093/aje/kwk052

33. Pallant J. SPSS survival manual. 5th ed. Berkshire: The McGraw-Hill companies; 2013.

34. Tabachnick B, Fidell L. Using multivariate statistics, 6th edition. Pearson education limited, 2014.

35. Swets J. Measuring the accuracy of diagnostic systems. Science. 1988; 240(4857):1285–93. https://doi.org/10.1126/science.3287615.

36. Polit DF, Beck CT. Nursing research: generating and assessing evidence for nursing practice 10th edition. Wolters Kluwer, 2017.

37. Berg-Nielsen T, Vikan A, Dahl A. Parenting related to child and parental psychopathology: a descriptive review of the literature. Clin Child Psychol Psychiatry. 2002;7(4):529–52. https://doi.org/10.1177/1359104502007004006.

38. Goodman S, Gotlib I. Risk for psychopathology in the children of depressed mothers: a developmental model for understanding mechanisms of transition. Psychol Rev. 1999;106(3):458–90.

39. Middeldorp C, Wesseldijk L, Hudziak J, Verhulst F, Lindauer R, Dieleman G. Parents of children with psychopathology: psychiatric problems and the association with their child's problems. Eur Child Adolesc Psychiatry. 2016; 25(8):919–27. https://doi.org/10.1007/s00787-015-0813-2.

40. Cummings E, Keller P, Davies P. Towards a family process model of maternal and paternal depressive symptoms: exploring multiple relations with child and family functioning. J Child Psychol Psychiatry. 2005;46(5):479–89. https://doi.org/10.1111/j.1469-7610.2004.00368.x.

41. McLauglin K, Gaderman A, Hwang I, Sampson N, Al-Hamzawi A, Andrade L. Parent psychopathology and offspring mental disorders: results from the WHO world mental health surveys. Br J Psychiatry. 2012;200(4):290–9. https://doi.org/10.1192/bjp.bp.111.101253.

42. Sijtsema J, Oldehinkel A, Veenstra R, Verhulst F, Ormel J. Effects of structural and dynamic family characteristics on the development of depressive and aggressive problems during adolescence. Eur Child Adolesc Psychiatry. 2014;23(6):499–513. https://doi.org/10.1007/s00787-013-0474-y.

43. Trimbos-institute. Modelbeschrijving FACT Jeugd. herziene versie. Utrecht: Trimbos-institute; 2013.

44. Henggeler S, Schoewald S, Borduin C, Rowland C, Cunningham P. Multisystemic therapy for antisocial behavior in children and adolescents 2th edition. New York: Guilford Press; 2009.

45. Chiariello M, Orvaschel H. Patterns of parent-child communication: relationship to depression. Clin Psychol Rev. 1995;15(5):395–407. https://doi.org/10.1016/0272-7358(95)00022-H.

46. National Institute for Health and Care Excellence. Psychosis and Schizophrenia in children and young people: Recognition and management, 2013. http://www.nice.org.uk/guidance. Accessed 3 July 2018.

47. National Institute for Health and Care Excellence. Bipolair disorder: the assessment and management of bipolar disorders in adults, children and young people in primary and secondary care, 2013. http://www.nice.org.uk/guidance. Accessed 3 July 2018.

48. National Institue for Health and Care Excellence. Antisocial behaviour and conduct disorders in children and young people: recognition and management. 2013. http://www.nice.org.uk/guidance. Accessed 3 july 2018.

49. National Institue for Health and Care Excellence. Depression in children and young people: identification and management. 2013. http://www.nice.org.uk/guidance. Accessed 3 july 2018.

50. Vijverberg R, Ferdinand R, Beekman A, van Meijel B. The effect of youth assertive community treatment: a systematic PRISMA review. BMC psychiatry. 2017;17:284. https://doi.org/10.1186/s12888-017-1501-1.

# 4

# Long-term psychiatric inpatients' perspectives on weight gain, body satisfaction, diet and physical activity: a mixed methods study

Susanna Every-Palmer[1,2]* (iD), Mark A. Huthwaite[1,2], Jane L. Elmslie[3], Eve Grant[2] and Sarah E. Romans[1]

## Abstract

**Background:** Obesity is a significant problem for people with serious mental illness. We aimed to consider body size from the perspective of long-stay psychiatric inpatients, focussing on: weight gain and its causes and impacts; diet and physical activity; and the perceived ability to make meaningful change in these domains.

**Method:** A mixed methods study with 51 long-term psychiatric forensic and rehabilitation inpatients using semi-structured interviews combined with biometric and demographic data.

**Results:** 94% of participants were overweight or obese (mean BMI 35.3, SD 8.1). They were concerned about their weight, with 75% of them attempting to lose weight. Qualitative responses indicated low personal effectiveness and self-stigmatisation. Participants viewed their weight gain as something 'done to them' through medication, hospitalisation and leave restrictions. A prevailing theme was that institutional constraints made it difficult to live a healthy life (*just the way the system is*). Many had an external locus of control, viewing weight loss as desirable but unachievable, inhibited by environmental factors and requiring a quantum of motivation they found hard to muster. Despite this, participants were thoughtful and interested, had sound ideas for weight loss, and wished to be engaged in a shared endeavour to achieve better health outcomes. Consulting people as experts on their experiences, preferences, and goals may help develop new solutions, remove unidentified barriers, and improve motivation.

**Conclusions:** The importance of an individualised, multifactorial approach in weight loss programmes for this group was clear. Patient-led ideas and co-design should be key principles in programme and environmental design.

**Keywords:** Obesity, Serious mental illness, Physical health, Physical activity, Schizophrenia, Health promotion

## Background

People with serious mental illnesses (SMI) such as schizophrenia, bipolar disorder and major depressive disorder, have poorer physical health and significantly reduced life expectancy compared with the general population [1]. Those with schizophrenia have a 2–3 fold increased standardised mortality ratio [1–4], a sobering fact aptly described as "the scandal of premature mortality" [5]. While the causes of this reduction in life span are multifactorial, there is little doubt that obesity and its complications (diabetes, heart disease, and hypertension) are significant contributors [6, 7].

However, amongst all the research on obesity and its correlates in SMI, very little traverses the experiences of those personally affected. A literature search we conducted in June 2017 revealed nearly 4000 articles containing the keywords 'psychiatric disorder' and 'obesity', but only a handful of qualitative studies containing personal accounts of those with SMI. The empirical evidence has incontrovertibly established a high prevalence of overweight and obesity *in* people with SMI [6–9], but the

* Correspondence: susanna.every-palmer@ccdhb.org.nz
[1]Department of Psychological Medicine, University of Otago Wellington, PO Box 7343, Wellington 6242, New Zealand
[2]Capital and Coast District Health Board, Wellington, New Zealand
Full list of author information is available at the end of the article

voices of people *with* SMI are lacking. The parlous physical health outcomes are well quantified, but what about effects of weight on self-esteem, confidence and stigma, and beliefs about causes, barriers and ideas for improved health and weight loss?

This apparent research gap is surprising, given the importance placed on patient-centred care and co-design in contemporary practice. Munk-Jorgensen and colleagues, for example, have noted the importance of involving patients in all stages of medical research, quoting the European Science Foundation [10].

The articles we identified covering mental health services users' experiences of weight included a 2011 review of studies on the perception of patients and/or nurses of health promotions targeting physical activity and eating habits [11]. This review found that in general, both mental health patients and nurses held positive views about health promotion but patients felt the ability to improve their physical health was beyond their control. Several barriers to health improvement were identified, including the mental illness itself, medication side effects, lack of support, finances, stigma and, additionally from the nurses only, poor motivation and unwillingness to participate.

Blanner Kristiansen and colleagues examined patients' and nurses' perspectives on health promotion [12] as part of systematic interventions aimed at reducing health risks in people with schizophrenia living in the community. The views of staff and patients were aligned, with perceived causes for poor physical health categorised into three clusters: lifestyle, the mental disorder and organisational issues. Both groups wanted less fragmentation of the 'treatment system' with physical health issues incorporated into routine psychiatric care.

The other papers also used qualitative methods to study health attitudes of people with SMI. Blomqvist and colleagues identified being seen as a whole human being (rather than a psychiatric patient) by self and others as the central theme in achieving a healthy lifestyle [13]. Sub-categories of this theme were having a normal everyday structure (healthy daily activities, sleep, diet), life events and social support, which provide motivation for healthy habits. Another Swedish study examined the lived experiences of people with SMI making or contemplating life style changes [14]. They found that the most helpful interventions focussed on individualised strengthening of the person's self-efficacy.

In an attempt to address the research gap, we have undertaken a mixed methods study exploring the experience of obesity and its correlates in a sample of long-term inpatients in New Zealand. Basic demographic and clinical data have been published already from an earlier project which quantified calorie intake, energy expenditure and sleep in the same cohort [15]. There we reported high calorie consumption with frequent non-nutritional eating

(junk food), excessive somnolence (median total sleep time > 9 h) and low levels of physical activity in this sample. This study seeks to understand the subjective perspective of our participants about their weight, diet, exercise regimes and self-esteem.

## Methods

We used a mixed methodology approach: cross sectional data collection to quantify obesity and thematic analysis to explore the related experiences of our participants.

Eligibility criteria were English-speaking adult patients (> 18) residing in regional New Zealand forensic and rehabilitation services who were competent to provide informed consent. While all the patients included in this study had serious mental illness, this was not specifically an inclusion criteria, rather a consequence of the sampling frame (having a SMI is essentially a prerequisite for long term psychiatric inpatient rehabilitation in New Zealand).

The treating team determined capacity, which was reconfirmed during the informed consent process. The research setting comprised five different units across two geographical sites. Three units were medium secure, one minimum secure and one was an unlocked unit. Residents had access to a general practitioner, gymnasium equipment, circuit training, a personal trainer, and occupational therapy programmes. Some but not all participants could use a swimming pool, yoga classes, walking and healthy lifestyle groups, cooking and shopping training. Meals were supplied by the hospital kitchen, but many residents purchased and consumed supplementary food.

### Data sources

Sociodemographic and clinical information was extracted from clinical records and from the participants and included diagnosis, age, gender, ethnicity, date of admission, admission BMI, current BMI, smoking status, medication, age of first treatment onset and whether people were under mental health compulsory treatment orders.

Participants were interviewed about their weight, diet, activity levels, their ability to change these things and the impact on their self-esteem, using structured and semi-structured interview schedules.

The semi-structured interview schedule had five main probes and canvassed views about weight, diet and exercise. Participants were asked to describe:

a) their feelings about their weight, how their weight had changed and what factors they saw as responsible for any weight change;
b) any efforts they were making to change their weight;
c) what changes, if any, they would make to their diet to maintain a healthy weight;

d) whether they used the exercise resources available and what their thoughts and feelings about these resources were;

e) how their physical activity differed in hospital compared to when they were living in the community.

The structured interview schedule collected demographic information and included the following three scale-based survey items:

a) likert-scale item relating to body dissatisfaction;

b) a three point scale on food volume (too much, right amount, not enough);

c) dichotomous questions on non-hungry eating (eating driven by emotional factors or food availability despite being satiated).

The interviews were structured in ways that previous experience suggested participants would be most comfortable; one-on-one interviews in a private space on the hospital campus with a researcher known by the participants. Each interview took approximately 40 min. The interviewer transcribed responses during the interviews; manual transcription was more acceptable to the participants than audio recording.

## Analysis

Data from the quantitative items were entered into Excel 2013 and SPSS version-21 (SPSS Inc. Chicago, Illinois, USA). Descriptive statistics used appropriate tests for the data type.

Analysis was conducted in accordance with Braun and Clarke's thematic approach [16]. Initially three researchers (SR, JE and MH) independently familiarized themselves with the interview transcripts. Data was then indexed in terms of similarity and contrast of content and initial codes were generated. These codes were then examined and discussed by the research team, moving back and forth between the data and the thematic coding, and were further condensed into themes and subthemes through this iterative process.

All recorded data was de-identified to preserve confidentiality.

## Ethics approval

The New Zealand Health and Disability Ethics Committee (reference 13/CEN/153) approved this study.

## Results

Fifty-one participants were recruited from a group of 87 eligible persons, a 59% response rate. They all had SMI, with onset of treatment (a proxy for illness onset) between 15 and 29 years previously. All participants had diagnoses of psychotic disorders, most commonly schizophrenia (78%), with diagnosis codes derived from data submitted to the national mental health database (PRIMHD) according to ICD 10 criteria. Most participants had been in hospital for over a year, and all but one were detained under a compulsory treatment order. Participant characteristics are summarised in Table 1.

## Weight

Obesity was the norm in our sample, with participants markedly heavier than the general population. Three quarters were obese with a mean BMI of 35.3 (SD 8.1), males 34.2 (SD 7.1), females 39.4 (SD 11.0, $p = 0.07$). Only three were of normal weight and none were underweight. The BMIs of our participants differed significantly from the national average. New Zealand has an obesity rate of 31.6% ($\chi^2 = 17.084$, df 1 $p < 0.0001$) and a mean BMI of 28.2 kg/m$^2$ (observed difference 7.1 kg/m$^2$, 95% CI 4.9–9.3, $p < 0.00001$).

Most participants reported gaining weight since starting antipsychotic medication (mean reported weight gain 33.4 kg).

## Personal views about weight

For causes of weight gain, 30 (60%) identified medication, 18 (36%) nominated food volume, 10 (20%) food type, 10 (20%) lack of exercise one illness and one smoking. One mentioned his use of synthetic cannabinoids as appetite stimulating (*'the munchies'*) leading to over-eating.

Some reported being surprised by the extent of their weight gain, feeling it did not make sense in the context of their personal circumstances:

*'Maybe a little bit of it is food but I don't eat that much, I hardly eat because I don't like the food here.'*

Only 21 (of 51) offered more than one cause of high body weight and none offered more than two (10: both food and medication, eight: food and lack of exercise, three: lack of exercise and medication). This suggests participants may hold a single cause (either-or) way of thinking about this issue.

While physical reasons predominated in response to survey questions about causes of weight gain, participants also had significant beliefs about psychological and environmental reasons underpinning their weight, which were strong themes in the semi-structured interviews.

## Weight and self-perception

Most people were unhappy with their weight. Three quarters (38/51) reported trying to lose weight. More than half worried about their body shape or appearance 'some to all of the time' (see Table 2). Over 60% reported being self-conscious and worried about their body shape

**Table 1** Participant characteristics

| Sociodemographic factors | |
|---|---|
| Age | Mean = 38 years (SD 10.4, range 19–68) |
| Gender | |
| Male | 40 (78%) |
| Female | 11 (22%) |
| Ethnicity | |
| New Zealand Pakeha | 15 (29%) |
| Māori | 33 (65%) |
| Pacific Island | 13 (26%) |
| Other | 3 (6%) |
| Relationship status | |
| Single | 40 (78%) |
| Married or de facto relationship | 4 (8%) |
| Separated or divorced | 6 (12%) |
| Widowed | 1 (2%) |
| Education | |
| No school leaving certificate | 33 (65%) |
| School certificate | 14 (27%) |
| Further higher qualifications | 4 (8%) |
| Illness-related factors | |
| Diagnosis (per ICD criteria) | |
| Schizophrenia | 40 (78%) |
| Schizoaffective disorder | 6 (12%) |
| Bipolar disorder (with psychotic features) | 2 (4%) |
| Other (unspecified psychosis etc.) | 3 (6%) |
| Legal status | |
| Voluntary inpatient order | 1 (2%) |
| Compulsory treatment order | 50 (98%) |
| Most common medications | |
| Clozapine | 25 (49%) |
| Non-clozapine antipsychotic | FGA = 4 (8%), SGA = 17 (33%), FGA + SGA = 4 (8%) |
| Mood stabiliser | 15 (29%) |
| Metformin | 23 (45%) |
| Statin | 15 (30%) |
| Mean age at onset of first treatment | 21.9 years (SD = 6.7) |
| Mean duration of treatment | 15.9 years (SD = 9.4) |
| Mean length of admission | 19.7 months (SD = 20.3) |

**Table 1** Participant characteristics *(Continued)*

| Weight | | |
|---|---|---|
| Mean BMI (kg/m²) | Our participants | New Zealand population [35] |
| All | 35.3 (SD 8.1) | 28.2 (SD 0.1) |
| Male | 34.2 (SD 7.1) | 28.1 (SD 0.2) |
| Female | 39.4 (SD 11.0) | 28.3 (SD 0.2) |
| World Health Organisation weight classification grading | Our participants | New Zealand population [35] |
| Normal weight range (BMI < 25) | 3 (6%) | 33.3% |
| Overweight (BMI 25–29.9) | 10 (20%) | 35.2% |
| Obesity Class I (BMI 30–34.9) | 10 (20%) | 18.9% |
| Obesity Class II (BMI 35–35.9) | 14 (28%) | 7.6% |
| Obesity Class III (BMI > 40) | 13 (26%) | 5.1% |
| Change in weight since admission | | |
| Weight gain (> 5 kg) | 24 (47.2%) | |
| Minimal change | 14 (27.8%) | |
| Weight loss (> 5 kg) | 13 (25%) | |

when they were with other people. A strong theme of shame and self-condemnation emerged for some, in which their weight triggered negative feelings about themselves. Comments included: *'being lazy'; 'being a pig and eating too much'* and *'being undisciplined'*.

Over-eating in response to emotional factors such as sadness or loneliness also emerged.

*'Depression—eating due to emotions as girls do.'*

*'Food, just wanting food—not being able to see my family.'*

This theme was reinforced by the survey questions on non-hungry eating (Table 3) in which almost half the participants (43%) endorsed eating in response to negative emotions. Females were significantly more likely to eat when emotionally distressed.

Not everyone was unhappy with their body size. A minority reported being comfortable with their current weight *'I'm happy how I am'; 'I want to be about 120kg but I want it to be muscle—I'm exercising in my room.'*

One male talked about the perceived advantages of being overweight in terms of personal protection and power, describing his weight gain as a deliberate strategy related to *'needing to protect myself, for advantage over others and to feel good. I wanted to be bigger than my brother.'*

### Weight loss strategies

For those trying to lose weight, 32 (63%) identified exercise and 16 (31%) dietary modifications as the means to achieve their goal, with twelve noting both strategies.

**Table 2** Body satisfaction

| Item | Positive response (some-all of the time) n (%), n = 42 | Male n (%) n = 31 | Female n (%) n = 11 | Significant difference between male and female |
|------|------|------|------|------|
| *Are you worried about your body shape or your appearance?* | 26 (62) | 20 (65) | 6 (55) | ns |
| *Do you think your body shape is worse than other people's: do you compare yourself negatively to others' body shape?* | 21 (50) | 15 (48) | 6 (55) | ns |
| *Do you become self-conscious and worried about your body shape when around other people?* | 26 (62) | 19 (61) | 7 (64) | ns |

## Diet

Most people (35/51) made suggestions for improvements in the hospital menu and in their own dietary choices. Thirty-one commented about some aspect of their food intake; these comments ranged from portion sizes to food type.

Suggestions included: *'eat more fruit', 'cut out bread', 'tick the medium size meal instead of large size', and 'cut down on my coke intake'.* Some recommended modifications to the hospital menus (*'maybe some better recipes – it's on a two-week rotation; getting more variety would be good', 'more vegetarian meals and [I wish] that the ones they serve were nicer'*).

Twenty-seven participants (56%) thought they were offered the right amount of food, 13 (26%) thought 'not enough' and nine (12%) 'too much food'. There was no statistical association between BMI and perception of food adequacy. Gender was not significant although none of the 10 women considered that they were being offered too much food.

## Physical activity

Most people were participating in some activities provided on the campus (e.g. playing table tennis, volleyball, swimming, joining the walking group, using the personal trainer). Seven specified 'using the gym'. Ten (21%) said that they used the courtyard daily. Nine indicated that no courtyard was available (one unit's courtyard was being renovated) and three needed staff to be available to access the space.

Eighteen participants, 14 men (45%) and four women (36%) said they used the personal trainer

regularly. Three indicated that they did not like to use weights and so did not work with the trainer. Some gave practical reasons for not using the personal trainer (three needed a referral, one had a conflicting appointment with the social worker at that time). Four indicated that the personal trainer was not available in their area.

There were some intriguing responses, which suggest underlying difficulties with working with the trainer, such as low motivation or frank, active psychotic symptomatology. Comments included: *'I don't want to see her', 'sick of that sort of thing', 'decided to stop going because of the voices'.* Some idiosyncratic plans for weight management included secrecy around exercise: *'I am on my own plan for my work out but it's a secret'* and *'[I'm] running in the shower'.*

## Activity levels in hospital compared to their community living

Forty participants (78%) said that they had been more active in the community than as inpatients and only nine indicated more activity in hospital. A number of the forensic patients spontaneously volunteered that they had been more active in prison. While this may be subject to recall bias, many provided credible information to illustrate their response with the following examples:

*'I only get to go out a certain number of times/hours compared to the community when you can go out any time.'*

*'Yeah - when in the community, I would usually walk around and up town to my mate's place everyday.'*

**Table 3** Eating when not hungry

| Questions | Yes (%) | Male Yes (%) | Female Yes (%) | Significant difference between male and female |
|-----------|---------|--------------|----------------|------------------------------------------------|
| *Do you have the urge to eat even when you're not hungry?* | 19 (45) | 14 (45) | 5 (45) | ns |
| *Do you find it hard to stop eating even when you are full?* | 16 (38) | 11 (35) | 5 (45) | ns |
| *Do you realise that you have eaten more than you intended to?* | 32 (76) | 24 (77) | 8 (73) | ns |
| *Do you eat more if there is food around?* | 28 (67) | 19 (61) | 9 (82) | ns |
| *Do you eat when you are emotionally stressed, upset, worried, tense or bored?* | 18 (43) | 10 (32) | 8 (72) | $\chi^2 = 5.4$, df 1 $p = 0.03$ |

*'I'm currently doing way less than when in community and in prison. There is nowhere to go to get out.'*

*'I used to run for an hour every day in prison. I've just started getting back into this.'*

*'You can't do what you want to do in here, but outside you can.'*

*'We do nothing in comparison to the outside where you're working and motivated.'*

## Barriers

Despite the options available for exercise, participants perceived significant barriers to weight management. People felt the highly regulated environment, with restrictions on personal autonomy, which one described as *'just the way the system is,'* contributed to both their weight gain and their inability to shift this weight. Some comments suggested an external locus of control and feelings of disempowerment. Other responses addressed systemic issues and including the restriction of movement, commenting on *'unfair treatment'*. Frequent reference was made to leave restrictions as a barrier to an active life.

Some participants specifically mentioned *'low motivation'*. Many described low self-efficacy to eat well or persevere with physical activity, with at least some showing self-awareness of these characteristics. *'Don't go [to the gym], cos I can't be stuffed,'* and *'I used to [meet with the personal trainer] but don't go anymore as I don't feel like it.'*

Participants identified obstacles that, in their view, made exercising difficult:

*'I sleep too much as the medication is too strong.'*

*'We don't have a ball.'*

*'I used to have leave to the courtyard but it got stopped 'cos I was getting high out there.'*

*'I have access for walks around [the courtyard] in the morning and when the weather is ok, we play volleyball. However, I have got holes in my shoes.'*

A number of comments showed the crucial importance of the socially interactive aspect of physical activity. *'I don't, 'cos no one else does.'*

*'I'd rather stay inside and see all the drama and action.'*

*'It's boring out there on my own.'*

## Discussion

This study focused on a particularly disadvantaged population: people with a mental illness serious enough that it necessitated a long period of inpatient psychiatric rehabilitation, the vast majority of whom were detained under compulsory mental health act legislation. This is a group whose opinions are seldom canvassed. In the review from Verhaeghe's group, only one ($n = 12$) of 14 studies of health attitudes in people with mental illness and their nurses had a specific inpatient focus [11]. The reviewed studies used qualitative methods, so our inpatient study with our combined quantitative and qualitative methods adds substantively to the existing literature.

### Participants were overweight and they cared about this

Obesity was a significant problem for our participants. Being overweight was not a selection criterion, but an overwhelming majority (94%) were overweight or obese. Participants were self-conscious and worried about their weight. Some described self-blame and self-disgust using derogatory epithets such as *pig* or *lazy* to described themselves. This group clearly carried society's high stigma about obesity [17], a double jeopardy when combined with the stigma of SMI. This seemed to lead to personal passivity and nihilism. These results differed from those of Minsky and colleagues who found that people with SMI underestimate their obesity [18]. They do align with the findings of Blanner Kristiansen's group that overweight was a paramount physical health problem for their participants [12].

### Overt and covert reasons for overweight

Thematic analysis of responses revealed participants implicated physical, psychological and social factors within the hospital as promoting and maintaining their weight gain. The physical factors were overt, explicitly identified by participants as causal factors for obesity, and included medication, diet, institutional restrictions and the sedentary lifestyle. Most participants viewed the combination of weight-promoting medication, inactive lifestyles, (most apparent in those patients with a higher security status and no leave), and diet as having potent effects on weight. They considered the inpatient environment inhibited incidental activity, such as active paid jobs, or walking in the community as a means of getting somewhere.

The psychological and social factors were more implicit and included loneliness, isolation, pleasure seeking and social isolation effects. Participants talked about using food to manage their feelings and as a substitute for other comforts. Narratives highlighted their lack of normal hedonic activities: warm, affectional bonds with close family members, including but not limited to sexual connectedness and recreation (socialising with friends, community activities, pursuit of hobbies and holidays and travel). The reduced access to previously used rewards such as alcohol may also be relevant. In a psychologically arid inpatient environment, food may have become overly important, becoming a substitute for other gratification sources.

A strong theme for the forensic participants was weight gain and reduced physical activity after moving from prison to hospital. Being fit and strong has high salience in custodial settings but less so in psychiatric hospitals. While medication and illness factors cannot be disentangled, social networks are known to influence weight status. The Framingham Heart study demonstrated that when a close social contact becomes obese, an individual's likelihood of similar weight gain increases by 171% [19]. In our setting, being surrounded by overweight people might change a person's tolerance for obesity and lead to imitation of weight promoting behaviours. Participants themselves clearly identified peers' behaviours as impacting on their own exercise regimes (I don't, 'cos no one else does). Eating habits may have been similarly influenced.

Overall, participants found the hospital's environmental constraints made living a healthy life difficult, and thought that changing this was beyond their control (just the way the system is). This may be a consequence of the well-recognised concept of institutionalisation, defined as "the impoverishment of feelings, thoughts, initiative and social activity" [20] which arises as a possible consequence of long term residence in a confined and controlled environment [21]. Social isolation and dependence on staff may result in the loss in belief of one's ability to act autonomously and in disempowerment. This is often compounded by illness-related factors. Maintaining the commitment and drive necessary for long-term weight loss is challenging for anyone, but even more so for those with SMI. Motivational deficit is a core negative symptom of schizophrenia [22]. Low motivation reduces the ability to predict future rewards, as well as the ability to appreciate or enjoy pleasurable experiences in the present (anhedonia) [23]. This may lead to an anhedonic drive to eat, with low motivation to change eating behaviours or physical activity.

Sørensen's research team [24] found people with SMI were more physically active if they possessed intrinsic motivation, held a cognitive self-schema of themselves as a physically active person, and found the activity to be enjoyable. Ussher and colleagues interviewed 120 people with SMI about physical activity preferences and barriers, and found a high level of interest in exercise but low 'self efficacy' (confidence in their ability) to exercise when sad or stressed [25]. Barriers included lack of support from family and friends, fatigue, illness, and bad weather. Medication sedation, weight gain, fear of unsafe conditions, fear of discrimination, lack of understanding, social and cultural factors (e.g., social isolation), and the physical environment and policy have also been identified as barriers [26, 27]. Our results echo those findings.

### Recommendations and future research

Holistic approaches, with individualised strengthening of self-efficacy have been recommended [13, 14]. Sørensen's construct of internal cognitive schemas, anchored but potentially mutable, seems useful [24]. If core beliefs of being lazy, greedy or weak could be reshaped through psychological interventions to become schemas of being active and healthy people, motivation could potentially be enhanced.

Further research could investigate "nudges" using behavioural economic approaches, focussing on interventions that make healthier choices seem easier and more rewarding. For example, present bias (overvaluing immediate costs and benefits and undervaluing future costs and benefits [28]) could be utilized with programmes that offer small, frequent (and therefore immediate) rewards for beneficial behaviours [29]. Such programmes targeted at weight loss, medication adherence and smoking cessation work in general community samples [30–32]. Newer technology such as fitness trackers warrants further investigation. For someone wanting to lose weight but struggling with motivation, the instant gratification of a daily steps tracker is more rewarding than deferred and subtle changes on the scales. More emphasis on the short and medium term benefits of exercise on mental health [33] may also be helpful.

Although staff at our research sites were cognisant and concerned about the health problems of residents, this does not suffice. While the services offered resources, many patients felt they were passive participants rather than active collaborators in choosing and using these resources. Targeting the obesogenic environment through lifestyle interventions for people with SMI has been shown to reduce waist circumference and metabolic risk in the short term, but sustaining these improvements is challenging and requires ongoing commitment [34]. Services need to think about how the environment can support healthy diets and physical activity—both deliberate (active healthy choices) and incidental (e.g. physical activity as a part of normal activities of daily living). Environmental (social and psychological) aspects are important. An inpatient environment with appealing, well-equipped accessible exercise and outdoor spaces designed by and for the users are necessary. Physical activity should be enjoyable and reflect the individual's preferences and include social features. Exercising with family, peers or support workers who embody healthy behaviour can be a powerful motivator and makes activities more fun and sustainable.

Therapeutic attention to the type, amount, and variety of food provided is also important, as is the emotional and psychological drivers of overeating.

The commonly held, oversimplified attribution of participants that weight gain had been 'done to' them by antipsychotic medication may lead to the view weight gain is inevitable and cannot be reversed without stopping treatment. This is potentially amenable with psychoeducation. Understanding that antipsychotic medication may promote appetite, but it is actually increased food consumption that leads to weight gain, allows for greater self-determination.

As a group, our participants were thoughtful and concerned about their health and weight, and when asked, were able to articulate clear, well-grounded ideas about their predicament, supporting the work of Blanner Kristiansen and her colleagues [12]. Participants had some very specific diet recommendations, such as more vegetarian options and greater variety than a static two week rotating menu. Our dietitian researcher (JE) liked the suggestion that large portion sizes not be routinely offered but only available on specific request.

## Limitations

As we drew our participants from only two hospital sites, findings may not be more widely generalizable. Similarly, the primary diagnosis for the majority of participants was schizophrenia; people with other diagnoses may have different experiences.

The study used a cross-sectional design, so it is not clear whether self-image and self-efficacy around health and well-being changes during extended inpatient stays. This should be studied specifically and could become an outcome metric for inpatient care.

Data saturation was not sought as all the interviews were conducted before the data analysis. Some emergent themes (such as the advantages of high body weight, for example as protection against victimisation from others) warrant further study. Some participants had lost some weight over their most recent admission, however in interviews these participants focussed more on their total weight gain since entering psychiatric services, rather than recent success in losing some of this gained weight. Re-interviewing this subgroup as to how they had lost weight and whether they had sustained this would have been of value.

## Conclusions

While we considered weight from the perspective of an inpatient group, many themes are more broadly applicable to mental health service users. Our participants were overweight, and cared about this, with 75% of them reporting attempts to lose weight. Self-blame and disgust were evident in some, alongside a reduced sense of

control and personal efficacy. Participants attributed weight gain to a combination of physical, psychological and social factors. A prevailing theme was that the institutional constraints made it difficult to live a healthy life, and that changing this was beyond their control.

Overall, given the interest and range of imaginative ideas about strategies for weight loss, participants showed themselves worthy and engaged collaborators in the quest for better health outcomes. Consulting people as experts on their experiences, preferences, and goals may help develop new solutions, remove unidentified barriers, and improve motivation.

Patient led ideas and co-design should be key principles in programme and environmental design.

**Abbreviations**
BMI: Body mass index; Df: Degrees of freedom; FGA: First generation antipsychotic; Kg: Kilogram; n: Number; ns: Not significant; SD: Standard deviation; SGA: Second generation antipsychotic; SMI: Serious mental illness

**Acknowledgements**
We thank those who generously gave their time to participate in this study.

**Funding**
This study was funded by a University of Otago Research Grant.

**Authors' contributions**
SE-P, MH and SER designed the study. EG collected the data. MH and SER did the initial analyses; JE undertook analysis of the food data. SER wrote the first draft of this report, SE-P the second and third drafts and all authors read and critically revised the manuscript, and approved the final version for publication.

**Consent for publication**
Not applicable.

**Competing interests**
All authors declare that they have no competing interests.

**Author details**
[1]Department of Psychological Medicine, University of Otago Wellington, PO Box 7343, Wellington 6242, New Zealand. [2]Capital and Coast District Health Board, Wellington, New Zealand. [3]University of Otago Christchurch, Christchurch, New Zealand.

## References

1. Fleischhacker WW, Cetkovich-Bakmas M, De Hert M, Hennekens CH, Lambert M, Leucht S, Maj M, McIntyre RS, Naber D, Newcomer JW. Comorbid somatic illnesses in patients with severe mental disorders: clinical, policy, and research challenges. J Clin Psychiatry. 2008;69(4):514.

2. Tiihonen J, Lönnqvist J, Wahlbeck K, Klaukka T, Niskanen L, Tanskanen A, Haukka J. 11-year follow-up of mortality in patients with schizophrenia: a population-based cohort study (FIN11 study). Lancet. 2009;374(9690):620–7.

3. Lahti M, Tiihonen J, Wildgust H, Beary M, Hodgson R, Kajantie E, Osmond C, Räikkönen K, Eriksson J. Cardiovascular morbidity, mortality and pharmacotherapy in patients with schizophrenia. Psychol Med. 2012;42(11): 2275–85.

4. Saha S, Chant D, McGrath J. A systematic review of mortality in schizophrenia: is the differential mortality gap worsening over time? Arch Gen Psychiatry. 2007;64(10):1123–31.

5. Thornicroft G. Physical health disparities and mental illness: the scandal of premature mortality. Br J Psychiatry. 2011;199(6):441–2.

6. Allison DB, Newcomer JW, Dunn AL, Blumenthal JA, Fabricatore AN, Daumit GL, Cope MB, Riley WT, Vreeland B, Hibbeln JR. Obesity among those with mental disorders: a National Institute of Mental Health meeting report. Am J Prev Med. 2009;36(4):341–50.

7. Hausswolff-Juhlin V, Bjartveit M, Lindström E, Jones P. Schizophrenia and physical health problems. Acta Psychiatr Scand. 2009;119(s438):15–21.

8. Holt RI, Peveler RC. Obesity, serious mental illness and antipsychotic drugs. Diabetes Obes Metab. 2009;11(7):665–79.

9. Newcomer JW. Antipsychotic medications: metabolic and cardiovascular risk. J Clin Psychiatry. 2007;68:8–13.

10. Munk-Jørgensen P, Blanner Kristiansen C, Uwawke R, Larsen J, Okkels N, Christiansen B, Hjorth P. The gap between available knowledge and its use in clinical psychiatry. Acta Psychiatr Scand. 2015;132(6):441–50.

11. Verhaeghe N, De Maeseneer J, Maes L, Van Heeringen C, Annemans L. Perceptions of mental health nurses and patients about health promotion in mental health care: a literature review. J Psychiatr Ment Health Nurs. 2011;18(6):487–92.

12. Blanner Kristiansen C, Juel A, Vinther Hansen M, Hansen AM, Kilian R, Hjorth P. Promoting physical health in severe mental illness: patient and staff perspective. Acta Psychiatr Scand. 2015;132(6):470–8.

13. Blomqvist M, Sandgren A, Carlsson IM, Jormfeldt H. Enabling healthy living: experiences of people with severe mental illness in psychiatric outpatient services. Int J Mental Health Nurs. 2018;27(1):236–46.

14. Lundström S, Ahlström BH, Jormfeldt H, Eriksson H, Skärsäter I. The meaning of the lived experience of lifestyle changes for people with severe mental illness. Issues Ment Health Nurs. 2017;38(9):717–25.

15. Huthwaite M, Elmslie J, Every-Palmer S, Grant E, Romans SE. Obesity in a forensic and rehabilitation psychiatric service: a missed opportunity? J Forensic Prac. 2017;19(4):269–77.

16. Braun V, Clarke V. Using thematic analysis in psychology. Qual Res Psychol. 2006;3(2):77–101.

17. Puhl RM, Heuer CA. The stigma of obesity: a review and update. Obesity. 2009;17(5):941–64.

18. Minsky S, Vreeland B, Miller M, Gara M. Concordance between measured and self-perceived weight status of persons with serious mental illness. Psychiatr Serv. 2013;64(1):91–3.

19. Christakis NA, Fowler JH. The spread of obesity in a large social network over 32 years. N Engl J Med. 2007;(357):370–9.

20. Liberakis E. Factors predisposing to institutionalism. Acta Psychiatr Scand. 1981;63(4):356–66.

21. Goffman E: Asylums: essays on the social situation of mental patients and other inmates: Garden City: Anchor Books; 1961.

22. Foussias G, Remington G. Negative symptoms in schizophrenia: Avolition and Occam's razor. Schizophrenia Bull. 2010;36(2):359–69.

23. Da Silva S, Saperia S, Siddiqui I, Fervaha G, Agid O, Daskalakis ZJ, Ravindran A, Voineskos AN, Zakzanis KK, Remington G, et al. Investigating consummatory and anticipatory pleasure across motivation deficits in schizophrenia and healthy controls. Psychiatry Res. 2017;254:112–7.

24. Sørensen M. Motivation for physical activity of psychiatric patients when physical activity was offered as part of treatment. Scand J Med Sci Sports. 2006;16(6):391–8.

25. Ussher M, Stanbury L, Cheeseman V, Faulkner G. Physical activity preferences and perceived barriers to activity among persons with severe mental illness in the United Kingdom. Psychiatr Serv. 2007;58(3):405–8.

26. McDevitt J, Snyder M, Miller A, Wilbur J. Perceptions of barriers and benefits to physical activity among outpatients in psychiatric rehabilitation. J Nurs Scholarsh. 2006;38(1):50–5.

27. Vancampfort D, Knapen J, Probst M, Scheewe T, Remans S, De Hert M. A systematic review of correlates of physical activity in patients with schizophrenia. Acta Psychiatr Scand. 2012;125(5):352–62.

28. O'Donoghue T, Rabin M. The economics of immediate gratification. J Behav Decis Making. 2000;13(2):233.

29. Loewenstein G, Asch DA, Friedman JY, Melichar LA, Volpp KG. Can behavioural economics make us healthier? Br Med J. 2012;344.

30. Volpp KG, John LK, Troxel AB, Norton L, Fassbender J, Loewenstein G. Financial incentive–based approaches for weight loss: a randomized trial. JAMA. 2008;300(22):2631–7.

31. Volpp KG, Loewenstein G, Troxel AB, Doshi J, Price M, Laskin M, Kimmel SE. A test of financial incentives to improve warfarin adherence. BMC Health Serv Res. 2008;8(1):272.

32. Volpp KG, Troxel AB, Pauly MV, Glick HA, Puig A, Asch DA, Galvin R, Zhu J, Wan F, DeGuzman J. A randomized, controlled trial of financial incentives for smoking cessation. N Engl J Med. 2009;360(7):699–709.

33. Gorczynski P, Faulkner G. Exercise therapy for schizophrenia. Cochrane Libr. 2010.

34. Looijmans A, Stiekema AP, Bruggeman R, van der Meer L, Stolk RP, Schoevers RA, Jörg F, Corpeleijn E. Changing the obesogenic environment to improve cardiometabolic health in residential patients with a severe mental illness: cluster randomised controlled trial. Br J Psychiatry. 2017; 211(5):296–303.

35. Ministry of Health. Understanding excess body weight: New Zealand health survey. Wellington: Ministry of Health; 2015.

# 5

# Related but different: distinguishing postpartum depression and fatigue among women seeking help for unsettled infant behaviours

Nathan Wilson[1], Karen Wynter[2,3], Jane Fisher[2,4] and Bei Bei[1]*

**Abstract**

**Background:** A growing body of evidence in relatively healthy populations suggests that postpartum depression and fatigue are likely distinct but related experiences. However, differentiating depression and fatigue in clinical settings remains a challenge. This study aimed to assess if depression and fatigue are distinct constructs in women with relatively high fatigue and psychological distress symptoms attending a residential program that assists with unsettled infant behaviour.

**Methods:** 167 women (age: $M = 34.26$, $SD = 4.23$) attending a private residential early parenting program completed the Depression Anxiety Stress Scale (DASS21-D), Fatigue Severity Scale (FSS) and self-report sleep variables before program commencement. Confirmatory Factor Analysis examined the associations between depression and fatigue latent factors.

**Results:** A two-factor model of separate but related depression and fatigue constructs provided a significantly better fit to the data than a one-factor model of combined depression and fatigue ($p < .001$). In the two-factor model, the depression and fatigue latent factors were moderately correlated (.41). Further predictive utility of this two-factor model was demonstrated as both depression and fatigue factors were independently predicted by worse self-reported sleep efficiency.

**Conclusions:** This study provides empirical evidence that for women attending a clinical service with relatively high fatigue and psychological distress, postpartum depression and fatigue remain separate but related experiences. These findings suggest that in women seeking clinical support in the postpartum period, both depression and fatigue need to be carefully assessed to ensure accurate diagnoses, and (b) whilst depression intervention may improve fatigue, targeted fatigue intervention may also be warranted.

**Keywords:** Postpartum, Depression, Fatigue, Postnatal, Confirmatory factor analysis, Depressive

## Background

Maternal depression and fatigue symptoms are both prevalent across the first two years after giving birth, with 10 to 20% reporting depressive symptoms and 40 to 60% reporting fatigue symptoms [1–3]. This may be at least partly due to the under-recognized nature of women's

caregiving work and the potential for occupational fatigue associated with the demands of infant caregiving [4]. Within this context, depression and fatigue can share complex bi-directional relationships. Fatigue is one of the most common symptoms of depression and part of the diagnostic criteria for depressive disorders [5, 6]. Several postpartum studies have reported significant positive univariate associations between depressive and fatigue symptoms within the first 32 weeks postpartum [7]. Depression and fatigue may also predict each other over time: across the first four years postpartum, depressive

* Correspondence: bei.bei@monash.edu
[1]Monash Institute of Cognitive and Clinical Neurosciences, School of Psychological Sciences, Monash University, 18 Innovation Walk, Clayton Campus, VIC 3800, Australia
Full list of author information is available at the end of the article

symptoms have been shown to predict future fatigue levels, and vice versa [8–10].

## Depression and fatigue in community samples of postpartum women

Given this close relationship between depression and fatigue, there has been a debate as whether they are distinct phenomena [11, 12]. In relatively healthy women in the postpartum period, evidence points to depression and fatigue being two different constructs [11, 13]. A qualitative study found that women with depressive symptoms reported symptoms such as feelings of emptiness and guilt that were not endorsed by non-depressed but fatigued women [14]. This is consistent with studies that identified clusters of women with high fatigue but not depressive symptoms [15, 16]. Two studies examined specific symptom constructs of postpartum depression and fatigue using confirmatory factor analysis (CFA) in community populations within the first year postpartum [11, 13] and one study also at four years postpartum [13]: both studies concluded that a two-factor model of related but separate latent factors of depression and fatigue provided a better fit to the data than a single combined factor at all time-points.

## What about women experiencing elevated postpartum fatigue and distress?

The differentiation of depression and fatigue symptoms has not been well examined in a clinical setting. Findings among healthy women may not generalise to those with elevated psychological distress and fatigue symptoms seeking clinical care. Depression and fatigue share many common features that can make them difficult to differentiate in clinical settings [14, 17]. For example, they may share similar indicators among women seeking clinical help, such as irritability, feeling overwhelmed, and impaired physical and cognitive functioning [13, 14, 18, 19]. Depression and fatigue can also share underlying causes such as sleep disturbance, physiological changes, or situational factors (e.g., unsettled infant behaviours; [12, 18, 20]). Together, these similarities in presentation and causes present a challenge in differentiating depression and fatigue and can lead to potential over-diagnosis of fatigue as depression [10, 13].

While there is evidence that fatigue and depression are related but separate constructs in healthy populations, it is possible that as depression and fatigue levels increase, they become less distinct and harder to differentiate [11, 17]. High fatigue symptoms may reduce self-care behaviours and pleasurable activities, which may contribute to low mood [11]. Conversely, it is also possible that distinct features of both depression and fatigue may become more apparent as symptom severity increases [11].

Better understanding of the relationship between depression and fatigue in mothers at risk for both conditions is of critical importance to clinical services for both assessment and treatment. It is currently routine practice in many postpartum settings to screen for depressive disorders, but the assessment of fatigue is not routine [6, 13]. If symptoms of fatigue and depression largely overlap, existing short screening measures of depressive symptoms may be sufficient, and treatments for postpartum depression may help both sets of symptoms [21]. However, if depression and fatigue remain distinct, then separate and more detailed assessment of both constructs could assist with more accurate diagnoses [13], and targeted interventions for depressive and fatigue symptoms may be warranted [22, 23].

## Current study

Unsettled infant behaviour occurs in ~ 25% of infants, and refers to persistent and inconsolable infant crying, resistance to soothing, short sleep intervals and frequent night awakenings [24]. Previous studies among women seeking support for unsettled infant behaviour have shown that many of these women experience elevated depression, anxiety, and fatigue symptoms [25–28]. Examining the profiles of these symptoms among women presenting at clinical services offering support for unsettled infant behaviour represents a unique opportunity to investigate whether depression and fatigue can be differentiated among women with elevated postpartum fatigue and psychological distress, and thereby address the previous lack of research in the relationship between depression and fatigue in clinical samples.

For this purpose, this study aimed to compare a one-factor model of combined depression and fatigue with a two-factor model of separate but related depression and fatigue. It was hypothesised that a two-factor model of related but separate depression and fatigue latent factors would provide a better fit for the data than a one-factor model, as is the case in community studies. To further demonstrate the predictive utility of the better fitting model, we explored the association(s) between the latent factor(s) and self-reported sleep efficiency given that sleep disturbance is related to both postpartum depression and fatigue [15, 29–33].

## Methods
### Study context and participants

Participants were women with infants aged up to 24 months who had been referred by medical practitioners to attend the Masada Private Hospital Early Parenting Centre (MPHEPC; Melbourne, Australia) for a residential early parenting program that assists with unsettled infant behaviour (for details on the intervention: [4, 24, 26, 34]). All women admitted to the MPHEPC between the 1st June 2015 and 12th October 2015 were invited to participate in the study with no exclusion criteria. Recruitment was carried out via advertisement on the MPHEPC website, a pamphlet in admission documentation, or by researchers on site. Participants completed a survey booklet on the first day of their admission before commencing treatment. The Avenue Hospital Research Ethics Committee (Trial 182) and Monash University Human Research Ethics Committee (CF15/1233) provided ethical approval. Written informed consent was obtained from all participants.

## Procedure

On the day of arrival to the MPHEPC, participants that expressed interest in the research project underwent an informed consent process and provided with a survey booklet that included the measures in this study. The survey booklet was returned to the researchers on site.

## Measures

### Demographics

Maternal and infant demographics were collected through self-report and medical records extraction (see Table 1).

### Depression

The Depression Anxiety Stress Scales Depression sub-scale (DASS21-D) [35] is a widely used 7-item measure of depressive symptoms during the last week. The DASS21-D has adequate validity and reliability for postpartum populations [11, 36]. For this study Cronbach's alpha was .88, Omega was 0.89, and Greatest Lower Bound was 0.92 [37].

### Fatigue

A revised five-item version of the Fatigue Severity Scale (FSS; [38]) was used to measure the interference of fatigue on functioning. The FSS is a widely used scale of fatigue severity and interference in chronic illness populations. Similar to findings in other chronic illness populations [39–42], the full nine-item FSS had several psychometric issues based on Rasch analysis [43]. The revised version (FSS-5R) was calculated from Items 4 to 8 of the original FSS with simplified response options (recoded from 1,234,567 to 1,112,345) and had improved psychometric properties [43]. Scale items are listed in Additional file 1: Table S1. For the FSS-5R, Cronbach's alpha was .87, Omega was .88, and Greatest Lower Bound was .89. Scores on the full FSS-9 were also used to calculate the proportion of women reporting fatigue severity above the suggested clinical cut-off (≥ 36) and for comparison with community studies in which the full scale was used.

**Table 1** Maternal and infant demographics (N = 167)

| Demographic Variable | n | % |
|---|---|---|
| Country of Birth: | | |
| Australia | 117 | 70.09 |
| Other | 48 | 28.74 |
| Language spoken at home: | | |
| Mainly English | 146 | 87.43 |
| English & other | 18 | 10.78 |
| Mainly other | 3 | 1.80 |
| Mental Health History: | | |
| Previous treatment[a] | 58 | 34.73 |
| No previous treatment | 109 | 65.27 |
| Relationship status: | | |
| Married | 144 | 86.23 |
| De facto (living together) | 21 | 12.57 |
| Separated | 1 | 0.60 |
| Single | 1 | 0.60 |
| Education Level: | | |
| University or higher university degree | 129 | 77.25 |
| Certificate/diploma/trade | 29 | 17.97 |
| Completed secondary school | 4 | 2.40 |
| Partial completion secondary school | 1 | 0.60 |
| Multiple Birth: | | |
| Single birth | 162 | 97.01 |
| Twins | 5 | 2.99 |
| Parity: | | |
| Primapara | 83 | 49.70 |
| Multipara | 58 | 34.73 |
| Infant Health: | | |
| Excellent | 84 | 50.30 |
| Very Good | 70 | 41.92 |
| Good | 9 | 5.39 |
| Fair | 2 | 1.20 |

*Note.* [a] Among the 58 who reported having received previous mental health treatment, 36 received treatment for depression, 38 for anxiety, and 5 for posttraumatic stress disorder

## Sleep quality

Sleep Efficiency (SE) represents overall sleep quality, and was calculated as the percentage of self-report total sleep time against time spent in bed over the past week. SE ranges from 0% (low) to 100% (high efficiency).

The following well-validated instruments were also used to characterise the overall psychological distress reported by the sample: Depression Anxiety Stress Scale Anxiety (DASS21-A) and Stress (DASS21-S) subscales [35]; Insomnia Severity Index (ISI; [44]); and the 6 item version of the Irritability Depression Anxiety Scale – Irritability subscale (IDA-I; [45]).

## Data analysis

Data analysis was conducted in Mplus Version 7.4 [46]. First, one-factor models of depression using the DASS21-D and fatigue using the FSS-5R were assessed separately to confirm the uni-dimensionality of each scale. Then, one- and two-factor models for depression and fatigue were conducted and compared. In the one-factor model, all depression and fatigue items loaded onto a single latent variable representing a single combined construct (see Fig. 1 below). In the two-factor model, items from the DASS21-D and the FSS-5R were separately loaded onto their respective latent variables; the depression and fatigue latent variables were allowed to be correlated (see Fig. 2). Thus, the two-factor model tests whether depression and fatigue are separate but correlated constructs [13].

Confirmatory factor analysis (CFA) analysis was conducted using diagonally weighted least squares (WLSMV) estimation [47]. The sample size ($N = 167$) had power of 0.80 to identify an effect size of 0.30 [48] and exceeded 10 observations per parameter [49]. The criteria for adequate model fit were: Chi-Square Test of Model Fit, Root Mean Square Error of Approximation (RMSEA) $\leq 0.05$, Comparative Fit Index (CFI) and Tucker-Lewis Index (TLI) > 0.9, and Weighted Root Mean Square Residual (WRMR) < 1.0 [50, 51]. Comparison of model fit was carried out using the Chi-Square difference test for WLSMV estimation. Discriminant validity of the two-factor model was also assessed by examining the standardised pattern and structure coefficients of the two-factor model of depression and fatigue [13, 52]. Discriminant validity is established if the difference in values of the pattern and structure coefficients is .2 or above [13]. Finally, the predictive utility of the better fitting model was assessed by adding SE as the predictor of the latent factor(s). As missing data were low (< 5%), they were handled using pairwise deletion. No model modifications were made.

## Results

During the 19-week recruitment period, 167 of the 380 women admitted to the MPHEPC (44%) completed the study. Maternal and infant demographics and descriptive statistics for the DASS21-D, FSS-5R and SE are reported in Table 1 and Table 2. Missing data were minimal: 1.1% for the DASS21-D, 0.3% for the FSS-5R, and 4.8% for SE. A correlation matrix of scale items is in Additional file 1: Table S2. Participants reported elevated depressive symptoms, with 50% reporting symptoms at or above the published cut off for mild depressive symptoms (DASS21-D $\geq 5$). Fatigue symptoms were also elevated, with 87% of women reporting fatigue severity above the suggested clinical cut-off ($\geq 36$) for the full FSS-9; scores were higher than those reported in a postpartum community population [22]. Scores on the other measures also point to an overall elevated level of distress in this sample. Forty-eight percent of women reported at least mild anxiety (DASS21-A $\geq 4$), 64% reported at least mild stress (DASS21-S $\geq 8$), and 46% reported insomnia symptoms in the clinical range (ISI $\geq 15$).

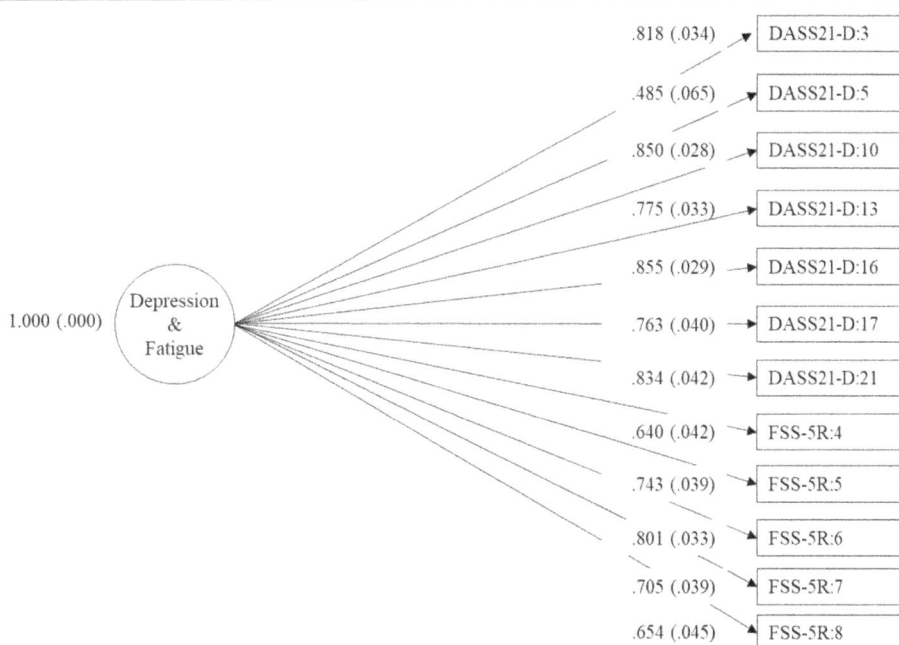

**Fig. 1** One-factor model of depression and fatigue. Note: Loadings are standardised

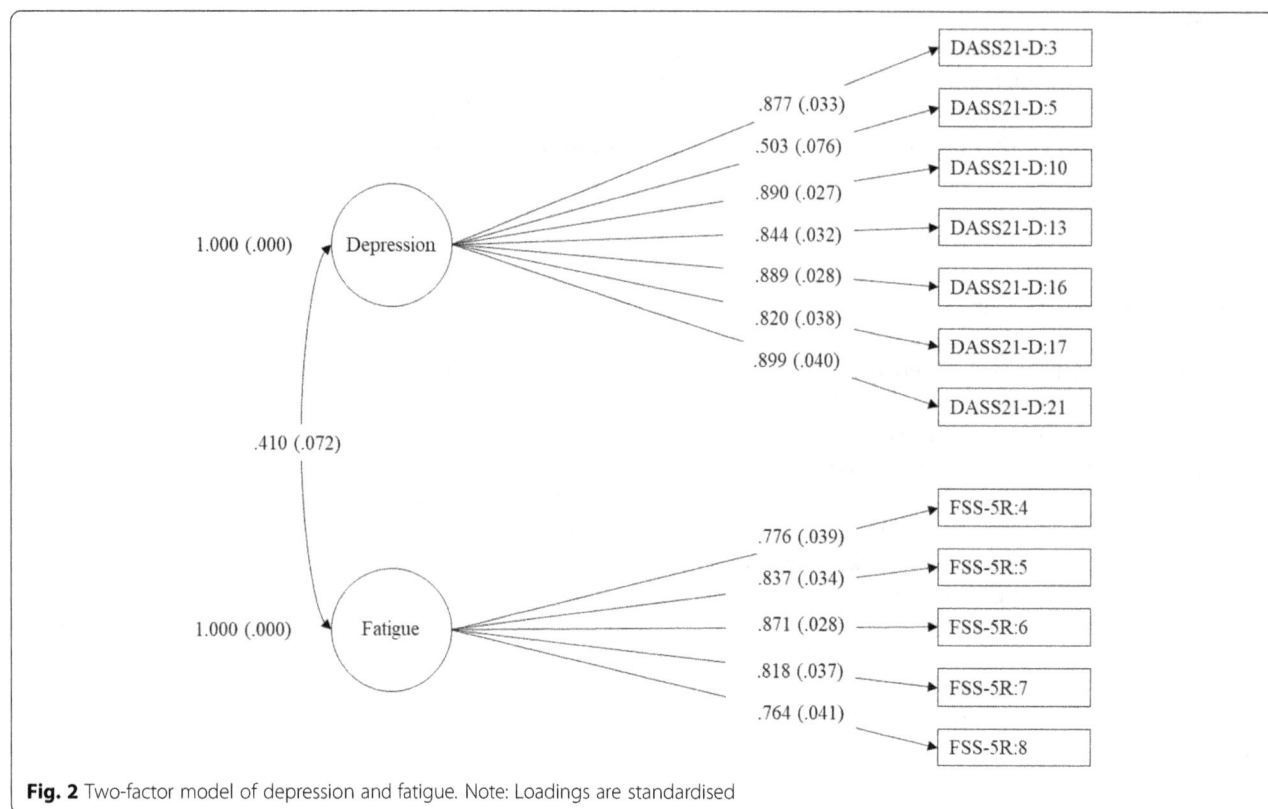

**Fig. 2** Two-factor model of depression and fatigue. Note: Loadings are standardised

## Confirmatory factor analysis

Separate models of the DASS21-D and FSS-5R both showed acceptable fit without modification (see Table 3). For both models, the standardised coefficients all significantly loaded onto the latent factor (all $p$-values < .001) and all exceeded .78 (see Table 4), except for DASS21-D Item 5. Therefore, both scales uni-dimensionally assessed the respective constructs.

**Table 2** Descriptive statistics ($N = 167$)

| Variable | $n$ | $M$ | $SD$ | Median | Min. | Max. |
|---|---|---|---|---|---|---|
| Maternal Age (years) | 167 | 34.26 | 4.23 | 34.00 | 24.00 | 49.00 |
| Infant Age (months) | 167 | 8.51 | 4.16 | 7.50 | 2.00 | 23.50 |
| FSS-9 | 163 | 47.92 | 8.85 | 49.00 | 21.00 | 63.00 |
| FSS-5R | 163 | 17.35 | 5.24 | 18.00 | 5.00 | 25.00 |
| DASS21-Depression | 162 | 5.12 | 3.81 | 5.00 | 0.00 | 18.00 |
| DASS21-Anxiety | 162 | 3.59 | 2.90 | 3.00 | 0.00 | 13.00 |
| DASS21-Stress | 158 | 9.71 | 4.11 | 9.00 | 0.00 | 20.00 |
| IDA-I | 165 | 7.28 | 3.92 | 7.00 | 1.00 | 18.00 |
| ISI | 165 | 13.76 | 5.13 | 14.00 | 1.00 | 28.00 |
| Sleep Efficiency (%) | 159 | 62.94 | 15.79 | 63.16 | 23.08 | 100.0 |

*Note. DASS21-D* Depression Anxiety Stress Scale, *FSS-9* Fatigue Severity Scale, *FSS-5R* Fatigue Severity Scale Revised 5-item version, *IDA-I* Irritability Depression Anxiety Scale – Irritability subscale 6 item version, *ISI* Insomnia Severity Index

The one-factor model with depression and fatigue items loading onto a single construct had a poor fit (see Table 3). All items loaded significantly on the single latent factor ($p < .001$) and the standardised coefficients ranged from 0.49 to 0.86 (see Table 4 and Fig. 1). The two-factor model of depression and fatigue as related but separate latent factors provided an acceptable and improved fit (see Table 3). The standardised coefficients for fatigue items on the fatigue latent factor and depression items on the depression latent factor were all significant ($p < .001$) (see Table 4 and Fig. 2). Compared to the one-factor model, the two-factor model provided a significantly better fit to the data, $\Delta\chi^2$ (1) = 67.50, $p < .001$. The correlation between the fatigue and depression latent factors in the two-factor model was 0.41 ($p < .001$).

The pattern and structure coefficients of the one and two-factor models are shown in Table 4. The differences between the structure and the fixed pattern coefficients ranged from 0.21 to 0.39 for both the depression and fatigue items, suggesting adequate discriminant validity.

In the better fitting two-factor model, SE was added as a simultaneous predictor of both the depression and fatigue latent factors. This model had an acceptable fit to the data without modification (see Table 3). Lower SE was associated with both higher depression ($p = .004$) and fatigue ($p < .001$), with no significant difference in the strength of these two paths, Wald $\chi^2$ (1) = 0.131, $p = .71$.

**Table 3** Fit Indices for models ($N = 167$)

| Model | $\chi^2$ | df | p | RMSEA [90% CI] | TLI | CFI | WRMR |
|---|---|---|---|---|---|---|---|
| Congeneric DASS21-D | 25.77 | 14 | .0277 | 0.071 [0.023, 0.113] | 0.992 | 0.995 | 0.583 |
| Congeneric FSS-5R | 14.38 | 5 | .0134 | 0.106 [0.044, 0.172] | 0.984 | 0.992 | 0.441 |
| One-factor model | 475.56 | 54 | <.0001 | 0.216 [0.199, 0.234] | 0.812 | 0.847 | 2.410 |
| Two-factor model | 136.28 | 53 | <.0001 | 0.097 [0.077, 0.117] | 0.962 | 0.970 | 0.987 |
| Two-factor model on SE | 147.72 | 63 | <.0001 | 0.092 [0.073, 0.111] | 0.956 | 0.964 | 0.965 |

Note. $\chi^2$ Chi-Square Test of Model Fit; CFI Comparative Fit Index, DASS21-D Depression Anxiety Stress Scale Depression subscale, FSS-5R Fatigue Severity Scale-Revised 5-item version, RMSEA Root Mean Square Error of Approximation, SE Sleep Efficiency, TLI Tucker-Lewis Index, WRMR Weighted Root Mean Square Residual

## Discussion

In this sample of women with elevated psychological distress and fatigue symptoms seeking support for un-settled infant behaviour, depression and fatigue symptoms are best considered as separate constructs that share a moderate correlation. Furthermore, both constructs were simultaneously predicted by a potential common cause (i.e., sleep efficiency), suggesting that the two-factor model may facilitate the understanding of the risk factors for both conditions. This study also supports the DASS21-D and a revised FSS-5R as uni-dimensional measures of depressive and fatigue symptoms in this population.

Findings from this study echo results from community postpartum populations where depression and fatigue were also found to be separate constructs [11, 13]. However, the correlation between the depression and fatigue latent

**Table 4** Pattern and structure standardised coefficients DASS21-D and FSS-5R

| Scale and Item | Congeneric model | One-factor model | Two-factor model[a] | | | |
|---|---|---|---|---|---|---|
| | | | Depression | | Fatigue | |
| | Pattern | Pattern | Pattern | Structure | Pattern | Structure |
| DASS21-D | | | | | | |
| Item 3 | 0.89 | 0.82 | 0.88 | 0.88 | 0.00[b] | 0.36 |
| Item 5 | 0.39 | 0.49 | 0.50 | 0.50 | 0.00[b] | 0.21 |
| Item 10 | 0.90 | 0.85 | 0.89 | 0.89 | 0.00[b] | 0.36 |
| Item 13 | 0.83 | 0.78 | 0.84 | 0.84 | 0.00[b] | 0.35 |
| Item 16 | 0.89 | 0.86 | 0.89 | 0.89 | 0.00[b] | 0.36 |
| Item 17 | 0.84 | 0.76 | 0.82 | 0.82 | 0.00[b] | 0.34 |
| Item 21 | 0.90 | 0.83 | 0.90 | 0.90 | 0.00[b] | 0.37 |
| FSS-5R | | | | | | |
| Item 4 | 0.79 | 0.64 | 0.00[b] | 0.32 | 0.78 | 0.78 |
| Item 5 | 0.83 | 0.74 | 0.00[b] | 0.34 | 0.84 | 0.84 |
| Item 6 | 0.86 | 0.80 | 0.00[b] | 0.36 | 0.87 | 0.87 |
| Item 7 | 0.81 | 0.71 | 0.00[b] | 0.34 | 0.82 | 0.82 |
| Item 8 | 0.78 | 0.65 | 0.00[b] | 0.31 | 0.76 | 0.76 |

Note: [a] In the two-factor model all correlations were free to be estimated, and factor variances were set to unity for model identification. [b] Parameters were fixed at 0.00. DASS21-D Depression Anxiety Stress Scale Depression subscale, FSS-5R Fatigue Severity Scale-Revised 5-item version; Values are standardised coefficients

factors in this study was smaller than the large associations seen in the two studies that applied CFA on non-clinical samples [11, 13]. This could be because in this study, depression levels while elevated are not severe based on cut-off scores, while fatigue levels are high based on cut-off scores, thus the difference between the two constructs may be more prominent. Alternatively, the lower correlation in this study could be due to differences in scales: the DASS21-D does not include any fatigue or somatic items, and the FSS-5R assesses fatigue interference rather than specific symptoms. This combination may have led to a weaker correlation between the two factors in this study compared to other combinations of scales. Nevertheless, the correlation between depression and fatigue in this study is comparable to that in other postpartum studies ($r = .30$ to .45; [10, 53–58]).

Our analyses on sleep efficiency serve as an example of many potential uses of the two-factor model in understanding common predictors and mechanisms. In this study, the findings were consistent with the literature linking self-report sleep disturbance with both postpartum fatigue and depressive symptoms [14, 15, 29–33].

### Limitations and strengths

As participants in this study were predominantly university-educated, born in Australia, and had the necessary resources to access privately funded treatment, this may limit the generalizability of our results. Also, despite overall high distress levels, depressive symptoms reported in our study were not severe. Thus, findings may not generalise to mothers meeting diagnostic criteria for a depressive disorder. A further limitation was that our sample comes from an ongoing clinical service that admits infants of 0–2 years, and infants in this study had an age range spanning 21.5 months. During this period, various psychological, biological and social factors may influence depression and fatigue. It is also possible that our sample could have included women with chronic health difficulties that contribute to their reported symptoms. Finally, given that the service we recruited from only admitted women with their infants, this paper did not examine the how potentially elevated mental health symptoms in partners [59] impact women's experiences and symptoms.

Nevertheless, this study represented a unique opportunity to investigate the relationship between depression and fatigue in a clinical postpartum population with elevated psychological distress and fatigue symptoms. Given the high prevalence of infant settling difficulties in the community, these results are likely to be relevant to a high proportion of women who have given birth in the last year or two [24]. Other strengths include a large sample size, a relatively high recruitment rate for a help-seeking population (44%), and the use of appropriate statistical modelling. A further strength of this study was that it serves as a demonstration of how a third construct such as sleep efficiency can influence both these constructs.

## Implications and conclusions

Theoretically, our findings add further support for the two-factor model of related but distinct postpartum depression and fatigue and show that depression and fatigue likely remain distinct constructs, even when mothers are experiencing elevated psychological distress and fatigue levels. By showing how sleep efficiency can be independently related to both the depression and fatigue factors, this study demonstrated the potential utility of the two-factor model for understanding other potential physiological, psychological, and situational factors that could underlie both conditions [12, 60].

Clinically, our results indicate that among women seeking support for unsettled infant behaviour, and perhaps more broadly, women who present to clinical services with high psychological distress and fatigue in the postpartum period, depression and fatigue symptoms need to be assessed and treated in their own right. Improved assessment and greater awareness that depression and fatigue are related but separate constructs could help prevent the diagnosis of fatigue symptoms as depressive symptoms [13, 14]. Given that fatigue is one of the DSM-5 diagnostic criteria for Major Depressive Disorder [5], some overlap between these two constructs is inevitable. However, more detailed assessment of both conditions will assist clinicians to determine whether impaired postpartum functioning is caused by depressive symptoms, fatigue symptoms, or a combination of both.

Women experiencing fatigue but not depression may benefit from targeted interventions for fatigue, rather than potentially more intensive pharmacological treatments or therapy that may be better suited for depression [13, 22, 23]. Residential early parenting programs that assist with unsettled infant behaviour have demonstrated efficacy in rapidly reducing fatigue and may be an appropriate treatment in this situation [27, 34].

## Additional file

> **Additional file 1: Table S1.** Summary of Items for FSS-5R and DASS21-D. **Table S2.** Means, standard deviations, and Pearson correlations for FSS-5R, DASS21-D and SE (N = 167). (DOCX 41 kb)

### Abbreviations
CFA: Confirmatory Factor Analysis; CFI: Comparative Fit Index (CFI); DASS21: Depression Anxiety Stress Scale; DSM-5: Diagnostic and Statistical Manual of Mental Disorders, 5th Edition; FSS-5R: Fatigue Severity Scale - Revised 5 item version; FSS-9: Fatigue Severity Scale; IDA-I: Irritability Depression Anxiety Scale – Irritability subscale, 6 item version; ISI: Insomnia Severity Index; MPHEPC: Masada Private Hospital Early Parenting Centre; RMSEA: Root Mean Square Error of Approximation; SE: Sleep Efficiency; TLI: Tucker-Lewis Index; WLSMV: Diagonally weighted least squares estimation; WRMR: Weighted Root Mean Square Residual

### Acknowledgements
The authors are grateful to the staff at Masada Private Hospital Early Parenting Centre for their collaboration in implementing this study; Olivia Chung, Hilary Brown and Hannah Gray for assisting with data collection and to the women who most generously contributed data. NW was supported by an Australian Government Research Training Program Scholarship, KW was supported by a Monash University Advancing Women's Research Success grant, and JF by a Monash Professorial Fellowship and the Jean Hailes Professorial Fellowship, which is supported by a grant to the Jean Hailes Foundation from the H and L Hecht Trust managed by Perpetual Trustees.

### Authors' contributions
NW, KW, JF and BB all contributed to study design, manuscript write-up, and approved the final manuscript. NW and KW carried out data collection. NW and BB conducted and reviewed the analyses, and wrote the first draft. All authors read and approved the final manuscript.

### Competing interests
NW has nothing to disclose. KW has nothing to disclose. JF reports personal fees from Masada Private Hospital, which is owned by Ramsay Healthcare, other from Global Public Health Unit, during the conduct of the study. BB has nothing to disclose.

### Author details
[1]Monash Institute of Cognitive and Clinical Neurosciences, School of Psychological Sciences, Monash University, 18 Innovation Walk, Clayton Campus, VIC 3800, Australia. [2]Global Public Health Unit, School of Public Health and Preventative Medicine, Monash University, Clayton, Victoria, Australia. [3]Centre for Quality and Patient Safety Research – Western Health Partnership, School of Nursing and Midwifery, Faculty of Health, Deakin University, Burwood, VIC, Australia. [4]Masada Early Parenting Centre, Masada Private Hospital, East St Kilda, VIC, Australia.

### References
1.   McGovern P, Dowd B, Gjerdingen D, Dagher R, Ukestad L, McCaffrey D, Lundberg U. Mothers' health and work-related factors at 11 weeks postpartum. Ann Fam Med. 2007;5(6):519–27.

2.  Parks PL, Lenz ER, Milligan RA, Han HR. What happens when fatigue lingers for 18 months after delivery? J Obstet Gynecol Neonatal Nurs. 1999;28(1): 87–93.

3.  Putnam KT, Wilcox M, Robertson-Blackmore E, Sharkey K, Bergink V, Munk-Olsen T, Deligiannidis KM, Payne J, Altemus M, Newport J, et al. Clinical phenotypes of perinatal depression and time of symptom onset: analysis of data from an international consortium. Lancet Psychiatry. 2017;4(6):477–85.

4.  Fisher JRW, Feekery C, Rowe H. Psycho-educational Early Parenting Interventions to Promote Infant Mental Health. In: Fitzgerald HE, Puura K, Tomlinson M, Paul C, editors. International Perspectives on Children and Mental Health. edn ed. Santa Barbara: ABC-CLIO; 2011. p. 205–36.

5.  American Psychiatric A: Diagnostic and statistical manual of mental disorders (DSM-5®): American psychiatric pub; 2013.

6.  Williamson JA, O'Hara MW, Stuart S, Hart KJ, Watson D. Assessment of postpartum depressive symptoms: the importance of somatic symptoms and irritability. Assessment. 2015;22(3):309–18.

7.  Badr H, Zauszniewski J. Meta-analysis of the predictive factors of postpartum fatigue. Appl Nurs Res. 2017;36(C):122–7.

8.  Bozoky I, Corwin EJ. Fatigue as a predictor of postpartum depression. J Obstet Gynecol Neonatal Nurs. 2002;31(4):436–43.

9.  Corwin EJ, Brownstead J, Barton N, Heckard S, Morin K. The impact of fatigue on the development of postpartum depression. J Obstet Gynecol Neonatal Nurs. 2005;34(5):577–86.

10. Giallo R, Gartland D, Woolhouse H, Brown S. "I didn't know it was possible to feel that tired": exploring the complex bidirectional associations between maternal depressive symptoms and fatigue in a prospective pregnancy cohort study. Arch Womens Ment Health. 2016;19(1):25–34.

11. Giallo R, Wade C, Cooklin A, Rose N. Assessment of maternal fatigue and depression in the postpartum period: support for two separate constructs. J Reprod Infant Psychol. 2011;29(1):69–80.

12. Milligan RA, Lenz ER, Parks PL, Pugh LC, Kitzman H. Postpartum fatigue: clarifying a concept. Sch Inq Nurs Pract. 1996;10(3):279–91.

13. Giallo R, Gartland D, Woolhouse H, Brown S. Differentiating maternal fatigue and depressive symptoms at six months and four years post partum: considerations for assessment, diagnosis and intervention. Midwifery. 2015; 31(2):316–22.

14. Runquist J. A depressive symptoms responsiveness model for differentiating fatigue from depression in the postpartum period. Arch Womens Ment Health. 2007;10(6):267–75.

15. Kuo S-Y, Yang Y-L, Kuo P-C, Tseng C-M, Tzeng Y-L. Trajectories of depressive symptoms and fatigue among postpartum women. J Obstet Gynecol Neonatal Nurs. 2012;41(2):216–26.

16. Wade C, Giallo R, Cooklin A. Maternal fatigue and depression: identifying vulnerability and relationship to early parenting practices. Adv Ment Health. 2012;10(3):277–91.

17. Jacobsen PB, Donovan KA, Weitzner MA. Distinguishing fatigue and depression in patients with cancer. Semin Clin Neuropsychiatry. 2003;8(4):229–40.

18. Runquist J. Persevering through postpartum fatigue. J Obstet Gynecol Neonatal Nurs. 2007;36(1):28–37.

19. Shahid A, Shen J, Shapiro CM. Measurements of sleepiness and fatigue. J Psychosom Res. 2010;69(1):81–9.

20. Kurth E, Kennedy HP, Spichiger E, Hösli I, Stutz EZ. Crying babies, tired mothers: what do we know? A systematic review. Midwifery. 2011;27(2): 187–94.

21. Cuijpers P, Brännmark JG, van Straten A: Psychological treatment of postpartum depression: a meta-analysis. J Clin Psychol 2008, 64(1): 103–118.

22. Giallo R, Cooklin A, Dunning M, Seymour M: The Efficacy of an Intervention for the Management of Postpartum Fatigue. In.; 2014.

23. Troy NW, Dalgas-Pelish P. The effectiveness of a self-care intervention for the management of postpartum fatigue. Appl Nurs Res. 2003;16(1):38–45.

24. Fisher JRW, Rowe H, Hiscock H, Jordan B, Bayer J, Colahan A, Amery V. Understanding and responding to unsettled infant behaviour. Aust Res Alliance Child Youth. 2011:1–60.

25. Bobevski I, Rowe H, Clarke DM, McKenzie DP, Fisher JRW. Postnatal demoralisation among women admitted to a hospital mother-baby unit: validation of a psychometric measure. Arch Womens Ment Health. 2015; 18(6):817–27.

26. Fisher JRW, Feekery CJ, Rowe-Murray HJ. Nature, severity and correlates of psychological distress in women admitted to a private mother-baby unit. J Paediatr Child Health. 2002;38(2):140–5.

27. Fisher JRW, Rowe H, Feekery C. Temperament and behaviour of infants aged 4–12 months on admission to a private mother-baby unit and at 1- and 6-month follow-up. Clin Psychol. 2004;8(1):15–21.

28. Giallo R, Rose N, Vittorino R. Fatigue, wellbeing and parenting in mothers of infants and toddlers with sleep problems. J Reprod Infant Psychol. 2011; 29(3):236–49.

29. Bei B, Coo S, Trinder J. Sleep and mood during pregnancy and the postpartum period. Sleep Med Clin. 2015;10(1):25–33.

30. Coo Calcagni S, Bei B, Milgrom J, Trinder J. The relationship between sleep and mood in first-time and experienced mothers. Behav Sleep Med. 2012; 10(3):167–79.

31. Gay CL, Lee KA, Lee S-Y. Sleep patterns and fatigue in new mothers and fathers. Biol Res Nurs. 2004;5(4):311–8.

32. Rychnovsky J, Hunter LP. The relationship between sleep characteristics and fatigue in healthy postpartum women. Womens Health Issues. 2009;19(1):38–44.

33. Thomas KA, Spieker S. Sleep, depression, and fatigue in late postpartum. MCN Am J Matern Child Nurs. 2016;41(2):104–9.

34. Fisher JRW, Feekery C, Rowe H. Treatment of maternal mood disorder and infant behaviour disturbance in an Australian private mothercraft unit: a follow-up study. Arch Womens Ment Health. 2004;7(1):89–93.

35. Lovibond PF, Lovibond SH: Manual for the depression, anxiety and stress scales (DASS). 1995.

36. Miller RL, Pallant JF, Negri LM. Anxiety and stress in the postpartum: is there more to postnatal distress than depression? BMC Psychiatry. 2006;6:12.

37. Peters G-JY. The alpha and the omega of scale reliability and validity: why and how to abandon Cronbach's alpha and the route towards more comprehensive assessment of scale quality. Eur Health Psychol. 2014;16(2):56–69.

38. Krupp LB, LaRocca NG, Muir-Nash J, Steinberg AD. The fatigue severity scale. Application to patients with multiple sclerosis and systemic lupus erythematosus. Arch Neurol. 1989;46(10):1121–3.

39. Lerdal A, Johansson S, Kottorp A, von Koch L: Psychometric properties of the fatigue severity scale: Rasch analyses of responses in a Norwegian and a Swedish MS cohort. Mult Scler 2010, 16(6):733–741.

40. Lerdal A, Kottorp A. Psychometric properties of the fatigue severity scale-Rasch analyses of individual responses in a Norwegian stroke cohort. Int J Nurs Stud. 2011;48(10):1258–65.

41. Mills R, Young C, Nicholas R, Pallant J, Tennant A. Rasch analysis of the fatigue severity scale in multiple sclerosis. Mult Scler. 2009;15(1):81–7.

42. Ottonello M, Pellicciari L, Giordano A, Foti C. Rasch analysis of the fatigue severity scale in Italian subjects with multiple sclerosis. J Rehabil Med. 2016; 48(7):597–603.

43. Wilson N, Wynter K, Fisher J, Bei B. Postpartum fatigue: assessing and improving the psychometric properties of the fatigue severity scale. Arch Womens Ment Health. 2018;21(4):471–4.

44. Bastien CH, Vallières A, Morin CM. Validation of the insomnia severity index as an outcome measure for insomnia research. Sleep Med. 2001; 2(4):297–307.

45. Snaith RP, Taylor CM. Irritability: definition, assessment and associated factors. Br J Psychiatry. 1985;147:127–36.

46. Muthén LK, Muthén BO: Mplus User's guide. Seventh edition. Los Angeles, CA: Muthén & Muthén,; 2012.

47. Li C-H. Confirmatory factor analysis with ordinal data: comparing robust maximum likelihood and diagonally weighted least squares. Behav Res Methods. 2016;48(3):936–49.

48. Soper DS: A-priori sample size calculator for structural equation models [software]. 2017.

49. Cappelleri JC, Jason Lundy J, Hays RD. Overview of classical test theory and item response theory for the quantitative assessment of items in developing patient-reported outcomes measures. Clin Ther. 2014;36(5): 648–62.

50. Hooper D, Coughlan J, Mullen M. Structural equation modelling: Guidelines for determining model fit. Electron J Bus Res Methods. 2008;6(1):53–60.

51. Yu C-Y. Evaluating cutoff criteria of model fit indices for latent variable models with binary and continuous outcomes. Los Angeles: University of California; 2002.

52. Thompson B. The importance of structure coefficients in structural equation modeling confirmatory factor analysis. Educ Psychol Meas. 1997;57(1):5–19.

53. Cheng CY, Pickler RH. Perinatal stress, fatigue, depressive symptoms, and immune modulation in late pregnancy and one month postpartum. ScientificWorldJournal. 2014;2014:652630.

54. Dennis C-L, Ross L. Relationships among infant sleep patterns, maternal fatigue, and development of depressive symptomatology. Birth. 2005; 32(3):187–93.

55. Elek SM, Hudson DB, Fleck MO. Couples' experiences with fatigue during the transition to parenthood. J Fam Nurs. 2002;8(3):221–40.

56. Gardner DL. Fatigue in postpartum women. Appl Nurs Res. 1991;4(2):57–62.

57. Lee S-Y, Grantham CH, Shelton S, Meaney-Delman D. Does activity matter: an exploratory study among mothers with preterm infants? Arch Womens Ment Health. 2012;15(3):185–92.

58. Song J-E, Chang S-B, Park S-M, Kim S, Nam C-M. Empirical test of an explanatory theory of postpartum fatigue in Korea. J Adv Nurs. 2010; 66(12):2627–39.

59. Wynter K, Wilson N, Thean P, Bei B, Fisher J. Psychological distress, alcohol use, fatigue, sleepiness, and sleep quality: an exploratory study among men whose partners are admitted to a residential early parenting service. Aust Psychol. 2018. p. 1–8. https://doi.org/10.1111/ap.12348.

60. Lenz ER, Pugh LC, Milligan RA, Gift A, Suppe F. The middle-range theory of unpleasant symptoms: an update. ANS Adv Nurs Sci. 1997;19(3):14–27.

# 6

# Polymorphisms in the human serotonin receptor 1B (HTR1B) gene are associated with schizophrenia: a case control study

Xi Xia, Mei Ding, Jin-feng Xuan, Jia-xin Xing, Hao Pang, Bao-jie Wang*⊙ and Jun Yao*

## Abstract

**Background:** Schizophrenia is associated with multiple neurotransmitter disorders, including serotonin (5-hydroxytryptamine, 5-HT). The neuromodulatory action of serotonin on brain function largely depends on the action of specific subtypes of serotonin receptors. The serotonin receptor 1B (HTR1B) gene has been proposed to play putative roles in the development of multiple emotional and psychiatric disorders.

**Methods:** To study the relationship of *HTR1B* polymorphisms and schizophrenia, gene information was drawn from a cohort of 310 schizophrenic patients (152 men and 158 women) and 313 healthy controls (153 men and 160 women) of northern Han Chinese descent. The χ2 test was used to compare allele and genotype distributions between case and control groups. The haplotype and linkage equilibrium were also assessed in two group comparisons.

**Results:** We detected 14 SNPs. Male patients were observed to have higher frequencies of the A-allele and AA+AG genotype at rs1778258 than female patients ($p = 0.012$ and $p = 0.015$, respectively). Both the A-allele and AA+AG genotype were associated with schizophrenia risk (OR = 1.986 and OR = 2.061, respectively), although the statistical significance of the genotype was lost after Bonferroni correction. Linkage analysis showed that rs17273700, rs11568817, rs9361234 and rs58138557 polymorphisms exhibit strong linkage disequilibrium (LD). In addition, schizophrenic patients show stronger linkage between 11,568,817 and rs130058 than healthy controls.

**Conclusions:** *HTR1B* polymorphisms are associated with schizophrenia in the northern Han Chinese population, which provides an etiological reference for schizophrenia.

**Keywords:** Schizophrenia, Single-nucleotide polymorphisms (SNPs), Serotonin receptor 1B (HTR1B)

## Background

Schizophrenia is a chronic disabling mental disorder affecting more than 21 million people worldwide, and is characterized by distortions in perception, thinking, emotions, sense of self and behavior. Common experiences include hearing voices and delusions (WHO2016). The etiology of schizophrenia is complicated, and genetic studies have had a guiding influence on schizophrenia research. A genome-wide association study (GWAS) suggested that schizophrenia is a complex polygenetic disease with over 80% heritability [1]. Numerous studies have focused on the neurotransmitters related to the pathogenesis of schizophrenia, including serotonin. Serotonin plays an import role in various brain activities including emotions, pain, assault, learning and memory [2].

The neuromodulatory action of serotonin on brain function largely depends on the actions of serotonin receptors, which comprise at least 14 different classes of subtypes [3]. HTR1B is a G-protein coupled receptor that activates a second messenger cascade to mediate inhibitory neurotransmission and regulate the release of serotonin, dopamine, and acetylcholine in the brain. HTR1B has been suggested to be associated with multiple emotional and psychiatric problems, including attention deficit hyperactivity disorder (ADHD) [4], antisocial behavior [5], aggressive behavior [6], bipolar disorder, anxiety/depression, schizophrenia [7, 8] and substance abuse [9]. It is also a common target for

---

* Correspondence: wangbj77@163.com; yaojun198717@163.com; 198717@163.com
School of Forensic Medicine, China Medical University, No. 77 Puhe Road, Shenbei New District, Shenyang 110122, China

psychotherapeutic drugs. The *HTR1B* gene is located on chromosome 6 at position 77,460,848–77,464,022 (GR Ch38.p7). It has been suggested that schizophrenic patients show increased *HTR1B* mRNA levels in the hippocampus. Simultaneous upregulation of *HTR1B* and downregulation of *HTR2A* could decrease GABAergic activity, which leads to an increased glutamatergic efferent in the hippocampus [7]. In previous studies, there were inconsistent results on the genetic association between *HTR1B* gene variations and schizophrenia. For example, rs2143823 is considered to be related to schizophrenia in Croatians [10]. However, there was no correlation between G861C and schizophrenia in Portuguese, German and Brazilian patients [11–13]. The associations between C129T, T371G, T655C, C705T, G861C, A1099G, G1120A and schizophrenia were also negative in mixed populations in the United States [14]. In addition, the *HTR1B* haplotype may be implicated in the gender discrepancy of schizophrenia in Spanish populations [15].

As the function of the coding regions has been studied extensively, SNPs located in regulatory regions were taken in to consideration. Prior studies addressing the association between schizophrenia and *HTR1B* polymorphisms in the Chinese Han population include only the 5′-untranslated (5'UTR) and coding regions, with little data concerning the 5′-promoter and 3′-regulatory regions. Therefore, we chose to investigate these regions to improve etiologic knowledge of this disease. Expanding sequences were investigated in our study, including a 2285 bp 5′-promoter region and a 1277 bp 3′-untranslated region, in the northern Han Chinese population to further explore the relationship between *HTR1B* and schizophrenia.

## Materials

### Subjects

Our sample comprised 310 schizophrenic patients (152 men and 158 women) and 313 genetically unrelated, healthy volunteers (153 men and 160 women), comprising a combined 623 individuals. All participants enrolled were of northern Han Chinese descent. Blood samples from schizophrenic patients were provided by the Third People's Hospital of Liaoning Province; those from healthy controls were supplied by the China Medical University's Forensic Evidence Department. Inclusion criteria included a diagnosis of schizophrenia by trained psychiatrists according to the Diagnostic and Statistical Manual of Mental Disorders, fourth edition (DSM-IV). Exclusion criteria included the presence of other psychiatric disorders. The results of patient questionnaires confirming no history nor present evidence of any psychiatric disorder and no history of mental disease for at least three prior generations were used to select healthy

controls. All subjects provided written informed consent prior to enrollment in this study.

### SNP selection

The following factors were considered for SNP selection: (1) as the function of the *HTR1B* coding region has been studied extensively, SNPs located within *HTR1B* regulatory regions were selected; (2) based on prior reports, we found that current knowledge of the association between schizophrenia and *HTR1B* polymorphisms in the Chinese Han population include the 5′ untranslated region (UTR), while the promoter and 3′ regulatory regions have not been well studied; and (3) according to the *HTR1B* polymorphism distribution, we selected SNPs with favorable polymorphisms (MAF ≥ 0.1). Considering that the regulatory effects of sequences that are distal to the coding region may be limited, we selected a 2285 bp 5′-promoter region and a 1277 bp 3′-untranslated region for SNP investigation.

### DNA isolation and genotyping

Genomic DNA was extracted by the phenol-chloroform method from whole blood [16]. A 2285 bp fragment in the 5′-promoter region and a 1277 bp fragment in the 3′-untranslated region were included in our analysis. Standard PCR was performed in a total reaction volume of 20 μl (adjusted with sterilized, deionized water) containing 2 μl genomic DNA as template (approximately 50 ng), 10 μl of 2 × GC Buffer, 0.2 μl (1 U) of Taq polymerase (Takara LA Taq, Dalian, China), 2 μl (3.75 nmol) of dNTPs, 1.5 μl (7.5 pmol) each of sense and antisense

**Table 1** SNPs (14 total) detected in the northern Han Chinese population

| SNP | Chr. pos. | Base change[1,2] | MAF | REGION |
|---|---|---|---|---|
| rs4140535 | 77,465,335 | − 1932 T > C | 0.375 | 5′near gene |
| rs1778258 | 77,464,492 | − 1089 G > A | 0.113 | 5′near gene |
| rs17273700 | 77,464,263 | − 860 T > C | 0.121 | 5′near gene |
| rs1228814 | 77,464,103 | −700 C > A | 0.166 | 5′near gene |
| rs11568817 | 77,463,665 | − 262 T > G | 0.116 | 5′UTR |
| rs130058 | 77,463,564 | −161 A > T | 0.077 | 5′UTR |
| rs6297 | 77,462,224 | *7 A > G | 0.112 | 3′UTR |
| rs3827804 | 77,462,215 | *16 G > A | 0.011 | 3′UTR |
| rs140792648 | 77,462,065 | *165_*166 Ins AG | 0.029 | 3′UTR |
| rs9361234 | 77,461,965 | *266 C > T | 0.113 | 3′UTR |
| rs183156887 | 77,461,962 | *269 C > A | 0.0064 | 3′UTR |
| rs76194807 | 77,461,898 | *333 G > T | 0.113 | 3′UTR |
| rs58138557 | 77,461,771 | *459_*460 Del GG | 0.115 | 3′UTR |
| rs13212041 | 77,461,407 | *824 A > G | 0.256 | 3′UTR |

[1]The A of the ATG start codon is designated as position 0
[2]An asterisk (*) indicates alterations in the coding region, which is 1173 bp in length

**Table 2** Allelic distributions of the 14 SNPs and their associations with schizophrenia

| SNP | Allele[1] | Genotype | Case (n=310) No. | Case Frequency | Control (n=313) No. | Control Frequency | p Value[2] Allele[1] | Codominant (AA/aa,Aa/aa,AA/Aa)[3] | | | Recessive | Dominant | Overdominant |
|---|---|---|---|---|---|---|---|---|---|---|---|---|---|
| rs4140535 | T | | 394 | 0.635 | 391 | 0.625 | 0.725 | 0.806 | 1.000 | 0.729 | 0.909 | 0.684 | 0.764 |
| | | CC | 44 | 0.142 | 46 | 0.147 | | | | | | | |
| | | CT | 138 | 0.445 | 143 | 0.457 | | | | | | | |
| | | TT | 128 | 0.413 | 124 | 0.396 | | | | | | | |
| rs1778258 | G | | 556 | 0.897 | 555 | 0.887 | 0.585 | 1.000 | 1.000 | 0.541 | 1.000 | 0.552 | 0.542 |
| | | AA | 4 | 0.013 | 4 | 0.013 | | | | | | | |
| | | AG | 56 | 0.181 | 63 | 0.201 | | | | | | | |
| | | GG | 250 | 0.806 | 246 | 0.786 | | | | | | | |
| rs17273700 | T | | 554 | 0.894 | 550 | 0.879 | 0.423 | 0.772 | 0.377 | 0.185 | 0.576 | 0.279 | 0.184 |
| | | CC | 7 | 0.023 | 5 | 0.016 | | | | | | | |
| | | CT | 52 | 0.168 | 66 | 0.211 | | | | | | | |
| | | TT | 251 | 0.810 | 242 | 0.773 | | | | | | | |
| rs1228814 | C | | 517 | 0.834 | 522 | 0.834 | 1.000 | 0.374 | 0.247 | 0.465 | 0.276 | 0.663 | 0.356 |
| | | AA | 13 | 0.042 | 8 | 0.026 | | | | | | | |
| | | AC | 77 | 0.248 | 88 | 0.281 | | | | | | | |
| | | CC | 220 | 0.710 | 217 | 0.693 | | | | | | | |
| rs11568817 | T | | 559 | 0.902 | 553 | 0.883 | 0.315 | 1.000 | 1.000 | 0.254 | 1.000 | 0.271 | 0.255 |
| | | GG | 5 | 0.016 | 5 | 0.016 | | | | | | | |
| | | GT | 51 | 0.165 | 63 | 0.201 | | | | | | | |
| | | TT | 254 | 0.819 | 245 | 0.783 | | | | | | | |
| rs130058 | T | | 49 | 0.079 | 48 | 0.077 | 0.916 | 0.686 | 0.816 | 0.434 | 1.000 | 0.449 | 0.816 |
| | | AA | 265 | 0.855 | 267 | 0.853 | | | | | | | |
| | | AT | 41 | 0.132 | 44 | 0.141 | | | | | | | |
| | | TT | 4 | 0.013 | 2 | 0.006 | | | | | | | |

**Table 2** Allelic distributions of the 14 SNPs and their associations with schizophrenia *(Continued)*

| SNP | Allele[1] | Genotype | Case (n=310) No. | Case Frequency | Control (n=313) No. | Control Frequency | p Value[2] Allele[1] | Codominant (AA/aa,Aa/aa,AA/Aa)[3] | | Recessive | Dominant | Overdominant |
|---|---|---|---|---|---|---|---|---|---|---|---|---|
| rs6297 | A | | 541 | 0.873 | 536 | 0.856 | 0.409 | 0.599 | 0.786 | 0.788 | 0.460 | 0.816 |
| | | AA | 237 | 0.765 | 231 | 0.738 | | | | | | |
| | | AG | 67 | 0.216 | 74 | 0.236 | | | | | | |
| | | GG | 6 | 0.019 | 8 | 0.026 | | | | | | |
| rs3827804 | A | | 8 | 0.013 | 7 | 0.011 | 0.802 | — | 0.800 | 0.800 | — | 0.800 |
| | | AG | 8 | 0.026 | 7 | 0.022 | | | | | | |
| | | GG | 302 | 0.974 | 306 | 0.978 | | | | | | |
| | | AA | 0 | 0.000 | 0 | 0.000 | | | | | | |
| rs140792648 | — | | 604 | 0.974 | 608 | 0.971 | 0.862 | — | 0.860 | — | 0.860 | 0.860 |
| | | —/— | 294 | 0.948 | 295 | 0.942 | | | | | | |
| | | —/AG | 16 | 0.052 | 18 | 0.058 | | | | | | |
| | | AG/AG | 0 | 0.000 | 0 | 0.000 | | | | | | |
| rs9361234 | C | | 559 | 0.902 | 555 | 0.887 | 0.408 | 1.000 | 1.000 | 1.000 | 0.364 | 0.349 |
| | | CC | 254 | 0.819 | 247 | 0.789 | | | | | | |
| | | CT | 51 | 0.165 | 61 | 0.195 | | | | | | |
| | | TT | 5 | 0.016 | 5 | 0.016 | | | | | | |
| rs183156887 | A | | 4 | 0.006 | 4 | 0.006 | 1.000 | — | 1.000 | 1.000 | — | 1.000 |
| | | AC | 4 | 0.013 | 4 | 0.013 | | | | | | |
| | | CC | 306 | 0.987 | 309 | 0.987 | | | | | | |
| | | AA | 0 | 0.000 | 0 | 0.000 | | | | | | |
| rs76194807 | T | | 79 | 0.127 | 71 | 0.113 | 0.486 | 0.725 | 0.242 | 0.340 | 0.725 | 0.242 |
| | | GG | 234 | 0.755 | 247 | 0.789 | | | | | | |
| | | GT | 73 | 0.235 | 61 | 0.195 | | | | | | |
| | | TT | 3 | 0.010 | 5 | 0.016 | | | | | | |

**Table 2** Allelic distributions of the 14 SNPs and their associations with schizophrenia (*Continued*)

| SNP | Allele[1] | Genotype | Case (n=310) | | Control (n=313) | | p Value[2] | | | | | | |
|---|---|---|---|---|---|---|---|---|---|---|---|---|---|
| | | | No. | Frequency | No. | Frequency | Allele[1] | Codominant (AA/aa,Aa/aa,AA/Aa)[3] | | | Recessive | Dominant | Overdominant |
| rs58138557 | GG | | 558 | 0.900 | 554 | 0.885 | 0.411 | 1.000 | 1.000 | 0.351 | 1.000 | 0.367 | 0.352 |
| | | –/– | 5 | 0.016 | 5 | 0.016 | | | | | | | |
| | | –/GG | 52 | 0.168 | 62 | 0.198 | | | | | | | |
| | | GG/GG | 253 | 0.816 | 246 | 0.786 | | | | | | | |
| rs13212041 | G | | 160 | 0.258 | 160 | 0.256 | 0.948 | 0.643 | 0.444 | 0.423 | 0.629 | 0.545 | 0.361 |
| | | AA | 171 | 0.552 | 179 | 0.572 | | | | | | | |
| | | AG | 118 | 0.381 | 108 | 0.345 | | | | | | | |
| | | GG | 21 | 0.068 | 26 | 0.083 | | | | | | | |

[1]The allele for each SNP indicated is that with the higher patient frequency.
[2]The significance levels of chi-squared tests for codominant, dominant, recessive and overdominant model were adjusted using the Bonferroni correction (significance level $p = 0.0036$).
[3]The SNP allele that is observed at a higher frequency in patients is designated A; the other allele is designated a.

primers. The primer sequences of the 5′-end fragment were 5′-TGGGTTTGTGCTTTATTGCCTT-3′ (sense), 5′-GGAGCAGAGGATAAGTTGGCTTG-3′ (antisense), and the primer sequences of the 3′-end fragment were 5′-CCCTTCTTCATCATCTCCCTAGTG-3′ (sense), 5′-ACCCCATTCCTCAATTGTGTAAG-3′ (antisense; Taihe Biotechnology Co., Beijing, China). PCR conditions for the 5′-end fragment were: 94 °C for 1 min; 35 cycles of 94 °C for 30 s, 58.4 °C for 30 s, and 72 °C for 1.5 min; then final extension at 72 °C for 7 min. PCR conditions for the 3′-end fragment were 94 °C for 1 min; by 35 cycles of 94 °C for 30 s, 60 °C for 30 s, 72 °C for 1 min; and extension at 72°Cfor 7 min. The Sanger double-chain termination method (Taihe Biotechnology Co., Beijing, China) was employed for DNA sequencing.

## Statistical analysis

Allele and genotype frequencies were calculated by direct counting. Haplotype blocks were determined by the confidence interval method in Haploview. Using this method, six 5′-promoter region SNPs were included in a haplotype block, while the eight 3′-promoter region SNPs were not included in a haplotype block. Thus, we performed analysis for haplotypes formed by the 6 SNPs in the block (namely, the 5′ block) and the remaining eight SNPs (designated the 3′ block) [17].

In order to test Hardy-Weinberg equilibrium (HWE) and construct haplotype blocks, linkage equilibrium (LD) analysis (D′ and $r^2$) were performed using Haploview version 4.2 software (Broad Institute, Cambridge, MA, USA) [18]. The $\chi^2$ test was used to estimate correlations between the variance of polymorphism frequency distribution and schizophrenia. Statistical significance was defined as $p < 0.05$ (two-tailed). Statistical analyses were performed using SPSS Software19.0 (IBM, Armonk, NY, USA). A Bonferroni correction was applied for multiple comparisons to control for type I error, and the $p$-value was divided by the total number of loci or haplotypes [17].

## Results

We identified 14 SNPs in the present study (Table 1). The genotype distribution was in accordance with Hardy-Weinberg equilibrium in the control group. A summary of allele and genotype frequencies is presented in Table 2. We found that male patients were observed to have a significantly higher A-allele frequency at rs1778258 than female patients ($p = 0.012$). The frequency of A-allele carriers (AA+AG genotype) among male patients was also significantly higher than among female patients ($p = 0.015$), although statistical significance was lost after Bonferroni correction. The presence of both the A-allele and AA+AG genotype increased schizophrenia risk (OR = 1.986 and OR = 2.061, respectively; Table 3).

**Table 3** The relationship between rs1778258 and schizophrenia according to biological sex

| Group | rs1778258 | Male | Female | p value[1] | OR | 95% CI |
|---|---|---|---|---|---|---|
| case | A | 41/304 | 23/316 | 0.012 | 1.986 | 1.161–3.398 |
| | AA+AG | 38/152 | 22/158 | 0.015 | 2.061 | 1.152–3.684 |
| control | A | 33/306 | 38/320 | 0.706 | 0.897 | 0.547–1.472 |
| | AA+AG | 38/153 | 22/160 | 0.891 | 0.945 | 0.550–1.622 |

[1]A significance level $p = 0.05$

We found no significant associations between any other SNPs and schizophrenia.

Via linkage disequilibrium (LD) analysis, rs11568817 was found to be in strong linkage disequilibrium with rs17273700, rs9361234 and rs58138557 in northern Han Chinese patients ($r^2 > 0.8$) [18]. We also found that, as compared to the healthy people, the linkage between rs11568817 and rs130058 in schizophrenic patients was more intense. Furthermore, LD analysis showed that the six 5′-promoter region SNPs are included in a haplotype using the confidence interval method, while the eight 3′-promoter region SNPs were not included in a haplotype block (Fig. 1). We next compared the frequencies of haplotypes formed by the six SNPs in block or the remaining eight SNPs between the patients and healthy people, and found that the haplotype frequency distributions for the 5′-promoter region C-G-C-A-G-A were significantly different among individuals in the case and control groups. ($p = 0.044$); however, statistical significance was lost after Bonferroni correction. No statistical differences between groups were observed for other haplotypes (Tables 4 and 5).

## Discussion

In the present study, we investigated *HTR1B* polymorphisms in 623 individuals of northern Han Chinese descent, including 310 schizophrenic patients and 313 healthy controls. We ultimately detected 14 SNPs. According to previously reported observations, no evidence regarding a relationship between *HTR1B* and schizophrenia was found in any allele or major haplotype for T-261G, -182INS/DEL-181, A-161 T, C129T and G861C in Han Chinese patients [19]. Our study showed consistent results regarding rs11568817 (T-261G) and rs130058 (A-161 T). When patients were grouped by gender, male patients were observed to have a significantly higher frequency of A-allele at rs1778258 than female patients ($p = 0.012$). Based on multiple comparisons of genotype effects, we inferred that the most probable mode of inheritance of rs1778258 is the dominant model [20]. The frequency of the AA+AG genotype in male patients was also significantly higher than in female patients ($p = 0.015$), although statistical significance was lost after Bonferroni correction. Both the A-allele and AA+AG

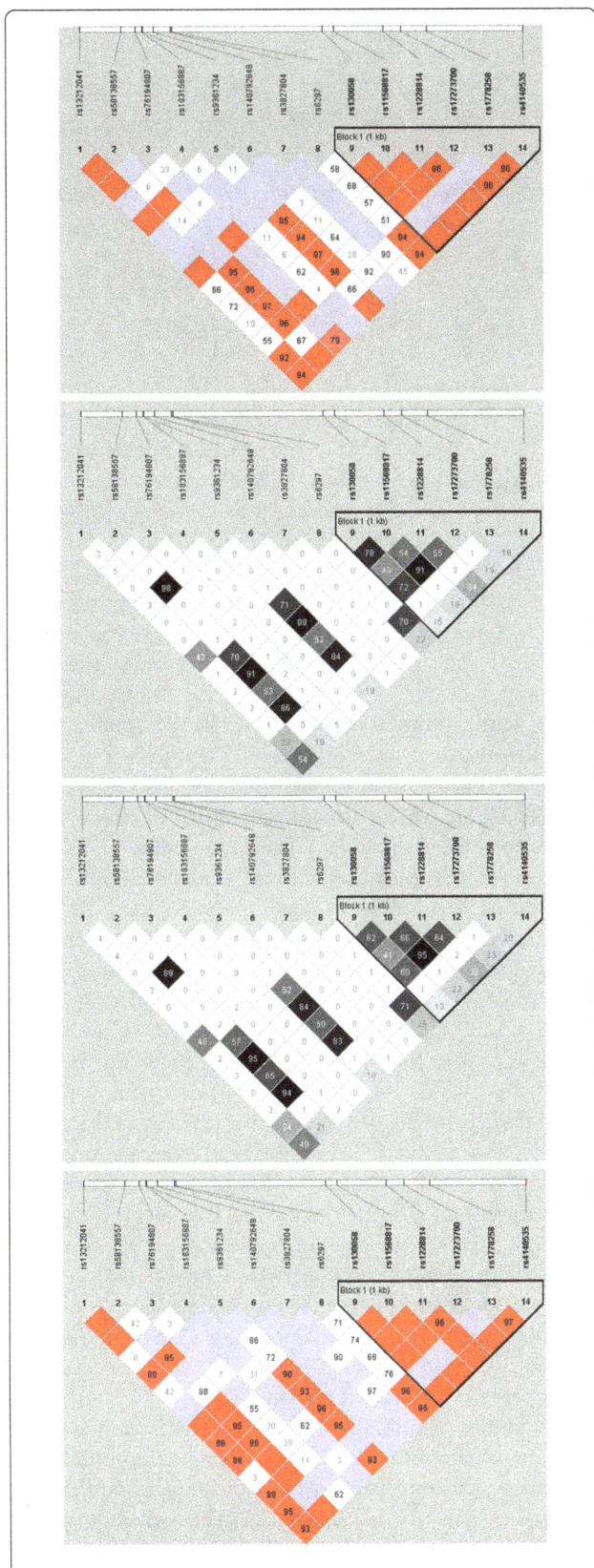

**Fig. 1** Linkage disequilibrium diagram of the 14 SNPs in HTR1B in the northern Han Chinese population. Cases D'. Cases r². Controls D'. Controls r². The number in the grid of the red-white diagram represents the D' value, the deep red grid represents D' 1, and the number in the grid of the black-white diagram represents the r² value

genotype were associated with increased risk of schizophrenia (OR = 1.986 and OR = 2.061, respectively). Thus, our study provides evidence that rs1778258 involved with gender variations in schizophrenia.

It is understood that sex differences exist in brain function as well as the vulnerability, incidence, manifestation, and treatment of numerous psychiatric diseases, which are determined by inherent biological differences between males and females. For instance, males show a higher propensity for Parkinson's disease, autism, attention deficit hyperactivity disorder (ADHD) and addiction. Females also show higher susceptibility to Alzheimer's disease and anxiety/depression [21]. Most studies have found the onset age of schizophrenia to be earlier in men than in women, although there is no sex difference in overall incidence of schizophrenia [22]. Men with schizophrenia also present with more cognitive disturbances and greater reductions in temporal lobe volume than women with schizophrenia [23]. Moreover, evidence also supports sex differences in serotonin neurotransmission and psychiatric disorders caused by malfunctions in the serotonin system. Such differences are not only due to hormonal regulation, but are also attributable genetic effects [21, 24]. It was previously reported that higher whole blood 5-HT levels in women than in men are influenced by multiple genes on chromosome 2, 6, and 17 [25]. In addition, the effects of sex hormones on serotonin regulation have also been reported. It has been shown that estradiol plays a protective role against the cognitive, positive, and negative symptom domains of schizophrenia [26]. Our results indicated that rs1778258 is associated with gender in schizophrenia. Since rs1778258 is located in the promoter region, it may have an influence on gene expression. Alternatively, there could be a functional site closely linked to rs1778258, and its variation thus could modify gene expression [27], which could have an influence on the serotonin system.

Previous genetic studies on schizophrenia have suggested that there is a gender-specific association between select dopamine genes and schizophrenia. Gender-specific associations between genotype and schizophrenia were also observed in GABAergic-mediated regulation of anterior cingulate cortex function. Male schizophrenic patients expressed significantly lower levels of GABA-Aα5, GABA-Aβ1, and GABA-Aε, while the expression of GABA-Aβ1 and GAD67 was significantly higher in female patients, as compared to sex-matched controls [28]. Since

**Table 4** The relationship between 5′-region haplotype and schizophrenia

| Haplotype | | | | | | | Case(n = 310) | | Control (n = 313) | | | | |
|---|---|---|---|---|---|---|---|---|---|---|---|---|---|
| 5′ rs4140535 | rs1778258 | rs17273700 | rs1228814 | rs11568817 | rs130058 | | N | F | N | F | p value[1] | OR | 95% CI |
| 1  T | G | T | C | T | A | | 391.840 | 0.632 | 389.998 | 0.623 | 0.770 | 1.040 | 0.827–1.309 |
| 2  C | A | T | C | T | A | | 62.620 | 0.101 | 70.112 | 0.112 | 0.583 | 0.898 | 0.627–1.288 |
| 3  C | G | T | C | T | A | | 58.900 | 0.095 | 58.844 | 0.094 | 1.000 | 0.011 | 0.692–1.477 |
| 4  C | G | C | A | G | T | | 48.980 | 0.079 | 48.202 | 0.077 | 0.916 | 1.033 | 0.683–1.564 |
| 5  C | G | T | A | T | A | | 39.060 | 0.063 | 30.048 | 0.048 | 0.266 | 1.334 | 0.817–2.176 |
| 6  C | G | C | A | G | A | | 11.780 | 0.019 | 25.040 | 0.040 | 0.044 | 0.474 | 0.236–0.953 |

[1]Significance level p = 0.01

it is known that these neurotransmitter systems are closely related [29], these differences may contribute to the gender-specific relationship between *HTR1B* polymorphisms and schizophrenia. Although sex differences are essential to study to fully understand the etiology of schizophrenia, unfortunately, few studies have been made regarding gender-specific associations between *HTR1B* and schizophrenia. The only association found to date was described in a Spanish population. The AAAC haplotype comprising rs6297, rs130058, rs1213366, and rs1213371 is significantly more frequent in female Spanish patients [15], which corroborates our finding that *HTR1B* genotype is related to gender in schizophrenia. It should be noted that rs1778258 was found to have a medium linkage with rs6297 (r² = 0.7) in our study. However, both rs1778258 and rs6297 were found to lack any direct functional effects. Other SNPs had not been found to be associated with schizophrenia, but still provide references for *HTR1B* gene polymorphisms in the northern Han Chinese population.

This study found that the frequency distributions of haplotype C-G-C-A-G-A in the 5′-promoter region are significantly different between patients and healthy controls (p = 0.044), but statistical significance was lost after Bonferroni correction. It has been proposed that the rs11568817 G-allele and rs130058 T-allele influence gene expression by modifying the binding of transcription factors (TFs). The rs11568817 G-allele does enhance transcriptional activity; conversely, rs130058 T-allele can reverse this [30]. In our study, only haplotypes C-G-C-A-G-T and C-G-C-A-G-A contained functional sites rs11568817 G-allele or rs130058 T-allele, but no significant differences were found between patients and healthy controls in either haplotype after Bonferroni correction (p = 0.916 and p = 0.044, respectively. We also found that the 3′ region contains a known functional SNP, rs13212041. KP Jensen et al. confirmed that the rs13212041 A-allele can combine with microRNA (miR-96) to induce mRNA repression, and that this microRNA-mediated mRNA silencing could be attenuated by rs13212041 G-allele [31]. Conner et al. found that men with low expression haplotypes are inclined to

present greater anger and hostility [27]. Although three known functional sites (rs11568817, rs130058, rs13212041) were found in our study, we discovered no direct associations between *HTR1B* and schizophrenia by haplotype. We hypothesize that the onset of schizophrenia could be affected by multiple functional sites, but their effects are counteracted [30]. Moreover, schizophrenia is associated with multiple neurotransmitters that have been noted to have physical and functional interactions [32]. Even these sites lead to changes in the serotonin system, but do not necessarily cause schizophrenia.

Our study showed that rs9361234, rs11568817 and rs17273700 are in strong linkage disequilibrium in the northern Han Chinese population. The linkage states of these SNPs are similar to those identified in Han Chinese populations in Beijing and southern China (1000 Genomes Project). We observed that rs58138557 was is intensely linked to rs9361234, rs11568817 and rs17273700 (Fig. 1). In addition, schizophrenic patients show stronger linkage between 11,568,817 and rs130058 than healthy controls (r² = 0.78 and r² = 0.62, respectively; Fig. 1). Linkage disequilibrium is related to population. For example, the linkage between rs11568817 and rs130058 in Han Chinese is weaker in northern China than in southern China based on the 1000 Genomes Project. This difference is also found in European and African-American populations [30]. Moreover, schizophrenia-associated genes vary among distinct ethnic populations [33]. Therefore, linkage disequilibrium of *HTR1B* could be associated with schizophrenia in northern Han Chinese peoples. This study presents information on the linkage state of *HTR1B* in schizophrenic patients of northern Han Chinese descent, and thereby provided references for the etiology of schizophrenia in different populations.

This study is limited by sample size and methods and, although we found that rs1778258 is related to gender in schizophrenia, unfortunately, the mechanism underlying this association was not addressed. This will require further exploration in the future. Because of the limitation of the candidate gene approach, caution must be taken in regards to the interpretation of the association we have observed. Since schizophrenia is a complex disease

**Table 5** The relationship between 3'-region haplotype and schizophrenia

| Haplotype | | | | | | | | | Case (n = 310) | | Control (n = 313) | | p value[1] | OR | 95% CI |
|---|---|---|---|---|---|---|---|---|---|---|---|---|---|---|---|
| 3' | rs6297 | rs3827804 | rs140792648 | rs9361234 | rs183156887 | rs76194807 | rs58138557 | rs13212041 | N | frequency | N | frequency | | | |
| 1 | A | G | A | C | C | G | T | A | 298.220 | 0.481 | 295.472 | 0.472 | 0.777 | 1.038 | 0.831–1.297 |
| 2 | A | G | A | C | C | G | T | G | 78.740 | 0.127 | 68.234 | 0.109 | 0.334 | 1.198 | 0.849–1.692 |
| 3 | G | G | A | C | C | G | T | G | 78.120 | 0.126 | 88.892 | 0.142 | 0.407 | 0.868 | 0.626–1.204 |
| 4 | A | G | A | C | C | T | T | A | 76.260 | 0.123 | 68.860 | 0.110 | 0.537 | 1.128 | 0.797–1.595 |
| 5 | A | G | A | T | C | G | A | A | 58.900 | 0.095 | 68.234 | 0.109 | 0.455 | 0.863 | 0.597–1.247 |
| 6 | A | G | T | C | C | G | T | A | 16.120 | 0.026 | 16.276 | 0.026 | 1.000 | 1.010 | 0.501–2.038 |
| 7 | A | A | A | C | C | G | T | A | 8.060 | 0.013 | 6.886 | 0.011 | 0.802 | 1.156 | 0.417–3.207 |

[1]Significance level = 0.0083

that is influenced by both genetic and environmental factors, both biological and psychological events experienced by individuals could have an impact on its onset. Thus, any associations cannot be fully explained by simply reducing them to a two-dimensional relationship between genetic variance and disease. We suggest that genetic background and behavioral events of enrolled patients should be taken into consideration [34]. Furthermore we will attempt to implement analysis of accurately defined phenotypes involving scale scores and treatment response, as well as the convergent analysis of genetic, serum and brain imaging markers.

## Conclusion

In this study, the *HTR1B* gene was found to be related to gender in schizophrenia, as the rs1778258 A-allele caused increased risk of schizophrenia in male patients. Linkage between rs11568817 and rs130058 is more intense in schizophrenic patients. Combining all results of this study, we assert that *HTR1B* has a putative relationship with schizophrenia in the northern Han Chinese population, which provides a reference schizophrenia etiology.

### Abbreviations

5-HT: 5-hydroxytryptamine; ADHD: Attention deficit hyperactivity disorder; DSM: Diagnostic Criteria of American Diagnostic and Statistical Manual of Mental Disorders; GWAS: Genome-wide association study; HTR1B: Serotonin receptor 1B; LD: Linkage disequilibrium; SNP: Single-nucleotide polymorphism; UTR: Untranslated region

### Acknowledgements

We acknowledge all patients who participated in this study. We thank Xue Wu, Fengling Xu, Yi Liu, Yongping Liu, Xicen Zhang for assistance in many aspects of this work. The final version of the manuscript has been edited by the editors of BioMed Proofreading LLC.

### Funding

Support has been provided by China Medical University. The funding body had no involvement with study design; data collection, analysis, or interpretation; or preparing the manuscript.

### Authors' contributions

BW conceived and designed this study. XX conducted the study, performed statistical analyses, and prepared the manuscript. JY revised the manuscript. MD, JX1, JX2, HP played important roles in interpreting the results and providing relevant assistance in conducting study. All authors read and approved the final manuscript.

### Consent for publication

Not applicable.

### Competing interests

The authors declare that they have no competing interests.

## References

1. Sullivan PF, Kendler KS, Neale MC. Schizophrenia as a complex trait: evidence from a meta-analysis of twin studies. Arch Gen Psychiatry. 2003; 60(12):1187–92.
2. Liy-Salmeron G, Meneses A. Role of 5-HT1-7 receptors in short- and long-term memory for an autoshaping task: intrahippocampal manipulations. Brain Res. 2007;1147:140–7.
3. Barnes NM, Sharp T. A review of central 5-HT receptors and their function. Neuropharmacology. 1999;38(8):1083–152.
4. Guimaraes AP, Schmitz M, Polanczyk GV, Zeni C, Genro J, Roman T, Rohde LA, Hutz MH. Further evidence for the association between attention deficit/hyperactivity disorder and the serotonin receptor 1B gene. J Neural Transm. 2009;116(12):1675–80.
5. Moul C, Dobson-Stone C, Brennan J, Hawes DJ, Dadds MR. Serotonin 1B receptor gene (HTR1B) methylation as a risk factor for callous-unemotional traits in antisocial boys. PLoS One. 2015;10(5):e0126903.
6. Hakulinen C, Jokela M, Hintsanen M, Merjonen P, Pulkki-Raback L, Seppala I, Lyytikainen LP, Lehtimaki T, Kahonen M, Viikari J, et al. Serotonin receptor 1B genotype and hostility, anger and aggressive behavior through the lifespan: the young Finns study. J Behav Med. 2013;36(6):583–90.
7. Lopez-Figueroa AL, Norton CS, Lopez-Figueroa MO, Armellini-Dodel D, Burke S, Akil H, Lopez JF, Watson SJ. Serotonin 5-HT1A, 5-HT1B, and 5-HT2A receptor mRNA expression in subjects with major depression, bipolar disorder, and schizophrenia. Biol Psychiatry. 2004;55(3):225–33.
8. Veldman ER, Svedberg MM, Svenningsson P, Lundberg J. Distribution and levels of 5-HT1B receptors in anterior cingulate cortex of patients with bipolar disorder, major depressive disorder and schizophrenia - an autoradiography study. European neuropsychopharmacology : the journal of the European College of Neuropsychopharmacology. 2017;27(5):504–14.
9. Cao J, LaRocque E, Li D: Associations of the 5-hydroxytryptamine (serotonin) receptor 1B gene (HTR1B) with alcohol, cocaine, and heroin abuse. American journal of medical genetics Part B, Neuropsychiatric genetics : the official publication of the International Society of Psychiatric Genetics 2013, 162B(2):169–176.
10. Pal P, Mihanovic M, Molnar S, Xi H, Sun G, Guha S, Jeran N, Tomljenovic A, Malnar A, Missoni S, et al. Association of tagging single nucleotide polymorphisms on 8 candidate genes in dopaminergic pathway with schizophrenia in Croatian population. Croatian medical journal. 2009;50(4): 361–9.
11. Ambrosio AM, Kennedy JL, Macciardi F, Coelho I, Soares MJ, Oliveira CR, Pato CN. Lack of association or linkage disequilibrium between schizophrenia and polymorphisms in the 5-HT1Dalpha and 5-HT1Dbeta autoreceptor genes: family-based association study. American journal of medical genetics Part B, Neuropsychiatric genetics : the official publication of the International Society of Psychiatr Genet. 2004;128B(1):1–5.
12. Rujescu D, Giegling I, Sato T, Moller HJ. Lack of association between serotonin 5-HT1B receptor gene polymorphism and suicidal behavior. American journal of medical genetics Part B, Neuropsychiatric genetics : the official publication of the International Society of Psychiatric Genetics. 2003; 116B(1):69–71.
13. Cordeiro Q, Vallada H. Lack of association between the G681C polimorphism in the 5-HT1D(beta) autoreceptor gene and schizophrenia. Arq Neuropsiquiatr. 2005;63(2B):380–2.
14. Sanders AR, Cao Q, Taylor J, Levin TE, Badner JA, Cravchik A, Comeron JM, Naruya S, Del Rosario A, Salvi DA, et al. Genetic diversity of the human serotonin receptor 1B (HTR1B) gene. Genomics. 2001;72(1):1–14.
15. Gilabert-Juan J, Ivorra JL, Tolosa A, Gratacos M, Costas J, Sanjuan J, Molto MD. Potential involvement of serotonin receptor genes with age of onset and gender in schizophrenia: a preliminary study in a Spanish sample. Psychiatry Res. 2011;186(1):153–4.
16. Kramvis A, Bukofzer S, Kew MC. Comparison of hepatitis B virus DNA extractions from serum by the QIAamp blood kit, GeneReleaser, and the phenol-chloroform method. J Clin Microbiol. 1996;34(11):2731–3.

Polymorphisms in the human serotonin receptor 1B (HTR1B) gene are associated...

61

17. Zhu F, Yan CX, Wang Q, Zhu YS, Zhao Y, Huang J, Zhang HB, Gao CG, Li SB. An association study between dopamine D1 receptor gene polymorphisms and the risk of schizophrenia. Brain Res. 2011;1420:106–13.

18. Barrett JC, Fry B, Maller J, Daly MJ. Haploview: analysis and visualization of LD and haplotype maps. Bioinformatics. 2005;21(2):263–5.

19. Duan S, Yin H, Chen W, Xing Q, chen Q, Guo T, Gao J, Li X, Gao R, Liu Z, et al. No association between the serotonin 1B receptor gene and schizophrenia in a case-control and family-based association study. Neurosci Lett. 2005;376(2):93–7.

20. Thakkinstian A, McElduff P, D'Este C, Duffy D, Attia J. A method for meta-analysis of molecular association studies. Stat Med. 2005;24(9):1291–306.

21. Ratnu VS, Emami MR, Bredy TW. Genetic and epigenetic factors underlying sex differences in the regulation of gene expression in the brain. J Neurosci Res. 2017;95(1–2):301–10.

22. Ochoa S, Usall J, Cobo J, Labad X, Kulkarni J. Gender differences in schizophrenia and first-episode psychosis: a comprehensive literature review. Schizophr Res Treat. 2012;2012:916198.

23. Bryant NL, Buchanan RW, Vladar K, Breier A, Rothman M. Gender differences in temporal lobe structures of patients with schizophrenia: a volumetric MRI study. Am J Psychiatry. 1999;156(4):603–9.

24. Gobinath AR, Choleris E, Galea LA. Sex, hormones, and genotype interact to influence psychiatric disease, treatment, and behavioral research. J Neurosci Res. 2017;95(1–2):50–64.

25. Weiss LA, Abney M, Cook EH Jr, Ober C. Sex-specific genetic architecture of whole blood serotonin levels. Am J Hum Genet. 2005;76(1):33–41.

26. Gogos A, Sbisa AM, Sun J, Gibbons A, Udawela M, Dean B. A role for estrogen in schizophrenia: clinical and preclinical findings. Int J Endocrinol. 2015;2015:615356.

27. Conner TS, Jensen KP, Tennen H, Furneaux HM, Kranzler HR, Covault J. Functional polymorphisms in the serotonin 1B receptor gene (HTR1B) predict self-reported anger and hostility among young men. American journal of medical genetics Part B, Neuropsychiatric genetics : the official publication of the International Society of Psychiatr Genet. 2010;153B(1):67–78.

28. Li R, Ma X, Wang G, Yang J, Wang C. Why sex differences in schizophrenia? Journal of translational neuroscience. 2016;1(1):37–42.

29. Di Giovanni G, Esposito E, Di Matteo V. Role of serotonin in central dopamine dysfunction. CNS neuroscience & therapeutics. 2010;16(3):179–94.

30. Duan J, Sanders AR, Molen JE, Martinolich L, Mowry BJ, Levinson DF, Crowe RR, Silverman JM, Gejman PV. Polymorphisms in the 5′-untranslated region of the human serotonin receptor 1B (HTR1B) gene affect gene expression. Mol Psychiatry. 2003;8(11):901–10.

31. Jensen KP, Covault J, Conner TS, Tennen H, Kranzler HR, Furneaux HM. A common polymorphism in serotonin receptor 1B mRNA moderates regulation by miR-96 and associates with aggressive human behaviors. Mol Psychiatry. 2009;14(4):381–9.

32. de Bartolomeis A, Buonaguro EF, Iasevoli F. Serotonin-glutamate and serotonin-dopamine reciprocal interactions as putative molecular targets for novel antipsychotic treatments: from receptor heterodimers to postsynaptic scaffolding and effector proteins. Psychopharmacology. 2013;225(1):1–19.

33. Ohi K, Shimada T, Yasuyama T, Uehara T, Kawasaki Y. Variability of 128 schizophrenia-associated gene variants across distinct ethnic populations. Transl Psychiatry. 2017;7(1):e988.

34. Drago A, Alboni S, Brunello N, De Ronchi D, Serretti A. HTR1B as a risk profile maker in psychiatric disorders: a review through motivation and memory. Eur J Clin Pharmacol. 2010;66(1):5–27.

# 7

# Demographic, psychosocial and clinical factors associated with postpartum depression in Kenyan women

Linnet Ongeri[1]* [iD], Valentine Wanga[2], Phelgona Otieno[1], Jane Mbui[1], Elizabeth Juma[1], Ann Vander Stoep[2] and Muthoni Mathai[3]

## Abstract

**Background:** Few longitudinal studies have examined associations between risk factors during pregnancy and mental health outcomes during the postpartum period. We used a cohort study design to estimate the prevalence, incidence and correlates of significant postpartum depressive symptoms in Kenyan women.

**Methods:** We recruited adult women residing in an urban, resource-poor setting and attending maternal and child health clinics in two public hospitals in Nairobi, Kenya. A translated Kiswahili Edinburgh Postpartum Depression Scale was used to screen for depressive symptoms at baseline assessment in the 3rd trimester and follow up assessment at 6–10 weeks postpartum. Information was collected on potential demographic, psychosocial and clinical risk variables. Potential risk factors for postpartum depression were evaluated using multivariate logistic regression analysis.

**Results:** Out of the 171 women who were followed up at 6–10 weeks postpartum, 18.7% (95% CI: 13.3–25.5) were found to have postpartum depression using an EPDS cut off of 10. In multivariate analyses, the odds of having postpartum depression was increased more than seven-fold in the presence of conflict with partner (OR = 7.52, 95% CI: 2.65–23.13). The association between antepartum and postpartum depression was quite strong but did not reach statistical significance (OR = 3.37, 95% CI: 0.98–11.64).

**Conclusions:** The high prevalence of significant postnatal depressive symptoms among Kenyan women underscores the need for addressing this public health burden. Depression screening and psychosocial support interventions that address partner conflict resolution should be offered as part of maternal health care.

**Keywords:** Postpartum depression, Antenatal depression, Psychosocial risk factors, Edinburgh postpartum depression scale

## Background

Perinatal depression is a public health concern worldwide with research showing a higher prevalence in low resource contexts [1, 2]. In high resource countries prevalence estimates of antepartum depression range from 7 to 15% [3, 4] while in low resource countries estimates ranging from 15 to 25% have been reported [1, 2]. Postpartum depression prevalence estimates also follow a similar pattern with estimates of nearly 10% in high resource countries [5] compared to 20% in low resource countries [1]. Estimates from East Africa are about 20% in the antepartum

period [6] and have been shown to range from 6 to 39% during the postpartum period [6, 7]. This wide range has been largely attributed to differences in assessment tools as well as study populations across the studies [1].

Perinatal depression, reflected in both clinical depression and significant depressive symptoms, carries adverse physical and psychological consequences for both the mother and child [8]. Antepartum depression has been linked to higher rates of spontaneous abortion, prolonged labour and operative deliveries in the untreated mother [9–11]. Poor birth outcomes like preterm births and low birth weight are also higher in women with antepartum depression [11–13]. In a recent Kenyan study antepartum depression was linked with pre-term delivery [14]. In the postpartum period, mothers with depression show poor

* Correspondence: linongeri@gmail.com; longeri@kemri.org
[1]Kenya Medical Research Institute, P.O. Box 54840 00200, Mbagathi Road, Nairobi, Kenya
Full list of author information is available at the end of the article

interaction with their infants with negative consequences to their child's cognitive and physical development [15–17]. Mothers with postpartum depression are more likely to display either intrusive or withdrawn interactive patterns [8]. The intrusive pattern is characterized by hostile affect, while withdrawn mothers are often disengaged and unresponsive. The consequences of these maternal response patterns are higher risk of dysregulated attention and arousal in the infant's cognitive development that can have adverse effects on affect regulation, learning and intelligence [11–13]. A large longitudinal study in sub Saharan found a 50% increase in new-born illnesses [18]. The effects of maternal depression are not limited to only the infancy stage but have been shown to persist into the toddler and adolescent stages of life. Longitudinal studies have shown higher risk of childhood disorders like ADHD and conduct disorders that may persist on into adolescence among children of depressed mothers [19, 20]. In a Kenyan study, mothers with postnatal depression were more likely to have underweight infants [21].

The prior mental health status of the mother is a strong determinant of postpartum depression. Specifically, a previous history of depression, presence of antepartum depression, experiencing stressful life events during pregnancy and low perceived levels of social support contribute to increased risk for postpartum depression [1, 22, 23]. Other contributors include obstetric complications, single marital status and low income [24]. Recent Kenyan studies have shown an exceptionally high prevalence of depression among mothers who are HIV positive (48%) [25], among pregnant adolescents (58%) [26] and in mothers with malnourished babies (66%) [14].

Identifying risk factors predisposing to postpartum depression is important especially in guiding proper screening for the condition. The authors have done substantial clinical work and research on depression in Kenya [25, 27], and have identified the need for further assessment of risk factors for PPD in this population. Moreover, research has shown that postpartum depression risk factors in low income countries are, to a large extent, influenced by culture [28]. This work is a step towards understanding risk factors for postpartum depression in the cultural context of Kenya. To date most of what we have learned about risk factors for postpartum depression in Sub-Saharan Africa has been generated with cross-sectional studies [29]. Because retrospective report of social and emotional factors is likely to be biased by current mental health status, prospective studies that assess risk factors during pregnancy and then mental health outcome during the postpartum period can yield stronger inferences. In a prior publication we reported univariate associations between postpartum depression and a broad spectrum of antepartum and postpartum risk factors [30]. In this study, we expand on the previous work by assessing multivariable associations with PPD.

The aims of the current study were to estimate the prevalence and incidence of significant postpartum depressive symptoms in a cohort of pregnant women residing in an urban resource poor setting in Nairobi, Kenya and to use multivariate analyses to determine the unique contributions of antenatal depression and selected demographic, psychosocial, and clinical factors to postpartum depression risk.

## Methods

### Study population and setting

Women were recruited from the outpatient waiting areas of maternal and child health (MCH) clinics associated with two major public hospitals (Mathari Teaching and Referral Hospital and Mbagathi District Hospital) in Nairobi, Kenya, between March and December 2014. The maternal and child health clinics offer both antenatal and postnatal care, including family planning and infant immunization. The majority of the women served by these two hospitals are from an urban, resource-poor catchment area.

### Participant recruitment and screening

Women were eligible if they were pregnant, between ages 18 and 49 years, and in their third trimester of pregnancy. Gestational age was verified using the patient attendance card. Since the study had a follow up time point to assess postpartum depression, participating women had to be willing to seek postnatal care at the same facility. Following registration at the MCH clinic, trained study nurses informed all attending women in their third trimester of the ongoing study. After giving an explanation of the study, a written informed consent was obtained from those who met the inclusion criteria.

### Ethics and consent

We obtained approval to carry out the study from the Kenya Medical Research Institute Ethics Review Board. We further got written permissions to carry out the research from the medical superintendents of the 2 facilities. We informed eligible participants that the study participation was voluntary, and information collected during the study would be used solely for the purposes of the study. Willing participants signed a written informed consent after detailed explanation of the study purpose.

### Assessment procedures

Demographic, psychosocial and clinical history data were collected using structured questionnaires during a face-to-face interview. Depression levels were assessed at baseline and again at 6–10 weeks postpartum using the Edinburgh Postpartum Depression Scale (EPDS). Nurses working at the facility administered the structured demographic, psychosocial and clinical questionnaires and the EPDS screening tool. The nurses were trained to conduct the interviews by the first author (LO) as part of a larger study to evaluate the feasibility and acceptability of integrating depression screening with the EPDS into Kenyan MCH clinics.

### Perinatal depression

The Edinburgh Postnatal Depression Scale (EPDS or EDS when used in the antenatal period) is the most widely used scale to screen for antepartum and postpartum depression symptoms in low and middle-income countries [31]. It is a 10-item questionnaire, with each item scored from 0 to 3; total scores range from 0 to 30. The scale has been validated for detection of depression in both antepartum and postpartum samples [32]. Prior to our data collection, the EPDS tool was translated and back translated through a rigorous process into Kiswahili language [33]. A cut off of 13 or more was set as an indication of antepartum depression, and a cut off of 10 or more was used to indicate postpartum depression, as recommended by Murray and Cox in the assessment for minor antepartum depression and minor postpartum depression, respectively [34].

### Factors investigated for association with postpartum depression

Demographic, psychosocial and clinical factors were selected based on a literature review of studies of maternal mental health. Demographic factors included age, marital status, religion, level of education and occupation of both the mother and her partner. Household income was assessed on the basis of the daily household food expenditure.

Psychosocial factors were assessed during the antenatal period using single items created by the authors. These included: relationship with the mother-in-law (*good, not good but can cope, bad and cannot cope, N/A*); conflict with the partner in the previous 12 months (*any verbal or physical, none, N/A*); partner's help with cooking, cleaning and/or childcare (*any, none, N/A*); and economic stress within the household during the pregnancy (*yes, no*).

Postnatal clinical factors assessed were mode of delivery (vaginal or cesarean), low birth weight, and nursery admission. A binary composite variable consisting of birth complications (yes/no) and birth outcome (baby alive/died) was created, such that 1 = birth complications present and/or mother lost baby, and zero otherwise.

For this analysis, we did not have a primary exposure of interest since our goal was to assess multiple risk factors. However, if we consider the exposure of antenatal depression, we had 72% power to detect a crude odds ratio for prenatal depression of 3.1 comparing women who had PPD and those who did not.

### Statistical analysis

The prevalence and incidence of postpartum depression and their 95% confidence intervals were determined. Incidence was calculated as the number of new cases of depression at the postnatal assessment divided by the number of postpartum person months contributed by all of the participating women. The 95% confidence interval around the incidence estimate was calculated using Fisher's exact test. Factors associated with postpartum depression were evaluated using multivariate logistic regression. We added variables in three successive steps. In step 1 we entered prenatal depression status and demographic variables; in step 2, we added the psychosocial variables, and in the final step, we added the postnatal clinical variables. All analyses were performed using R version 3.1.2, and significance level evaluated at 5%.

### Results

Of the 215 women who were eligible for enrollment, seven refused to participate due to time constraints (four women) and the need to obtain permission from their partners before enrollment (three women). An additional 20 women were excluded because they did not plan to continue with postnatal care (including vaccination and family planning) in the same facility. A total of 188 women were included in the study. Seventeen women were lost to follow-up after antenatal assessment, 10 of whom reported to have moved to their rural home and hence not willing to continue as study participants, the rest could not be traced on phone despite 3 attempts to reach them thus 171 were assessed postpartum (Fig. 1).

The prevalence of significant depressive symptoms at 6–10 weeks postpartum was 18.7% (95% CI: 13.3–25.5). The cumulative incidence of postpartum depression (PPD) among the 140 women who did not have antenatal depression was 21 new cases or 15.0% (95% CI: 0.10–0.22).

The distribution of most demographic variables was comparable between those with and without PPD. Most women were married (91% vs. 87% of those with and without PPD, respectively), had at least secondary education (69% vs. 74%), and were Catholic or Protestant (78% vs. 88%). The median age of women in both groups was 25 years. Larger variations were seen in number of children and family income. Of women with PPD, 6% had three or more children, compared to 24% of women without PPD. Of women with PPD, 56% had a monthly family income of Kenyan Shillings (KES) 24,000 or less, compared to 36% of women without PPD (Table 1).

Of women with and without PPD, 56% and 63%, respectively, reported having a good relationship with their mother-in-law, and 53% and 71% reported that their partners were helping with childcare, cooking, and/or cleaning. Women with PPD were more likely to report

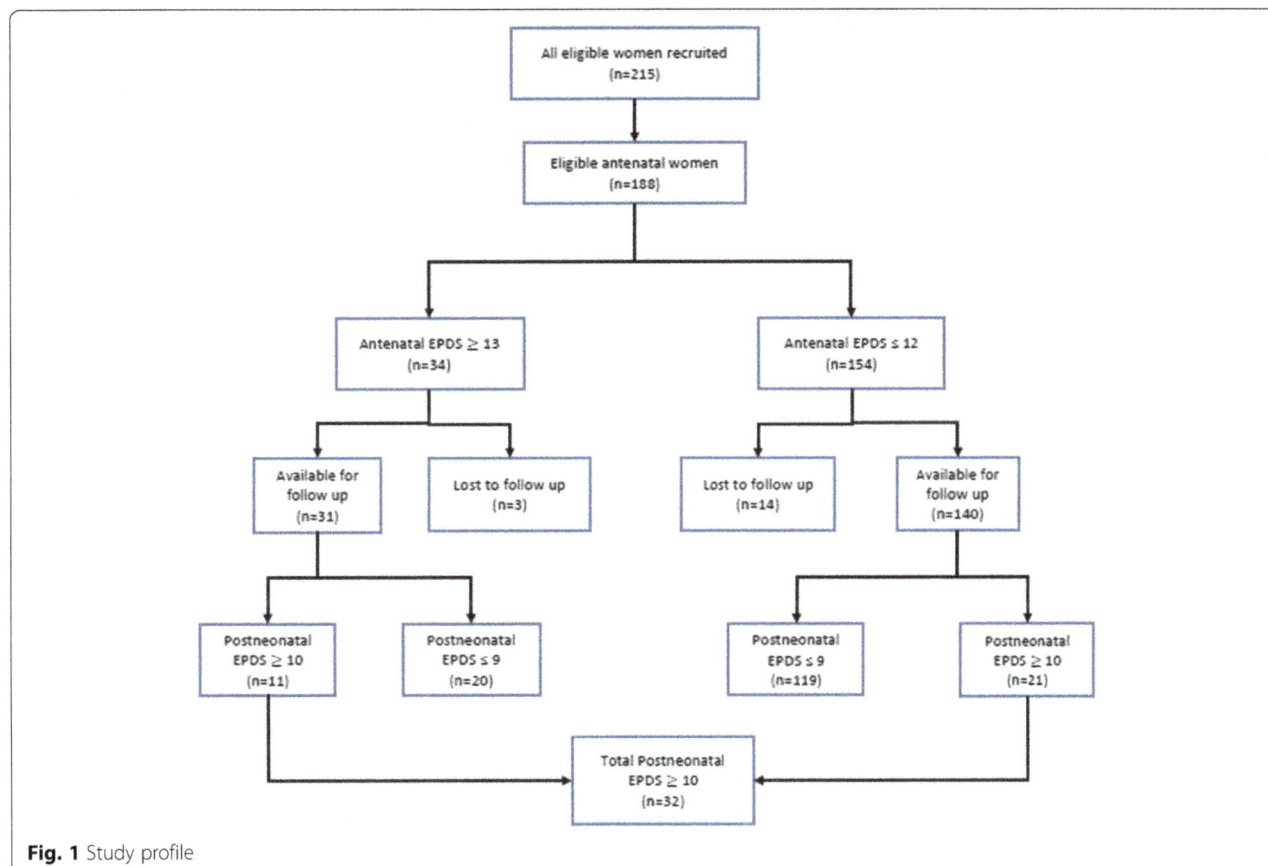

**Fig. 1** Study profile

having recent economic stress and conflict with partner than those without PPD (53% vs. 30% and 56% vs. 15%, respectively) (Table 2).

Most women had vaginal delivery (84% and 81% of those with and without PPD, respectively), delivered babies of normal birth weight (88% and 91%), and did not report a history of the baby being unwell (84% and 83%). However, the distribution of reported birth complications and nursery admission between women with and without PPD differed; women with PPD were more likely to report birth complications (34% vs 16%) and nursery admission (16% vs 9%) (Table 3). Among all the risk factors assessed in Tables 1, 2 and 3, only number of children, antepartum depression, economic stress and conflict with partner had statistically significant associations with PPD status.

In a multivariate analysis adjusted for demographic variables (education, marital status, family income, parity and maternal age) the estimated odds ratio (OR) of PPD comparing those with and without antepartum depression was 2.83 (95% CI: 1.10–7.34, p-value: 0.029). In step 2 when psychosocial risk factors (economic stress, conflict with partner, relationship with partner's mother and partner helping with childcare) were taken into account, this odds ratio was attenuated to 2.50 (95% CI: 0.79–7.77) and was

not statistically significant (p-value: 0.112). Further adjustment for postnatal clinical factors in step 3 yielded a somewhat stronger, but still not statistically significant, association between PPD and antepartum depression: OR = 3.37 (95% CI: 0.98–11.64, p-value = 0.05) (Table 4).

After adjusting for demographic variables and antepartum depression, two psychosocial factors, economic stress and conflict with partner, were found to be positively associated with PPD (OR = 2.73 (95% CI: 1.02–7.50, p-value = 0.046) and OR = 7.12 (95% CI: 2.62–20.67, p-value < 0.001), respectively). Having a good relationship with the mother-in-law and having a partner who helped with housework and childcare were associated with lower odds of postpartum depression (OR = 0.69 (95% CI: 0.24–1.95, p-value = 0.474) and OR = 0.49 (95% CI: 0.17–1.46, p-value = 0.197), respectively); however, neither reached statistical significance.

In the final analyses in which postnatal clinical factors were evaluated in addition to demographic variables, psychosocial risk factors and antepartum depression, the odds ratio comparing mothers who had babies with low birth weight to those with normal birth weight was 1.31 (95% CI: 0.19–6.95, p-value = 0.764). Similarly, the odds ratio of PPD comparing mothers who had birth complications or death of baby at birth to those whose babies were alive at

**Table 1** Demographic Characteristics of Participants

| Variable | Postpartum depression | |
|---|---|---|
| | Yes (n = 32) | No (n = 139) |
| Age in years; median (IQR) | 25.5 (22.8, 28.0) | 25.0 (22.5, 29.0) |
| Marital status; n (%) | | |
| Never married/Separated | 3 (9) | 18 (13) |
| Married | 29 (91) | 121 (87) |
| Highest level of education; n (%) | | |
| ≤ Primary | 10 (31) | 36 (26) |
| Secondary | 17 (53) | 62 (45) |
| Tertiary (college/university) | 5 (16) | 41 (29) |
| Religion; n (%) | | |
| Catholic | 8 (25) | 44 (32) |
| Protestant | 17 (53) | 78 (56) |
| Other | 7 (22) | 17 (12) |
| Monthly Family Income in KES; n (%) | | |
| ≤ 24,000 | 18 (56) | 50 (36) |
| > 24,100 | 14 (44) | 89 (64) |
| Number of children¥ | | |
| 0–1 | 10 (31) | 54 (39) |
| 2 | 20 (63) | 51 (37) |
| 3–5 | 2 (6) | 34 (24) |

¥ = p-value < 0.02; *IQR* interquartile range, *KES* Kenyan Shillings
(1 USD = 100KES);
number of children including newborn

**Table 2** Psychosocial Risk Factors for Postpartum Depression

| Variable; n (%) | Postpartum depression | |
|---|---|---|
| | Yes (n = 32) | No (n = 139) |
| Antepartum depression¥ | | |
| Yes | 11 (34) | 20 (14) |
| No | 21 (66) | 119 (86) |
| Relationship with partner's mother | | |
| Good | 18 (56) | 87 (63) |
| Other* | 14 (44) | 52 (47) |
| Economic stress¥ | | |
| Yes | 17 (53) | 42 (30) |
| No | 15 (47) | 97 (70) |
| Conflict with partner**,¥ | | |
| Physical/verbal | 18 (56) | 21 (15) |
| No conflict | 14 (44) | 118 (85) |
| Partner helping with cooking, cleaning and child care | | |
| Yes | 17 (53) | 99 (71) |
| No | 15 (47) | 40 (29) |

¥ = p-value < 0.02; *Other includes bad or not applicable; **Conflict with
partner during previous 12 months

**Table 3** Postnatal Clinical Risk Factors for Postpartum
Depression

| Variable; n (%) | Postpartum depression | |
|---|---|---|
| | Yes (n = 32) | No (n = 139) |
| Mode of Delivery | | |
| Vaginal | 27 (84) | 112 (81) |
| Caesarean Section | 5 (16) | 27 (19) |
| Reported birth complications | | |
| Present | 11 (34) | 22 (16) |
| Absent | 21 (66) | 117 (84) |
| Low birth weight | | |
| Yes | 4 (12) | 13 (9) |
| No | 28 (88) | 126 (91) |
| Nursery admission | | |
| Yes | 5 (16) | 12 (9) |
| No | 27 (84) | 127 (91) |
| Birth outcome | | |
| Alive | 27 (84) | 133 (96) |
| Baby died | 5 (16) | 6 (4) |

birth and had no birth complications was 2.71 (95% CI:0.74–9.93, p-value = 0.127). On the contrary, vaginal delivery and nursery admission were associated with lower odds of PPD (OR = 0.53 (95% CI: 0.15–2.03) and OR = 0.73 (95% CI: 0.11–4.03), respectively). In these adjusted analyses, none of the birth outcomes was statistically significantly associated with postpartum depression. However, conflict with partner was still positively associated with postpartum depression - the odds ratio comparing women who reported having conflict with partner to those who reported no conflict with partner was 7.52 (95% CI: 2.65–23.13, p-value < 0.001).

## Discussion

This study used multivariate analysis to highlight factors associated with postpartum depression in the first prospective study in a sample of Kenyan women recruited from antenatal clinics. The study showed the perinatal period to be a time of high risk for significant depressive symptoms with prevalence of PPD estimated at 18.7% (95% CI: 13.3–25.5). This estimate is within the range of prior prevalence estimates reported in sub-Saharan Africa (6.1–34.7) [6, 35] where poverty, intimate partner violence and HIV infection have been implicated as major contributors [36–39]. In this study, the antepartum risk factors that had the strongest independent associations with postpartum depression included depression during the antepartum period, as well as self-reported conflict with partner and economic stress. However, in multivariate analyses, the magnitude of the effect size for the association between antepartum and postpartum remained

**Table 4** Logistic regression results for Risk Factors for Postpartum Depression (N = 171)

| Variable (Reference category) | 1[a] | 2[a] | 3[a] |
| --- | --- | --- | --- |
| Antepartum depression (No) | 2.83 (1.09–7.20)* | 2.50 (0.79–7.77) | 3.37 (0.98–11.64) |
| Relationship with partner's mother good (other) | | 0.69 (0.24–1.95) | 0.83 (0.28–2.53) |
| Economic stress (No) | | 2.73 (1.02–7.50)* | 2.54 (0.89–7.43) |
| Conflict with partner (No conflict) | | 7.12 (2.62–20.67)* | 7.52 (2.65–23.13)* |
| Partner helping with child care (No) | | 0.49 (0.17–1.46) | 0.66 (0.20–2.16) |
| Mode of delivery (C-section) | | | 0.53 (0.15–2.03) |
| Low birth weight (No) | | | 1.31 (0.19–6.95) |
| Nursery admission (No) | | | 0.73 (0.11–4.03) |
| Birth complications/outcome (No/baby alive) | | | 2.71 (0.74–9.93) |

[a]OR (95% confidence interval): adjusted for education, marital status, family income, parity and maternal age; *p-value < 0.05

large, based on the point estimate, but did not reach statistical significance. Findings from a recent meta-analysis report conducted on over 14,000 women found depression during pregnancy as one of the strongest predictors of postpartum depression [40] . One large cohort study in Ghana similarly reported antenatal depression as the strongest determinant of postnatal depression [41].Similar longitudinal studies that evaluated depression in pregnancy, as well as in the postpartum period, have found a strong association between postpartum depression and both antepartum depression and history of exposure to violence and conflict [29, 42, 43], as well as having a non-supportive husband [22, 32, 35, 38]. In addition to partner conflict, we asked women to evaluate the relationship with their mother in law. While we did not find a statistically significant association between postpartum depression and relationship with mother-in-law, this may be explained by the fact that our study focused on an urban population cohort. Urban settings differ from rural settings where communal living that includes the mother in law is the norm.

Numerous previous studies have shown that strong social support networks evidenced by good interpersonal relationships enhance resilience to stress and hence contribute immensely to protecting the individual from developing depression [44–47]. A supportive husband and a marital relationship with less friction play a part in promoting a strong social support system for the mother. Sustained perceived pressure from economic stress has been found to elevate cortisol levels and hence contribute towards vulnerability for developing depression [48–50]. A study examining the interaction of economic stress and postpartum family support on cortisol levels found women who reported good family support had lower levels of cortisol compared to women with low family support, even those with underlying high perceived economic stress. These findings indicate that having a supportive partner can buffer the detrimental effects of economic stress [51].

Prior research has shown that obstetric and infant-related clinical factors such as intrapartum hemorrhage, prolonged labor and bad outcome of the baby confers a small increased risk of developing postpartum depression [52–54], once demographic and psychosocial factors are adjusted for. However, these clinical factors did not contribute significantly to a higher likelihood of depression among mothers in our study. This further underscores the important contributions of psychosocial factors to postpartum depression risk.

The finding that nearly one in five women reported significant postpartum depressive symptoms in this Kenyan study suggests the need for post-partum depression screening. Our study also suggests that screening for partner conflict during the prenatal period could help to identify pregnant women at risk of later depression. However, screening programs are recommended only in circumstances where women who screen positive have access to follow-up interventions. Rahman et al. (2014) [55] conducted a systematic review of evidence regarding effectiveness of interventions to address common perinatal mental disorders in low and middle income countries. Robust effects on maternal depression were reported in a study of Pakistani mothers with depression who received a multi-modal intervention delivered by trained lay providers that included elements of cognitive behavior therapy, active listening, support for strengthening the mother-infant relationship, and mobilization of family support [56] . Because of the high prevalence of depression in pregnant women and new mothers, the adverse consequences of maternal depression to the health and well-being to mothers and infants, and the availability of screening tools and empirically supported interventions, conditions are rife for prioritizing perinatal depression screening and intervention in low resource settings. Results of our study highlight intervention targets that would be salient for reducing the burden of postpartum depression in Kenyan women.

## Study limitations

One limitation of our study was the small number of women evaluated. While several of the factors that we evaluated, such as the mother having a good relationship with her mother-in-law and her partner helping with child-rearing, were associated with lower odds of post-partum depression, small sample size contributed to wide confidence intervals around odds ratio estimates. In addition, information about the HIV status of mothers was not available – the prevalence of postpartum depression has been shown previously to be high in Kenyan women who are HIV positive [25]. Furthermore, the follow-up assessment for our study was conducted between 6 and 10 weeks after the birth of the infant. However, the risk of postpartum depression remains high up to 24 weeks postpartum. Our study did not include women who had depression onset after 10 weeks.

We administered the EPDS which has been validated [35] and used extensively worldwide. However, since we conducted our study in 2014, a 9-item perinatal depression screening tool has been developed in Kenya that incorporates local idioms and shows high sensitivity and specificity (0.90/0.90) vis a vis meeting DSM-5 diagnostic criteria for major depression [57]. The authors of this study reported considerably lower sensitivity and specificity (0.70/0.72) for the EPDS at the optimal cutoff. Our study was conducted in an urban setting. Thus, caution is warranted in generalizing our findings to rural areas where access to pre- and post-natal care may be more limited, and social support within the community may be stronger. Finally, as this was part of a larger study to confirm feasibility of integrating EPDS depression screening in maternal and child health clinics, we did not include a concurrent use of a diagnostic tool to confirm depression diagnosis.

## Conclusions

To our knowledge this is the first study to evaluate risk factors for postpartum depression prospectively in an urban cohort of Kenyan women. Our results are consistent with prior research conducted in other settings showing antepartum depression, economic stress, and conflict with partner as predictors of postpartum depression and underscore the need for addressing the public health burden of these interrelated problems. To build upon our study findings, we recommend that more multi-wave cohort studies be conducted in Kenya. Future studies should include longer post-partum follow-up periods and utilize the recently validated Kenyan Perinatal Depression Screen, more refined tools for measuring partner conflict and support, and larger population samples that include women from rural settings.

**Abbreviations**
ADHD: Attention Deficit Hyperactivity Disorder; EDS: Edinburgh Depression Scale; EPDS: Edinburgh Postpartum Depression Scale; HIV: Human Immunodeficiency Virus; KES: Kenyan Shillings; MCH: Maternal and Child Health; PPD: Postpartum depression

**Acknowledgements**
The authors are grateful to Francis Creed, for his help in editing the manuscript, and the mothers who participated in the study.

**Funding**
This research was supported by a grant from the Kenya Medical Research Institute.

**Authors' contributions**
LO designed the study, trained the nurses who conducted the interviews with participants and wrote the first draft of the paper. VW conducted the statistical analyses and wrote the methods and results section of the paper. PO, JM and EJ participated in study design and implementation. AVS wrote and edited the first and subsequent drafts of the manuscript. MM revised the manuscript and made valuable suggestions. All authors reviewed and approved the final version of the manuscript.

**Consent for publication**
Not applicable.

**Competing interests**
The authors declare that they have no competing interests.

**Author details**
¹Kenya Medical Research Institute, P.O. Box 54840 00200, Mbagathi Road, Nairobi, Kenya. ²University of Washington, Jefferson St. Seattle WA 98104, Nairobi 908, Kenya. ³University of Nairobi, P.O. Box 30197, Off Ngong Road, Nairobi, Kenya.

**References**
1. Gelaye B, Rondon MB, Araya R, Williams MA. Epidemiology of maternal depression, risk factors, and child outcomes in low-income and middle-income countries. The lancet Psychiatry. NIH Public Access; 2016 [cited 2017 Mar 6];3: 973–82. Available from: http://www.ncbi.nlm.nih.gov/pubmed/27650773
2. Fisher J, Cabral de Mello M, Patel V, Rahman A, Tran T, Holton S, et al. Prevalence and determinants of common perinatal mental disorders in women in low- and lower-middle-income countries: a systematic review. Bull World Health Organ 2012 [cited 2017 Mar 6];90:139–149H. Available from: http://www.who.int/entity/bulletin/volumes/90/2/11-091850.pdf
3. Evans J, Heron J, Francomb H, Oke S, Golding J. Cohort study of depressed mood during pregnancy and after childbirth. BMJ. 2001 [cited 2015 May 1]; 323:257–60. Available from: http://www.pubmedcentral.nih.gov/articlerender.fcgi?artid=35345&tool=pmcentrez&rendertype=abstract
4. Grote NK, Bridge JA, Gavin AR, Melville JL, Iyengar S, Katon WJ. A meta-analysis of depression during pregnancy and the risk of preterm birth, low birth weight, and intrauterine growth restriction. Arch Gen Psychiatry. NIH

Public Access; 2010 [cited 2017 Mar 6];67:1012–24. Available from: http://www.ncbi.nlm.nih.gov/pubmed/20921117

5.  Gavin NI, Gaynes BN, Lohr KN, Meltzer-Brody S, Gartlehner G, Swinson T. Perinatal Depression. Obstet Gynecol [Internet]. 2005 [cited 2017 Mar 7];106:1071–83. Available from: http://www.ncbi.nlm.nih.gov/pubmed/16260528

6.  Nakku JEM, Nakasi G, Mirembe F. Postpartum major depression at six weeks in primary health care: prevalence and associated factors. Afr Health Sci. Makerere University Medical School; 2006 [cited 2017 mar 7];6:207–14. Available from: http://www.ncbi.nlm.nih.gov/pubmed/17604509.

7.  Kaida A, Matthews LT, Ashaba S, Tsai AC, Kanters S, Robak M, et al. Depression during pregnancy and the postpartum among HIV-infected women on antiretroviral therapy in Uganda. J Acquir Immune Defic Syndr. 2014 [cited 2015 Dec 6];67 Suppl 4:S179–87. Available from: http://www.pubmedcentral.nih.gov/articlerender.fcgi?artid=4251908&tool=pmcentrez&rendertype=abstract.

8.  Muzik M, Borovska S. Perinatal depression: implications for child mental health. Ment Health Fam Med. Radcliffe Publishing and Wonca; 2010 [cited 2017 mar 7];7:239–47. Available from: http://www.ncbi.nlm.nih.gov/pubmed/22477948.

9.  Chung TK, Lau TK, Yip AS, Chiu HF, Lee DT. Antepartum depressive symptomatology is associated with adverse obstetric and neonatal outcomes. Psychosom Med. [cited 2017 Mar 7];63:830–4. Available from: http://www.ncbi.nlm.nih.gov/pubmed/11573032

10. Bonari L, Pinto N, Ahn E, Einarson A, Steiner M, Koren G. Perinatal risks of untreated depression during pregnancy. Can J Psychiatr. 2004 [cited 2015 Apr 29];49:726–35. Available from: http://www.ncbi.nlm.nih.gov/pubmed/15633850

11. Waters CS, Hay DF, Simmonds JR, van Goozen SHM. Antenatal depression and children's developmental outcomes: potential mechanisms and treatment options. Eur Child Adolesc Psychiatry. 2014 [cited 2017 Mar 7];23:957–71. Available from: http://www.ncbi.nlm.nih.gov/pubmed/25037152

12. Surkan PJ, Kennedy CE, Hurley KM, Black MM. Maternal depression and early childhood growth in developing countries: systematic review and meta-analysis. Bull World Health Organ. 2011 [cited 2017 Mar 7];89:608–615E. Available from: http://www.ncbi.nlm.nih.gov/pubmed/21836759

13. Lefkovics E, Baji I, Rig?? J. Impact of maternal depression on pregnancies and on early attachment. Infant Ment Health J. 2014 [cited 2017 Mar 7];35:354–65. Available from: http://www.ncbi.nlm.nih.gov/pubmed/25798487

14. Kingi Mochache,Kumar Manasi, Muthoni Mathai GO. Depression in Pregnancy and Preterm delivery. A prospective cohort study among women attending antenatal clinic at Pumwani maternity hospital. In: University of Nairobi; 2016.

15. O'Connor TG, Monk C, Burke AS. Maternal affective illness in the perinatal period and child development: findings on developmental timing, mechanisms, and intervention. Curr Psychiatry Rep. 2016 [cited 2017 Mar 7];18:24. Available from: http://www.ncbi.nlm.nih.gov/pubmed/26830882

16. Stein A, Craske MG, Lehtonen A, Harvey A, Savage-McGlynn E, Davies B, et al. Maternal cognitions and mother–infant interaction in postnatal depression and generalized anxiety disorder. J Abnorm Psychol 2012 [cited 2017 Mar 7];121:795–809. Available from: http://www.ncbi.nlm.nih.gov/pubmed/22288906

17. Vameghi R, Amir Aliakbari S, Sajjad H, Sajedi F, Alavimajd H. Correlation Between Mothers' Depression and Developmental Delay in Infants Aged 6–18 Months. Glob J Health Sci. 2015 [cited 2017 Mar 7];8:11. Available from: http://www.ncbi.nlm.nih.gov/pubmed/26652078

18. Weobong B, Ten Asbroek AHA, Soremekun S, Manu AA, Owusu-Agyei S, Prince M, et al. Association of Antenatal Depression with adverse consequences for the mother and newborn in rural Ghana: findings from the DON population-based cohort study. Fischer G, editor. PLoS One. Public Library of Science; 2014 [cited 2018 Apr 20];9:e116333. Available from: http://dx.plos.org/10.1371/journal.pone.0116333

19. Whelan YM, Leibenluft E, Stringaris A, Barker ED. Pathways from maternal depressive symptoms to adolescent depressive symptoms: the unique contribution of irritability symptoms. J Child Psychol Psychiatry. 2015 [cited 2017 Mar 7];56:1092–100. Available from: http://www.ncbi.nlm.nih.gov/pubmed/25665134

20. Closa-Monasterolo R, Gispert-Llaurado M, Canals J, Luque V, Zaragoza-Jordana M, Koletzko B, et al. The effect of postpartum depression and current mental health problems of the mother on child behaviour at eight years. Matern Child Health J]. 2017 [cited 2017 Mar 7]; Available from: http://www.ncbi.nlm.nih.gov/pubmed/28188472

21. Madeghe BA, Kimani VN, Vander Stoep A, Nicodimos S, Kumar M. Postpartum depression and infant feeding practices in a low income urban settlement in Nairobi-Kenya. BMC Res Notes. BioMed Central; 2016 [cited 2017 Mar 7];9:506. Available from: http://www.ncbi.nlm.nih.gov/pubmed/27931248

22. Robertson E, Grace S, Wallington T, Stewart DE. Antenatal risk factors for postpartum depression: a synthesis of recent literature. Gen Hosp Psychiatry [Internet]. 2004 [cited 2017 May 10];26:289–95. Available from: http://www.ncbi.nlm.nih.gov/pubmed/15234824

23. Manikkam L, Burns JK. Antenatal depression and its risk factors: an urban prevalence study in KwaZulu-Natal. S Afr Med J. 2012 [cited 2015 Mar 20];102:940–4. Available from: http://www.ncbi.nlm.nih.gov/pubmed/23498042

24. Stewart DE, Robertson FE, Phil M, Dennis C-L, Grace SL, Wallington T. Postpartum Depression: Literature Review of Risk Factors and Interventions. ©University Heal Netw Women's Heal Progr. 2003 [cited 2017 Mar 6]; Available from: http://www.who.int/mental_health/prevention/suicide/lit_review_postpartum_depression.pdf?ua=1.

25. Yator O, Mathai M, Vander Stoep A, Rao D, Kumar M. Risk factors for postpartum depression in women living with HIV attending prevention of mother-to-child transmission clinic at Kenyatta National Hospital, Nairobi. AIDS Care. 2016 [cited 2017 Mar 7];28:884–9. Available from: https://www.tandfonline.com/doi/full/10.1080/09540121.2016.1160026

26. Olecha JO, of Nairobi U. Depression and Psychosocial Risk Factors Associated with Pregnant Adolescents Mixed Method Study Based at Kangemi Health Centre, Nairobi. 2016 [cited 2017 Aug 7]. Available from: http://erepository.uonbi.ac.ke/bitstream/handle/11295/97483/Osok_Depression and Psychosocial Risk Factors Associated With Pregnant Adolescentsmixed Method Study Based at Kangemi Health Centre%2CNairobi.pdf?sequence=1&isAllowe.

27. Polkovnikova-Wamoto A, Mathai M, Stoep A Vander, Kumar M. "Haven of safety" and "secure base": a qualitative inquiry into factors affecting child attachment security in Nairobi, Kenya. Vulnerable Child Youth Stud. 2016 [cited 2018 May 1];11:286–96. Available from: https://www.tandfonline.com/doi/full/10.1080/17450128.2016.1201237

28. Wittkowski A, Gardner PL, Bunton P, Edge D. Culturally determined risk factors for postnatal depression in Sub-Saharan Africa: a mixed method systematic review. J Affect Disord. 2014 [cited 2018 Apr 18];163:115–24. Available from: http://linkinghub.elsevier.com/retrieve/pii/S0165032713008811

29. Sawyer A, Ayers S, Smith H. Pre- and postnatal psychological wellbeing in Africa: a systematic review. J Affect Disord. 2010 [cited 2016 Jan 11];123:17–29. Available from: http://www.ncbi.nlm.nih.gov/pubmed/19635636

30. Ongeri L, Otieno P, Mbui J, Juma E, Mathai M. Antepartum Risk Factors for Postpartum Depression: A Follow up Study among Urban Women Living in Nairobi, Kenya. J Pregnancy Child Heal. OMICS International; 2016 [cited 2017 May 12];03:1–8. Available from: https://www.omicsgroup.org/journals/antepartum-risk-factors-for-postpartum-depression-a-follow-up-study-amongurban-women-living-in-nairobi-kenya-2376-127X-1000288.php?aid=81579

31. Cox JL, Holden JM, Sagovsky R. Detection of postnatal depression. Development of the 10-item Edinburgh Postnatal Depression Scale. Br J Psychiatry. 1987 [cited 2015 Mar 16];150:782–6. Available from: http://www.ncbi.nlm.nih.gov/pubmed/3651732

32. Gibson J, McKenzie-McHarg K, Shakespeare J, Price J, Gray R. A systematic review of studies validating the Edinburgh Postnatal Depression Scale in antepartum and postpartum women. Acta Psychiatr Scand. 2009 [cited 2015 Jan 28];119:350–64. Available from: http://www.ncbi.nlm.nih.gov/pubmed/19298573

33. Kumar M, Ongeri L, Mathai M, Mbwayo A. Translation of EPDS Questionnaire into Kiswahili: Understanding the Cross-Cultural and Translation Issues in Mental Health Research. J pregnancy child Heal. 2015 [cited 2015 May 21];2. Available from: http://www.pubmedcentral.nih.gov/articlerender.fcgi?artid=4399496&tool=pmcentrez&rendertype=abstract.

34. Murray L, Carothers AD. The validation of the Edinburgh post-natal depression scale on a community sample. Br J Psychiatry. 1990;157:288–90.

35. Cooper PJ, Tomlinson M, Swartz L, Woolgar M, Murray L, Molteno C. Post-partum depression and the mother-infant relationship in a south African peri-urban settlement. Br J Psychiatry. 1999 [cited 2015 Apr 29];175:554–8. Available from: http://www.ncbi.nlm.nih.gov/pubmed/10789353

36. Hartley M, Tomlinson M, Greco E, Comulada WS, Stewart J, le Roux I, et al. Depressed mood in pregnancy: prevalence and correlates in two Cape Town peri-urban settlements. Reprod Health [Internet]. 2011 [cited 2015 Mar 29];8:9. Available from: http://www.pubmedcentral.nih.gov/articlerender.fcgi?artid=3113332&tool=pmcentrez&rendertype=abstract.

37. Dibaba Y, Fantahun M, Hindin MJ. The association of unwanted pregnancy and social support with depressive symptoms in pregnancy: evidence from rural Southwestern Ethiopia. BMC Pregnancy Childbirth. 2013 [cited 2015 Mar 29];13:135. Available from: http://www.pubmedcentral.nih.gov/articlerender.fcgi?artid=3716614&tool=pmcentrez&rendertype=abstract

38. Owoeye AO, Aina OF, Morakinyo O. Risk factors of postpartum depression and EPDS scores in a group of Nigerian women. Trop Doct [Internet]. 2006 [cited 2018 Mar 21];36:100–3. Available from: http://journals.sagepub.com/doi/10.1258/004947506776593341

39. Chibanda D, Mangezi W, Tshimanga M, Woelk G, Rusakaniko S, Stranix-Chibanda L, et al. Postnatal Depression by HIV Status Among Women in Zimbabwe. J Women's Heal. 2010 [cited 2018 May 1];19:2071–7. Available from: http://www.ncbi.nlm.nih.gov/pubmed/20849286

40. Robertson E, Grace S, Wallington T, Stewart DE. Antenatal risk factors for postpartum depression: a synthesis of recent literature. Gen Hosp Psychiatry. 2004 [cited 2017 Mar 6];26:289–95. Available from: http://linkinghub.elsevier.com/retrieve/pii/S0163834304000398

41. Weobong B, Ten Asbroek AH, Soremekun S, Danso S, Owusu-Agyei S, Prince M, et al. Determinants of postnatal depression in rural Ghana: findings from the Don population based cohort study. Depress Anxiety. 2015 [cited 2018 Apr 20];32:108–19. Available from: http://www.ncbi.nlm.nih.gov/pubmed/24272979

42. Milgrom J, Gemmill AW, Bilszta JL, Hayes B, Barnett B, Brooks J, et al. Antenatal risk factors for postnatal depression: A large prospective study. J Affect Disord. 2008 [cited 2017 May 10];108:147–57. Available from: http://www.ncbi.nlm.nih.gov/pubmed/18067974

43. Kirkan TS, Aydin N, Yazici E, Akcali Aslan P, Acemoglu H, Daloglu AG. The depression in women in pregnancy and postpartum period: a follow-up study. Int J Soc Psychiatry. 2014 [cited 2015 Feb 26]; Available from: http://www.ncbi.nlm.nih.gov/pubmed/25069455

44. Ozbay F, Johnson DC, Dimoulas E, Morgan CA, Charney D, Southwick S, et al. Social support and resilience to stress: from neurobiology to clinical practice. Psychiatry (Edgmont). Matrix Medical Communications; 2007 [cited 2017 may 10];4:35–40. Available from: http://www.ncbi.nlm.nih.gov/pubmed/20806028.

45. Saligheh M, Rooney RM, McNamara B, Kane RT. The relationship between postnatal depression, sociodemographic factors, levels of partner support, and levels of physical activity. Front Psychol. Frontiers Media SA; 2014 [cited 2017 May 10];5:597. Available from: http://www.ncbi.nlm.nih.gov/pubmed/25071618

46. Urquia ML, Pulver A, Heaman MI, Ray JG, Daoud N, O'Campo P. Partner Disengagement from Pregnancy and Adverse Maternal and Infant Outcomes. J Women's Heal. 2017 [cited 2017 May 10];26:234–40. Available from: http://www.ncbi.nlm.nih.gov/pubmed/27860534

47. Patel V, Rodrigues M, DeSouza N. Gender, Poverty, and Postnatal Depression: A Study of Mothers in Goa, India. Am J Psychiatry. 2002 [cited 2017 May 10];159:43–7. Available from: http://www.ncbi.nlm.nih.gov/pubmed/11772688

48. Mastorakos G, Ilias I. Maternal and fetal hypothalamic-pituitary-adrenal axes during pregnancy and postpartum. Ann N Y Acad Sci. 2003 [cited 2017 May 12];997:136–49. Available from: http://www.ncbi.nlm.nih.gov/pubmed/14644820

49. Björntorp P, Rosmond R. Hypothalamic origin of the metabolic syndrome X. Ann N Y Acad Sci. 1999 [cited 2017 May 12];892:297–307. Available from: http://www.ncbi.nlm.nih.gov/pubmed/10842670

50. McEwen BS. The neurobiology of stress: from serendipity to clinical relevance. Brain Res. 2000 [cited 2017 may 12];886:172–89. Available from: http://www.ncbi.nlm.nih.gov/pubmed/11119695

51. Jewell SL, Luecken LJ, Gress-Smith J, Crnic KA, Gonzales NA. Economic Stress and Cortisol Among Postpartum Low-Income Mexican American Women: Buffering Influence of Family Support. Behav Med. NIH Public Access; 2015 [cited 2017 May 12];41:138–44. Available from: http://www.ncbi.nlm.nih.gov/pubmed/26332931

52. Nolte S, Wong D, Latchford G, Boyle O, Anaenugwu A. Amphetamines for schizophrenia. In: Nolte S, editor. Cochrane Database Syst Rev. Chichester, UK: John Wiley & Sons, Ltd; 2004 [cited 2016 Dec 3]. p. CD004964. Available from: http://www.ncbi.nlm.nih.gov/pubmed/15495131

53. Sentilhes L, Gromez A, Clavier E, Resch B, Descamps P, Marpeau L. Long-term psychological impact of severe postpartum hemorrhage. Acta Obstet Gynecol Scand. 2011 [cited 2016 Mar 9];90:615–20. Available from: http://www.ncbi.nlm.nih.gov/pubmed/21370999

54. Mei Z, Huang M. [Association of psychological factors with post-partum hemorrhage and labor duration]. Nan Fang Yi Ke Da Xue Xue Bao. 2006 [cited 2016 mar 9];26:1203–4. Available from: http://www.ncbi.nlm.nih.gov/pubmed/16939922.

55. Rahman A, Fisher J, Bower P, Luchters S, Tran T, Yasamy MT, et al. Interventions for common perinatal mental disorders in women in low- and middle-income countries: a systematic review and meta-analysis. Bull World Health Organ. 2013 [cited 2015 Mar 30];91:593–601I. Available from: http://www.pubmedcentral.nih.gov/articlerender.fcgi?artid=3738304&tool=pmcentrez&rendertype=abstract.

56. Stewart RC, Umar E, Kauye F, Bunn J, Vokhiwa M, Fitzgerald M, et al. Maternal common mental disorder and infant growth--a cross-sectional study from Malawi. Matern Child Nutr. 2008 [cited 2018 Mar 21];4:209–19. Available from: http://doi.wiley.com/10.1111/j.1740-8709.2008.00147.x

57. Green EP, Tuli H, Kwobah E, Menya D, Chesire I, Schmidt C. Developing and validating a perinatal depression screening tool in Kenya blending Western criteria with local idioms: A mixed methods study. J Affect Disord. 2018 [cited 2018 Apr 18];228:49–59. Available from: http://www.ncbi.nlm.nih.gov/pubmed/29227955

# 8

# Successfully treating 90 patients with obsessive compulsive disorder in eight days: the Bergen 4-day treatment

Gerd Kvale[1,2], Bjarne Hansen[1,2], Thröstur Björgvinsson[3,4], Tore Børtveit[1], Kristen Hagen[1,5], Svein Haseth[6], Unn Beate Kristensen[7], Gunvor Launes[8], Kerry J. Ressler[3,4], Stian Solem[1,9*], Arne Strand[10], Odile A. van den Heuvel[1,11] and Lars-Göran Öst[1,12]

## Abstract

**Background:** Oslo University Hospital, Norway, had by autumn 2016, accumulated a waiting list of 101 patients with obsessive-compulsive disorder (OCD) who had a legal right to receive treatment by a specialized OCD team. In this challenging situation, the Bergen OCD-team suggested to solve the problem by offering all patients an option for the rapid Bergen 4-day treatment (B4DT). The B4DT is an individual treatment delivered during four consecutive days in a group of six patients with the same number of therapists. The approach has previously shown a post-treatment response rate of 90% and a 3-month remission rate of 70%.

**Methods:** Ninety-seven of the wait-list patients were available for the scheduled time slots, and 90 received the 4-day format during 8 days (45 patients each week). The therapists were recruited from 22 different specialized OCD-teams from all over Norway, and 44 (68%) had not previously delivered the 4-day format.

**Results:** Post-treatment; 91.1% of the patients were classified as responders, and 72.2% were in remission. At 3-month follow-up; 84.4 were classified as responders and the remission rate was 67.7%. Oslo University Hospital now offers the 4-day treatment as standard treatment for OCD.

**Conclusions:** We conclude that the B4DT is an acceptable and potentially effective OCD-treatment.

**Keywords:** Obsessive-compulsive disorder, OCD, 4-day treatment, Exposure

## Background

In Norway, all patients with obsessive-compulsive disorder (OCD) are granted empirically supported treatment by a specialized OCD-team [1], and 30 teams have been established since 2012. At Oslo University Hospital (OUH) the consequence of this new rule of granted treatment was a tripling of patients from 2014 to 2016, and more than 100 patients were waiting for treatment by the end of 2016. The most probable reason is that many more OCD-patients than previously applied for treatment when they realized they might be granted empirically supported treatment. While OUH employed a protocol for individual

exposure and response prevention (ERP) [2] where patients typically are treated over 12–16 weeks, the OCD-team at Haukeland University Hospital, Bergen, has developed a novel treatment format where ERP is delivered during just four consecutive days. Despite the relatively brief treatment, the Bergen 4-day treatment (B4DT) has been shown to yield a good outcome [3–5]. At post-treatment assessment the proportion of responders varied from 83% [4] to 93.8% [5] with a weighted mean of 89.4%. At 6- or 12-month follow-up the mean response rate was 82.4%. The post-treatment remission rate varied between 73.8% [4] and 77.1% [3] with a weighted mean of 76.0%, and at follow-up the average rate was 69.7%. Also, the 4-day format has shown to be acceptable for the patients and has a 'low drop-out rate; 0.7% (only 1 out of 142 patients; [3–5]. However, these studies have

* Correspondence: stian.solem@ntnu.no
[1]Haukeland University Hospital, OCD-team, 5021 Bergen, Norway
[9]Department of Psychology, Norwegian University of Science and Technology, Trondheim, Norway
Full list of author information is available at the end of the article

had small sample sizes ($N$ = 35, 42, and 65) so larger trials are warranted.

There are a few published studies on concentrated ERP for OCD (using Yale-Brown Obsessive Compulsive Scale as primary outcome measure) but no randomized trial comparing it to weekly sessions of ERP. Franklin et al. [6] and Abramowitz et al. [7] published uncontrolled effectiveness studies on concentrated ERP using 15 2 hour sessions over 4 weeks and 12 sessions of 90 min over 4 weeks, respectively. Hiss et al. [8] and Lindsey et al. [9] published efficacy studies using 19 sessions of 90 min over 4 weeks and 15 2 hour sessions over 3 weeks, respectively. Finally, there are two non-randomized comparison trials involving concentrated ERP. Abramowitz et al. [10] compared 15 2 hour sessions over 3 weeks with 15 sessions over 8 weeks (twice weekly) and found that the concentrated treatment yielded a significantly higher proportion of recovered patients post-treatment but not at 3-month follow-up. Storch et al. [11] compared 14 sessions of 90 min over 3 weeks with 14 weekly sessions and found no significant differences at post- or at 3-month follow-up assessment. Combining the Y-BOCS data for these six studies ($N$ = 266) yielded a weighted mean at pre-treatment of 26.2 (SD 4.9) and at post-treatment of 11.9 (6.9), with a within-group effect size (Cohen's $d$) of 2.42. This can be compared to 2.06 for standard ERP in the meta-analysis by Öst et al. [12]. Thus, previous versions of concentrated ERP have used daily sessions of 90 or 120 min over 3–4 weeks, which is quite different to the B4DT, consisting of four sessions of 3–8 h across four consecutive days. Since longer versions of concentrated ERP seem to yield somewhat better effects than standard ERP it is possible that our highly concentrated version yields even better effects.

The leader of the Bergen OCD-team (GK) was made aware of the treatment delay problem at OUH and suggested offering the 4-day treatment to patients on the waiting list, which OUH accepted. The 4-day treatment is best described as "individual treatment in a group setting" since the ratio between therapist and patients is 1:1 in groups which usually range from three to six patients. In order to treat 100 patients, eight parallel groups during two separate weeks would be needed. It was decided to offer OCD-therapists from the other specialized OCD-teams in Norway the opportunity to participate, and by doing so to start their training in the 4-day format. This logistically demanding project of treating 100 OCD-patients in 8 days was initiated during the spring of 2017. The present paper reports on the results.

Based on the outcomes of three previous effectiveness studies from our team [3–5] we predicted that the outcome of the present study would be equally good since the disorder and treatment were the same. Also, because the three previous studies [3–5] on the B4DT were all carried out with, to a large extent new therapists, we expected that the B4DT would be effective also with a substantial number of new therapists. Thus, the present study can be seen as an example of systematic replication [13] having the purpose to test the outcome when a large number of OCD-patients are treated at a new clinic by new therapists.

## Methods

### Participants and procedure

In Norway, OCD-patients with a principal DSM-5 diagnosis of OCD [14] are entitled to empirically supported treatment from an outpatient OCD-team. In February 2017, the 101 patients on the OUH waitlist were offered the 4-day treatment. Inclusion criteria were a diagnosis of OCD and patients had to be fluent in Norwegian. Exclusion criteria included suicidality, psychosis, and active substance abuse. Patients declining would receive standard care at OUH. Four were unable to attend due to school obligations, work, and a prescheduled vacation and 97 patients were scheduled (see flow chart in Fig. 1).

Patients referred to OUH had all been diagnosed with OCD (by a psychiatrist or clinical psychologist at the OUH OCD-team) and severity of OCD had been assessed with a Y-BOCS interview before being placed on the waiting list. Diagnoses were assessed using the MINI International Neuropsychiatric Interview [15]. For the present study, patients on the waiting list were formally referred to the OCD-team in Bergen, and they were re-assessed before starting treatment by using the OCD entry questions from DSM-5 as well as another Y-BOCS interview. This re-assessment was necessary as some patients had been waiting for treatment for many months. When formally referred to Bergen, patients were asked to complete a number of questionnaires administrated online (see measures) prior to the treatment, and to complete these questionnaires post-treatment as well as at 3-month follow-up.

Y-BOCS at post-treatment, as well as at 3-month follow-up, were conducted over the phone by specially trained clinical psychologists who worked at other clinics and were not involved in the treatment. At 3-month follow-up, 20% of the sample was randomly selected to be re-interviewed within 1 week by another independent psychologist. The inter-rater reliability, Intra Class Coefficient (3.1) = 0.93, was excellent.

The treatment was conducted in Oslo by bringing in therapists from all over Norway. Three of the 97 patients became ill (two with flu, one with a minor bleeding during pregnancy). One patient turned out to have severe language problems, and three were misdiagnosed (one had OCD-like symptoms which turned out to be

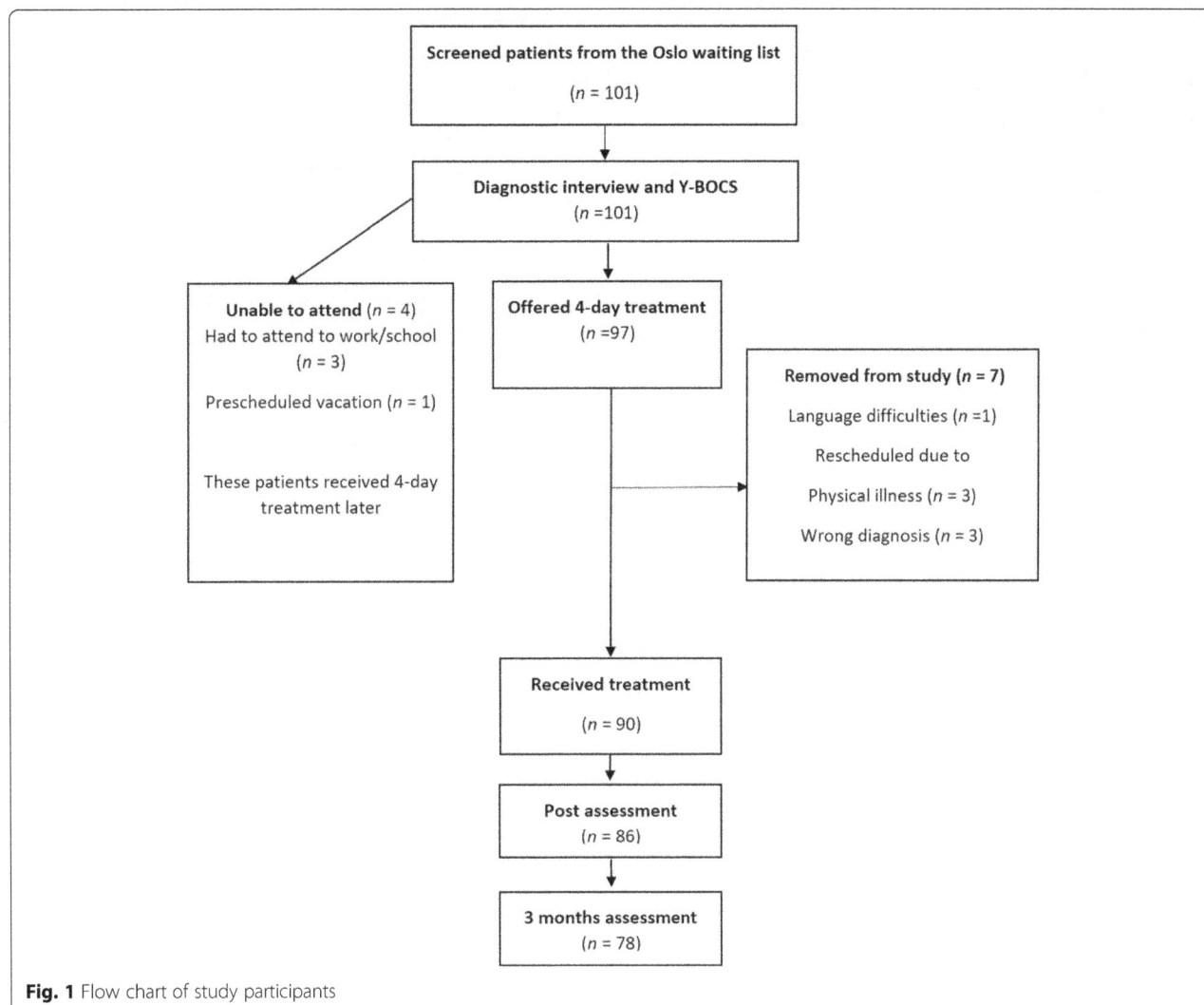

**Fig. 1** Flow chart of study participants

due to a neurological disorder; one was preparing for a transsexual operation and the OCD-like symptoms were related to this, and one patient had a primary diagnosis of generalized anxiety disorder). Thus, the number of OCD patients who received the 4-day treatment was 90. All of these patients completed treatment so the attrition rate was 0%.

### Demographics
Mean age was 32.7 ($SD$ = 9.7), 57% were women, and 58% single. A total of 78% were either working or studying, whereas 22% received different social benefits. Mean years of education was 12.6 ($SD$ = 3.5). Thirty-two patients reported to have family members with OCD (see Table 1 for details).

### OCD severity and comorbidity
Mean pre-treatment score on the Yale-Brown Obsessive Compulsive Scale (Y-BOCS) was 26.16 ($SD$ = 3.37), 77% had severe OCD (Y-BOCS score of 24–38), and 23% had

a moderate OCD (Y-BOCS score of 18–23). A total of 86.7% had received previous treatment trials, but none of the patients had received CBT for OCD with including ERP procedures. Patients with previous therapy trials ($M$ = 26.25, $SD$ = 3.47) did not differ significantly from treatment naïve ($M$ = 25.45, $SD$ = 2.62), $t(88)$ = 0.73, $p$ = .47. A total of 56 patients (62%) had one or more co-morbid disorders (see Table 1 for details).

### Pharmacological treatment
Forty patients used psychotropic medications: 35 used antidepressants, one antiepileptic medication, eight antipsychotics, four stimulants, five anxiolytics, three hypnotics, and one received drug assisted treatment for substance abuse. Patients with and without psychotropic medication did not differ on Y-BOCS scores, $t(88)$ = .014, $p$ = .99, GAD-7 scores $t(88)$ = .41 $p$ = .69, or PHQ-9 scores, $t(88)$ = 1.10, $p$ = .27, at pre-treatment.

No changes were applied to medication, but the patients were informed that the use of anxiolytics was

**Table 1** Demographic and diagnostic characteristics of the sample (*N* = 90)

| Demographics | n (%)/ M (SD) | Comorbidity | |
|---|---|---|---|
| Age | 32.70 (9.72) | GAD | 27 (30.0%) |
| Years of education | 12.60 (3.46) | Depression | 20 (22.2%) |
| Female gender | 51 (56.7%) | Bipolar | 1 (1.1%) |
| Single | 52 (57.8%) | Panic | 14 (15.5%) |
| Working | 51 (56.7%) | Tourette | 2 (2.2%) |
| Studying | 19 (21.1%) | Specific phobia | 4 (4.4%) |
| Social benefits | 20 (22.2%) | Social phobia | 11 (12.2%) |
| Previous treatment | 79 (87.8%) | BDD | 1 (1.1%) |
| Psychotropic meds | 40 (44.4%) | Health anxiety | 2 (2.2%) |
| GAF-S (0–100) | 51.73 (5.50) | Anorexia | 1 (1.1%) |
| GAF-F (0–100) | 57.54 (9.96) | Bulimia | 2 (2.2%) |
| Age at OCD onset | 15.47 (6.55) | ADHD | 1 (1.1%) |
| Years with OCD | 16.12 (10.40) | | |

*Note: GAF* general assessment of functioning, *GAD* generalized anxiety disorder, *BDD* body dysmorphic disorder, *ADHD* attention deficit hyperactivity disorder

prohibited during and after the 4-day treatment. Patients were not receiving other treatment during the treatment period.

### Preparing the patients for treatment

In order to ensure standardized information, patients received written information and watched a video presenting the outline of the 4-day treatment https://www.youtube.com/watch?v=nqx8knpy3i4 as well as a 6 minute description of the treatment made in 2014 by and broadcasted on Norwegian national TV (NRK) https://www.youtube.com/watch?v=ZRSExyZ3GPg. After accepting the treatment offer, they watched the following video describing the 4-day treatment in more detail https://www.youtube.com/watch?v=1Fnxt0_ljpY&t=1s.

The patients' expectations of treatment outcome and evaluation of the treatment credibility, were assessed with an adapted version of the Borkovec and Nau [16] *Reaction to treatment scale* (0–100%). A score below 100% on any of the four questions was taken as an opportunity to clarify possible misunderstandings. The patients were instructed to suggest exposure tasks, and as guidance they were told that "exposures that their OCD would appreciate the least" often were the most relevant. During the week before treatment, the group leader (see below) called each patient and performed a standard interview, focusing on clarifying possible misunderstandings and ensuring that the patients understood that they were required to prepare exposure tasks.

### Staffing the groups

In order to be able to treat 100 patients, two time slots were selected with eight groups of six patients in each. Therapists from 22 different OCD-teams in Norway wanted to participate, as well as a Scandinavian-speaking American colleague and three Icelandic psychologists. Therapists with the most extensive OCD-experience were given priority, as were therapists from teams that would be able to participate in both time-slots. When possible, the groups were staffed with 50% of qualified 4-day therapists, or therapists with at least one prior experience with the 4-day treatment. In order to qualify as a 4-day therapist he or she must have participated in a minimum of two 4-day groups and demonstrated competency in the exposure procedure evaluated independently by two 4-day experts. All group leaders had acted as therapists in minimum of six groups. In the Oslo case, group leaders did not have responsibility for a given patient, but rather was responsible to ensure that all therapists and patients received the necessary supervision, intervention, and assistance. In each group, one of the therapists also acted as "second in command". Furthermore, each group had a person taking care of the logistics. In total, 66 therapists (including group leader) participated, 61 of them twice, and 44 of them without prior experience with the 4-day format.

### Preparing the therapists for the 4-day treatment and logistic

Groups were scheduled from Tuesday to Friday, and therapists met the day before for 8 hours in preparation, including introduction to the psychoeducation and a detailed outline of the 4-day treatment, given by the developers, Bjarne Hansen (BH) and Gerd Kvale (GK). Prior to this, all therapists received the same introduction to the 4-day treatment as the patients. The therapists also received all relevant information regarding their patients. GK and BH had daily meetings with each group leader and "second in command" to ensure that potential challenges were dealt with in accordance with the 4-day protocol.

Groups were located at different places at the OUH, minimizing external disturbances related to the number of parallel groups. Also, a centrally located "control center" led by GK and BH and staffed with support personnel was established.

### Treatment

The first of the 4 days (approximately 3 h) was allocated to psychoeducation and to prepare individual exposure tasks. The two middle days were dedicated to individually tailored and therapist assisted exposure training (8–10 h each day) in a wide range of OCD-relevant settings.

The main feature of the 4-day treatment is to teach the patients to actively approach whatever elicits the relevant anxiety or discomfort, and to help them systematically use the anxiety and discomfort as a cue to "LEan into The anxiety" (LET-technique) instead of employing obvious or subtle avoidance. Typically, the therapist serves as a coach in the beginning, gradually leaving more responsibility to the patients. The therapists work as a team, which means that the patients are not necessarily working with the same therapist during the 2 days of exposure (see below). Rather, the team leaders allocate and reallocate therapists (during frequent and brief team-meetings) to ensure that the patients who are struggling are assisted by the most experienced therapists.

The exposures were interspaced with brief group meetings where each participant reported on how they were doing, especially on how they were practicing the LET-technique. The patients had individual exposure tasks for the afternoon and evenings, and reported progression back to the therapist with the last contact typically being at 9 p.m. Relatives and friends were invited to a psycho-educative meeting (one for each group) in the afternoon of day 3. The last day "lessons learnt" were summarized and plans for the next 3 weeks of self-administered exposures were made. The patients were informed how to contact the health care provider if an emergency situation should occur. The next 3 weeks, the patients were encouraged to report online every day on how they were practicing the LET-technique. The clinicians read the reports, without being in contact with the patients.

Three months after treatment, patients were invited to an individual session (30 min, conducted by the Oslo team) where their experiences in the period following treatment were discussed, and the principles of the LET-technique repeated. No exposure work was conducted in this session.

## Measures

*Yale-Brown Obsessive Compulsive Scale, Y-BOCS*; [17, 18] a semi-structured clinical interview that consists of 10 items (each 0–4) covering the severity of both obsessions and compulsions, and is a standard approach to assess OCD severity. The psychometric properties of the interview are well established. Y-BOCS has been found to be sensitive to change after treatment (e.g., 8).

*Patient Health Questionnaire-9, PHQ-9*; [19] is a frequently used self-administered screening instrument consisting of nine questions each rated on a 0–3 scale. A score of 10 or more is indicative of a depressive disorder [20]. The psychometric properties of the instrument are sound [20].

*Generalized Anxiety Disorder scale, GAD-7*; [20] is a self-administered screening instrument for symptoms of generalized anxiety consisting of seven items each rated on a 0–3 scale. The psychometric properties for the instrument are good [20].

## Benchmarking

As is customary in effectiveness studies we compared the mean Y-BOCS score and remission rate of the present sample and the average for published effectiveness studies on ERP. In order to do a fair comparison, we selected studies that had short-term follow-up assessment (3–6 months post-treatment) as in the present study, and used any format of ERP. The following studies were included in the benchmarking analysis [21, 22, 23–25] comprising a total of 381 patients fulfilling DSM-IV criteria for OCD.

## Statistical analyses

Statistical analyses were performed with SPSS version 24.0. Repeated measures ANOVA for Y-BOCS was conducted using pre-treatment, post-treatment, and follow-up scores. Effect sizes were calculated with Cohen's $d$, defined as (Mpre – Mpost)/SDpre.

Treatment response was calculated based on the international consensus criteria [26] which requires a $\geq$ 35% reduction of the individual patient's pre-treatment Y-BOCS score in order to be classified as a *clinically relevant response*. A patient is classified as *remitted* if the post-treatment Y-BOCS score is $\leq$12 points. For Y-BOCS scores there were no missing data at pre-treatment, whereas data were missing for four patients at post-treatment and 12 at follow-up. For PHQ-9 one case was missing at pre-treatment and 10 at post-treatment. For GAD-7 there were 2 patients with missing data at pre-treatment and 10 at post-treatment. Missing data were replaced using the expectation-maximization method of SPSS, version 24. The method was chosen to allow for repeated measures ANOVA. All data presented are an integrated part of the 4-day standard quality control procedure.

## Results
### Primary measures

Table 2 displays the results for Y-BOCS at pre-treatment, post-treatment, and 3-month follow-up. Repeated measures ANOVA (Wilks' Lambda) found a significant effect of time, $F(2) = 428.94$, $p < .001$, partial Eta squared = .91. Mauchly's test of sphericity was not significant ($p = .263$). A large effect size was observed with a Cohen's $d$ of 4.6 both at post-treatment and at follow-up. There were no significant changes in symptoms from post-treatment to follow-up assessment ($p = .82$).

**Table 2** Means, standard deviations and effect sizes (Cohen's *d*) for symptoms of OCD, anxiety, and depression

|          | M     | SD   | *d*  |
|----------|-------|------|------|
| Y-BOCS   |       |      |      |
| Pre      | 26.16 | 3.37 |      |
| Post     | 10.54 | 4.61 | 4.63 |
| 3 months | 10.68 | 6.31 | 4.59 |
| GAD-7    |       |      |      |
| Pre      | 11.88 | 4.88 |      |
| Post     | 8.80  | 4.49 | 0.63 |
| PHQ-9    |       |      |      |
| Pre      | 11.75 | 5.36 |      |
| Post     | 8.34  | 4.59 | 0.64 |

*Note: N = 90. d = (Mpre – Mpost)/SDpre*

### Clinically significant change in OCD-severity

At post-treatment, 91.1% of the patients had responded (≥35% improvement) and 72.2% were in remission (≥35% reduction and Y-BOCS score of ≤12). At 3-month follow-up, 84.4% had responded, and 67.8% were in remission.

Table 3 shows the clinical improvement at post-treatment and 3-month follow-up for the individual patients. Of the 65 patients who were in remission at post-treatment, 51 patients (78.5%) were classified as in remission at follow-up. Of the 17 patients who were classified as responders at post-treatment, 6 had become remitted at follow-up, 9 remained as a responder whereas 2 had deteriorated to the category of no change. Of the 8 patients who were classified as unchanged at post-treatment, 4 were in remission at follow-up, and 4 remained unchanged.

Clinically significant change was also calculated for the two severity subgroups. For the moderate subgroup, 76.2% were classified as remitted at post-treatment and 23.8% showed no change. At follow-up 81.0% were remitted, 4.8% responded, and 14.3% showed no change. For the severe/extreme subgroup; 71.0% were remitted at post-treatment while 24.6% responded, and 4.3% showed no change. At follow-up 63.8% were remitted, 20.3% responded, and 15.9% showed no change.

**Table 3** Comparison of clinical improvement rates at post-treatment and follow-up

|           | 3 months follow-up |           |           |       |
|-----------|--------------------|-----------|-----------|-------|
|           | Remission          | Responded | Unchanged | Total |
| Post      |                    |           |           |       |
| Remission | 51                 | 6         | 8         | 65    |
| Responded | 6                  | 9         | 2         | 17    |
| Unchanged | 4                  | 0         | 4         | 8     |
| Total     | 61                 | 15        | 14        | 90    |

Remission rates at post-treatment were not significantly different between the two severity subgroups, $\chi^2$ (1) = 0.22, *p* = .64. The same was true at follow-up, $\chi^2$ (1) = 2.18, *p* = .14.

### Depression and generalized anxiety

There were also significant decreases in symptoms of depression and generalized anxiety from pre- to post-treatment, equal to moderate effect sizes of .64 and .63 respectively (see Table 4).

### Comparison with our previous studies

Table 5 shows a comparison of the Y-BOCS data between the present study and our previous three studies [3–5] carried out in Bergen. The present sample of OCD-patients starts at the same severity level as the previous samples and has very similar post-treatment and 3-month follow-up results. There are no significant differences on Y-BOCS between the present and the previous samples at any time point.

### Benchmarking

Table 6 shows the comparison between the present sample and standard ERP from published uncontrolled effectiveness studies. The Oslo patients, treated with the Bergen 4-day treatment, had a significantly higher mean Y-BOCS score at pre-treatment. However, both at post-treatment and at 3-month follow-up their means were significantly lower than the average for the published effectiveness studies. The remission rate was also significantly higher for the Oslo patients than for the patients in the effectiveness studies.

### Discussion

The joint effort to erase the waiting list of more than 100 OCD-patients at Oslo University Hospital during 8 days worked well. In comparison, during the entire year of 2016 OUH was able to treat 70 patients. Ninety-one percent of the 90 patients treated with the 4-day format responded at post-treatment, and 68% were in remission at three-month follow-up.

**Table 4** Severity of anxiety and depression at pre-treatment, post-treatment, and 3-months follow-up

|          | GAD-7       |             | PHQ-9       |             |
|----------|-------------|-------------|-------------|-------------|
| Severity | Pre         | Post        | Pre         | Post        |
| None     | 5 (5.6%)    | 13 (14.4%)  | 6 (6.7%)    | 15 (16.7%)  |
| Mild     | 22 (24.4%)  | 43 (47.8%)  | 25 (27.8%)  | 42 (46.7%)  |
| Moderate | 37 (41.1%)  | 24 (26.7%)  | 32 (35.6%)  | 25 (27.8%)  |
| Severe   | 26 (28.9%)  | 10 (11.1%)  | 27 (30.0%)  | 8 (8.9%)    |

*Note: Pre Pre-treatment, Post Post-treatment. Cut-offs used for both GAD-7 and PHQ-9 were 0–4 (none), 5–9 (mild), 10–14 (moderate), 15 and above (severe)*

**Table 5** Comparison the 4-day treatment studies on Y-BOCS scores (M and SD)

| Study | | | | |
|---|---|---|---|---|
| Time point | Havnen (2014) | Havnen (2017) | Hansen (2018) | Present study |
| N: | 35 | 42 | 65 | 90 |
| Pre | 26.1 (4.3) | 25.7 (4.3) | 25.8 (4.7) | 26.2 (3.4) |
| Post | 9.0 (4.8) | 10.8 (3.9) | 10.2 (5.1) | 10.5 (4.6) |
| 3 months | 10.6 (7.0) | — | 10.5 (5.9) | 10.7 (6.3) |
| 6 months | 10.3 (5.7) | 12.2 (6.4) | — | — |
| 1 year | — | — | 10.6 (7.0) | — |
| 4 years | 9.9 (7.4) | | | |

*Note*: The 4-year time point pertain to the combination of the Havnen et al. 2014 and 2017 studies

The results from Oslo are basically the same as reported on the 4-day format in our previous effectiveness studies [3–5]. Furthermore, we have documented that the changes are maintained at 1-year follow-up [5] and at 4-year follow-up [27]. Compared to standard ERP treatment approaches, the 4-day format has a number of potential advantages. It has a low declining rate and attrition rate. Moreover, this treatment may have a significantly larger response rate and remission rate at post-treatment compared to standard ERP in effectiveness studies.

In the present study we demonstrated that we were able to upscale, and to help 90 moderately to severely affected OCD-patients in 8 days; 45 in each 4-day slot. This was done as a part of the public mental health care, with no selection of patients.

The 4-day format is often labelled "individual treatment in a group setting" indicating that the ratio between therapists and patients is 1:1. Basically, this means that each therapist is able to treat one patient in less than a week, which probably is highly cost-effective. All the participating therapists were experienced in treating patients with OCD using CBT, but 67% of them had

**Table 6** Comparison between the Bergen 4-day treatment and standard ERP in effectiveness studies

| | Bergen 4-day | | Effectiveness | | Statistic |
|---|---|---|---|---|---|
| | N | M (SD) | N | M (SD) | t-test (p) |
| Y-BOCS | | | | | |
| Pre | 90 | 26.2 (3.4) | 381 | 24.4 (5.4) | 3.02 (=.0026) |
| Post | 90 | 10.5 (4.6) | 374 | 18.2 (7.0) | 9.93 (<.0001) |
| 3 months | 90 | 10.7 (6.3) | 317 | 16.2 (8.1) | 5.95 (<.0001) |
| Remission | | | | | Fisher's test |
| Post | 90 | 72.2% | 110 | 35.5% | p < .0001 |
| 3 months | 90 | 67.8% | 110 | 45.5% | p = .0017 |

*Note*: Data for effectiveness studies were taken from uncontrolled studies of ERP having 3–6 month follow-up. N indicates the total number of participants across these studies. Remission was calculated as ≥35% reduction of pre-treatment Y-BOCS scores and ≤ 12 on post and follow-up Y-BOCS

previously not worked with the 4-day format and the clear majority of the therapists had never worked together before. Since each group is staffed with as many therapists as patients, the format serves as a good opportunity to work side-by-side with, and observe experienced 4-day therapists, and to get hands-on supervision. While model learning with hands-on supervision is an obvious approach for physicians who are going to learn surgery or any other medical discipline, it is rare in the mental health care. It is a unique experience to be able to observe six patients with OCD going through major changes in only 4 days. After the Oslo experience, all teams involved have asked to be fully trained in order to deliver the 4-day format.

There are different limitations of the current study. Evaluations of this treatment format has so far only been tested using open trial designs, which do not compare the effect of treatment with other established treatments or placebo control. A RCT is necessary to draw definitive conclusions about the efficacy and specificity of the 4-day treatment. Also, participants had not previously received evidence based treatment for OCD. This could limit generalizability of the findings. However, the present study was aimed at ordinary OCD-patients, not those who are treatment resistant. The study design and study population could be possible explanations for the good results. Another possible explanation is that the current concentrated format is different from that used in previous studies of concentrated treatment. They have used daily sessions of 90–120 min across 3–4 weeks, while we used 4 days and 3–8 h sessions. Longer sessions in highly concentrated ERP could yield better effects than standard ERP. Another issue concerns missing data as 13% of participants did not provide data at follow-up.

The present study tentatively indicates that the 4-day treatment can yield good outcome at another site than the originators' place of work. Whether it works as well for other research groups and in other countries remains to be tested in future studies. However, the treatment is currently being tested in Iceland and an uncontrolled pilot study [28] obtained equally good effects as the original studies in Norway [3–5].

This approach has been developed as an integrated part of the specialist health care with severely affected patients and with virtually no bias in the selection of cases that are offered the treatment. Since clinical changes that are achieved during a very brief window of time are large, seen in a large majority of patients, and to a large extent are maintained at follow-up, we argue that the 4-day treatment might offer a unique longitudinal and nearly experimental approach to study basic mechanisms of brain plasticity. Because no other factors apart from treatment are of influence during the 4 days of intervention, it is an ideal setting for studies using functional magnetic resonance brain imaging (fMRI) or biomarkers of e.g. epigenetic changes to elucidate functional and structural changes on a number of different explanatory levels [29, 30]. This is an interesting area for future research which should be pursued.

## Conclusions
In sum, the Bergen 4-day treatment for OCD showed promising results. Future studies should test this treatment format using a RCT design.

## Abbreviations
DSM: Diagnostic and statistical manual of mental disorders; ERP: Exposure and response prevention; fMRI: Functional magnetic resonance imaging; GAD-7: Generalized Anxiety Disorder-7; LET: Lean into The anxiety; OCD: Obsessive-compulsive disorder; OUH: Oslo University Hospital; PHQ-9: Patient health questionnaire-9; SCID: Structured clinical interview; Y-BOCS: Yale-Brown obsessive-compulsive scale

## Acknowledgments
The authors would like to thank all participants in the study as well as therapists and the assessment team.

## Authors' contributions
GK and BH designed the study. KH, SS, and L-GÖ conducted statistical analyses. GK, BH, KH, ThB, TB, SH, UBK, and GL supervised the treatment. AS represented the OCD patient organization and helped with planning and organizing the study. KJR and OAH helped with interpretation and revising the manuscript. All authors participated with drafting and revising the manuscript.

## Consent for publication
Not applicable.

## Competing interests
The authors declare that they have no competing interests.

## Author details
[1]Haukeland University Hospital, OCD-team, 5021 Bergen, Norway. [2]Department of Clinical Psychology, University of Bergen, Bergen, Norway. [3]McLean Hospital, Belmont, MA, USA. [4]Harvard Medical School, Boston, MA, USA. [5]Molde Hospital, Molde, Norway. [6]Nidaros DPS, Division of Psychiatry, St. Olav University Hospital, Trondheim, Norway. [7]Oslo University Hospital, Oslo, Norway. [8]Sørlandet Sykehus, Kristiansand, Norway. [9]Department of Psychology, Norwegian University of Science and Technology, Trondheim, Norway. [10]Norwegian OCD-foundation, Ananke, Oslo, Norway. [11]Department of Psychiatry and Department of Anatomy & Neurosciences, VU university medical center (VUmc), Amsterdam, The Netherlands. [12]Department of Psychology, Stockholm University, Stockholm, Sweden.

## References
1. Kvale G, Hansen B. Dissemination and intensifying evidence-based treatment for OCD: Norway is in the lead. Nordic Psychiat. 2014;3(1):14–5.
2. Foa EB, Yadin E, Lichner TK. Exposure and response prevention for OCD: therapist guide. London: Oxford University Press; 2012.
3. Havnen A, Hansen B, Öst L-G, Kvale G. Concentrated ERP delivered in a group setting: an effectiveness study. J Obsessive-Compulsive Relat Disord. 2014;3(4):319–24 https://doi.org/10.1016/j.jocrd.2014.08.002.
4. Havnen A, Hansen B, Öst LG, Kvale G. Concentrated ERP delivered in a group setting: a replication study. Behav Cogn Psychother. 2017;45(5):1–7 https://doi.org/10.1017/S1352465817000091.
5. Hansen B, Hagen K, Öst L-G, Solem S, Kvale G. The Bergen 4-day OCD treatment delivered in a group setting: 12-month follow-up. Front Psychol. 2018;9:369 https://doi.org/10.3389/fpsyg.2018.00639.
6. Franklin ME, Abramowitz JS, Kozak MJ, Levitt J, Foa EB. Effectiveness of exposure and ritual prevention for obsessive-compulsive disorder: randomized compared with nonrandomized samples. J Consult Clin Psychol. 2000;68:594–602. https://doi.org/10.1037/0022-006X.68.4.594.
7. Abramowitz JS, Tolin DF, Diefenbach GJ. Measuring change in OCD: sensitivity of the obsessive-compulsive scale-revised. J Psychopathol Behav Assess. 2005;27:317–24. https://doi.org/10.1017/s10862-005-2411-y.
8. Hiss H, Foa EB, Kozak MJ. Relapse prevention program for treatment of obsessive-compulsive disorder. J Consult Clin Psychol. 1994;62(4):801–8 https://doi.org/10.1037/0022-006X.62.4.801.
9. Lindsay M, Crino R, Andrews G. Controlled trial of exposure and response prevention in obsessive-compulsive disorder. Br J Psychiat. 1997;171:135–9 https://doi.org/10.1192/bjp.171.2.135.
10. Abramowitz JS, Foa EB, Franklin ME. Exposure and ritual prevention for obsessive-compulsive disorder: effects of intensive versus twice-weekly sessions. J Consult Clin Psychol. 2003;71(2):394–8 http://psycnet.apa.org/doi/10.1037/0022-006X.71.2.394.
11. Storch EA, Merlo LJ, Lehmkuhl H, Geffken GR, Jacob M, Ricketts E, Murphy TK, Goodman WK. Cognitive-behavioral therapy for obsessive-compulsive disorder: a non-randomized comparison of intensive and weekly approaches. J Anxiety Disord. 2008;22:1146–52 https://doi.org/10.1016/j.janxdis.2007.12.001.
12. Öst L-G, Havnen A, Hansen B, Kvale G. Cognitive behavioral treatments of obsessive-compulsive disorder. A systematic review and meta-analysis of studies published 1993-2014. Clin Psychol Rev. 2015;40:156–69 https://doi.org/10.1016/j.cpr.2015.06.003.
13. Barlow D, Nock MK, Hersen M. Single case experimental designs: strategies for studying behavior change (3rd ed.). Boston, MA: Pearson; 2009.
14. American Psychiatric Association. Diagnostic and statistical manual of mental disorders. 5th ed. Washington, DC: American Psychiatric Publishing; 2013.
15. Sheehan DV, Lecrubier Y, Sheehan KH, Amorim P, Janavs J, Weiller E, et al. The mini-international neuropsychiatric interview (M.I.N.I.): the development and validation of a structured diagnostic psychiatric interview for DSM-IV and ICD-10. J Clin Psychiat. 1998;59(Suppl. 20):22–33.
16. Borkovec TD, Nau SD. Credibility of analogue therapy rationales. J Behav Ther Exp Psychiatry. 1972;3(4):257–60 https://doi.org/10.1016/0005-7916(72)90045-6.
17. Goodman WK, Price LH, Rasmussen SA, Mazure C, Delgado P, Heninger GR, et al. The Yale-Brown obsessive compulsive scale. II. Validity. Arch Gen Psychiatry. 1989;46(11):1012–6 https://doi.org/10.1001/archpsyc.1989.01810110054008.
18. Goodman WK, Price LH, Rasmussen SA, Mazure C, Fleischmann RL, Hill CL, et al. The Yale-Brown obsessive compulsive scale. I. Development, use, and reliability. Arch Gen Psychiatry. 1989;46(11):1006–11 https://doi.org/10.1001/archpsyc.1989.01810110048007.
19. Kroenke K, Spitzer RL, Williams JB, Lowe B. The patient health questionnaire somatic, anxiety, and depressive symptom scales: a systematic review. Gen Hosp Psychiatry. 2010;32(4):345–59 https://doi.org/10.1016/j.genhosppsych.2010.03.00614.

20. Spitzer RL, Kroenke K, Williams JB, Lowe B. A brief measure for assessing generalized anxiety disorder: the GAD-7. Arch Int Med. 2006;166(10):1092–7 https://doi.org/10.1001/archinte.166.10.1092.

21. Boschen MJ, Drummond LM. Community treatment of severe, refractory obsessive-compulsive disorder. Behav Res Ther. 2012;50(3):203–9. https://doi.org/10.1016/j.brat.2012.01.002.

22. Håland ÅT, Vogel PA, Lie B, Launes G, Pripp AH, Himle JA. (2010). Behavioural group therapy for obsessive-compulsive disorder in Norway. An open community-based trial. Behav. Res. Ther. 2010;48(6):547–54. https://doi.org/10.1016/j.brat.2010.03.005.

23. Himle JA, Rassi S, Haghigthatgou H, Krone KP, Nesse RM, Abelson J. Group behavioral therapy of obsessive-compulsive disorder: seven-vs. twelve-week outcomes. Depress Anxiety. 2001;13(4):161–5 https://doi.org/10.1002/(ISSN)1520-6394.

24. Tolin DF, Maltby N, Diefenbach GJ, Hannan SE, Worhunsky P. Cognitive–behavioral therapy for medication nonresponders with obsessive–compulsive disorder. a wait-list-controlled open trial J Clin Psychiat. 2004;65(7):922–31 https://doi.org/10.4088/JCP.v65n0708.

25. Tolin DF, Hannan S, Maltby N, Diefenbach GJ, Worhunsky P, Brady RE. A randomized controlled trial of self-directed versus therapist-directed cognitive-behavioral therapy for obsessive-compulsive disorder patients with prior medication trials. Behav Ther. 2007;38:179–91 https://doi.org/10.1016/j.beth.2006.07.001.

26. Mataix-Cols D, Fernandez dela Cruz L, Nordsletten AE, Lenhard F, Isomura K, Simpson HB. Towards an international expert consensus for defining treatment response, remission, recovery and relapse in obsessive-compulsive disorder. World Psychiatry. 2016;15(1):80–1 https://doi.org/10.1002/wps.20299.

27. Hansen B, Kvale G, Hagen K, Havnen A, Öst L-G. The Bergen 4-day format for OCD: four years follow-up of concentrated ERP in a clinical mental health setting. Cogn Behav Ther. in press. https://doi.org/10.1080/16506073.2018.1478447.

28. Davíðsdóttir SD, Sigurjónsdóttir O, Ludvigsdóttir SJ, Hansen B, Laukvik IL, Hagen K, Björgvinsson T, Kvale G. Implementation of the Bergen 4-day treatment for OCD in Iceland. Clin Neuropsychiatry. in press. http://www.clinicalneuropsychiatry.org/.

29. Thorsen AL, van den Heuvel OA, Hansen B, Kvale G. Neuroimaging of psychotherapy for obsessive-compulsive disorder: a systematic review. Psychiatry Res Neuroimaging 2015;233(3):306–313: https://doi.org/10.1016/j.comppsych.2016.11.011.

30. van den Heuvel OA, van Wingen G, Soriano-Mas C, Alonso P, Chamberlain SR, Nakamae T, et al. Brain circuitry of compulsivity. Eur Neuropsychopharmacol. 2016;26(5):810–27 https://doi.org/10.1016/j.euroneuro.2015.12.005.

# 9

# Application of the ICD-11 classification of personality disorders

Bo Bach[1*] and Michael B First[2]

## Abstract

**Background:** The ICD-11 classification of Personality Disorders focuses on core personality dysfunction, while allowing the practitioner to classify three levels of severity (Mild Personality Disorder, Moderate Personality Disorder, and Severe Personality Disorder) and the option of specifying one or more prominent trait domain qualifiers (Negative Affectivity, Detachment, Disinhibition, Dissociality, and Anankastia). Additionally, the practitioner is also allowed to specify a Borderline Pattern qualifier. This article presents how the ICD-11 Personality Disorder classification may be applied in clinical practice using five brief cases.

**Case presentation:** (1) a 29-year-old woman with Severe Personality Disorder, Borderline Pattern, and prominent traits of Negative Affectivity, Disinhibition, and Dissociality; (2) a 36-year-old man with Mild Personality Disorder, and prominent traits of Negative Affectivity and Detachment; (3) a 26-year-old man with Severe Personality Disorder, and prominent traits of Dissociality, Disinhibition, and Detachment; (4) a 19-year-old woman with Personality Difficulty, and prominent traits of Negative Affectivity and Anankastia; (5) a 53-year-old man with Moderate Personality Disorder, and prominent traits of Anankastia and Dissociality.

**Conclusions:** The ICD-11 Personality Disorder classification was applicable to five clinical cases, which were classified according to Personality Disorder severity and trait domain qualifiers. We propose that the classification of severity may help inform clinical prognosis and intensity of treatment, whereas the coding of trait qualifiers may help inform the focus and style of treatment. Empirical investigation of such important aspects of clinical utility are warranted.

**Keywords:** ICD-11, Classification, Personality disorder, Severity, Trait

## Background

Personality Disorder is important to all health care practitioners because it is a prevalent condition that applies to approximately 12% of the general community [1], 25% of primary care patients [2], and at least 50% of psychiatric outpatients [3]. This potentially complicates the relationship between patients and health care professionals, increases the risk of premature mortality, and results in a huge cost to society [4]. However, research highlights significant problems with the ICD-10 and DSM-IV/DSM-5 categorical approaches to Personality Disorder diagnostics, including arbitrary diagnostic thresholds, extensive overlap among categories, lack of evidence for 10 distinct categories, and insufficient clinical utility [4–6]. In

comparison to the assessment of other mental disorders, assessment of Personality Disorders is more difficult in routine clinical practice. Reviewing the 79 DSM criteria for 10 disorders (plus 15 criteria of conduct disorder) is cumbersome and requires specialized training. In response to these shortcomings, the 11th edition of the International Classification of Diseases (ICD-11) adopts a dimensional approach to the classification of Personality Disorders that focuses on global level of severity and five trait qualifiers [7]. The present article aims to introduce and illustrate how the ICD-11 Personality Disorder classification may be applied in clinical practice using five brief cases with different diagnostic features.

### Rationale of the ICD-11 classification of personality disorders

The ICD-11 nomenclature for Personality Disorders [8] focuses on the impairment of self and interpersonal personality functioning, which may be classified according to

* Correspondence: bbpn@regionsjaelland.dk; bobachsayad@gmail.com
[1]Center of Excellence on Personality Disorder, Psychiatric Research Unit, Region Zealand, Slagelse Psychiatric Hospital, Fælledvej 6, Bygning 3, 4200 Slagelse, Denmark
Full list of author information is available at the end of the article

degree of severity ("Personality Difficulty", "Mild Personality Disorder", "Moderate Personality Disorder", and "Severe Personality Disorder"). Furthermore, the diagnosis may also be specified with one or more prominent trait qualifiers (Negative Affectivity, Detachment, Dissociality, Disinhibition, and Anankastia), which contribute to the impairment in personality functioning. Unlike the polythetic ICD-10 criteria for Personality Disorders (e.g., five out of nine criteria) which set the disorder/non-disorder threshold based on the number of criteria that are met, the ICD-11 diagnostic requirements for Personality Disorders base the diagnosis on a global evaluation of personality functioning. Given that personality functioning might be impaired in various ways, the trait qualifiers are available to describe the specific pattern of traits that contribute to the global personality dysfunction. The general diagnostic requirements for Personality Disorder are presented in Table 1, the guidelines for determination of the level of severity are presented in Tables 2, 3 and 4 and the five trait domain qualifiers are elucidated in Table 5. In addition to specifying Personality Disorder severity and stylistic trait qualifiers, the user is also allowed to code substhreshold Personality Difficulty and a Borderline Pattern qualifier (see Table 6).

As shown in Table 2 and 3, the classification of severity aligns with the psychodynamic tradition of personality organization [9, 10] as well as scientifically valid models of core Personality Disorder features [11–15]. Importantly, research shows that much of the predictive and prognostic value in Personality Disorder assessment can be derived from such a core dimension [13, 16]. A classification according to severity

**Table 1** General diagnostic requirements

• An enduring disturbance characterized by problems in functioning of aspects of the self (e.g., identity, self-worth, accuracy of self-view, self-direction), and/or interpersonal dysfunction (e.g., ability to develop and maintain close and mutually satisfying relationships, ability to understand others' perspectives and to manage conflict in relationships).
• The disturbance has persisted over an extended period of time (> 2 years).
• The disturbance is manifest in patterns of cognition, emotional experience, emotional expression, and behaviour that are maladaptive (e.g., inflexible or poorly regulated).
• The disturbance is manifest across a range of personal and social situations (i.e., is not limited to specific relationships or social roles), though it may be consistently evoked by particular types of circumstances but not others.
• The patterns of behaviour characterizing the disturbance are not developmentally appropriate and cannot be explained primarily by social or cultural factors, including socio-political conflict.
• The symptoms are not due to the direct effects of a medication or substance, including withdrawal effects, and are not better explained by another Mental and Behavioural Disorder, a Disease of the Nervous System, or another health condition.
• The disturbance is associated with substantial distress or significant impairment in personal, family, social, educational, occupational or other important areas of functioning.

*Note.* Adapted from the ICD-11 Clinical Descriptions and Diagnostic Guidelines for Personality Disorder.

**Table 2** Aspects of personality functioning that contribute to severity determination in Personality Disorder

Degree and pervasiveness of disturbances in functioning of aspects of the self:
• Stability and coherence of one's sense of identity (e.g., extent to which identity or sense of self is variable and inconsistent or overly rigid and fixed).
• Ability to maintain an overall positive and stable sense of self-worth.
• Accuracy of one's view of one's characteristics, strengths, limitations.
• Capacity for self-direction (ability to plan, choose, and implement appropriate goals).

Degree and pervasiveness of interpersonal dysfunction across various contexts and relationships (e.g., romantic relationships, school/work, parent-child, family, friendships, peer contexts):
• Interest in engaging in relationships with others.
• Ability to understand and appreciate others' perspectives.
• Ability to develop and maintain close and mutually satisfying relationships.
• Ability to manage conflict in relationships.

Pervasiveness, severity, and chronicity of emotional, cognitive, and behavioral manifestations of the personality dysfunction:
Emotional manifestations
   ○ Range and appropriateness of emotional experience and expression.
   ○ Tendency to be emotionally over- or underreactive.
   ○ Ability to recognize and acknowledge unwanted emotions (e.g., anger, sadness).
Cognitive manifestations
   ○ Accuracy of situational and interpersonal appraisals, especially under stress.
   ○ Ability to make appropriate decisions in situations of uncertainty.
   ○ Appropriate stability and flexibility of belief systems.
Behavioural manifestations
   ○ Flexibility in controlling impulses and modulating behaviour based on the situation and consideration of the consequences.
   ○ Appropriateness of behavioural responses to intense emotions and stressful circumstances (e.g., propensity to self-harm or violence).

The extent to which the dysfunctions in the above areas are associated with distress or impairment in personal, family, social, educational, occupational or other important areas of functioning.

*Note.* Adapted from the ICD-11 Clinical Descriptions and Diagnostic Guidelines for Personality Disorder

also provides information for guiding intensity of clinical management and treatment [10, 17, 18].

Finally, as shown in Table 5, the deliniation of five trait domain qualifiers aligns with other empirically-derived dimensional schemes, including the cross-culturally replicated Five-Factor Model [19–21] and the DSM-5 Alternative Model of Personality Disorders [22–24]. The ICD-11 trait domain qualifiers not only provide scientifically sound and homogenous building blocks of personality psychopathology but also clinical information for selecting type and focus of treatment [25–28].

## Application of the ICD-11 model in clinical practice

At a basic level, the ICD-11 classification allows the clinician the option of rapid assessment of personality functioning. As such, a practitioner should be able first

**Table 3** Essential features of Personality Disorder severity

| Mild Personality Disorder | Moderate Personality Disorder | Severe Personality Disorder |
|---|---|---|
| Disturbances affect some areas of personality functioning but not others (e.g., problems with self-direction in the absence of problems with stability and coherence of identity or self-worth; see Table 2), and may not be apparent in some contexts. | Disturbances affect multiple areas of personality functioning (e.g., identity or sense of self, ability to form intimate relationships, ability to control impulses and modulate behaviour; see Table 2). However, some areas of personality functioning may be relatively less affected. | There are severe disturbances in functioning of the self (e.g., sense of self may be so unstable that individuals report not having a sense of who they are or so rigid that they refuse to participate in any but an extremely narrow range of situations; self view may be characterized by self-contempt or be grandiose or highly eccentric; see Table 2). |
| There are problems in many interpersonal relationships and/or in performance of expected occupational and social roles, but some relationships are maintained and/or some roles carried out. | There are marked problems in most interpersonal relationships and the performance of most expected social and occupational roles are compromised to some degree. Relationships are likely to be characterized by conflict, avoidance, withdrawal, or extreme dependency (e.g., few friendships maintained, persistent conflict in work relationships and consequent occupational problems, romantic relationships characterized by serious disruption or inappropriate submissiveness). | Problems in interpersonal functioning seriously affect virtually all relationships and the ability and willingness to perform expected social and occupational roles is absent or severely compromised. |
| Specific manifestations of personality disturbances are generally of mild severity (see examples in Table 4). | Specific manifestations of personality disturbance are generally of moderate severity (see examples in Table 4). | Specific manifestations of personality disturbance are severe (see examples in Table 4) and affect most, if not all, areas of personality functioning. |
| Is typically not associated with substantial harm to self or others. | Is sometimes associated with harm to self or others. | Is often associated with harm to self or others. |
| May be associated with substantial distress or with impairment in personal, family, social, educational, occupational or other important areas of functioning that is either limited to circumscribed areas (e.g., romantic relationships; employment) or present in more areas but milder. | Is associated with marked impairment in personal, family, social, educational, occupational or other important areas of functioning, although functioning in circumscribed areas may be maintained. | Is associated with severe impairment in all or nearly all areas of life, including personal, family, social, educational, occupational, and other important areas of functioning. |

*Note.* The diagnostic guideline should be accompanied with the examples provided in Table 4. Adapted from the ICD-11 Clinical Descriptions and Diagnostic Guidelines for Personality Disorder. All five levels of personality functioning are described and exemplified in Additional file 1

to identify the presence or absence of Personality Disorder, then its severity, and, if appropriate, one or more prominent trait qualifiers that contribute to the expression of personality dysfunction. Accordingly, the procedure for classification of ICD-11 Personality Disorder is fairly similar to the procedure of diagnosing ICD-10 F32 Depressive episode which has three levels of severity (*mild, moderate,* and *severe*), and which may, if appropriate, be further qualified by additional codes for individual features. For example, F32.11 Moderate depressive episode with somatic syndrome or F32.3 Severe depressive episode with psychotic symptoms.

**Classification of personality disorder severity replaces comorbidity**
Because the ten different types of categorical Personality Disorder diagnoses no longer exist in the ICD-11 classification, the practitioner has no choice but to assess Personality Disorder itself rather than focussing the assessment on overlapping and heterogenous polythetic categories (see Tables 1 and 2) [4]. Accordingly, instead of the classification into ten types, the ICD-11 can be said to involve a subclassification into three categories of severity, which cannot

co-exist with one another (i.e., a patient cannot have a Mild Personality Disorder while also having a Severe Personality Disorder). Thus, the ICD-11 classification eradicates the excessive comorbidity characterizing the different ICD-10 Personality Disorder categories. However, the clinician still has the option of indicating the presence of a Personality Disorder without specifying its severity (i.e., "severity unspecified"). The specified severity threshold for yielding a Personality Disorder diagnosis (at least "mild" severity) is explained in Table 3 and exemplified in Table 4. Thus, the definition of "mild" severity may also be employed as a screener for presence or absence of Personality Disorder.

**The option of coding subthreshold personality difficulty**
In addition to the Personality Disorder diagnosis (in the chapter on Mental and behavioral disorders), clinicians have the option of indicating the presence of Personality Difficulty. Personality Difficulty is not considered to be a mental disorder per se, but is availble for clinical use and is located in the section of the ICD-11 classification for non-disease entities that constitute factors influencing health status and encounters with health services. Personality Difficulty is somewhat akin to the ICD-10 non-disorder category Z73.1

**Table 4** Examples of specific disturbances in personality functioning

| Mild Personality Disorder | Moderate Personality Disorder | Severe Personality Disorder |
| --- | --- | --- |
| The individual's sense of self may be somewhat contradictory and inconsistent with how others view them. | The individual's sense of self may become incoherent in times of crisis. | The individual's self-view is very unrealistic and typically is highly unstable or internally contradictory. |
| The individual has difficulty recovering from injuries to self-esteem. | The individual has considerable difficulty maintaining positive self-esteem or, alternatively, has an unrealistically positive self-view that is not modified by evidence to the contrary. | The individual has serious difficulty with regulation of self-esteem, emotional experience and expression, and impulses, as well as other aspects of behaviour (e.g., perseveration, indecision). |
| The individual's ability to set appropriate goals and to work towards them is compromised; the individual has difficulty handling even minor setbacks. | The individual exhibits poor emotion regulation in the face of setbacks, often becoming highly upset and giving up easily. Alternatively, the individual may persist unreasonably in pursuit of goals that have no chance of success. | The individual is largely unable to set and pursue realistic goals. |
| The individual may have conflicts with supervisors and co-workers, but is generally able to sustain employment. | The individual may exhibit little genuine interest in or efforts toward sustained employment. | The individual is unwilling or unable to sustain regular work due to lack of interest or effort, poor performance (e.g., failure to complete assignments or perform expected roles, unreliability), interpersonal difficulties, or inappropriate behaviour (e.g., fits of temper, insubordination). |
| The individual's limitations in the ability to understand and appreciate others' perspectives create difficulties in developing close and mutually satisfying relationships. | Major limitations in the ability to understand and appreciate others' perspectives hinder developing close and mutually satisfying relationships. | The individual's interpersonal relationships, if any, lack mutuality; are shallow, extremely one-sided, unstable, and/or highly conflictual, often to the point of violence. |
| There may be estrangement in some relationships, but relationships are more commonly characterized by intermittent or frequent, minor conflicts that are not so severe that they cause serious and long-standing disruption. Alternatively, relationships may be characterized by dependence and avoidance of conflict by giving in to others, even at some cost to themselves. | Problems in those relationships that do exist are common and persistent; may involve frequent, serious, and volatile conflict; and typically are quite one-sided (e.g., very strongly dominant or highly submissive). | Family relationships are absent (despite having living relatives) or marred by significant conflict. The individual has extreme difficulty acknowledging unwanted emotions (e.g., does not recognize or acknowledge experiencing anger, sadness, or other emotion). |
| Under stress, there may be some distortions in the individual's situational and interpersonal appraisals but reality testing remains intact. | Under stress there are marked distortions in the individual's situational and interpersonal appraisals. There may be mild dissociative states or psychotic-like beliefs or perceptions (e.g., paranoid ideas). | Under stress, there are extreme distortions in the individual's situational and interpersonal appraisals. There are often dissociative states or psychotic-like beliefs or perceptions (e.g., extreme paranoid reactions). |

*Note.* The examples should be accompanied with the diagnostic guideline provided in Table 3. Adapted from the ICD-11 Clinical Descriptions and Diagnostic Guidelines for Personality Disorder. All five levels of personality functioning are described and exemplified in Additional file 1

"accentuation of personality traits" which is a subcategory of the Z73 "Problems Related to Life-Management Difficulty" in the chapter "Factors Influencing Health Status and Contact with Health Services".

Like a Personality Disorder diagnosis, Personality Difficulty is characterized by relatively stable difficulties (e.g., at least 2 years). Such difficulties are associated with some problems in functioning which are insufficiently severe to cause notable disruption in social, occupational, and interpersonal relationships and that may be limited to specific relationships or situations. Problems with emotions, cognitions, and behaviors are only expressed intermittently (e.g., during times of stress) or at low intensity. In contrast to Mild Personality Disorder, the individual with Personality Difficulty only has some intermittent or low intensity personality-related problems (e.g., in circumscribed risk situations), but not to the extent that it compromises the individual's ability to

keep a job, initiate and maintain friendships, and have somewhat satisfactory intimate relationships.

For example, a patient with eating disorder may have personality difficulties of rigid perfectionism (i.e., Anankastia) while maintaining a strong social network and making slow but steady progress towards finishing an education. Another patient with resistant anxiety symptoms may have difficulties of anxiousness (i.e., Negative Affectivity) but otherwise be viewed as a treasured friend and collegue. In both cases, the specified patterns of Personality Difficulty reveal specific vulnerabilities. Taken together, when most appropriate a code of Personality Difficulty may be applied to the patient with noteworthy but not prominent personality problems.

### Personality trait qualifiers

One or more stylistic trait qualifiers may be coded if they are prominent in the personality makeup of the

**Table 5** Trait domain qualifiers that contribute to the expression of personality dysfunction

| Trait domain | Core definition | Specific features |
|---|---|---|
| Negative Affectivity | A tendency to experience a broad range of negative emotions with a frequency and intensity out of proportion to the situation. | Anxiety, anger, worry, fear, vulnerability, hostility, shame, depression, pessimism, guilt, low self-esteem, and mistrustfulness. For example, once upset, such individuals have difficulty regaining their composure and must rely on others or on leaving the situation to calm down. |
| Detachment | A tendency to maintain interpersonal distance (social detachment) and emotional distance (emotional detachment) | *Social detachment* including avoidance of social interactions, lack of friendships, and avoidance of intimacy. *Emotional detachment* including being reserved, aloofness, and limited emotional expression and experience. For example, such individuals seek out employment that does not involve interactions with others. |
| Dissociality | Disregard for the rights and feelings of others, encompassing both self-centeredness and lack of empathy. | *Self-centeredness* including entitlement, grandiosity, expectation of others' admiration, and attention-seeking. *Lack of empathy* including being deceptive, manipulative, exploiting, ruthless, mean, callous, and physically aggressive, while sometimes taking pleasure in others' suffering. For example, such individuals respond with anger or denigration of others when they are not granted admiration. |
| Disinhibition | A tendency to act rashly based on immediate external or internal stimuli (i.e., sensations, emotions, thoughts), without consideration of potential negative consequences. | Impulsivity, distractibility, irresponsibility, recklessness, and lack of planning. For example, such individuals may be engaged in reckless driving, dangerous sports, substance use, gambling, and unplanned sexual activity. |
| Anankastia | A narrow focus on one's rigid standard of perfection and of right and wrong, and on controlling one's own and others' behaviour and controlling situations to ensure conformity to these standards. | *Perfectionism* including concern with rules, norms of right and wrong, details, hyper-scheduling, orderliness, and neatness. *Emotional and behavioral constraint* including rigid control over emotional expression, stubbornness, risk-avoidance, perseveration, and deliberativeness. For example, such individuals may stubbornly redo the work of others because it does not meet their standards. |

*Note.* Adapted from the ICD-11 Clinical Descriptions and Diagnostic Guidelines for Personality Disorder, which include a more detailed description of the trait domain qualifiers

individual diagnosed with Personality Disorder or Personality Difficulty. Yet, it is important to recognize that the trait qualifiers are not like categories or syndromal diagnoses, but instead denote stylistic dimensions that contribute to the expression of the personality dysfunction. However, for the purpose of coding, the prominent trait qualifiers can only be indicated as present or absent even though they exist on a continuum. Essentially, the overall severity of personality dysfunction (i.e., *mild, moderate,* and *severe*) reflects the degree to which the prominent traits have an impact on the patient's self- and interpersonal functioning [29], which is illustrated in a figure for each of the five cases. Thus, Severe Personality Disorder is likely to be associated with several trait domain qualifiers, whereas Mild Personality Disorder may be associated with the presence of only one trait qualifier. In other words, complexity of trait domain qualifiers may often reflect the severity of the Personality Disorder. However, in some cases an individual may have a Severe Personality Disorder and manifest only one prominent trait qualifier (e.g., Dissociality causing severe danger towards others).

### Borderline pattern qualifier
As presented in Table 6, the ICD-11 classification of Personality Disorders also includes the option of specifying

a *Borderline Pattern Qualifier.* Like the trait qualifiers, the Borderline Pattern qualifier is considered optional and can be used in combination with the trait qualifiers (e.g., *Moderate Personality Disorder, with Borderline Pattern, with Negative Affectiviy, Disinhibition, and Dissociality*). Unlike the trait qualifiers, the Borderline Pattern Qualifier is operationalized as requiring at least 5 out of 9 polythetic features adapted from the DSM-5 criteria for Borderline Personality Disorder. It has been suggested that this qualifier may serve as a familiar indicator for choosing psychotherapeutic treatment consistent with established theory and treatment manuals.

### Onset and stability of personality disorder
As presented in Table 1, the personality disturbance must have persisted over an extended period of time (> 2 years). Elements of Personality Disorder tend to first appear in childhood or adolescence and continue to be manifest into adulthood. However, while ICD-10 states that Personality Disorders tend to be stable over time, the ICD-11 guideline explicitly states that Personality Disorders are only "relatively" stable after young adulthood, and may change such that a person who had a Personality Disorder during young adulthood no longer has one by middle age. In some cases, a person who earlier did not have a diagnosable Personality

**Table 6** Borderline pattern qualifier

The Borderline pattern qualifier may be applied to individuals whose pattern of personality disturbance is characterized by a pervasive pattern of instability of interpersonal relationships, self-image, and affects, and marked impulsivity, as indicated by five (or more) of the following:
- Frantic efforts to avoid real or imagined abandonment.
- A pattern of unstable and intense interpersonal relationships, typically characterized by alternating between extremes of idealization and devaluation.
- Identity disturbance, manifested in markedly and persistently unstable self-image or sense of self.
- Impulsivity manifested in potentially self-damaging behaviours (e.g., risky sexual behaviour, reckless driving, excessive alcohol or substance use, binge eating).
- Recurrent episodes of self-harm (e.g., suicide attempts or gestures, self-mutilation).
- Emotional instability due to marked reactivity of mood. Fluctuations of mood may be triggered either internally (e.g., by one's own thoughts) or by external events. As a consequence, the individual experiences intense dysphoric mood states, which typically last for a few hours but may last for up to several days.
- Chronic feelings of emptiness.
- Inappropriate intense anger or difficulty controlling anger manifested in frequent displays of temper (e.g., yelling or screaming, throwing or breaking things, getting into physical fights).
- Transient dissociative symptoms or psychotic-like features (e.g., brief hallucinations, paranoia) in situations of high affective arousal.

Other manifestations of Borderline pattern, not all of which may be present in a given individual at a given time, include the following:
- A view of the self as inadequate, bad, guilty, disgusting, and contemptible.
- An experience of the self as profoundly different and isolated from other people; a painful sense of alienation and pervasive loneliness.
- Proneness to rejection hypersensitivity; problems in establishing and maintaining consistent and appropriate levels of trust in interpersonal relationships; frequent misinterpretation of social signals.

*Note.* Adapted from the ICD-11 Clinical Descriptions and Diagnostic Guidelines for Personality Disorder

Disorder, may develop one later in life. Sometimes, emergence of Personality Disorder in older adults may be related to the loss of social supports that had previously helped to compensate for personality disturbance.

### Features of psychoticism and level of severity

In contrast to the DSM-5 Section II and Section III approaches, the ICD-11 classification does not provide any code for Schizotypal Personality Disorder or Psychoticism because such features are coded within Schizophrenia and other primary psychotic disorders. However, as shown in Tables 3 and 4, the ICD-11 classification of Personality Disorder severity may be based on whether the patient experiences "dissociative states or psychotic-like beliefs or perceptions" and/or is "highly eccentric", which may resemble certain features of Schizotypal Personality Disorder. This is consistent with the traditional structural approach to classification of personality organization (e.g., high, middle, and low borderline levels) [9, 10], in which the lowest and most severe level may involve transient psychotic states. In other words, the ICD-11 approach classifies the capacity for reality testing (i.e., accuracy of situational and interpersonal appraisals) according to level of Personality Disorder severity and not as a distinct type or trait domain. However, as shown

in Table 6, the *Borderline Pattern qualifier* also involves "Transient dissociative symptoms or psychotic-like features (e.g., brief hallucinations, paranoia) in situations of high affective arousal," which is consistent with the established DSM-IV/5 construct of Borderline Personality Disorder.

### How to operationalize the ICD-11 personality disorder diagnosis?

After having ensured that the general diagnostic requirements for Personality Disorder are met (Table 1), the user may select one of three different diagnostic codes according to Personality Disorder severity (Table 3), followed by the option of coding one or more prominent trait qualifiers (Table 5). Additionally, the Borderline Pattern qualifier may also be applied if the clinical description matches this pattern (Table 6). As in the ICD-10, the relevant information may be gathered from clinical interviews and observations, review of clinical records, and/or informant reports.

Assessment tools are curently being developed to assist clinicians and researchers in the assessment of Personality Disorder diagnosis according to ICD-11. In the meantime, diagnostic information obtained from assessment tools developed for the DSM-5 AMPD model can be used for making an ICD-11 dimensional Personality Disorder diagnosis. For example, the Structured Clinical Interview for the DSM-5 Alternative Model of Personality Disorders (SCID-AMPD) operationalizes personality functioning according to the DSM-5 Level of Personality Functioning Scale (LPFS) along with the 25 DSM-5 trait facets [30]. The LPFS score along with the 25-facet personality profile can be converted into an ICD-11 Personality Disorder diagnosis using a "cross walk" as described in Table 7.

**Table 7** ICD-11 "Cross Walk" for DSM-5 Alternative Model of Personality Disorders

| ICD-11 Severity of Personality Dysfunction | DSM-5 Criterion A: Level of Personality Functioning |
| --- | --- |
| None | 0) No impairment (Healthy Functioning) |
| Personality Difficulty | 1) Some impairment |
| Mild Personality Disorder | 2) Moderate impairment |
| Moderate Personality Disorder | 3) Severe impairment |
| Severe Personality Disorder | 4) Extreme impairment |
| | |
| ICD-11 Trait Domain Qualifiers | DSM-5 Criterion B: Trait Domains |
| Negative Affectivity | Negative Affectivity |
| Detachment | Detachment |
| Disinhibition | Disinhibition |
| Dissociality | Antagonism |
| Anankastia | [Rigid Perfectionism and Perseveration][a] |

*Note.* The threshold for a Personality Disorder diagnosis is a t least Mild Personality Disorder (ICD-11) or Moderate impairment of personality functioning (DSM-5)
[a]These are facets from the domains of (low) Disinhibition and (high) Negative Affectivity, respectively

Accordingly, SCID-AMPD Module I evaluates three levels of Personality Disorder impairment (the two lower levels comprise subthreshold for diagnosis and healthy functioning, respectively) [31], which translate into the ICD-11 classification of Mild Personality Disorder, Moderate Personality Disorder, and Severe Personality Disorder as illustrated in Table 7. Likewise, the SCID-AMPD Module II evaluates DSM-5 trait facets and domains [30], which may be translated into ICD-11 trait domain qualifiers directly (see Table 7) or deliniated by means of an algorithm for trait facets measured with the Personality Inventory for DSM-5 (PID-5)[1] [32]. Finally, the ICD-11 trait domain qualifiers may also be derived from available ICD-10 categorical Personality Disorder information using the "cross walk" presented in Table 8 [22].

For clinical screening and research purposes, self-report measures have been developed to deliniate severity of personality dysfunction and prominent trait qualifiers. For example, the Level of Personality Functioning Scale – Brief Form 2.0 (LPFS-BF) [33, 34] efficiently measures impairment of self- and interpersonal functioning consistent with the ICD-11 diagnostic guidelines. The Personality Inventory for ICD-11 (PiCD) is a 60-item self-report or informant-report instrument, which describes the five ICD-11 domains [19]. Finally, as previously asserted, the ICD-11 domains may also be deliniated using an empirically established algorithm for using the ratings on the Personality Inventory for DSM-5 (PID-5) to determine the ICD-11 trait domain qualifiers [32].

## Case presentation

The following five cases demonstrate how the ICD-11 Personality Disorder classification may be applied to individuals with varying severity of personality dysfunction and configurations of trait qualifiers. All five cases meet the general diagnostic requirements for Personality Disorder, except for Case 4 (Fig. 4) whose clinical presentation is only characterized by subthreshold Personality Difficulty.

Case 1 (Fig. 1) is a 29-year-old women, who has a history of numerous serious suicide attempts resulting in repeated hospitalizations, multiple treatment providers, and medication trials typically with little to no benefit. She has been diagnosed with ICD-10 F60.3 Emotionally unstable Personality Disorder, but her clinical presentation is also complicated by substance abuse (i.e., cannabis and amphetamine), eating disorder, panic attacks, aggressive/impulsive behaviors leading to a total loss of reliable friends, and severe self-harm that has endangered her life. During her childhood she was verbally and physically abused by her mother, and sexually abused by two of her mother's male acquantances; she never knew her dad. Under stress she suffers from trauma-related dissociative states including symptoms of depersonalization and psychotic-like voices telling her to punish herself or vanish from the

present reality, though, she is mostly aware that the voices only exist in her mind. When experiencing minor defeats or perceived rejection, she responds with feelings of self-loathing or anger. Due to excessive mistrust of other people, her ability to form intimate relationships and capacity for empathy is severely compromised, and she has no idea what to do with her life or what she has to offer. Apart from experiencing mistrust, emptiness, and anger, she occasionally uses ingratiation and charm in her attempts to have her need for warmth and approval met. As displayed in the figure, Case 1's (Fig. 1) clinical presentation is classified as *Severe Personality Disorder* (e.g., serious difficulty with regulation of emotional experience, self-esteem, and impulses with a past history and future expectation of severe harm to self, psychotic-like perceptions, and she lacks reliable friends) with prominent trait qualifiers of *Negative Affectivity* (e.g., experiences negative emotions that are out of proportion to the situation including shame, mistrustfulness, and anger), *Disinhibition* (e.g., tendency to act impulsively in response to immediate stimuli in a harmful manner), and *Dissociality* (e.g., mistrust-related aggression and tendency to manipulate or seduce others). In this case *Moderate Personality Disorder* does not apply because Case 1 (Fig. 1) is not even able to maintain a few friendships or a regular job, and her self-injuries have caused long-term damage and endangered her life. Additionally, Case 1's (Fig. 1) diagnosis may be further elucidated using the Borderline Pattern qualifier as indicated by nearly all of the features presented in Table 6.

Case 2 (Fig. 2) is a 36-year-old man with a history of panic attacks and recurrent depressive episodes. He is intelligent and sensitive but has not managed to finish any degree after high school. A psychiatric evaluation at an outpatient psychotherapy unit concluded that his personality features met ICD-10 criteria for F60.6 Avoidant Personality Disorder and F60.7 Dependent Personality Disorder. Case 2 (Fig. 2) grew up in a home with poor resources and a family climate characterized by emotional and physical neglect along with some emotional abuse by both parents. During adolescence, he suffered from loneliness, insecurity, poor self-worth, and self-defeating behaviors such as letting peers take advantage of him. He virtually had no friends in school and he generally felt anxious, shy, and unaccepted among peers. Accordingly, he was prone to act as an underdog or people-pleaser. These features were preserved in adulthood in terms of social withdrawal and intimacy avoidance in order not to feel criticized, ashamed, or rejected. However, today he maintains a permanent job and a couple of relationships beyond his two brothers. As displayed in the figure, Case 2's (Fig. 2) clinical presentation is classified as *Mild Personality Disorder* (e.g., some distortions in interpersonal appraisal, difficulty maintaining positive

**Table 8** Tentative ICD-10 "Cross Walk" for ICD-11 Trait Domain Qualifiers

| ICD-10 Category | ICD-11 Qualifier | Specific ICD-11 Trait Features |
|---|---|---|
| F60.0 Paranoid | Negative Affectivity | Mistrustfulness, anger, bitterness, tendency to hold grudges; may become overwrought over real or perceived slights or insults from others. |
| | Detachment | Emotional and interpersonal distance; avoidance of close friendships. |
| F60.1 Schizoid | Detachment | Do not enjoy intimacy or social interactions and are not particularly interested in sexual relations; aloofness, emotional unexpressiveness, non-reactive to negative and positive events, with a limited capacity for enjoyment. |
| | low Negative Affectivity | Absence of emotional intensity and sensitivity. |
| F60.2 Dissocial | Dissociality | Lack of empathy including callous, deceptive, manipulative, exploiting, mean, ruthless, and physically aggressive behavior, and may sometimes take pleasure in inflicting pain or harm. |
| | Disinhibition | Impulsivity, irresponsibility, recklessness, and lack of planning without regard for risks or consequences. |
| | low Negative Affectivity | Absence of vulnerability, shame, and anxiety. |
| F60.3 Emotionally unstable | Negative Affectivity | Poor emotion regulation including being overreactive to criticism, problems, and setbacks; low frustration tolerance; often experiencing and displaying multiple emotions simultaneously or vacillate among a range of emotions in a short period of time. Once upset, it is difficult to regain composure. |
| | Disinhibition | Impulsivity associated with e.g., substance use, unplanned sexual activity, and sometimes deliberate self-harm; lack of planning. |
| | Dissociality | Sometimes being mean and physically aggressive. |
| F60.4 Histrionic | Dissociality | Expectation of others' admiration and attention-seeking behaviours to ensure being the center of others' focus. |
| | Disinhibition | Easily distracted by extraneous stimuli, such as others' conversations and tend to scan the environment for more enjoyable options. Acts rashly based on whatever is attractive at the moment. Focus on immediate feelings and sensations. |
| | Negative Affectivity | Emotional lability including being overreactive to external events; often experiences and displays multiple emotions simultaneously. |
| | low Detachment | Reversed emotional and social detachment including avoidance of social interactions, limited emotional expression and experience. |
| F60.5 Anankastic | Anankastia | Perfectionism including hyper-scheduling, planfulness, orderliness, and neatness. Behavioral constraint including control over emotional expression, stubbornness, risk-avoidance, perseveration, and deliberativeness. |
| | low Disinhibition | Reversed irresponsibility, lack of Planning, and impulsivity. |
| | Negative Affectivity | Worry, anxiety, and negativistic attitudes involving rejection of other's suggestions or advice. |
| F60.6 Anxious (avoidant) | Negative Affectivity | Anxiety, vulnerability, fear, shame, and low self-esteem/confidence including avoidance of situations and activities that are judged too difficult. |
| | Detachment | Avoidance of social interactions and intimacy, seek out employment that does not involve interactions with others, and even refuse promotions if it would entail more interaction with others. |
| | low Dissociality | Reversed self-centeredness: attention-seeking behaviours to ensure being the center of others' focus; believing that one has have many admirable qualities, that one's accomplishments are outstanding, that one will achieve greatness, and that others should admire one. |
| F60.7 Dependent | Negative Affectivity | Anxiety, vulnerability, and low self-confidence including dependency, which may be manifested in frequent reliance on others for advice, direction, and other kinds of help. |
| | low Dissociality | Excessive prosocial behavior and absence of self-centeredness: lack of concern about own needs, desires, and comfort, while those of others are overly considered. |
| F60.8 Other: Narcissistic | Dissociality | Grandiosity, a sense of entitlement, believing that they have many admirable qualities, that they have or will achieve greatness, and that others should admire them. |
| | Negative affectivity | Dysregulated self-esteem, which may involve envy of others' abilities and indicators of success; the individual can become overwrought over real or perceived slights or insults. |

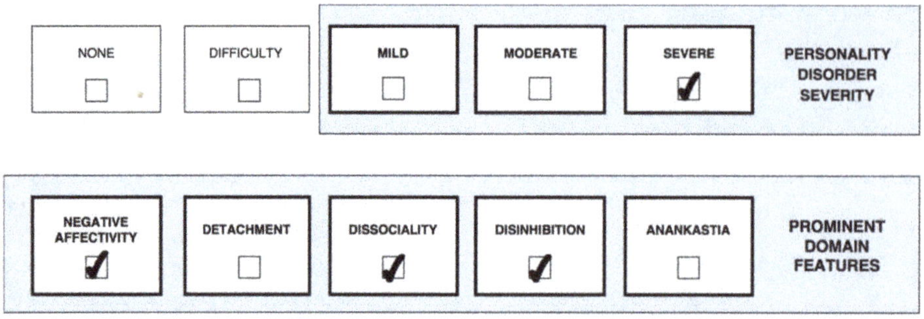

**Fig. 1** Severe Personality Disorder with Borderline Pattern and prominent traits of Negative Affectivity, Dissociality, and Disinhibition

self-esteem, is highly submissive in relationships but at least some healthy relationships and occupational roles are maintained) with prominent features of *Negative Affectivity* (e.g., anxiety, shame, low self-esteem, vulnerability, and depression depressivity) and *Detachment* (e.g., avoidance of social interactions). Notably, when Case 2 (Fig. 2) was younger, he would probably have been classified as *Moderate Personality Disorder* because he virtually had no friends; but he has improved since then as he now maintains a stable job and at least a couple of relationships.

Case 3 (Fig. 3) is a 26-year-old man incarcerated for brutal violence (e.g., purposely injured a shop owner with a blunt instrument just to get his money). Although he claimed to feel no suffering from any symptoms or dysfunction, he sought rehabilitation for his dependency on cocaine which had caused him certain problems while imprisoned including withdrawal symptoms and symptoms of intoxication (e.g., tremor and dry mouth). A psychiatric evaluation concluded that his personality features met ICD-10 criteria for F60.2 Dissocial Personality Disorder including some characteristic psychopathic (e.g., callousness and exploitativeness) and narcissistic (e.g., entitlement) features as well as recklessness without concern for others' safety. Case 3 (Fig. 3) did not recall much from his childhood and appeared aloof and emotionally detached while mentioning that his father was extremely physically abusive towards him and his mother. He did not experience anything

positive from friendships, unless they could provide him with certain favors. Moreover, he was not ashamed of admitting that he did not care about harming others, but was rather proud of it, and he generally never felt any emotional or physical pain nor remorse. Case 3's (Fig. 3) clinical presentation is classified as *Severe Personality Disorder* (e.g., past history and future expectation of severe harm to others, friendships have no genuine value to him, and self-view is characterized by entitlement) with prominent features of *Dissociality* (e.g., callousness, exploitation of others, and entitlement), *Disinhibition* (e.g., recklessness with no regard for others' safety), and some *Detachment* (e.g., aloofness). In this case *Moderate Personality Disorder* would not apply because Case 3 (Fig. 3) is not even interested in maintaining a single friendship and the risk of dangerous harm to others is not just "sometimes" but "often" taking place.

Case 4 (Fig. 4) is a 19-year-old highschool student, who was referred for treatment of ICD-10 F41.2 mixed anxiety and depressive disorder along with symptoms of anorexia nervosa, which she had previously been treated for in a private adolescent psychiatric clinic. Case 4 (Fig. 4) is from a relatively stable familiy, where the father works as physician and the mother as dentist. She has always been good at school and at finishing her duties in the home. Even though her parents have been busy with their own careers, they have persistently encouraged her to play the piano at different occasions and excel at horse riding competitions

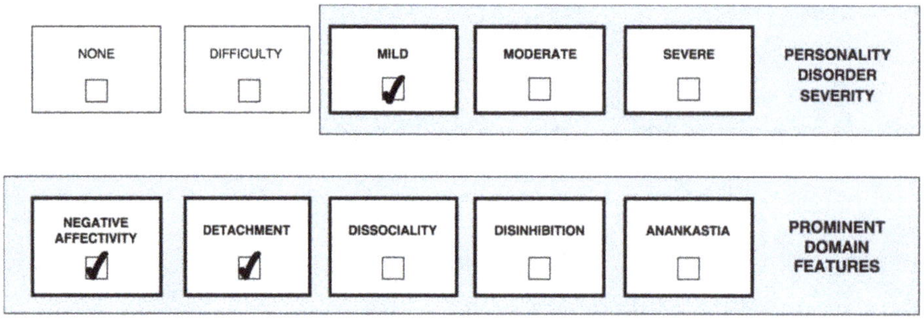

**Fig. 2** Mild Personality Disorder with prominent traits of Negative Affectivity and Detachment

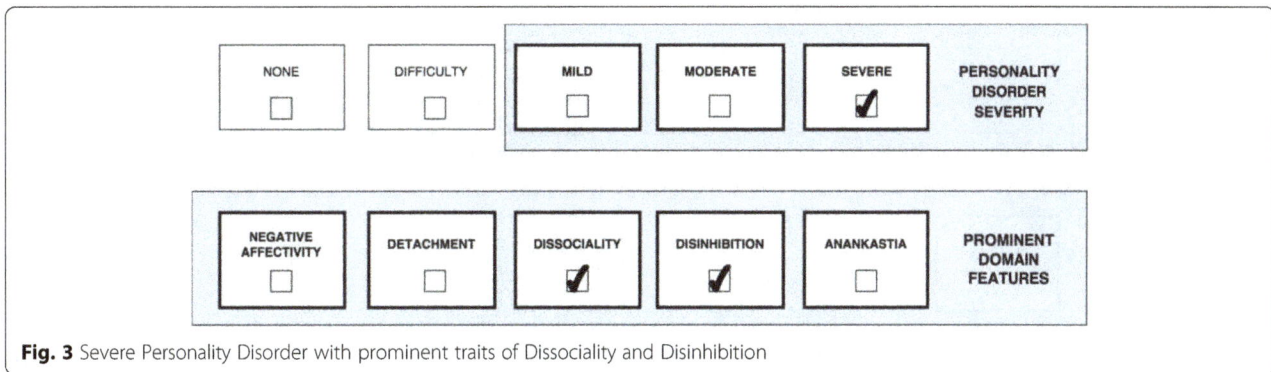

**Fig. 3** Severe Personality Disorder with prominent traits of Dissociality and Disinhibition

because they knew and expected that she was good at that. For that reason, her father never responded positively when she performed very well, whereas he showed disaoppointment if she did not get an A at her exams. While she was 13 her world fell apart as she discovered her father having an affair with another woman from his workplace, and she started overperforming in school and in sport while gradually developing eating disorder symptoms (restricting food leading to abnormally low weight) and even more unrelenting standards. However, she managed to maintain satisfying relationships with her friends as well as her mother and siblings. Case 4's (Fig. 4) clinical presentation is primarily classified as *Anorexia Nervosa* in the context of *Personality Difficulty* (i.e., some long-standing difficulties in her way of thinking about the self and the world, including unrelenting standards, which are insufficiently severe to cause notable disruption in school and most relationships) with prominent features of *Negative Affectivity* (e.g., depressivity, shame, and anxiety) and *Anankastia* (e.g., perfectionism, concern with meeting obligations, perseveration, deliberatetiveness, and tight control of own emotional expression). In this case *Mild Personality Disorder* would not apply because Case 4's (Fig. 4) habitual personality issues are not leading to any notable psychosocial impairment, whereas her problems are mainly attributable to other current mental problems.

Case 5 (Fig. 5) is a 53-year-old highly skilled and well-groomed accountant who has worked for several companies during his carreer. At his current job, Case 5 (Fig. 5) was referred to a psychologist at the company's HR department. Overall his personality characteristics were consistent with the ICD-10 Personality Disorder diagnoses F60.5 Anankastic Personality Disorder and F60.8 Other: Narcissistic Personality Disorder. Since adolescence, Case 5 (Fig. 5) has been more or less preoccupied with order, details, rules, and organization, including excessive pedantry and stubbornness. He always knew the "right" solution to most problems, and felt more capable of solving complicated things than nearly anyone else. Furthermore, he felt more important and entitled than most other people, and turned hostile when this was not recognized by others. Therefore, at work he has been reluctant to collaborate with others or to delegate "important" tasks to others, unless they submit to exactly his way of doing it. Colleagues and other people who know him well describes him as officious, supercilious, high-handed, unimaginative, intrusive, petty-minded, meddlesome, and nosy. An ex-wife has called Case 5 (Fig. 5) "a narcissist", whereas he refers to her as "too vulnerable and unintelligent". For those reasons he has not been able to maintain his occupational positions due to conflicts with superiors and emotional abuse of co-workers who he perceives as less efficient than himself. According to his account of things, it was

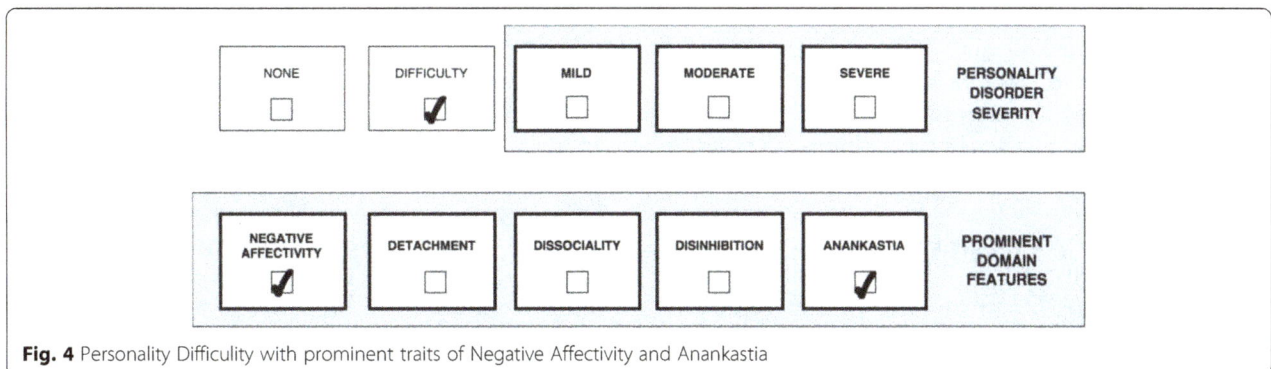

**Fig. 4** Personality Difficulty with prominent traits of Negative Affectivity and Anankastia

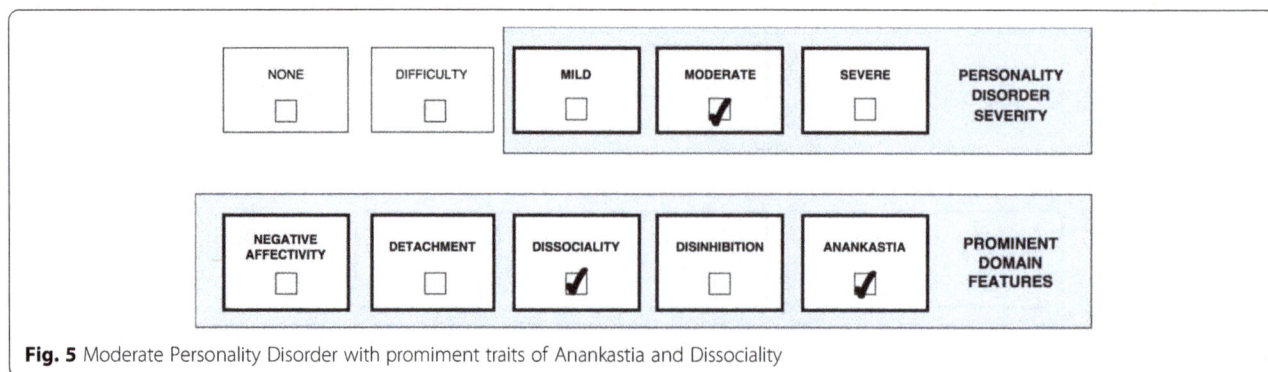

**Fig. 5** Moderate Personality Disorder with prominent traits of Anankastia and Dissociality

his decision to leave the different companies during his career simply because they were not professional enough. According to ICD-11 guidelines, Case 5's (Fig. 5) clinical presentation may be classified as *Moderate Personality Disorder* (e.g., a compromized capacity for understanding and appreciating others' perspectives, work relationships are disrupted, and persistent conflicts result in emotional harm to others) with prominent traits of *Anankastia* (e.g., stubbornness, orderliness, and perfectionism) and *Dissociality* (e.g., entitlement, grandiosity, lack of empathy, meanness, and hostility). In this case, *Severe Personality Disorder* does not apply because while Case 5's (Fig. 5) intimate and occupational relationships have been disrupted by frequent conflicts, he is still able to maintain work productivity and at least some relationships for a certain period of time. Likewise, *Mild Personality Disorder* does not apply because he is virtually incapable of or unwilling to sustain employment due to interpersonal issues, and he does not have any positive/healthy relationships not even with family members.

## Discussion

The ICD-11 approach changes the structure and process of diagnosing a Personality Disorder by focusing attention on the universal features of personality dysfunction including a classification of severity. Such a classification system has the advantage of simplifying the process of identifying a Personality Disorder. For example, the practitioner does not have to rule out the presence of a Personality Disorder by determining that none of the nine ICD-10 categories are present. Moreover, the ICD-11 classification is likely to have greater clinical utility because placing severity of personality functioning at the center of the diagnostic process can help service providers to distinguish those patients who have the greatest level of disturbance from those who do not, and thereby help services to target their interventions more effectively [13, 18].

The parsimoniousness of the ICD-11 classification may also frustrate some clinicians who desire a more detailed conceptualization of the patient's personality stucture. Accordingly, in comparison to the nine categories in ICD-10

or the 25 facets in the DSM-5 AMPD model, the ICD-11's five trait domains may be viewed as insufficiently detailed for describing all the subtle nuances of the patient's personality. Yet, when all trait qualifier combinations are taken into account, the number of diagnostic constellations provides information for a more detailed clinical conceptualization. For example, when describing features of the ICD-10 diagnosis *Avoidant Personality Disorder*, the clinician may use the ICD-11 code *Mild Personality Disorder with prominent features of Negative Affectivity* (i.e., anxiousness and poor self-esteem) *and Detachment* (i.e., social withdrawal and intimacy avoidance). However, the ICD-11 classification does not accommodate a coding of the specific subfeatures or facets as in the DSM-5 AMPD model where *Avoidant Personality Disorder* may be described in terms of *anxiousness, withdrawal,* and *intimacy avoidance*. In any case, preliminary research suggests that the five ICD-11 trait domains explain a substantial amount of variance in all Personality Disorder categories [22, 35–38]. From this empirical perspective, little information (i.e. variance) seems lost in the transition from the 10 familiar Personality Disorder types to 5 trait domain qualifiers. However, this empirical reality may not necessarily be noticed by practitioners when using this new approach for the first time, and communication remains a central purpose of a diagnostic system.

The ICD-11 classification allows the clinician to apply as many trait domain qualifiers as necessary to portray the clinical reality and dynamics of personality functioning, which offers more unique diagnostic profiles in various combinations. For example, the trait domain qualifier of *Negative Affectivity* applies to both Case 1 and Case 2 (Figs 1 and 2) but with a substantially distinct "flavour" in each case due to the influence of co-occuring trait qualifiers. This is acknowledged in the ICD-11 guidelines, which indicates that the manifestation of one prominent trait is largely dependent on the presence of other traits. Accordingly, Case 1 (Fig. 1) is likely to experience "externalizing" features of *Negative Affectivity* (e.g., anger and contempt) due to her co-occuring Dissociality, whereas Case 2 (Fig. 2) is likely to experience "internalizing" features of *Negative Affectivity* (e.g., depression, anxiety, guilt) due to his co-occuring Detachment.

## Application of severity and traits in clinical treatment

In contrast to the ICD-10 Personality Disorder categories, the ICD-11 classification separates common features of personality dysfunction (e.g, capacity for self-direction and ability to understand others' perspectives) from specific features of personality traits (e.g., impulsivity and attention seeking). This is consistent with research suggesting that severity of Personality Disorder tends to change or fluctuate while personality trait patterns tend to be relatively stable [6, 13, 16, 17]. From a treatment-perspective, traits tend to be resistant to change, whereas the severity of impairment related to the trait is less resistant to change. In other words, patients (and people in general) tend to stay essentially who they are, even if successful treatment helps them adapt who they are to their environment more effectively. Therefore, treatment should target what the Personality Disorder *does* to the patient (i.e., severity), as we cannot really change what it is (i.e., traits). For example, we estimated that Case 2's (Fig. 2) disorder previously would have been classified as *Moderate Personality Disorder with prominent features of Negative Affectivity and Detachment* because he virtually had no friends beforehand. Due to his improvement he now maintains a stable job and at least a couple of relationships, and for that reason his disorder is now only classified as *Mild Personality Disorder* but still with the pattern of *Negative Affectivity* and *Detachment*. Likewise, an urgent goal of treating Case 1 (Fig. 1) would involve helping her regulate emotions in a less destructive manner so that her diagnosis may be changed from *Severe Personality Disorder* to *Moderate Personality Disorder* without getting rid of her basic style of *Negative Affectivity, Dissociality*, and *Disinhibition*. Similarly, a major goal of treating Case 3 (Fig. 3) would involve providing him with skills that may prevent him from being dangerous to others, and thereby changing his level of impairment from *Severe Personality Disorder* to *Moderate Personality Disorder*, while his dissocial core traits basically remain the same.

*Level of severity* tells the clinician important information about level of risk, prognosis, and treatment intensity, and it provides a variable for the assessment of change common to all individuals with a Personality Disorder diagnosis [13, 17]. Accordingly, the more severe a patient's personality pathology, the greater the risk there is for extreme or problematic behavior (e.g., harm to self or others, treatment dropout, criminal issues, and psychotic-like symptoms) and the less optimistic the clinician can be for a smooth treatment with rapid and enduring gains [17]. Individuals with *Severe Personality Disorder* may need more intense treatments, such as hospitalization or multimodal approaches (e.g., combined group and individual). For example, Case 1 (Fig. 1)

(*Severe Personality Disorder with prominent features of Negative Affectivity, Disinhibition, and Dissociality; Borderline Pattern qualifier*) would need a more intensive treatment program than Case 2 (Fig. 2) (*Mild Personality Disorder with prominent features of Negative Affectivity and Detachment*).

*Trait domain qualifiers* can be said to contribute to the more individual expression of personality dysfunction. For example, one patient may show impairment of the capacity for interpersonal functioning. Yet, it makes a great difference whether this impairment is related to being very dominant (e.g., *Dissociality*) or being overly submissive (e.g., *Negative Affectivity and Detachment*). Those two different trait expressions inform different treament foci and style. Moreover, knowing the patient's prominent traits is useful for establishing a favorable treatment alliance, providing psychoeducation, increasing the patient's self-knowledge, planning realistic treatment goals, and matching therapy to the patient's personality (e.g., group therapy or individual therapy) [26]. Importantly, traits may also mirror habitual defensive- or coping responses (e.g., Detachment as a defense against shame or fears of being hurt by others) [28, 39, 40]. Therefore, traits may play an important role for improving the patient's personality functioning.

## Conclusion

In this article we illustrated the application of the ICD-11 classification using five different cases in which we took all aspects of the diagnostic guidelines into account. The ICD-11 Personality Disorder classification was found applicable to the five clinical cases, which were classified according to Personaity Disorder severity and trait domain qualifiers. We propose that the classification of severity may help inform clinical prognosis and intensity of treatment, whereas the classification of trait qualifiers may help inform the focus and style of treatment. Empirical research is warranted to investigate such important aspects of clinical utility. Moreover, future empirical research should evaluate perceived ease of use, utility for communication with patients and professionals, and inter-rater reliability. Finally, it seems vital to investigate whether practitioners across all WHO member countries can use the classification in a reliable manner despite substantial diversity in culture and professional resources.

## Endnotes

[1]The PID-5 is a 220-item self-report or informant-report inventory developed for the assessment of the trait criterion of the AMPD model (different versions of PID-5 are freely available from psychiatry.org).

## Additional file

> **Additional file 1:** Essential features and examples of ICD-11 levels of personality disturbance, including "None" and "Personality Difficulty". (PDF 114 kb)

### Abbreviations
AMPD: Alternative Model of Personality Disorders; DSM: Diagnostic and Statistical Manual of Mental Disorders; ICD: International Classification of Diseases; LPFS: Level of Personality Functioning Scale; LPFS-BF 2.0: Level of Personality Functioning Scale – Brief Form 2.0; PiCD: Personality Inventory for ICD-11; PID-5: Personality Inventory for DSM-5; SCID-AMPD: Structured Clinical Interview for DSM-5 Alternative Model of Personality Disorders

### Acknowledgements
We owe thanks to Geoffrey M. Reed and the ICD-11 Personality Disorder Work Group for paving the way for this work.

### Funding
Grants have been received from the Health Scientific Research Fund of Region Zealand.

### Authors' contributions
BB drafted the manuscript and MF provided substantial contributions and critical feedback. Both authors read and approved the final manuscript.

### Consent for publication
Demographic and other patient specific information has been de-identified for each case.
Written informed consent was obtained from the patient for publication of this case report. A copy of the written consent is available for review by the editor of this journal.

### Competing interests
The authors are involved in developing a structured interview to assess the ICD-11 classification of Personality Disorder.
Author Bo Bach is currently acting as an Associate Editor for BMC Psychiatry.

### Author details
[1]Center of Excellence on Personality Disorder, Psychiatric Research Unit, Region Zealand, Slagelse Psychiatric Hospital, Fælledvej 6, Bygning 3, 4200 Slagelse, Denmark. [2]Department of Psychiatry, New York State Psychiatric Institute, Columbia University, New York, NY, USA.

### References
1.  Torgersen S. Epidimiology. In: Widiger TA, editor. The Oxford handbook of personality disorders. 1st edition. Oxford University press; 2013. p. 186.
2.  Moran P, Jenkins R, Tylee A, Blizard R, Mann A. The prevalence of personality disorder among UK primary care attenders. Acta Psychiatr Scand. 2000;102:52–7.
3.  Beckwith H, Moran PF, Reilly J. Personality disorder prevalence in psychiatric outpatients: a systematic literature review. Personal Ment Health. 2014;8:91–101.
4.  Tyrer P, Reed GM, Crawford MJ. Classification, assessment, prevalence, and effect of personality disorder. Lancet. 2015;385:717–26.
5.  Widiger TA, Trull TJ. Plate tectonics in the classification of personality disorder. Am Psychol. 2007;62:71–83.
6.  Clark LA. Assessment and diagnosis of personality disorder: perennial issues and an emerging reconceptualization. Annu Rev Psychol. 2007;58:227–57.
7.  Reed GM. Progress in developing a classification of personality disorders for ICD-11. World Psychiatry. 2018;17:227–8.
8.  WHO. ICD-11 Clinical Descriptions and Diagnostic Guidelines for Mental and Behavioural Disorders. 2018. https://gcp.network/en/private/icd-11-guidelines/disorders.
9.  Doering S, Burgmer M, Heuft G, Menke D, Bäumer B, Lübking M, et al. Reliability and validity of the German version of the structured interview of personality organization (STIPO). BMC Psychiatry. 2013;13:210.
10. Caligor E, Kernberg OF, Clarkin JF, Yeomans FE. Psychodynamic therapy for personality pathology: treating self and interpersonal functioning. Arlington: American Psychiatric Publishing; 2018.
11. Sharp C, Wright AGC, Fowler JC, Frueh BC, Allen JG, Oldham J, et al. The structure of personality pathology: both general ('g') and specific ('s') factors? J Abnorm Psychol. 2015;124:387–98.
12. Morey LC, Bender DS, Skodol AE. Validating the proposed diagnostic and statistical manual of mental disorders, 5th edition, severity indicator for personality disorder. J Nerv Ment Dis. 2013;201:729–35.
13. Clark LA, Nuzum H, Ro E. Manifestations of personality impairment severity: comorbidity, course/prognosis, psychosocial dysfunction, and 'borderline' personality features. Curr Opin Psychol. 2018;21:117–21.
14. Williams TF, Scalco MD, Simms LJ. The construct validity of general and specific dimensions of personality pathology. Psychol Med. 2018;48:834–48.
15. Hopwood CJ, Malone JC, Ansell EB, CA S, Grilo CM, McGlashan TH, et al. Personality assessment in DSM-5: empirical support for rating severity, style, and traits. J Personal Disord. 2011;25:305–20.
16. Wright AGC, Hopwood CJ, Skodol AE, Morey LC. Longitudinal validation of general and specific structural features of personality pathology. J Abnorm Psychol. 2016;125:1120–34.
17. Crawford MJ, Koldobsky N, Mulder R, Tyrer P. Classifying personality disorder according to severity. J Personal Disord. 2011;25:321–30.
18. Bach B. Treating comorbid depression and personality disorders in DSM-5 and ICD-11. Lancet Psychiatry. in press. https://doi.org/S2215-0366(18)30351-1.
19. Oltmanns JR, Widiger TA. A self-report measure for the ICD-11 dimensional trait model proposal: the personality inventory for ICD-11. Psychol Assess. 2017;30(2):154–69.
20. Widiger TA, Simonsen E. Alternative dimensional models of personality disorder: finding a common ground. J Personal Disord. 2005;19:110–30.
21. Mulder RT, Newton-Howes G, Crawford MJ, Tyrer PJ. The central domains of personality pathology in psychiatric patients. J Personal Disord. 2011;25:364–77.
22. Bach B, Sellbom M, Skjernov M, Simonsen E. ICD-11 and DSM-5 personality trait domains capture categorical personality disorders: finding a common ground. Aust New Zeal J Psychiatry. 2018;52:425–34.
23. American Psychiatric Association. Diagnostic and statistical manual of mental disorders 5th edition (DSM-5). Arlington: American Psychiatric Publishing, Inc.; 2013.
24. Lotfi M, Bach B, Amini M, Simonsen E. Structure of DSM-5 and ICD-11 personality domains in Iranian community sample. Personal Ment Health. 2018;95:86–95.
25. Bagby RM, Gralnick TM, Al-Dajani N, Uliaszek AA. The role of the five-factor model in personality assessment and treatment planning. Clin Psychol Sci Pract. 2016;23:365–81.
26. Bach B, Presnall-Shvorin J. Using DSM-5 and ICD-11 personality traits in clinical treatment. In: Gratz KL, Lejuez C, editors. Cambridge: Cambridge Handbook of Personality Disorders: Cambridge University Press; in press.
27. Bach B, Kongerslev MT. Personality dynamics in Schema therapy and the forthcoming ICD-11 classification of personality disorder. Eur J Pers. https://doi.org/10.1002/per.2174.
28. Bach B, Bernstein DP. Schema therapy conceptualization of personality functioning and traits in ICD-11 and DSM-5. Curr Opin Psychiatry. https://doi.org/10.1097/YCO.0000000000000464.
29. Olajide K, Munjiza J, Moran P, O'Connell L, Newton-Howes G, Bassett P, et al. Development and psychometric properties of the standardized assessment of severity of personality disorder (SASPD). J Personal Disord. 2018;32:44–56.
30. Skodol AE, First MB, Bender DS, Oldham JM, Module II. Structured clinical interview for personality traits. In: First MB, Skodol AE, Bender DS, Oldham JM, editors. Structured clinical interview for the DSM-5 alternative model for personality disorders (SCID-AMPD). Arlington: American Psychiatric Association; 2018.
31. Bender DS, Skodol A, First MB, Oldham J, Module I. Structured clinical interview for the level of personality functioning scale. In: First M, Skodol A, Bender D, Oldham J, editors. Structured clinical interview for the DSM-5

alternative model for personality disorders (SCID-AMPD). Arlington: American Psychiatric Association; 2018.

32. Bach B, Sellbom M, Kongerslev M, Simonsen E, Krueger RF, Mulder R. Deriving ICD-11 personality disorder domains from dsm-5 traits: initial attempt to harmonize two diagnostic systems. Acta Psychiatr Scand. 2017; 136:108–17.

33. Bach B, Hutsebaut J. Level of personality functioning scale–brief form 2.0: utility in capturing personality problems in psychiatric outpatients and incarcerated addicts. J Pers Assess. https://doi.org/10.1080/00223891.2018.1428984.

34. Bach B, Anderson JL. Patient-reported ICD-11 personality disorder severity and DSM-5 level of personality functioning. J Personal Disord. 2018. https://doi.org/10.1521/pedi_2018_32_393.

35. Fossati A, Krueger RF, Markon KE, Borroni S, Maffei C. Reliability and validity of the personality inventory for DSM-5 (PID-5): predicting DSM-IV personality disorders and psychopathy in community-dwelling Italian adults. Assessment. 2013;20:689–708.

36. Morey LC, Benson KT, Skodol AE. Relating DSM-5 section III personality traits to section II personality disorder diagnoses. Psychol Med. 2016;46:647–55.

37. Hopwood CJ, Thomas KM, Markon KE, Wright AGC, Krueger RF. DSM-5 personality traits and DSM-IV personality disorders. J Abnorm Psychol. 2012; 121:424–32.

38. Sellbom M, Sansone RA, Songer DA, Anderson JL. Convergence between DSM-5 section II and section III diagnostic criteria for borderline personality disorder. Aust N Z J Psychiatry. 2014;48:325–32.

39. Huprich SK. Moving beyond categories and dimensions in personality pathology assessment and diagnosis. Br J Psychiatry. https://doi.org/10.1192/bjp.2018.149.

40. Granieri A, La Marca L, Mannino G, Giunta S, Guglielmucci F, Schimmenti A. The relationship between defense patterns and DSM-5 maladaptive personality domains. Front Psychol. 2017;8:1–12.

# 10

# The future disposition Inventory-24: reliability and validity estimates in a large sample of Chinese University students

Lu Yuan[1], Dong-Fang Wang[2], Bob Lew[3], Augustine Osman[4] and Cun-Xian Jia[1]*

## Abstract

**Background:** This study was designed to assess the factor structure, internal consistency reliability, and preliminary psychometric properties of the Chinese version of the Future Disposition Inventory-24 (FDI-24) in a large sample of Chinese university students.

**Methods:** We translated the English version of the Future Disposition Inventory-24 (FDI-24) into Chinese and examined its factor structure, estimates of internal consistency reliability, and psychometric properties in a representative sample of university students. In particular, students ($N = 2,074$) from two universities in Shandong Province in China were identified using the multi-stage stratified sampling method. In addition to the FDI-24, we collected preliminary data using self-report instruments that included the Beck Hopelessness Scale (BHS) and a general sociodemographic information questionnaire.

**Results:** The results of the internal consistency reliability estimates were adequate regarding the scores on the three FDI-24 subscales: Cronbach's alpha = .89–.97, Omega total = .85–.96, Revelle's Omega total = .88–.96, the greatest lower bound (GLB) = .89–.96 and Coefficient $H$ = .86–.94. Bivariate correlation analyses showed evidence for criterion and discriminant validity. The 3-factor oblique-Geomin-rotation solution accounted for 62.92% of the total variance in the exploratory factor analysis (EFA). The exploratory structural equation modeling (ESEM) result showed that the 3-factor model provided adequate fit statistics for the sample data: the robust comparative fit index (R-CFI) was .959, robust Tucker Lewis index (R-TLI) was .946 and robust root mean square error of approximation (R-RMSEA) was .090.

**Conclusion:** The FDI-24 has a satisfactory factor structure, reliability estimates, and satisfactory evidence of concurrent validity estimates for students with different demographic and cultural backgrounds. The FDI-24 holds promise for use in future investigations with Chinese students.

**Keywords:** Reliability, Validity, Future disposition Inventory-24, Hopelessness, Suicide

## Background

Suicide remains an important public mental health concern for Western and non-Western nations. In particular, as reported by the World Health Organization (WHO) in 2014 [1], among young people aged 15–29 years, suicide remains the second leading cause of death globally. In China, in particular, suicide-related behaviors tend to be acute and serious mental health problems among young adults [1]. To date, a majority of the studies in the existing suicide literature tend to focus on psychopathology or risk factors, such as mood disorders [2, 3], anxiety disorders [4], and specific constructs, including hopelessness [5, 6], anger [7, 8], and loneliness [9, 10].

Hopelessness has been identified as a critical risk factor in the assessment of suicidal intentions and behaviors among students [11]. In recent years, several self-report instruments have been designed for the assessment of risk factors that are associated with suicide-related behaviors. As an example, according to

* Correspondence: jiacunxian@sdu.edu.cn
[1]Department of Epidemiology, School of Public Health, Shandong University & Shandong University Center for Suicide Prevention Research, Jinan, Shandong, China
Full list of author information is available at the end of the article

Beck's hopelessness theory of suicide, hopelessness is generally conceptualized as a pessimistic attitude or expectation about future life events; that is, it is generally considered one of the core cognitive vulnerability factors for suicide [12]. Indeed, previous studies have shown that prolonged and severe feelings of hopelessness may lead to high incidents of suicide-related behaviors [13]. Additionally, hopelessness has been identified as a moderator or mediator of the association between various psychological symptoms and suicide-related behaviors, even extending significantly beyond depression in predicting the severity of suicidal intent [14–16]. Furthermore, findings from theories such as strain theory of suicide [17] have demonstrated that individuals experiencing intolerable pain, hopelessness, and psychological strain might engage in high-risk suicide-related behaviors (e.g., suicide attempts). Therefore, it is of great significance to continue to evaluate the role of the hopelessness construct in assessing suicide-related behaviors.

In the past few years, self-report instruments have been developed and validated for the purpose of screening or assessing the hopelessness construct. As a notable example, the Beck Hopelessness Scale (BHS), developed 40 years ago, has been widely used to measure feelings of hopelessness in clinical and nonclinical samples [18–21]. Recently, however, Gutierrez and Osman [22] have argued for the inclusion of both risk and protective factors simultaneously in the assessment of suicide-related behaviors. Although some items regarding future prospects and pessimistic statements are included in the BHS, only a single dimension with a mix of positively worded (e.g., "I look forward to the future with hope and enthusiasm") and negatively worded (e.g., "My future seems dark") items underlies this given scale. We assume that the multiple aspects of positive and negative thinking may be differentially associated with hopelessness in individuals [23, 24]. To derive a total scale score for the BHS, nine of the positively worded items are reverse-scored (see comments by [25, 26]). It has also been noted that the BHS lacks content specificity for the assessment of suicide-related behaviors [27].

One self-report instrument receiving increasing attention in the extant literature in the assessment of future-related events is the Future Disposition Inventory–24 (FDI-24) [28]. In particular, the FDI-24 is designed to address some of the substantive psychometric limitations of existing self-report instruments, such as the BHS. In brief, the FDI-24 conceptualizes future events in terms of a *future disposition* along three correlated domains. The Positive domain of the FDI-24 focuses on responses such as optimism, plans, satisfaction with the future and determination in handling difficulties. The Negative domain focuses on feelings of worry,

cognitive rigidity and life dissatisfaction, and the Suicide Orientation domain comprises suicidal rumination, ideation and the wish to die. Each item is scored on a 5-point Likert-type scale, ranging from 1 (*not at all true of me*) to 5 (*extremely true of me*). None of the 24 items is reverse-scored. Successfully used in some Western studies, the factor structure of the FDI-24 has been established, and its strong psychometric properties in adult and adolescent samples have been accepted [29–31]. However, it is unknown whether this instrument can be used to evaluate the construct of *future disposition* among university students in China. Thus, the specific aims of the current study were as follows. First, we examined the replicability of the 3-factor oblique solution of the FDI-24 in a large convenience sample of nonclinical participants. Second, we confirmed the structure of the final solution in the second half of the sample (referred to as *cross-validation* for purposes of the analyses). Third, we evaluated evidence of internal consistency reliability for scores on each domain. Fourth, we assessed the differential correlates of the FDI-24 domains.

## Methods
### Sample and procedure
Using a multi-stage stratified sampling procedure, the study participants consisted of a sample of undergraduate students recruited from two convenient large public medical universities in Jinan City, Shandong Province, eastern China. We selected two similar faculty colleges as the primary sampling unit from each university. Stratified on the basis of grade, three or four classes from each grade were randomly selected to be the secondary sampling units. Grade selection ranged from freshman to senior, with consideration of students' absence for hospital internships. All students in the sampled classes present on the day of the survey were invited to complete the questionnaires. Professionals trained in instrument use and validation supervised the in-class survey administration (i.e., paper-pencil). In addition to the demographic questionnaire, the participants completed the Chinese versions of the Beck Hopelessness Scale [32] and the FDI-24. Of the 2,197 self-report questionnaires that were handed out, 2,074 were completed with no missing items on any of the study instruments. The sample, including 1,368 female students and 706 male students, had a mean age of 19.79 ± 1.39 years (female, mean age = 19.75 ± 1.33; male, mean age = 19.86 ± 1.50). The sample consisted of 574 (27.7%) freshmen, 521 (25.1%) sophomores, 619 (29.8%) juniors, and 369 (17.4%) seniors. In terms of ethnic composition, most of the participants were Han Chinese (1939, 93.5%), and 135 (6.5%) were from minority races. Before attending college, 1015 (48.9%) of them lived in an urban area, and 1059 (51.1%) lived in a

rural environment. Preliminary analyses showed no statistically significant differences between separate units on demographic variables, such as gender, age, nationality, academic level and residency, all $p$ values > .05.

### Future disposition inventory (FDI-24): Chinese version

Because this instrument has not been used previously with Chinese samples, the initial goal was to construct a Chinese version. Accordingly, we invited two bilingual experts specialized in mental health to guide the translation process of the FDI-24 instructions and items. To ensure appropriate and equivalent meanings and clarity of expressions, one expert translated all 24 items and instructions from English into Chinese, and the other expert translated the Chinese items and instructions back into English without being provided with the original instrument [33, 34]. After several rounds of discussion and revision, the final Chinese version of the instrument (i.e., retaining all 24 items) was adopted for use in the current study.

### The Beck hopelessness scale (BHS)

The BHS is a 20-item self-report instrument that is designed to assess negative attitudes about future events. Thus, it is considered a theoretically valid instrument for evaluating criterion validity estimates of scores on the FDI-24. Due to its development and good construct validation, this instrument has been widely used and translated into various languages. The instrument has strong estimates of test-retest reliability and construct validity in Chinese samples [32]. In brief, the BHS includes nine positively worded items and 11 negatively worded items concerning negative attitudes about the future. The total score of 20 items (each of which ranges from 1 to 5 points, with reverse scoring) is usually derived to evaluate levels of the hopelessness construct; higher total scores represent extreme levels of hopelessness. Used as a criterion-related validation instrument in the current study, the estimate of internal consistency of the BHS score for the study sample was adequate (Cronbach's alpha = .90; average inter-item correlation [AIC] = .314).

### Statistical methods

The Cronbach's alpha, Omega coefficients, Coefficient $H$ and the greatest lower bound (GLB) procedures were used with the sample data to evaluate the estimate of internal consistency for scores on the self-report instruments.

Pearson correlations between scores on the BHS and the three domains of the FDI-24 were computed to examine the evidence for criterion-related validity. Based on the FDI-24 score distribution, a $t$-test was used to compare differences in the mean scores between extreme groups (the groups with the top 27% of scores and the bottom 27% of scores, respectively) [35, 36], and

the method of Cohen's $d$ was applied to compute the discriminating power of subscales and to distinguish ability at different levels. These methods, used in a general student population, were able to distinguish extreme values to help define the high-scoring group members with a disposition of future thinking.

Participants were randomly divided into two groups by statistical software to evaluate further evidence for construct validity. Specifically, Exploratory Factor Analysis (EFA) was conducted with data obtained from one group, and Confirmatory Factor Analysis (CFA) was used with data from the other group. Finally, we retested the whole sample in fitting a confirmatory 3-factor model by exploratory structural equation modeling (ESEM; implemented in the Mplus 7.4 statistical software). The coefficient calculation was available in R packages. Considering the non-normal distribution of the scale item scores, we adopted the method of maximum likelihood means-adjusted estimator (Robust) to conduct the analyses. The $x^2/df$ value, robust comparative fit index (R-CFI), robust Tucker Lewis index (R-TLI), robust root-mean-square error of approximation (R-RMSEA), and its 95% $CI$ were used to assess fit estimates for the 1-factor, 2-factor, and 3-factor solutions [37].

All statistical significance levels were set at a $p$ value of .05.

### Ethics approval and consent to participate

The study was overseen by and obtained signed ethics approval from the institutional review board of the Ethics Committee at the School of Public Health, Shandong University (No. 20161103). All study participants gave voluntary verbal consent to participate in the anonymous survey after receiving an explanation of the study design and reading the questionnaire instructions prior to responding.

## Results
### Reliability

The Cronbach's alphas for each scale score of the FDI-24 were high (.89–.97), indicating good internal consistency reliability (see Table 1) [38]. Measures of reliability alongside Cronbach's alpha, Omega coefficients, the greatest lower bound (GLB) and Coefficient $H$ were reported on the three subscales, performing well in assessing the reliability of scales. The corrected item-total correlations beyond .30 are acceptable based on an empirical study [39], as shown in Table 2, although the correlations for each scale were higher than what we expected. Specifically, the range was .741 to .828 for the Positive Focus scale items, .737 to .884 for the Suicide Orientation scale items, and .629 to .853 for the Negative Focus scale items, respectively. Taken together, all correlation coefficient values were statistically significant ($p < .001$).

**Table 1** Internal consistency of dimension-total scores of the future disposition inventory-24

| Dimension | Items | Mean ± SD | a | ω | Revelle's ω | GLB | H |
|---|---|---|---|---|---|---|---|
| Positive focus | 8 | 30.96±7.26 | 0.94 | 0.92 | 0.94 | 0.94 | 0.92 |
| Suicide orientation | 8 | 12.17±7.00 | 0.97 | 0.96 | 0.96 | 0.96 | 0.94 |
| Negative focus | 8 | 16.48±6.30 | 0.89 | 0.85 | 0.88 | 0.89 | 0.86 |

*a*: Cronbach's alpha; *ω*: Omega total; Revelle's *ω* = Revelle's Omega total; GLB: the Greatest Lower Bound; *H*: Coefficient *H*

### Criterion validity

The Beck Hopelessness Scale (BHS) total scale score was used as the criterion measure in our analyses. It might weaken the effects of opposite directions to evaluate global future attitudes, thoughts and feelings using just a single orientation of an inventory. Thus, for a better understanding of the correlations between scores on the BHS total scale and the FDI-24 subscales, we conducted separate correlation analyses with the specific FDI-24 scales' scores. Consequently, we found that the Positive Focus scale score was negatively and significantly associated with the BHS total scale score ($r = -.53$, $p < .001$). The Negative Focus scale score was positively and significantly associated with the BHS total scale score ($r = .49$, $p < .001$). The Suicide Orientation scale score was also positively and significantly associated with the BHS total scale score ($r = .40$, $p < .001$), suggesting evidence for adequate criterion validity of scores on the FDI-24 scales.

### Discrimination

An independent samples *t*-test was used to compare the different means between the high- and low-scoring

**Table 2** Internal consistency of item-dimension scores of the future disposition inventory-24

| Abbreviated content items | Mean ± SD | r |
|---|---|---|
| Positive focus | | |
| 1. I expect things to turn out better. | 4.08±1.14 | .809 |
| 2. I plan to work harder to make things better. | 4.03±1.11 | .828 |
| 5. I plan to deal better with most of the setbacks. | 3.61±1.19 | .747 |
| 7. I expect to enjoy the results or outcomes of all my hard work. | 3.90±1.17 | .794 |
| 10. I remain determined to deal better with demands on me. | 3.84±1.13 | .823 |
| 11. I expect to be happier and more content with my life. | 3.99±1.12 | .822 |
| 13. I plan to look at the positive side of my life. | 3.74±1.12 | .783 |
| 15 I intend to succeed in working through most personal problems. | 3.77±1.16 | .741 |
| Suicide orientation | | |
| 3. I think that by ending my life, all problems will go away. | 1.63±1.14 | .737 |
| 6. I think life is not worth living. | 1.58±1.08 | .830 |
| 8. I think things will get better if I were dead. | 1.51±1.03 | .865 |
| 9. I think people would be better off without me. | 1.57±1.12 | .798 |
| 17. I sometimes wish I were dead. | 1.52±1.06 | .873 |
| 18. I think I would be better off dead. | 1.45±1.03 | .884 |
| 22. I wish I could succeed at attempts to kill myself. | 1.42±0.98 | .816 |
| 23. I have nothing to lose by ending my life. | 1.48±1.05 | .808 |
| Negative focus | | |
| 4. I worry that things will never go well. | 1.76±1.10 | .665 |
| 12. I get confused and uncertain. | 2.49±1.15 | .853 |
| 14. I doubt whether things will ever get better. | 2.39±1.14 | .697 |
| 16. I have a hard time imagining that things will ever get better for me. | 1.80±1.13 | .691 |
| 19. I wonder whether I would ever be satisfied. | 2.34±1.20 | .629 |
| 20. I fear that I will run into more difficulties. | 2.16±1.14 | .762 |
| 21. All I can see ahead of me are hardships. | 1.68±1.03 | .730 |
| 24. I often doubt whether I will ever have control. | 1.86±1.15 | .765 |

groups. For the Positive Focus scale of FDI-24 inventory data, we observed that the mean of the group with the top 27% of scores (27.41 ± 6.29) was significantly lower than that of the group with the bottom 27% of scores (30.57 ± 8.10, $p < .001$). As expected, similar results were obtained when the analyses were undertaken with the other two specific FDI-24 subscales scores (See Table 3). A percentage of 27% was used because this value was able to maximize differences in normal distributions while providing enough cases for analysis. Cohen's $d$ as a measure of group differences was also reported in the result, displaying acceptable discriminating power of each scale.

### Construct validity

The items in the Chinese version of the FDI-24 were first analyzed using the oblique-Geomin-rotation procedure. The results of Bartlett's Test of Sphericity and the Kaiser-Meyer-Olkin (KMO) test ($x^2 = 17260$, $p < .001$ and the KMO = .942) showed that the present sample was well suited for factor analysis. Based on the results of the screen plot and the criterion of eigenvalues greater than 1, the three-factor solution was retained, accounting for 62.92% of the total variance.

We used the recommended cutoff score of .50 or higher to guide detailed interpretations of the item-factor loadings [40]. In the scale designer's initial analysis, the pattern of loadings on each domain was eight items [28]. However, using a cutoff score of .50 or higher, we found that, in EFA, Item 4 ("I worry that things will never go well for me no matter what I do") from the Negative Focus factor had a high loading on the Suicide Orientation factor, at .624. Furthermore, Item 16 ("I have a hard time imagining that things will ever get better for me in the future") had a loading that was lower than expected on the Negative Focus factor. For the Suicide Orientation factor, we found that Item 22 ("I wish I could succeed at attempts to kill myself") and Item 23 ("I feel I have nothing to lose by ending my life") had higher loadings on the Negative Focus factor than on the expected Suicide Orientation factor (see Table 4).

We conducted confirmatory factor analysis (CFA) to confirm the fit of the three-factor model with the second sample data. Table 5 shows fit estimates for the different structural models, providing support for the construct validity of the correlated three-factor model. Regarding the CFA factor loadings, each factor was composed of

eight items, similar to the original solution. The range of the standardized factor loadings for each factor is presented: .714 to .934 for Positive Focus, .789 to .969 for Suicide Orientation, and .508 to .848 for Negative Focus (see Table 4).

The ESEM fit indices of the 3-factor model also indicated adequate fit of the model to the sample data in Table 5. As shown in Table 6, most of the items had adequate loadings on the proposed original factors [28], while Items 4, 16 and 23 had higher loadings on factors other than the original.

As expected, the correlation between the Positive Focus factor and the Suicide Orientation factor was negative and high at −.569. The correlation between the Suicide Orientation factor and the Negative Focus factor was positive and high at .873. The correlation between the Positive Focus factor and the Negative Focus factor was negative and moderate at −.372.

### Discussion

In this study, the main findings are as follows. First, the Future Disposition Inventory-24 (FDI-24) domains had satisfactory internal consistency reliability estimates in a sample of Chinese students with different cultural backgrounds. Second, we found, using scores on the Beck Hopelessness Scale (BHS), that the FDI-24 scale scores had acceptable criterion validity. Third, the estimate of discrimination, assessed by examining scores between high- and low-scoring groups, could be considered adequate. Fourth, evaluation of the three-factor model with conventional goodness-of-fit statistics showed replicability of the three-factor solution of the items in the study samples, providing support for construct validity.

Although we found that the FDI-24 evaluated the same three domains of the future disposition construct for the Chinese-speaking students, minor differences were observed between these groups on four of the FDI-24 items. For the Chinese-speaking students, factor loadings of two future suicide orientation items (i.e., Items 22 and 23) were high on the Negative Focus scale for the future (e.g., worry about the future). It should also be noted that two of the Negative Focus items (Items 4 and 16) had loadings of .40 or higher on the Suicide Orientation scale in the EFA and ESEM (see Tables 4 and 6). However, when the 3-factor oblique model was examined in the validation sample, we found that all four of these items (Items 4, 16, 22,

**Table 3** Discriminant validity of the future disposition inventory-24

| Dimension | High 27% Mean ± SD | Low 27% Mean ± SD | t-value | p-value | Cohen's d |
|---|---|---|---|---|---|
| Positive focus | 27.41 ± 6.29 | 30.57 ± 8.10 | -7.677 | <.001 | -.436 |
| Suicide orientation | 9.18 ± 2.51 | 19.11 ± 9.28 | -26.337 | <.001 | -1.461 |
| Negative focus | 12.47 ±3.22 | 23.65 ± 5.44 | -44.453 | <.001 | -2.501 |

**Table 4** Factor loadings from the exploratory and confirmatory factor analyses

| | EFA($n_1$=1037) | | | CFA($n_2$=1037) | | |
| | 1 | 2 | 3 | 1 | 2 | 3 |
|---|---|---|---|---|---|---|
| | Factor1 | | | Factor1 | | |
| 1 | 0.733 | -0.443 | 0.237 | 0.928 | | |
| 2 | 0.754 | -0.393 | 0.186 | 0.934 | | |
| 5 | 0.741 | 0.014 | -0.079 | 0.740 | | |
| 7 | 0.771 | -0.089 | -0.029 | 0.799 | | |
| 10 | 0.846 | 0.060 | -0.145 | 0.867 | | |
| 11 | 0.833 | -0.004 | -0.135 | 0.841 | | |
| 13 | 0.767 | 0.017 | -0.167 | 0.800 | | |
| 15 | 0.750 | 0.009 | -0.090 | 0.714 | | |
| | Factor2 | | | | Factor2 | |
| 3 | -0.030 | 0.737 | 0.114 | | 0.789 | |
| 6 | -0.090 | 0.743 | 0.196 | | 0.892 | |
| 8 | -0.124 | 0.828 | 0.122 | | 0.915 | |
| 9 | -0.101 | 0.754 | 0.130 | | 0.867 | |
| 17 | -0.079 | 0.735 | 0.295 | | 0.936 | |
| 18 | -0.101 | 0.743 | 0.290 | | 0.969 | |
| 22 | -0.248 | 0.445 | 0.523 | | 0.937 | |
| 23 | -0.220 | 0.451 | 0.525 | | 0.897 | |
| | | | Factor3 | | | Factor3 |
| 4 | -0.057 | 0.624 | 0.213 | | | 0.841 |
| 12 | 0.079 | 0.158 | 0.501 | | | 0.561 |
| 14 | 0.082 | 0.178 | 0.569 | | | 0.625 |
| 16 | -0.106 | 0.473 | 0.395 | | | 0.825 |
| 19 | 0.112 | -0.132 | 0.781 | | | 0.508 |
| 20 | -0.028 | 0.022 | 0.809 | | | 0.680 |
| 21 | -0.121 | 0.281 | 0.623 | | | 0.848 |
| 24 | -0.102 | 0.244 | 0.633 | | | 0.808 |

EFA = Exploratory Factor Analysis; CFA = Confirmatory Factor Analysis; n1 and n2 were two random sample

**Table 5** Fit estimates for the different structural models in EFA, CFA and ESEM

| | $x^2$ | df | R-CFI | R-TLI | R-RMSEA | R-RMSEA 95% CI |
|---|---|---|---|---|---|---|
| Exploratory Factor Analysis (EFA) | | | | | | |
| 1-factor | 6824.335[a] | 252 | 0.852 | 0.837 | 0.159 | (0.155-0.162) |
| 2-factor | 2845.755[a] | 229 | 0.941 | 0.929 | 0.105 | (0.102-0.108) |
| 3-factor | 1848.354[a] | 207 | 0.963 | 0.951 | 0.087 | (0.084-0.091) |
| Confirmatory Factor Analysis (CFA) | | | | | | |
| 3-factor | 2618.928[a] | 249 | 0.945 | 0.939 | 0.096 | (0.093-0.099) |
| Exploratory Structural Equation Modeling (ESEM) | | | | | | |
| 1-factor | 13558.135[a] | 252 | 0.846 | 0.832 | 0.160 | (0.157-0.162) |
| 2-factor | 5775.137[a] | 229 | 0.936 | 0.923 | 0.108 | (0.106-0.110) |
| 3-factor | 3713.35[a] | 207 | 0.959 | 0.946 | 0.090 | (0.088-0.093) |

$x^2$ Chi-square test value, df degree of freedom, R-CFI robust comparative fit index, R-TLI robust Tucker Lewis index, R-RMSEA robust root-mean-square error of approximation, CI confidence interval, [a]p<.05

**Table 6** Factor loadings from the Exploratory Structural Equation Modeling (ESEM)

| | ESEM(n=2074) | | |
| --- | --- | --- | --- |
| | 1 | 2 | 3 |
| | Factor1 | | |
| 1 | 0.731 | -0.462 | 0.272 |
| 2 | 0.742 | -0.427 | 0.223 |
| 5 | 0.742 | 0.028 | -0.108 |
| 7 | 0.774 | -0.074 | -0.036 |
| 10 | 0.851 | 0.024 | -0.121 |
| 11 | 0.833 | -0.004 | -0.118 |
| 13 | 0.776 | 0.027 | -0.173 |
| 15 | 0.754 | 0.032 | -0.081 |
| | Factor2 | | |
| 3 | -0.002 | 0.733 | 0.145 |
| 6 | -0.109 | 0.742 | 0.183 |
| 8 | -0.081 | 0.826 | 0.143 |
| 9 | -0.093 | 0.746 | 0.153 |
| 17 | -0.095 | 0.745 | 0.266 |
| 18 | -0.143 | 0.737 | 0.273 |
| 22 | -0.293 | 0.425 | 0.517 |
| 23 | -0.228 | 0.449 | 0.497 |
| | Factor3 | | |
| 4 | -0.046 | 0.602 | 0.255 |
| 12 | 0.098 | 0.177 | 0.511 |
| 14 | 0.087 | 0.218 | 0.539 |
| 16 | -0.095 | 0.494 | 0.363 |
| 19 | 0.098 | -0.122 | 0.765 |
| 20 | -0.003 | 0.008 | 0.817 |
| 21 | -0.130 | 0.289 | 0.598 |
| 24 | -0.080 | 0.245 | 0.638 |

and 23) had high, positive and significant loadings. Accordingly, we did not exclude any of the FDI-24 items in the analyses. Future measurement invariance investigations with independent American and Chinese samples might identify specific items that are considered as country specific.

The present study is the first to examine the psychometric properties of the FDI-24 in a sample of Chinese university students. As with the American student samples, we found that most of the item-total correlations for three domains of the FDI-24 were greater than .70. In particular, in a study by Osman and colleagues [28], the reliability estimates for the three subscales' scores were moderate to high (i.e., ranging from .86 to .93). Ballard et al. [31] also reported good internal consistency reliability estimates of .86 and .89 for two domains of the FDI-24 among undergraduate psychology students. Likewise, high reliability estimates of the scale scores

were reported for military personnel samples in the United States [41]. An additional strength of the current study relates to the use of data from a large sample of study participants. In addition, systematic steps that involved the use of both exploratory and confirmatory procedures were undertaken to address the specific goals of the study.

Despite the strengths noted, several limitations were also prominent. First, the findings need to be replicated in other Western and non-Western clinical and nonclinical samples. Second, all the study participants were college-age students who presented with low to moderate risk factors for suicide-related behaviors. It might have been useful to screen study participants for suicide-related behaviors, including the frequency of suicide ideation, history of suicide threats, and other forms of psychopathology. It is worth noting, however, that the sample was composed of medical students, who tend to present with higher prevalence rates of depression and anxiety symptoms as well as higher levels of psychological distress than in the general population [42]. Despite these limitations, this is the first study to demonstrate acceptable internal consistency reliability and validity estimates of FDI-24 scores in Chinese university students. These findings support the adequacy of the psychometric properties of the FDI-24 scale scores in Chinese culture.

## Conclusion

The reliability and validity of the FDI-24 were supported by the data from a large Chinese university student sample. More studies with nationwide samples are needed to replicate current findings and to further examine other psychometric properties of the FDI-24.

## Abbreviations

AIC: (average inter-item correlation); BHS: Beck Hopelessness Scale; CFA: Confirmatory Factor Analysis; EFA: Exploratory Factor Analysis; ESEM: Exploratory Structural Equation Modeling; FDI-24: Future Disposition Inventory-24; KMO: Kaiser-Meyer-Olkin; NF: Negative Focus; PF: Positive Focus; R-CFI: Robust comparative fit index; R-RMSEA: Robust root-mean-square error of approximation; R-TLI: Robust Tucker Lewis index; SO: Suicide Orientation

## Acknowledgements
We would like to thank the teachers and staff from the School of Public Health and Medicine, Shandong University and Shandong University of Traditional Chinese Medicine for providing support. We also thank all of the participants in this study.

## Authors' contributions
BL, AO and CXJ conceptualized and designed the study and coordinated the survey process. DFW contributed to the data collection. LY analyzed the data and wrote the first draft of the manuscript. CXJ supervised the study and critically revised the manuscript. All authors carried out the study and approved the paper.

## Consent for publication
Not applicable.

## Competing interests
The authors declare that they have no competing interests.

## Author details
[1]Department of Epidemiology, School of Public Health, Shandong University & Shandong University Center for Suicide Prevention Research, Jinan, Shandong, China. [2]Department of Preventive Medicine, School of Basic Medical Sciences, Shandong University of Traditional Chinese Medicine, Changqing, Jinan, Shandong, China. [3]Department of Social Psychology, Faculty of Human Ecology, Putra University of Malaysia, Serdang, Selangor, Malaysia. [4]Department of Psychology, One UTSA Circle, The University of Texas at San Antonio, San Antonio, TX, USA.

## References
1. Phillips MR, Li XY, Zhang YP. Suicide rates in China, 1995-99. Lancet (London, England). 2002;359:835–40.
2. Conner KR, McCarthy MD, Bajorska A, Caine ED, Tu XM, Knox KL. Mood, anxiety, and substance-use disorders and suicide risk in a military population cohort. Suicide Life Threat Behav. 2012;42(6):699–708.
3. Chapman CL, Mullin K, Ryan CJ, Kuffel A, Nielssen O, Large M. Meta-analysis of the association between suicidal ideation and later suicide among patients with either a schizophrenia spectrum psychosis or a mood disorder. Acta Psychiatr Scand. 2015;131(3):162–73.
4. Hill RM, Castellanos D, Pettit JW. Suicide-related behaviors and anxiety in children and adolescents: a review. Clin Psycho Review. 2011;31(7):1133–44.
5. Chang EC. Hope and hopelessness as predictors of suicide ideation in Hungarian college students. Death Studies. 2017;41(7):455-60.
6. Bagge CL, Lamis DA, Nadorff M, Osman A. Relations between hopelessness, depressive symptoms and suicidality: mediation by reasons for living. J Clin Psychol. 2014;70(1):18–31.
7. Daniel SS, Goldston D, Erkanli A, Franklin JC, Mayfield AM. Trait anger, anger expression, and suicide attempts among adolescents and young adults: a prospective study. J Clin Child Adolesc Psychol. 2009;40(5):91–9.
8. Hawkins KA, Hames JL, Ribeiro JD, Silva C, Joiner TE, Cougle JR. An examination of the relationship between anger and suicide risk through the lens of the interpersonal theory of suicide. J Psychiatr Res. 2014;50(1):59–65.
9. Lasgaard M, Goossens L, Elklit A. Loneliness, depressive symptomatology, and suicide ideation in adolescence: cross-sectional and longitudinal analyses. J Abnorm Child Psychol. 2011;39(1):137–50.
10. Stravynski A, Boyer R. Loneliness in relation to suicide ideation and parasuicide: a population-wide study. Suicide Life Threat Behav. 2001;31(1):32–40.
11. Lester D. Hopelessness in undergraduate students around the world: a review. J Affect Disord. 2013;150(3):1204–8.
12. Beck AT, Weissman A, Lester D, Trexler L. The measurement of pessimism: the Beck hopelessness scale. J Consult Clin Psychol. 1974;42(6):861–5.
13. Beck AT, Steer RA, Kovacs M, Garrison B. Hopelessness and eventual suicide: a 10-year prospective study of patients hospitalized with suicidal ideation. Am J Psychiatry. 1985;142(5):559–63.
14. Kovacs M, Beck AT, Weissman A. Hopelessness: an indicator of suicidal risk. Suicide. 1975;5(2):98.
15. Beck AT, Kovacs M, Weissman A. Hopelessness and suicidal behavior: an overview. JAMA. 1975;234(11):1146–9.
16. Qiu T, Klonsky ED, Klein DN. Hopelessness predicts suicide ideation but not attempts: a 10-year longitudinal study. Suicide Life Threat Behav. 2017;47(6):718-22.
17. Zhang J. A strain theory of suicide. Hauppauge. New York: Nova Science; 2012.
18. Zhang W, Jia C, Hu X, Qiu H, Liu X. Beck hopelessness scale: psychometric properties among rural Chinese suicide attempters and non-attempters. Death studies. 2015;39(7):442–6.
19. Dozois DJ, Covin R. The Beck depression inventory-II (BDI-II), Beck hopelessness scale (BHS), and Beck scale for suicide ideation (BSS), vol. 2. Hoboken, NJ: John Wiley & Sons Inc; 2004.
20. Mcmillan D, Gilbody S, Beresford E, Neilly L. Can we predict suicide and non-fatal self-harm with the Beck hopelessness scale? A meta-analysis. Psychol Med. 2007;37(6):769–78.
21. Beck AT, Steer RA, Beck JS, Newman CF. Hopelessness, depression, suicidal ideation, and clinical diagnosis of depression. Suicide Life Threat Behav. 1993;23(2):139–45.
22. Gutierrez PM, Osman A, Kopper BA, Barrios FX, Bagge CL. Suicide risk assessment in a college student population. J Couns Psychol. 2000;47(4):403–13.
23. MacLeod AK, Tata P, Tyrer P, Schmidt U, Davidson K, Thompson S. Hopelessness and positive and negative future thinking in parasuicide. Br J Clin Psychol. 2005;44(Pt 4):495–504.
24. Goodby E, MacLeod AK. Future-directed thinking in first-episode psychosis. Br J Clin Psychol. 2016;55(2):93–106.

25. Herche J, Engelland B. Reversed-polarity items and scale unidimensionality. J Acad Mark Sci. 1996;24(4):366.

26. Rodebaugh TL, Woods CM, Heimberg RG. The reverse of social anxiety is not always the opposite: the reverse-scored items of the social interaction anxiety scale do not belong. Behav Ther. 2007;38(2):192–206.

27. Young MA, Halper IS, Clark DC, Scheftner W, Fawcett J. An item-response theory evaluation of the Beck hopelessness scale. Cognit Ther Res. 1992; 16(5):579–87.

28. Osman A, Gutierrez PM, Barrios F, Wong JL, Freedenthal S, Lozano G. Development and initial psychometric properties of the University of Texas at san Antonio future disposition inventory. J Clin Psychol. 2010; 66(4):410–29.

29. Jahn DR, Cukrowicz KC, Mitchell SM, Poindexter EK, Guidry ET. The mediating role of perceived burdensomeness in relations between domains of cognitive functioning and indicators of suicide risk. J Clin Psychol. 2015;71(9):908–19.

30. Bryan CJ, Ray-Sannerud B, Morrow CE, Etienne N. Guilt is more strongly associated with suicidal ideation among military personnel with direct combat exposure. J Affect Disord. 2013;148(1):37–41.

31. Ballard ED, Patel AB, Ward M, Lamis DA. Future disposition and suicidal ideation: mediation by depressive symptom clusters. J Affect Disord. 2015; 170(170C):1–6.

32. Kong YY, Zhang J, Jia SH, Zhou L. Reliability and validity of the Beck hopelessness scale for adolescent. Chin Ment Health J. 2007;21(10):686–9.

33. Guillemin F, Bombardier C, Beaton D. Cross-cultural adaptation of health-related quality of life measures: literature review and proposed guidelines. J Clin Epidemiol. 1993;46(12):1417.

34. Sperber AD, Devellis RF, Boehlecke B. Cross-cultural translation: methodology and validation. J Cross-Cult Psychol. 1994;25(4):501–24.

35. Huang Q, Wang X, Chen G. Reliability and validity of 10-item CES-D among middle aged and older adults in China. Chin. J. Health Psychol. 2015;7:1036–41.

36. Shen Q, Jiang S. Life meaning and well-being in adolescents. Chin Ment Health J. 2013;27(8):634–40.

37. Schermelleh-Engel K, Moosbrugger H, Müller H. Evaluating the fit of structural equation models: tests of significance and descriptive goodness-of-fit measures. Methods of Psychological Research (online). 2003;8(2):23–74.

38. Bland JM, Altman DG. Statistics notes: Cronbach's alpha. BMJ. 1997;314:572.

39. Nunnally JC. Psychometric theory (2nd edition). New York: McGraw-Hill; 1978.

40. Fornell C, Larcker DF. Evaluating structural equation models with unobservable variables and measurement error. J Mark Res. 1981;18(1):39–50.

41. Bryan CJ, Ray-Sannerud BN, Morrow CE, Etienne N. Optimism reduces suicidal ideation and weakens the effect of hopelessness among military personnel. Cognit Ther Res. 2013;37(5):996–1003.

42. Dyrbye LN, Thomas MR, Shanafelt TD. Systematic review of depression, anxiety, and other indicators of psychological distress among U.S. and Canadian medical students. Acad Med. 2006;81(4):354–73.

# 11

# Meaningful connections in dementia end of life care in long term care homes

Lynn McCleary[1]* ⓘ, Genevieve N Thompson[2], Lorraine Venturato[3], Abigail Wickson-Griffiths[4], Paulette Hunter[5], Tamara Sussman[6] and Sharon Kaasalainen[7]

## Abstract

**Background:** Most persons with dementia die in long term care (LTC) homes, where palliative approaches are appropriate. However, palliative approaches have not been widely implemented and there is limited understanding of staff and family experiences of dying and bereavement in this context.

**Method:** This descriptive qualitative study explored family and staff experiences of end of life and end of life care for persons with dementia in LTC homes. Eighteen focus groups were conducted with 77 staff members and 19 relatives of persons with dementia at four LTC homes in four Canadian provinces.

**Results:** Three themes emerged: *knowing the resident*, the understanding that *they are all human beings*, and the *long slow decline and death* of residents with dementia.

**Discussion:** Intimate knowledge of the person with dementia, obtained through longstanding relationships, was foundational for person-centred end of life care. Health care aides need to be included in end of life care planning to take advantage of their knowledge of residents with dementia. There were unmet bereavement support needs among staff, particularly health care aides. Persons with dementia were affected by death around them and existing rituals for marking deaths in LTC homes may not fit their needs. Staff were uncomfortable answering relatives' questions about end of life.

**Conclusions:** Longstanding intimate relationships enhanced end of life care but left health care aides with unmet bereavement support needs. Staff in LTC homes should be supported to answer questions about the trajectory of decline of dementia and death. Further research about residents' experiences of deaths of other residents is needed.

**Keywords:** Palliative care, Nursing homes, Death, Bereavement, Illness trajectory

## Background

The prevalence of dementia is increasing dramatically with population aging. Dementia, a class of neurodegenrative diseases, is characterized by progressive deterioration and decline in cognition and functioning. In late stages of dementia, the person is completely dependent on care providers. Although community-based care for dementia is more common than it once was, in North America most people with dementia die in long term care (LTC) homes [1].

Lack of access to palliative care is a problem for persons with dementia, who are less likely than people with cancer to be referred to palliative care despite a similar burden of suffering [2]. In recent years, increased attention has been paid to the need for better end of life and palliative care for persons with dementia. The European Association for Palliative Care (EAPC) white paper on palliative care for persons with dementia affirmed that because dementia is a terminal condition, with care focused on maintaining and improving quality of life, palliative care is appropriate for dementia [3].

A palliative approach includes attending to comfort needs, psychosocial needs, spiritual needs, symptom management, and advanced care planning. The focus is on quality of life of the person with dementia and their family or informal carers [4]. It is congruent with the person centred approach of good dementia care [5, 6].

Literature on end of life care and dementia in LTC is emerging, particularly in the areas of advance care

* Correspondence: lmccleary@brocku.ca
[1]Department of Nursing, Brock University, St. Catharines, Canada
Full list of author information is available at the end of the article

planning [7, 8] and pain and symptom management [2, 9], with less research about psychosocial and spiritual aspects of palliative care.

There is some evidence of suboptimal palliative care for persons with dementia in LTC homes [2, 10]. In their synthesis of evaluations of programs to improve palliative care in LTC homes, Goodman and colleagues concluded that "for people with dementia living and dying in care homes uncertainty is an inevitable and integral part of end of life care" [27, 11]. Uncertainty means that it is difficult to predict death or recognize when someone with dementia is nearing end of life. Additional challenges for staff and families include lack of recognition of dementia as a life-limiting illness and the high prevalence of comorbid conditions in end stage dementia [2, 11, 12].

Emerging evidence indicates that comprehensive programs that include staff training and tools to support practice change can improve end of life in LTC homes [11, 13, 14]. This literature also highlights the importance of a holistic palliative approach that attends to the psychosocial and spiritual needs of staff and families as the resident dies and in their bereavement [15]. Better understanding of staff and family experiences of end of life and end of life care of persons with dementia in LTC homes is essential for implementing holistic palliative care programs. The purpose of this study was to describe family and staff experiences of end of life and end of life care of persons with dementia in LTC homes. Specifically, we explored how care near the end of life is provided, what facilitates this care, and challenges experienced by staff and families.

## Method

This descriptive qualitative study was conducted as a sub study during baseline data collection for a multi-site investigation of a program to enhance end of life care in LTC homes [16]. The research was approved by five university Research Ethics Boards. The study was conducted in four LTC homes in four Canadian provinces. The homes have between 50 and 284 beds and between 14 and 58 deaths per year. Two have segregated dementia units.

Multiple focus groups were conducted at each LTC home. Four focus groups were conducted with relatives of residents of the LTC homes, one at each site. Family participants were recruited through a combination of flyers, email letters, posters, and through the Family Councils of the LTC homes. Thirteen staff focus groups were held (3 or 4 in each LTC home). Staff were recruited through information sessions at staff meetings and posters in the LTC homes inviting staff to participate. All participants provided written informed consent.

Focus groups lasted between 30 min and about an hour and were audiorecorded and transcribed verbatim.

The interview guides prompted discussion about end of life practices in the LTC home; compassion and comfort in end of life care; staff comfort with providing end of life care, including barriers, facilitators, and learning needs; and family expectations of end of life care. Staff focus groups included discussion of experiences talking about end of life with residents and families, while family focus groups discussed experiences talking with staff about end of life. Participants were asked about the impact of dementia as the various topics were discussed.

Thematic analysis [17] was conducted beginning with reading and rereading the transcripts and preliminary discussion of the data (LM, GT, LV). Initial data coding, collating codes into emergent themes, and comparison of findings within and between staff and family focus group transcripts, was conducted by the first author, followed by discussion of and confirmation of themes and discussion of the meaning of findings by three authors (LM, GT, LV).

## Results

### Sample

Between 4 and 5 family members attended each family focus group, resulting in 19 family participants. Their relatives had been living in the LTC home for an average of 4.5 years (SD = 4.5; range, less than 1 to 13 years). A description of the family member sample is presented in Table 1.

Between 3 and 13 staff members attended each staff focus group, resulting in 77 staff participants. The average number of years employed at the LTC home was 8.9 (SD = 7.8; range, less than 1 to 38 years). A description of the staff sample is presented in Table 2.

**Table 1** Family participant characteristics (N = 19)

| Characteristic | N | % |
|---|---|---|
| Sex | | |
|   Female | 14 | 73.7 |
|   Male | 5 | 26.3 |
| Kin relationship to resident | | |
|   Child | 14 | 73.7 |
|   Spouse | 2 | 10.5 |
|   Sibling | 1 | 5.3 |
|   Other | 2 | 10.5 |
| Age in years | | |
|   45 to 54 | 1 | 5.3 |
|   55 to 64 | 8 | 42.1 |
|   65 to 74 | 7 | 36.8 |
|   75 to 84 | 2 | 10.5 |
|   85 or older | 1 | 5.3 |

**Table 2** Staff participant characteristics (N = 77)

| Characteristic | N | % |
|---|---|---|
| Sex | | |
| Female | 69 | 89.6 |
| Male | 7 | 9.1 |
| Missing | 1 | 1.3 |
| Age | | |
| Under 25 | 2 | 2.6 |
| 25 to 34 | 11 | 14.3 |
| 35 to 44 | 17 | 22.1 |
| 45 to 54 | 24 | 31.2 |
| 55 to 64 | 16 | 20.8 |
| 65 and older | 7 | 9.1 |
| Profession | | |
| Health care aide | 26 | 33.8 |
| Nurse (registered nurse, registered practical nurse, licensed practical nurse) | 22 | 28.6 |
| Allied Health Professional | 13 | 16.9 |
| Housekeeping and Dietary Staff | 8 | 10.4 |
| Manager | 5 | 6.5 |
| Support Staff | 3 | 3.9 |
| Employment Status | | |
| Full time | 56 | 72.7 |
| Part time | 18 | 23.4 |
| No response | 3 | 3.9 |
| Completed Some Palliative Education or Training | | |
| Yes | 47 | 61.0 |
| No | 26 | 33.8 |
| No response | 4 | 5.2 |

## Themes

Three themes emerged: (1) the importance of knowing the resident; (2) they are all human beings; and (3) long slow decline and death in dementia. Following is an elaboration of each theme and the sub-themes within them.

### Knowing the resident

That LTC staff have an intimate knowledge of the person with dementia emerged as significant to both staff and family participants. This theme reflects the importance to participants that staff know the person with dementia intimately. Knowing the person with dementia allowed staff to provide comfort and compassion when the person with dementia could not communicate through words. Knowing the person with dementia was a result of the long time that staff spent working with the person. Staff thought that when persons with dementia were admitted within a few months of their eventual death, staff did not have enough time to get to know the person, making it more difficult to provide person-centred end of life care. There were three sub-themes within this theme: time for staff to come to know the resident intimately; time to establish a relationship; and consistent staffing.

### Time to know the resident intimately

As a result of time spent caring for the person with dementia, health care aides, dietary aides, and activation recreation staff knew the person with dementia intimately. They knew their routines, their preferences for food and beverages, their facial expressions, what position they preferred for sleeping, and what comforted them. This intimate knowledge made it easier to provide comfort and to overcome communication challenges with persons with dementia, especially when the dying person was unresponsive either because of being in late stages of dementia or because death was near. Knowing the person intimately was important to staff and to families. As one son described:

> You have to get to know them personally... and obviously as you get to know that person, then I think you can provide that compassionate care because you know what their needs are. (Family ID 1)

Knowing the resident intimately allowed staff greater ability to detect subtle changes, particularly in regard to pain. Providing adequate pain management at the end of life was critically important to staff and family participants. Staff reported that it was difficult to assess pain of persons with dementia. Health care aides and family participants thought that knowledge of the person with dementia contributed positively to pain assessment and management. A health care aide described:

> Even the dementia residents do not tell you they are in pain, you can see it in their face that they are in pain. (Staff ID 14)

### Time to establish relationships

This theme emerged primarily from descriptions provided by families and health care aides, as well as from supervisors' descriptions and observations about health care aides, dietary aides, and activity and recreation staff. For health care aides, working with a resident with dementia over many months or even years meant that they had established close relationships. Health care aides viewed themselves as an extension of the resident's family and described their relationships as family-like or friendships. For some, these relationships made it easier to be compassionate at the end of life. Health care aides described that the person with dementia reacts differently to them during end of life, depending on the relationship that is established and the quality of their relationship. These close relationships were reported to result in persons with dementia, even when mostly unresponsive, being able to recognize the staff member's presence and be comforted by it. Two health care aides discussed this:

> First health care aide: I work on the dementia units. Most of our seniors when they get to the point when they are dying, they don't talk much. They don't really know much about what's going on. But, yet, you do see some responses to being there with them. (Staff ID 20)

> Interviewer: Yeah.

> Second health care aide: Whether it's they relax more, or they will cling to your hand, or start mumbling, or kind of sing quietly. (Staff ID 21)

These longstanding close relationships also meant that the loss of the relationship when the resident died could be felt deeply. Health care aides spoke about experiencing sadness, loss, and grief when residents with dementia die. They discussed the importance of maintaining relationships after a resident or health care aide was transferred to another unit, especially being able to visit before the resident died. A health care aide explained:

> It's kind of sad when you suddenly, you didn't even have a visit. So, if you have a last visit on their last day, you say goodbye. It feels okay. (Staff ID 18)

Staff experiences of grief and need for time to mourn were recognized by family participants and by supervisor participants. However, some health care aides felt unsupported by their supervisors, who did not acknowledge the meaning of the death and loss for them. For some health care aides, it was very important to attend a resident's funeral or funeral home visitation, especially if they felt particularly close to the resident. It was uncommon for them to be provided with time to attend funerals or visitations.

### Consistent staffing

For both family and staff participants, having time to know the person with dementia and time to establish relationships was linked to consistent staffing. Families thought that staff consistently working on the same units made it possible for staff to attend to and notice signs of distress or agitation that might indicate pain or

fear. Staff and managers who worked in a LTC home where staff did not rotate between units thought that this staffing practice was important both for achieving intimate knowledge of their residents and for residents being comfortable with staff. A manager explained:

> Here you come in say year one and group one (of residents) and year ten you are in group one. They always have, and that's really helpful with dementia because they get to recognize them. (Staff ID 23)

### They are all human beings

This theme reflects staff and family views about what they referred to as the "human" experience of end of life and grief for persons with dementia. There were three sub-themes; the first was persons with dementia deserving good end of life care; the second, person centred end of life care for residents with dementia; and the third, living with death around them.

### Persons with dementia deserve good end of life care

When asked about differences in providing end of life care for persons with dementia compared to residents who do not have dementia, staff were consistently very quick to respond that it does not matter whether the dying person has dementia. This seemed to be related to staff values for equity and good end of life care; that everyone deserves comfort and compassion at the end of their life. Staff often referred to the dementia diagnosis not defining the person, that people with dementia are "still human" or "all human beings." Family participants expressed hope that end of life care would be similar for those with and without dementia.

### Providing person centred end of life care for residents with dementia

In further discussion, staff and family described some unique aspects of end of life care for persons with dementia, as compared to residents who do not have dementia. These related to time and effort to provide nursing care, the impact of behavioral symptoms of dementia, and the importance of touch for persons with dementia.

**Time and effort** Staff explained that care takes more time when someone is dying, even more so when the person has dementia and cannot express their needs verbally. Nurses and health care aides referred to needing to use their knowledge of the person and go through more of "a process of figuring out what comforts them" (Staff ID 67) when the dying person has dementia. A health care aide discussed and explained the challenge of positioning a resident and the importance of teamwork:

Two person [care] is good, especially the dementia person. When they are dying it is very hard for us. For resident also it's very hard. So, if two person, we can consult each other to put position that would be best for her. And always we keep an eye on how he or she is doing. (Staff ID 16)

Extra time and effort was also needed for communication with and reassuring the person with dementia at end of life. A health care aide explained:

If they are palliative, until they are unresponsive, sometimes just knowing that you might have to repeat things so many times to them about their condition and what you are going to do .... It seems like you have to give even more reassurance and repeat yourself more often to answer their questions more frequently because they do tend to forget what you say to them or maybe respond in a different manner than someone else might, who does not have dementia. (Staff ID 65)

Family participants also thought that end of life care would take more time with a resident who had dementia. Time that, in many cases, they thought staff did not have.

**Behavioural symptoms** Staff and family participants explained that if the person with dementia has "aggressive" behaviours, then it is more challenging for staff to be compassionate. As a health care aide explained:

Depends on what behaviours they have, unfortunately. If somebody comes in and they are aggressive with us from day one until the day they pass away, like, I don't particularly like getting physically hit. It makes it harder to spend that quality time with them. (Staff ID 20)

A daughter expressed similar thoughts about staff interactions with residents who have behavioural symptoms:

If they don't have training or understanding how to deal with it, most people, just by human nature, I think, are going to try and back off. (Staff ID 5)

**Touch** For staff and family participants, touch was described as an important way of demonstrating compassion and care for anyone who is dying, especially for persons with dementia. A manager explained:

Touch can sometimes be that final way of connecting when the words don't make sense any more. Or I can't even see you or if I'm seeing this cup and I don't even know what it is. Just the presence and touching. (Staff ID 25)

**Living with death around them**
Family and staff participants described persons with dementia noticing deaths of other residents, being affected by the deaths, and experiencing grief. Family participants described LTC home residents as living with death around them. There were differing opinions among family participants about how to acknowledge deaths. Some thought it might not be good to tell their relatives that someone had died, others thought that the residents with dementia needed support when someone in the LTC home died. A son described his father noticing and being affected by the death of a resident he did not know well:

Well, you know, he doesn't even know the fellow. But, you know, he's only been here a few days and hasn't even met the fellow. But, you know, just knowing this is kind of his last home. It bothered him. (Family ID 6)

A daughter, discussing what it was like when a roommate died, recounted:

Even if the roommate had dementia, you know, they're still... you can still get little flashes of insight ... having someone die in your room would be very upsetting. Because my Dad did have a roommate die. He was aware of it. (Staff ID 17)

According to staff participants, persons with dementia know when someone dies, they feel the loss, need support, and, for the most part, are not supported in their grief. As one staff participant explained:

You remember when (resident's name) died and (resident's name) got so upset. So, the residents build relationships with each other, right. They get close. But when you have dementia, you still have closeness. (Staff ID 15)

Several of the homes recognized deaths of residents by posting memorial lists of names or photographs of residents who died. This was not viewed as sufficient support for residents with dementia. As described by a staff participant:

There is very little support for the roommate or the friends of the person who has passed away. Like, it's all informal, right? (Staff ID 20)

One home had a practice of recognizing a resident's death by putting a rose at the person's place in the dining room at a meal the day after the person dies. At the meal, there would be a brief acknowledgement of the person's death and a prayer. This practice was seen by family participants as a good way to recognize and support their relatives' grieving.

## Long slow decline and death

This theme reflects staff and family views about the long slow decline and death of the person with dementia. There were three sub-themes in this theme: prolonged losses; uncertainty for families about the dementia illness trajectory; and death as a release from misery.

### Prolonged losses and decline

Family participants talked about the prolonged suffering of their relatives and the multiple losses they experienced. They viewed the LTC home as the "end of the line," as one daughter described it (Family ID 7). Another family participant explained: "People in long term care are gradually dying very slowly" (Family ID 18).

There were varying opinions about what this means for families when their relative dies. Some family participants thought that compared to death of a relative from another cause, the prolonged losses and decline experienced with dementia might make death worse for families. A daughter anticipated that her grief may be easier than grief associated with death from other causes:

> We lived with my Mom in long term care for so many years and watched the slow decline with dementia. It's like we... we've started saying goodbye a long time ago, so the final breath isn't, won't be as traumatic as maybe a sudden death would be. (Family ID 15)

Some staff and family participants referred to persons with dementia as "already lost" (Staff ID 23), "not being the same person" (Family ID 6), or that "they are not really alive the way they should be" (Family ID 8) by the time late stages of dementia and end of life occurred. This was more common among registered nursing staff than health care aides, who also reported closer relationships with residents with dementia. This perceived loss of the person to dementia prior to death, was seen as resulting in some family members not being there when the person with dementia died. A recreation therapist described an experience:

> I have sat with a resident while he was passing away as long as I could before. Just because the family had said. It wasn't here. The family has said that I lost my father years ago, I don't need to be here. (Staff ID 75)

### Family uncertainty about the dementia illness trajectory

While staff participants thought that some families viewed their relative as already lost or gone, they also found that families are often not ready for their relative's decline and uncertain about the trajectory of decline associated with dementia. Staff thought that understanding this decline would help families anticipate and accept death. A nurse explained:

> We have people with dementia, families are expecting them to be behaving and acting the same way they used to six months ago or even sometimes, when they were at home. And there are slow, gradual changes. And they are thinking, well the individual can't hear. That is what the problem is. The problem is not that the hearing has deteriorated, it is that the information processing has changed and they are not ready to accept that. They want the hearing issue dealt with. (Staff ID 66)

Similarly, family participants described how important it was to understand dementia and the course of illness. They needed answers to their questions about how much longer their relative would live. They wanted to know what death would be like and what kind of care their relative would receive as death neared. For some, there was a perception that staff were not comfortable with these discussions. As described by a sibling of a resident:

> To me, helping people understand, really, really understand what an end of life process is. It just. Then there still seems to be an incredible amount of reluctance on the provider's side to even talk about that. Because it's not necessarily a pretty process. It seems like the general belief is it's better for people to be surprised by it or whatever. I don't know what the hell it is but and because of that people don't properly prepare. (Family ID 10)

Staff participants explained that it was difficult to answer families' questions about resident comfort, how long the person had to live, or when death could be expected. A health care aide described being "totally outside my comfort zone" (Staff ID 21) when interacting with families of residents with dementia who are dying. A nurse described being comfortable with families, attributing this to interacting with and coming to know families over time on a dementia unit.

### Death is a release from misery

Family participants described the long process of decline as suffering. Many staff viewed death of a person with dementia as a release from suffering and misery. This suffering included the losses that the person experienced over the course of dementia and their experiences of behavioural and psychological symptoms of dementia. A health care aide described the relief she felt when someone died:

> You feel sorry for them. The aggressive person. ... But it's good they can go peacefully. (Staff ID 28)

Staff participants reported that families were usually, but not always, grateful that their relative had been released from suffering.

A health care aide explained:

> I think it is kind of more comforting for the family, though. Like, if ... their death had been caused by the dementia. You know what I mean. They had just been continually declining and it is almost, they feel like they are not suffering anymore ... sometimes I think family are happy to know that they are in a better place. (Staff ID 73)

Some staff thought that their relative's death might be a relief from stress for families but that some families were not ready to let go. A nurse explained:

> I think sometimes family members are more, not in every case, but family members are more willing to let go and to almost. There is almost a positive anticipation. Not sure if you would agree. But, sometimes I guess there is a lot of stress and challenges when a family member is suffering dementia and, so, maybe that arises out of a sense of there being relief. (Staff ID 77)

## Discussion

Close intimate relationships between staff and residents were seen as vital for providing end of life care and overcoming challenges related to the person with dementia's diminished communication ability. These findings have implications for implementing palliative approaches to end of life care for persons with dementia in LTC homes. The person centred care approach that is advocated in dementia care continued to be relevant at end of life. Relationships, valuing people with dementia, and treating people as individuals are core tenants of person centred care [18] and were evident in the *knowing the resident* and *they are all human beings* themes. This is consistent with the principles of palliative care and the European Association for Palliative Care (EAPC) white paper on dementia [3]. However, there are varying opinions about the value of a palliative approach in advanced dementia care [4]. Efforts to adopt palliative care approaches should build on commonalities between good palliative and end of life care and the person centred care approaches that are already used in LTC homes [5, 6].

When implementing palliative care with persons with dementia in LTC homes, training and education can help staff to see the link between end of life care practices and the person centred care approaches they value and are already using.

Pain management is notoriously challenging with persons with dementia, particularly at the end of life [2]. Pain and agitation are common among persons with dementia at the end of life, and pain interventions are underutilized [2, 9, 19]. Staff and families thought that intimate knowledge of the person with dementia made it easier to know when a dying person with dementia was in pain and respond to signs of pain, agitation, or distress. Health care aides were confident about recognizing pain. The close relationship between the health care aides and residents, the health care aides' intimate knowledge of the person, and their ability to recognize subtle indicators of discomfort and distress should be leveraged to improve pain management. However, inadequate acknowledgement and support of health care aides' ability to detect pain and advocate for residents is a barrier to improving pain management in LTC [20]. Health care aides' opinions are frequently dismissed, and they are not included in case conferences where pain management is discussed [21]. Implementing comprehensive palliative care programs such as the Gold Standard Framework in Care Homes can result in improved collaboration between nursing staff and health care aides [13], potentially paving the way to incorporating health care aides' intimate knowledge of dying residents with dementia in their pain management.

The amount of time that a person with dementia lives in a LTC home varies by jurisdiction from months to several years [22]. In Canada length of stay at time of death in LTC homes is decreasing [23]. This trend may impact end of life care for residents with dementia. In this study, staff indicated that when there was a shorter length of stay, they did not feel the same connection to and knowledge of the needs, preferences and essence of who the dying resident is.

The advantages that close relationships and intimate knowledge bestow on end of life care come at a cost for staff, especially for health care aides. This is consistent with previous research where staff described family-like relationships and grief associated with end of life care of persons with dementia [24, 25] and points to the importance of supporting staff grief and bereavement [15]. However, previous research has identified issues of inadequate support for staff related to grief and emotional needs [24–27]. The close relationships between staff and residents with dementia are not acknowledged when residents die and there is not enough time for staff to grieve [25]. Similarly, health care aides in a previous study received support in their grief from their peers but not from supervisors [27].

Administrators and supervisors recognized the need to support staff after residents died. Managers' concern about staff wellbeing after residents die supports feasibility of increasing support from supervisors. End of life education and support needs vary depending on staff role [28]. Supervisors who are aware that health care aides may be less likely than other staff to view the person with dementia as "already gone" prior to death may be better able to support their grief and purposefully check in with and acknowledge grief when a resident with dementia dies.

Supporting staff as residents deteriorate and after their deaths is an important part of end of life dementia care [15]. Some LTC homes had rituals to acknowledge the death of a resident; rituals that could play a role in acknowledging and supporting staff grief, such as memorial photographs, having a staff honor guard when the resident's body leaves the building, and memorial services. These practices and others, such as providing emotional support through regular discussions about recent deaths, have been identified as positive [29, 30]. However, for some staff, rituals in the LTC home were insufficient and it was important to be able to attend the deceased resident's funeral or visitation. This was rarely possible. While resources are limited in LTC homes, supporting staff grief and need to participate in funeral rituals would be consistent with and demonstrate value for the relationships staff form with residents with dementia.

Several writers have discussed death as "hidden" in LTC homes [27, 31]. This aspect of the culture of LTC homes is relevant to our findings about the impact of death on surviving residents with dementia in LTC homes and family need for information about the illness trajectory of dementia. Consistent with recent research, staff and family participants identified unmet support needs for residents with dementia when a fellow resident died [32]. Posting a memorial name or photograph was seen as inadequate, especially for residents with dementia. The ceremonial marking of a resident's death by placing a rose at their dining table and praying at a meal shortly after the resident died seemed to be meaningful to staff and seen as positive for residents. Long term care homes should consider adapting and implementing this practice.

Helping families to understand the trajectory of decline and death in dementia is important in LTC homes. Family recognition of dementia as a terminal illness is associated with better resident comfort at end of life [33]. Family participants seemed to understand dementia as a terminal illness. However, they did not understand the trajectory of decline of dementia and some wanted to know what death would be like. Relatives of persons with moderate to severe dementia living in LTC homes have been found to misunderstand the terminal nature of dementia, the trajectory of decline, and what death would be like, even after the disease process has been explained to them [31, 34]. In recent research, bereaved relatives indicated that they would have appreciated receiving verbal and written information about the course of dementia and end of life [35]. Thus, there is a need to provide information in a variety of formats and repeatedly, and for staff to convey openness to answering questions about decline and death.

Some family participants perceived staff discomfort with answering [8] questions about death and the illness trajectory, consistent with previous findings [36]. These perceptions are likely accurate; staff reported being uncomfortable answering families' questions about decline and death. Health care providers' limited knowledge of the death process and the dementia illness trajectory have been identified in the literature [37] and LTC home staff have attributed their reluctance to discuss end of life with relatives of persons with dementia to lack of confidence [26]. Additionally, in LTC homes, uncertainty about when death is imminent for residents with advanced dementia is common [11]. Together, these findings support a need to provide staff with education about the trajectory of dementia, the challenges of recognizing when someone is dying, and the death process.

Limited skills for discussing emotion-laden topics or limited understanding of the therapeutic value of such discussions may also play a role in staff discomfort answering families' questions and discussing death. Staff may benefit from knowing that coming to understand the dementia illness trajectory relieves families [38]. End of life education for health care workers should include communication skills training and practice talking to relatives about decline and death of a person with dementia. Understanding that grief and distress are common for family of persons in the late stages of dementia [15, 35] may enhance staff's ability to respond to families. There is some evidence that such approaches have been effective in palliative care settings [39].

Methodological strengths of this study include the number of focus groups and diversity in the sample with respect to the LTC homes and the staff participants. LTC homes were purposefully sampled to include for-profit and not-for-profit homes, in different provinces, which vary in terms of funding and regulations for LTC homes. Diversity in the staff sample with respect to professional designation and job category meant that various staff perspectives and experiences were included. The inclusion of family and staff participants allowed us to compare their perspectives. The sample may be biased towards people who strongly value end of life care and this may be associated with some characteristics that were reported to be associated with experiences and challenges in the provision of end of life care.

The findings suggest opportunities to support end of life care for persons with dementia in LTC homes. It is important to acknowledge and support the value of relationships, the time it takes to establish relationships, and the grief experienced by staff who provide care. Health care aides' intimate knowledge of persons with dementia should be incorporated in interprofessional pain management interventions. Residents with dementia are not immune to grief and loss when other residents die. Further research about their needs is required. Existing rituals within LTC homes may need to be enhanced. Families want and need information about the dementia illness trajectory and end of life. Education and training for staff to be confident in providing this information and answering families' questions is needed.

## Abbreviations
EAPC: European Association for Palliative Care; LTC: Long term care

## Acknowledgements
The authors thank staff and family members who generously provided their time and explanations of their experiences to us and our research assistants who contributed to interviewing and transcribed the data.

## Funding
Canadian Institutes of Health Research Grant No. 337678, Ontario Ministry of Health and Long Term Care (Grant No. 06718), Saskatchewan Health Research Foundation (Grant No. 3316), Manitoba Health Research Council (Grant No. PHE-141804), Alberta Innovates Health Solutions (Grant No. 10012108), and Extendicare Canada. The funders provided funding based on the research grant application. They had no role in the design of the study; data collection, analysis and interpretation; or writing the manuscript. Brock University Open Access Publishing Fund supported the costs of open access publication.

## Authors' contributions
TS and SK planned and designed the study. All authors acquired the data. LM analysed and interpreted the data. GT & LV reviewed the analysis. LM drafted the manuscript. All authors commented on drafts of the manuscript. All authors reviewed and suggested revisions for the final manuscript. All authors contributed and approved the final manuscript.

## Consent for publication
Not applicable.

## Competing interests
The authors declare that they have no competing interests.

## Author details
[1]Department of Nursing, Brock University, St. Catharines, Canada. [2]College of Nursing, University of Manitoba, Winnipeg, Canada. [3]Faculty of Nursing, University of Calgary, Calgary, Canada. [4]Faculty of Nursing, University of Regina, Regina, Canada. [5]Department of Psychology, St. Thomas More College, University of Saskatchewan, Saskatoon, Canada. [6]School of Social Work, McGill University, Montreal, Canada. [7]School of Nursing, McMaster University, Hamilton, Canada.

## References
1. Reyniers T, Deliens L, Pasman HR, Morin L, Addington-Hall J, Frova L, Houttekier D. International variation in place of death of older people who died from dementia in 12 European and non-European countries. JAMDA. 2015;16(2):165–71. https://doi.org/10.1016/j.jamda.2014.11.003.
2. Dempsey L, Dowling M, Larkin P, Murphy K. The unmet palliative care needs of those dying with dementia. Int J Palliat Nurs. 2015;21(3):126–33. https://doi.org/10.12968/ijpn.2015.21.3.126.
3. van der Steen JT, Radbruch L, Hertogh CMPM, de Boer ME, Hughes JC, Larkin P…, Volicer L. White paper defining optimal palliative care in older people with dementia: a Delphi study and recommendations from the European Association for Palliative Care. Palliative Med. 2014;28(3):197–209. https://doi.org/10.1177/0269216313493685.
4. Sampson E, van den Noortgate N, van der Steen JT. Palliative care of patients with dementia and pain. In: Gibson SJ, Lautenbacher S, editors. Pain in Dementia. Philadelphia: Lippincott Williams & Wilkins; 2017. p. 293–304.
5. Hughes JC, Jolley D, Jordan A, Sampson EL. Palliative care in dementia: issues and evidence. Adv Psychiatr Treat. 2007;13:251–60. https://doi.org/10.1192/apt.bp.106.003442.
6. Kydd A, Sharp B. Palliative care and dementia – a time and place? Maturitas. 2016;84(5):5–10. https://doi.org/10.1016/j.maturitas.2015.10.007.
7. Beck E, McIlfatrick S, Hasson F, Leavey G. Health care professionals' perspectives of advance care planning for people with dementia living in long-term care settings: a narrative review of the literature. Dementia. 2017;16:486–512. https://doi.org/10.1177/1471301215604997.
8. Jones K, Birchley G, Huxtable R, Clare L, Walter T & Dixon J. End of life care: a scoping review of experiences of advance care planning for people with dementia. Dementia 2016; 0;1–21. https://doi.org/10.1177/1471301216676121.
9. Hendriks SA, Smalbrugge M, Galindo-Garre F, Hertogh CMPM, van der Steen JT. From admission to death: prevalence and course of pain, agitation, and shortness of breath, and treatment of these symptoms in nursing home residents with dementia. JAMDA. 2015;16:475–81. https://doi.org/10.1016/j.jamda.2014.12.016.
10. Mitchell SL, Kiely DK, Hamel MB. Dying with advanced dementia in the nursing home. Arch Intern Med. 2004;164(3):321–6. https://doi.org/10.1001/archinte.164.3.321.
11. Goodman C, Froggatt K, Amador S, Mathie E, Mayrhofer A. End of life care interventions for people with dementia in care homes: addressing uncertainty within a framework for service delivery and evaluation. BMC Palliat Care. 2015;14(1):42. https://doi.org/10.1186/s12904-015-0040-0.
12. Hill SR, Mason H, Poole M, Vale L, Robinson L. What is important at the end of life for people with dementia? The views of people with dementia and their care partners. Int J Geriatr Psych. 2017;32:1037–45. https://doi.org/10.1002/gps.4564.
13. Badger F, Plumridge G, Hewiston A, Shaw K, Thomas K, Clifford C. An evaluation of the impact of the gold standards framework on collaboration in end-of-life care in nursing homes. A qualitative and quantitative evaluation. Int J Nurs Stud. 2012;49(5):586–95. https://doi.org/10.1016/j.ijnurstu.2011.10.021.
14. Kinley J, Stone L, Dewey M, Levy J, Stewart R, McCrone P, Sykes N, Hansford P, Begum A, Hockley J. The effect of using high facilitation when implementing the gold standards framework in care homes programme: a cluster randomised controlled trial. Palliat Med. 2014;28(9):1099–109. https://doi.org/10.1177/0269216314539785.
15. Jones L, Candy B, Davis S, Elliott M, Gola A, Harrington J, Kupeli N, Lord K, Moore K, Scott S, Vickerstaff V, Omar R, King M, Leavey G, Nazareth I, Sampson E. Development of a model for integrated care at the end of life

in advanced dementia: a whole systems UK-wide approach. Palliat Med. 2016;30(3):279–95. https://doi.org/10.1177/0269216315605447.

16. Kaasalainen S, Sussman T, Neves P, Papaioannou A. Strengthening a palliative approach in long-term care (SPA-LTC): a new program to improve quality of living and dying for residents and their family members. J Am Med Dir Assoc. 2016;17(3):B21. https://doi.org/10.1016/j.jamda.2015.12.067.

17. Braun V, Clarke V. Using thematic analysis in psychology. Qual Res Psychol. 2006;3:77–101. https://doi.org/10.1177/1471301215604997.

18. Hunter PV, Hadjistavropoulos T, Kaasalainen S. A qualitative study of nursing assistants' awareness of person-centred approaches to dementia care. Ageing Soc. 2015;36:1211–37. https://doi.org/10.1017/S0144686X15000276.

19. Hendriks SA, Smalbrugge M, Hertogh CMPM, van der Steen JT. Dying with dementia: symptoms, treatment, and quality of life in the last week of life. J Pain Symptom Manag. 2014;47:710–20. https://doi.org/10.1016/j.jpainsymman.2013.05.015.

20. Kaasalainen S, Brazil K, Coker E, Ploeg J, Martin-Misener R, Donald F, Burns T. An action-based approach to improving pain management in long-term care. Can J Aging. 2010;29:503–17. https://doi.org/10.1017/S0714980810000528.

21. Jansen BDW, Brazil K, Passmore P, Buchanan H, Maxwell D, McIlfatrick SJ, Parsons C. Exploring healthcare assistants' role and experience in pain assessment and management for people with advanced dementia towards the end of life: a qualitative study. BMC Palliat Care. 2017;16:6. https://doi.org/10.1186/s12904-017-0184-1.

22. Kelly A, Conell-Price J, Covinsky K, Cenzer IS, Chang A, Boscardin WJ, Smith AK. Lengths of stay for older adults residing in nursing homes at the end of life. J Am Geriatr Soc. 2010;58:1701–6. https://doi.org/10.1111/j.1532-5415.2010.03005.x.

23. Ontario Long Term Care Association. This is long term care 2016. Toronto, ON: Author. Retrieved September 18, 2017 from https://www.oltca.com/OLTCA/Documents/Reports/TILTC2016.pdf.

24. Lawrence V, Samsi K, Murray J, Harari D, Banerjee S. Dying well with dementia: qualitative examination of end-of-life care. Brit J Psychiat. 2011;199:417–22. https://doi.org/10.1192/bjp.bp.111.093989.

25. Livingston G, Pitfield C, Morris J, Manela M, Lewis-Holmes E, Jacobs H. Care at the end of life for people with dementia living in a care home: a qualitative study of staff experience and attitudes. Int J Geriatr Psych. 2012;27:643–50. https://doi.org/10.1002/gps.2772.

26. Goddard C, Stewart F, Thompson G, Hall S. Providing end-of-life care in care homes for older people: a qualitative study of the views of care home staff and community nurses. J Appl Gerontol. 2013;32(1):76–95. https://doi.org/10.1177/0733464811405047.

27. Marcella J, Kelley ML. "Death is part of the job" in long-term care homes: supporting direct care staff with their grief and bereavement. SAGE Open. 2015. https://doi.org/10.1177/2158244015573912.

28. Kaasalainen S, Sussman T, Bui M, Akhtar-Danesh N, Laporte RD, McCleary L, O'Leary J. What are the differences among occupational groups related to their palliative care-specific educational needs and intensity of interprofessional collaboration in long-term care homes? BMC Palliat Care. 2017;16:33. https://doi.org/10.1186/s12904-017-0207-y.

29. Schulz M. Taking the lead: Supporting staff in coping with grief and loss in dementia care. Health Manage Forum. 2017;30(1):16–9. https://doi.org/10.1177/0840470416658482.

30. Wickson-Griffiths A, Kaasalainen S, Brazil K, McAiney C, Crawshaw D, Turner M, Kelley ML. Comfort care rounds: a staff capacity-building initiative in long-term care homes. J Gerontol Nurs. 2015;41(1):42–8. https://doi.org/10.3928/00989134-20140611-01.

31. Sarabia-Cobo CM, Pérez V, de Lorena P, Nuñez MJ, Domínguez E. Decisions at the end of life made by relatives of institutionalized patients with dementia. Appl Nurs Res. 2016;31:e6–e10. https://doi.org/10.1016/j.apnr.2016.02.003.

32. Sussman T, Kaasalainen S, Mintzberg S, Sinclair S, Young L, Ploeg J, Mc Kee M. Broadening the purview of comfort to improve palliative care practices in LTC. Can J Aging. 2017;36(3):306–17.

33. van Uden N, Van den Block L, van der Steen JT, Onwuteaka-Philipsen BD, Vandervoort A, Vander Stichele R, Deliens L. Quality of dying of nursing home residents with dementia as judged by relatives. Int Psychogeriatr. 2013;25:1697–707. https://doi.org/10.1017/S1041610213000756.

34. Thompson GN, Roger K. Understanding the needs of family caregivers of older adults dying with dementia. Palliat Support Care. 2014. https://doi.org/10.1017/S1478951513000461.

35. Moore K, Davis S, Gola A, Harrington J, Kupeli N, Vickerstaff V, King M, Leavet G, Nazareth I, Jones L, Sampson E. Experiences of end of life amongst family carers of people with advanced dementia: longitudinal cohort study with mixed methods. BMC Geriatr. 2017;17(1):135. https://doi.org/10.1186/s12877-017-0523-3.

36. Thompson GN, McClement S, Menec V, Chochinov H. Understanding bereaved family member's dissatisfaction with end-of-life care in nursing homes. J Gerontol Nurs. 2012;12:223–31. https://doi.org/10.3928/00989134-20120906-94.

37. Karascony S, Chang E, Johnson A, Good A, Edenborough M. Measuring nursing assistants' knowledge, skills and attitudes in a palliative approach: a literature review. Nurs Educ Today. 2015;35:1232–9. https://doi.org/10.1016/j.nedt.2015.05.008.

38. Hansen L, Archbold PG, Stewart B, Westfall UB, Ganzini L. Family caregivers making life-sustaining treatment decisions: Factors associated with role strain and ease. J Gerontol Nurs. 2005;31:28–35. https://doi.org/10.3928/0098-9134-20051101-08.

39. Barnes S, Gardiner C, Gott M, Payne S, Chady B, Small N, Seamark D, Halpin D. Enhancing patient-professional communication about end-of-life issues in life-limiting conditions: a critical review of the literature. J Pain Symptom Manag. 2012;44:866–79. https://doi.org/10.1016/j.jpainsymman.2011.11.009.

# 12

# Association between depression and the risk for fracture: a meta-analysis and systematic review

Lei Qiu[1,2], Qin Yang[1], Na Sun[1], Dandan Li[1], Yuxin Zhao[1], Xiaotong Li[1], Yanhong Gong[1], Chuanzhu Lv[3,4*] and Xiaoxv Yin[1*]

## Abstract

**Background:** Several studies have suggested that depression is associated with an increased risk for fracture; however, the results are conflicting. This study aimed to conduct a meta-analysis of cohort studies assessing the association between depression and the risk for fracture.

**Methods:** Relevant studies were identified by a search of Web of Science, PubMed, Embase, China National Knowledge Infrastructure and WanFang database to Feb 2018. Cohort studies on the relationship between depression and the risk for fracture in the general population were included in the meta-analysis. Data collection was in accordance with the Meta-analysis of Observational Studies in Epidemiology (MOOSE) guidelines, and the quality of the included studies was assessed using the Newcastle–Ottawa scale. Two independent investigators screened the abstracts and full texts of the studies, extracted data, and assessed the quality of the study. Either a fixed-effect or random-effects model was used to compute the pooled risk estimates when appropriate.

**Results:** In total, 16 cohort studies with 25 independent reports that included 414,686 participants during a follow-up duration of 3–14 years were included in the analysis. The pooled hazard ratio (HR) for total fracture was 1.24 (95% confidence interval [CI]: 1.14–1.35; $P < 0.001$ for heterogeneity; random-effects model). In the subgroup analyses conducted in terms of study region, the pooled HR for the studies conducted in Europe was higher (HR: 1.76; 95% CI: 1.44–2.17; $P = 0.792$ for heterogeneity) than that in America and Asia, with a significant difference between the groups ($P = 0.036$).

**Conclusion:** The results of our meta-analysis suggest that depression is prospectively associated with a significantly increased risk for fracture, which may have substantial implications, both clinical and preventive.

**Keywords:** Depression, Fracture, Meta-analysis

## Background

Osteoporotic fracture is a critical health problem worldwide because it causes severe pain, disability, decreased quality of life, and increased mortality and health costs [1, 2]. More than one-third of women and approximately one-tenth of men aged 50 years will sustain a major osteoporotic fracture in their remaining lifetime [3]. Similar to fracture, depression was a common disorder

in modern society, with a high prevalence among the general population [4]. The lifetime incidence of depression is approximately 16% among adults in the United States [5]. Globally, the total number of individuals with depression was around 300 million in 2015, which is equivalent to 4.4% of the world's population [6].

During the past decades, several studies have assessed the association between depression and the risk for fracture. However, the results were conflicting [7–9]. Some studies have reported that depression, was often complicated with decreased bone mineral density (BMD) and bone loss and is associated with a significant increased risk in fracture, but other studies have not found such

* Correspondence: lvchuanzhu677@126.com; yxx@hust.edu.cn
[3]Department of Emergency, The Second Affiliated Hospital of Hainan Medical University, Haikou 571199, People's Republic of China
[1]School of Public Health, Tongji Medical College, Huazhong University of Science and Technology, 430030 Wuhan, People's Republic of China
Full list of author information is available at the end of the article

risk. A previous meta-analysis pooled results from 10 studies published before 2009 as a secondary analysis and showed the association between depression and an increased risk for fracture [10]. However, this previous study had several limitations. First, the potential sources of heterogeneity were not explored, with limited description on heterogeneity across studies. Second, its subgroup analysis was limited to sex and whether the study controlled for the use of antidepressants and lack of subgroup analyses stratified by other important study and participant characteristics. For example, because the prevalence of depression varied in different regions, investigating the geographical region differences in the depression–fracture association is of interest. In addition, more studies conducted in various countries have been published in recent years, which allowed for a more detailed analysis of the relationship between depression and the risk for fracture. Given the limitations of previous review and the recent publication of numerous large cohort studies, it is necessary for us to assess the effect of depression on the risk for fractures via an updated meta-analysis based on cohort studies.

## Methods
### Search strategy
This review was conducted in accordance with the Meta-analysis of Observational Studies in Epidemiology (MOOSE) guidelines [11], with reference to the Preferred Reporting Items for Systematic Reviews and Meta-analyses (PRISMA) [12]. A literature search on prospective or retrospective cohort studies showing the association between depression and fracture in Web of Science, PubMed, Embase, China National Knowledge Infrastructure (CNKI) and WanFang database was conducted from inception to February 2018.

The following search terms were used to identify relevant citations: ("depression" [Mesh] or "depressive disorder" [Mesh] or "depressive disorder, major" [Mesh] or "mood disorders" [Mesh]) and ("fractures, bone" [Mesh] or "fracture" or "bone fracture") along with ("cohort studies" or "longitudinal studies" or "follow-up studies"). In addition, the reference lists of the original and relevant review articles were also assessed to further identify relevant studies. Papers published in English or Chinese were considered.

### Selection criteria
Studies were included in the meta-analysis based on the following inclusion criteria: (1) the cohort comprised non-institutionalized adults; (2) the exposure of interest was depression; (3) the outcome was fracture; (4) the risk estimates with the corresponding 95% confidence intervals (CI) of depression related to fracture were reported. Studies were excluded if (1) the study had a case

control design or retrospective design; (2) Reviews, letters, commentaries were excluded; (3) Lack of any information that allowed to calculate effect estimates and corresponding 95% CI. For cohorts with several reports, we tried using data from non-overlapping follow-up periods of each report, or publications with the longest follow-up periods were selected.

### Data extraction and quality assessment
We extracted the following information from each eligible study: last name of the first author, year of publication, country where the study was performed, number of participants, characteristics of the participants (sex, age range, and mean age), follow-up time, depression measures, fracture type, and covariates adjusted in the multivariable analysis.

Quality assessment was performed according to the Newcastle–Ottawa scale (NOS) [13], which is a nine-point scale allocating points based on the quality of selection (0–4 points), comparability (0–2 points), and the outcomes of the study participants (0–3 points). In the NOS, poor, fair, and good quality were scored 0–3, 4–6, and 7–9, respectively. Two investigators (L.Q and Q.Y) independently performed the literature search, selected eligible studies and assessed their quality, and extracted data; disagreements or uncertainties were resolved via discussion with an additional investigator (X.X.Y).

### Statistical analysis
Hazard ratio (HRs) and their 95% CI were used to quantify the association between depression and fracture, and the reported relative risk (RRs) were considered equivalent to HRs. Any study results stratified by sex and fracture type were considered as independent reports. The heterogeneity of HRs across the studies was evaluated using the Cochran Q test ($P$ value < 0.10 was considered an indication of statistically significant heterogeneity) and the $I^2$ statistic (values of 25%, 50%, and 75% representing low, moderate, and high heterogeneity, respectively) [14, 15]. A fixed-effect model was used if no or low heterogeneity was detected; otherwise, the random-effects model was adopted [16].

Subgroup and sensitivity analyses were conducted to explore potential heterogeneity across studies, and the differences among subgroups were tested via meta-regression analysis. Publication bias was assessed via visual inspection of the funnel plot and using the Begg [17] and Egger tests [18]. The Duval and Tweedie nonparametric trim-and-fill method was used to adjust the potential publication bias [19]. Data were statistically analyzed with STATA version 11.0 (StataCorp, College Station, Texas, the USA). All statistical tests were two-sided with a 0.05 significance level.

## Patient involvement

No Patients were involved in determining the research question or the outcome measures or in developing plans for the design or implementation of the study. In addition, no patients were required to provide advice on the interpretation or writing of the results. There were no plans of disseminating the research results to the study participants or the relevant patient population.

## Results

### Literature search

Initially, we retrieved 209, 677 and 568 citations from Web of Science, PubMed, and Embase, respectively. After removing duplicates and reviewing the titles and abstracts, we identified 87 potentially relevant articles. After assessing the full text of articles that may be relevant, 16 eligible studies met the inclusion criteria and were finally included in our meta-analysis. The results of literature search and selection are presented in Fig. 1.

### Study characteristics

Additional file 1: Table S1 shows the main characteristics of the 16 cohort studies that were published between 1999 and 2017 and included in the present study. The quality assessment scores of all the studies ranged from 6 to 9, with an average score of 7.6. The size of the cohorts ranged from 482 to 139,110, with a total of 414,686 participants, of which 105,298 were men and 309,388 were women, and the follow-up durations ranged from 3 to 14 years. Of the 16 studies, most were from America (eight studies) or European countries (five

studies). Meanwhile, one study was conducted in Australia [20] and two in Taiwan [8, 21]. Nine studies comprised both men and women, with four reporting results that were based on sex group, two studies included men only [22, 23], and five studies involved only women [20, 24–27]. In most of the studies, depression was assessed using self-reported symptom scales, and in three studies, the condition was confirmed based on the physician's diagnosis [8, 21, 28]. With regard to fracture types, only five studies reported about any fracture [7, 20, 23, 26, 29], and only four studies were about hip fracture [8, 9, 27, 30]. Moreover, only two studies reported about nonvertebral fracture [22, 31], and one on vertebral fracture [21]. The remaining four studies were about two or more types of fracture [24, 25, 28, 32]. Adjusted HRs could be determined in all studies. The following confounding factors were adjusted: smoking status (nine studies), BMD (six studies), physical activity (five studies), and use of antidepressants (five studies).

### Association between depression and risk for fracture

Results from the random-effects meta-analysis of depression and the risk for fracture are presented in Fig. 2. Among the 25 reports from the 16 studies (which were stratified by sex and fracture type and were considered independent reports), most showed a positive association between depression and fracture incidence (i.e., HR $> 1.00$), of which 11 were statistically significant. The pooled HR was 1.24 (95% CI: 1.14–1.35), with substantial heterogeneity across studies ($P = 0.000$, $I^2 = 56.5\%$).

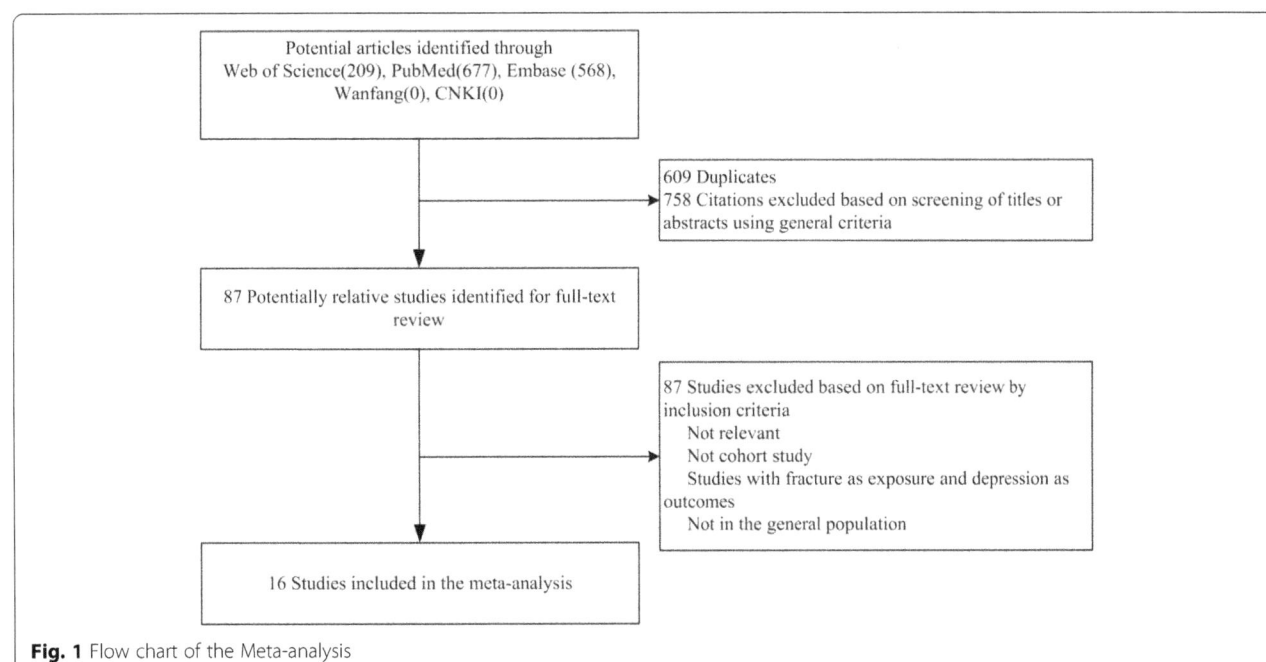

**Fig. 1** Flow chart of the Meta-analysis

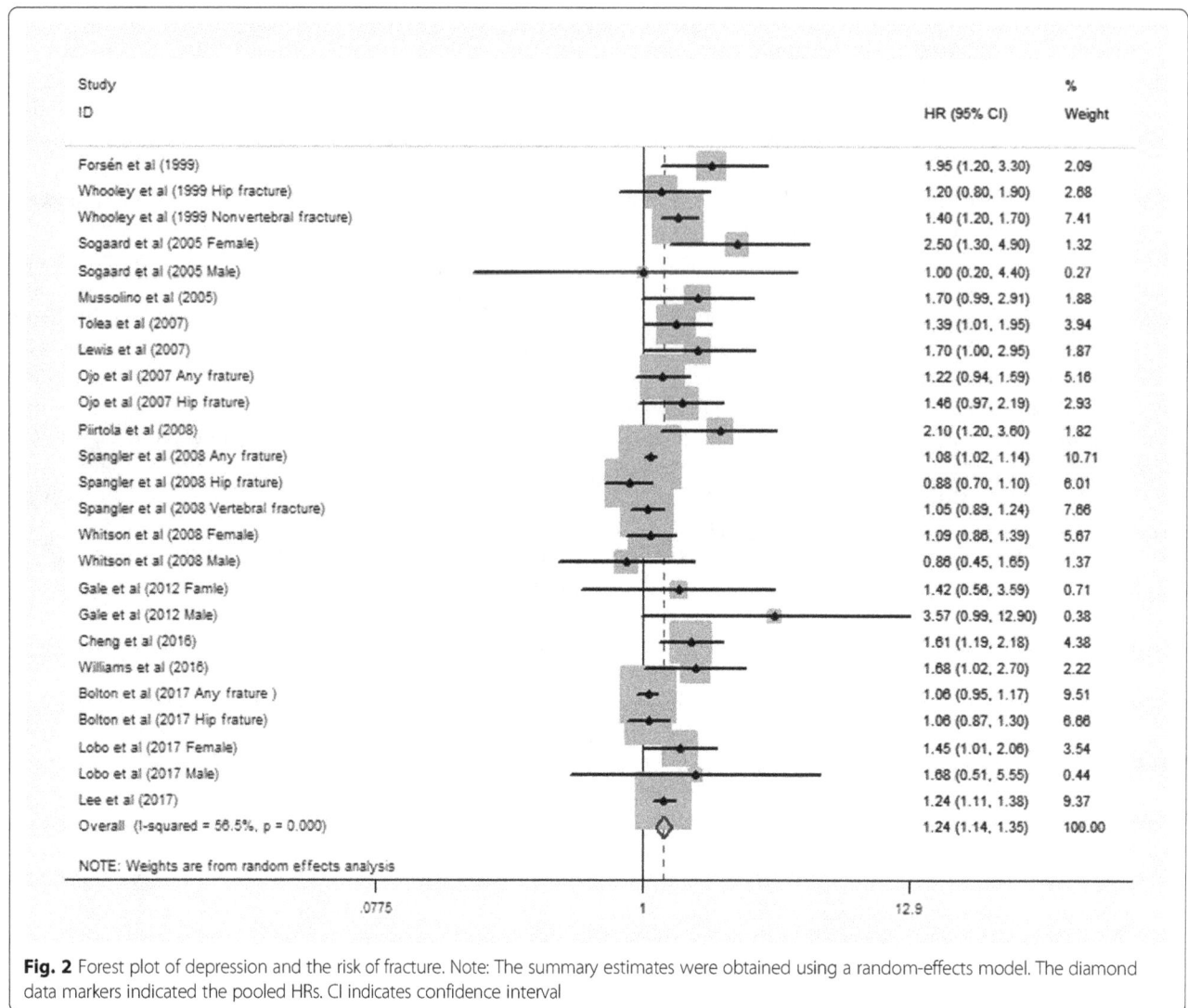

**Fig. 2** Forest plot of depression and the risk of fracture. Note: The summary estimates were obtained using a random-effects model. The diamond data markers indicated the pooled HRs. CI indicates confidence interval

## Subgroup analyses

Table 1 shows the results from the subgroup analyses examining the stability of the primary results and to explore the latent source of potential heterogeneity. Low-to-moderate heterogeneities were observed in most subgroups. Depression was associated with an increased risk for fracture in all subgroups (HR > 1.00). The increased risk was more evident in the groups with a relatively small study sample ($n < 5000$). When applying study regional categories, the pooled HR for the studies conducted in European countries was higher (HR: 1.76; 95% CI: 1.44–2.17; $n = 9$) than that in America and Asia, with a statistically significant difference ($P = 0.036$). No significant difference was found between the groups in terms of other variables.

## Publication bias

To examine the impact of a single study on the results, we omitted a study at each turn and pooled the results of the remaining studies. The pooled HR did not substantially change, ranging from 1.24 (95% CI: 1.14–1.35) to 1.29 (95% CI: 1.19–1.42). Visual inspection of the funnel plot revealed some asymmetry (Fig. 3). The Egger test suggested publication bias. However, the Begg test did not (Egger, $P = 0.000$; Begg, $P = 0.018$). We used the trim-and-fill method to assess the impact of any potential publication bias, and results showed that eight studies may be needed to obtain funnel plot symmetry for fracture (Fig. 4). By using the trim-and-fill method, the corrected HR was 1.14 (95% CI: 1.05–1.24; random-effects model, $P = 0.003$). Therefore, the pooled HR did not substantially change after the correction for potential publication bias.

## Discussion

Data from 16 cohort studies with 25 independent reports about 414, 686 participants were used, and our meta-analysis showed that depression was associated

**Table 1** Subgroup analyses on the association of depression and fracture risk

| | No. of report[a] | HR (95% CI) | Q-Statistic | P value for heterogeneity | $I^2$ (%) | P value between groups |
|---|---|---|---|---|---|---|
| Fracture Type | | | | | | |
| Any fracture | 9 | 1.16 (1.05–1.29) | 15.74 | 0.073 | 42.8 | 0.834 |
| Hip fracture | 10 | 1.31 (1.08–1.59) | 19.75 | 0.011 | 59.5 | |
| Nonvertebral fracture | 4 | 1.51 (1.23–1.85) | 3.28 | 0.351 | 8.5 | |
| vertebral fracture | 2 | 1.16 (1.00–1.36) | 2.7 | 0.100 | 63.5 | |
| Sex | | | | | | |
| Male | 6 | 1.59 (1.11–2.29) | 6.36 | 0.273 | 21.4 | 0.429 |
| Female | 12 | 1.23 (1.09–1.39) | 29.87 | 0.002 | 63.2 | |
| Mixed | 7 | 1.22 (1.08–1.37) | 12.83 | 0.046 | 53.2 | |
| Mean age at baseline | | | | | | |
| < 65 | 11 | 1.15 (1.05–1.26) | 27.07 | 0.003 | 63.1 | 0.050 |
| > =65 | 14 | 1.36 (1.22–1.50) | 13.81 | 0.387 | 5.9 | |
| Study region | | | | | | 0.036 |
| America | 14 | 1.13 (1.05–1.22) | 22.95 | 0.042 | 43.4 | |
| Europe, Australia | 9 | 1.76 (1.44–2.17) | 4.67 | 0.792 | 0 | |
| Asia | 2 | 1.36 (1.06–1.73) | 2.53 | 0.112 | 60.5 | |
| Duration of follow-up | | | | | | |
| < 10 | 17 | 1.23 (1.10–1.38) | 35.61 | 0.003 | 55.1 | 0.679 |
| > =10 | 8 | 1.28 (1.11–1.47) | 17.89 | 0.012 | 60.9 | |
| Type of depression measure | | | | | | |
| Self-reported scales | 21 | 1.29 (1.16–1.44) | 45.44 | 0.001 | 56.0 | 0.469 |
| physician diagnoses | 4 | 1.18 (1.03–1.36) | 9.59 | 0.023 | 68.6 | |
| Sample size | | | | | | |
| < 5000 | 9 | 1.44 (1.25–1.66) | 5.76 | 0.674 | 0.0 | 0.049 |
| > =5000 | 16 | 1.18 (1.08–1.29) | 38.78 | 0.001 | 61.3 | |
| Control BMD in models | | | | | | |
| Yes | 10 | 1.15 (1.03–1.29) | 19.87 | 0.019 | 54.7 | 0.109 |
| No | 15 | 1.36 (1.20–1.54) | 29.9 | 0.008 | 53.2 | |
| Control for antidepressants use | | | | | | |
| Yes | 7 | 1.19 (1.03–1.39) | 12.52 | 0.051 | 52.1 | 0.513 |
| No | 18 | 1.28 (1.15–1.42) | 42.31 | 0.001 | 59.8 | |
| Control for smoking | | | | | | |
| Yes | 16 | 1.22 (1.08–1.38) | 30.01 | 0.012 | 50 | 0.637 |
| No | 9 | 1.28 (1.14–1.44) | 20.23 | 0.009 | 60.5 | |
| Control for physical activity | | | | | | |
| Yes | | 1.19 (1.01–1.41) | 18.03 | 0.012 | 61.2 | 0.404 |
| No | | 1.24 (1.44–1.35) | 28.79 | 0.025 | 44.4 | |

Note: [a]Four articles reported their results by sex group and four articles by type of fracture; there are 25 reports from 16 articles;*BMD* bone mineral density; *CI* confidence interval; *HR* Hazard ratio; Q-Statistic, Cochrane Q statistic; $I^2$, the percentage of total variation due to heterogeneity among studies

with a significantly increased risk for fracture. In addition, the associations remained statistically significant in the groups adjusted for fracture type, sex, study region, and other studies and characteristics of the participants; therefore, our results are robust and suggest that depression is prospectively associated with a significantly increases risk of fracture.

Our results showed that the pooled HR was 1.24 (95% CI: 1.14–1.35), which was slightly higher than that of a previous meta-analysis of 10 studies published before

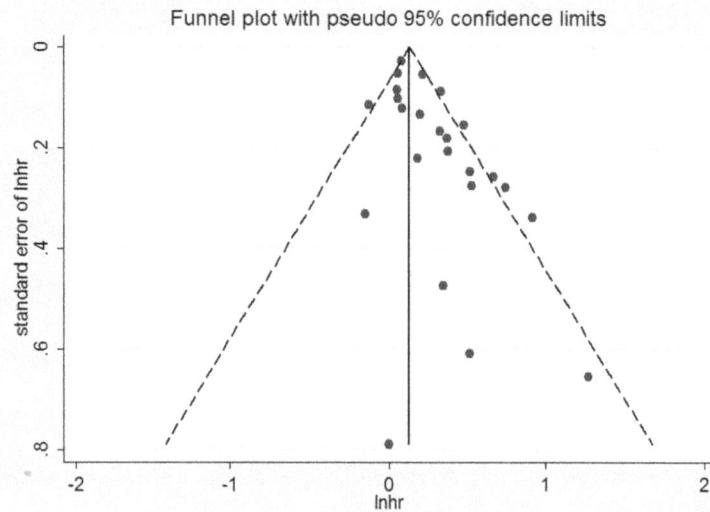

**Fig. 3** Funnel plot for studies on depression and fracture risk. Note: The horizontal line represents the summary effect estimates, and the dotted lines are pseudo 95% confidence intervals

2009 (HR: 1.17; 95% CI: 1.00–1.36) [10]. The current meta-analysis included 25 independent reports with sample sizes that are 4 times larger, which significantly enhanced statistical power and provided more accurate and comprehensive estimates of the association between depression and the risk for fracture. More importantly, compared with the previous meta-analysis, heterogeneity was thoroughly assessed, and subgroup analyses were conducted.

Our subgroups analyses identified an important finding. That is, the associations between depression and fractures varied between populations when subgroups analyses conducted by continents. The association was stronger in individuals from European countries than those from America and Asia. This may be attributed to the variation in health care systems in different geographic regions, availability of health services and other factors that are currently unknown. Since the studies included in the current meta-analysis were conducted in high-income countries(areas), such as those in Europe, North America, and Taiwan (research from Asian countries included only two studies conducted in Taiwan), these results should be

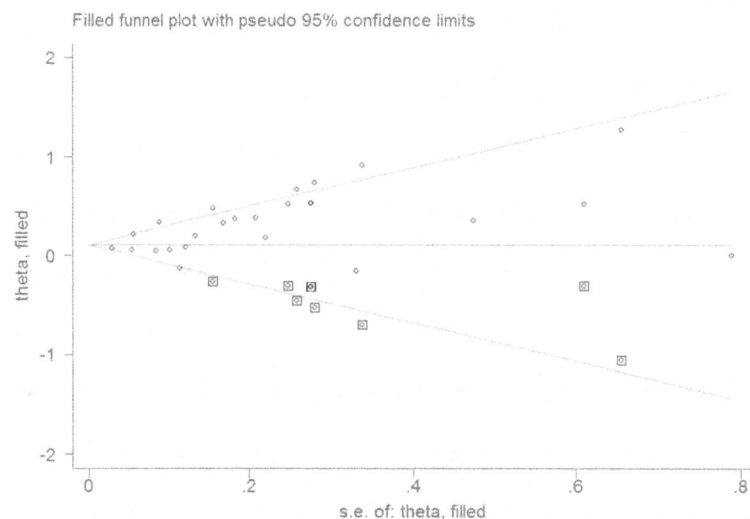

**Fig. 4** Filled funnel plot of HR from studies that investigated the association between depression and fracture risk. Note: The circles alone are real studies and the circles enclosed in boxes are "filled" studies. The horizontal line represents the summary effect estimates, and the diagonal lines represent pseudo- 95% CI limits

cautiously generalized to developing countries. To apply this finding to a wider population, more studies must be conducted in other populations from Asia, Africa, and South America.

Depression may contribute to fracture via several possible mechanisms. First, depressive disorders are associated with the deregulation of the hypothalamic–pituitary–adrenocortical axis [33], chronic low-grade inflammatory response [34, 35], and increased oxidative and nitrosative stress [36]. These neuroendocrine and inflammatory effects caused by depressive disorders had implications for osteoporosis, which ultimately increased the risk for fracture [37, 38]. Second, some studies have shown that neuropathological lesions in certain regions of the brain in patients with depressive disorders can influence these patients' balance, judgment, gait, and coordination, thus increasing the likelihood of falls, which in turn increases the risk for fracture [21, 39, 40]. Third, depression was associated with other major comorbidities, such as hypertension [41, 42] and diabetes [43]; these comorbidities were considered as risk factors for fracture, which were confirmed in two recent meta-analyses [44, 45]. Lastly, epidemiological findings showed that antidepressants, in particular selective serotonin reuptake inhibitors, may have direct effects on bone metabolism and decreased bone strength [46, 47], thereby increasing the risk for fracture [48]. However, the role of antidepressants should be cautiously interpreted because drug use can be a sign of severe depression, and numerous studies lacked information about the dose and duration of drug use.

This meta-analysis has several limitations. First, a moderate level of heterogeneity across studies was observed, which might result from the differences in the characteristics of the participants, sample sizes, depression measures, and statistical adjustments for potential confounders. Although moderate heterogeneities were still observed in some subgroups, the pooled HRs consistently showed positive associations in all subgroups and the prediction interval remained significant. Second, the funnel plot indicated a possible publication bias; however, the trim-and-fill method was used to correct the bias, which did not materially change the positive association. Third, we conducted only limited subgroups analyses because most original studies included in this meta-analysis did not adjust for other confounders such as social-economic status, medical comorbidities or ethnicity; information about these factors was not provided in most original reports. Finally, because the measurement of depression was mainly based on self-reported symptom scales, misclassification of exposure was inevitable, and this might bias the actual association between depression and fracture.

## Conclusion

In conclusion, this meta-analysis provides strong evidence that depression is significantly associated with an increased risk of fracture, particularly in individuals in Europe. Given the high prevalence of depression and osteoporotic fractures in the general population, the observed association between depression and fractures have substantial implications, both clinical and preventive. Mental health is closely related to bone health. It is greatly important for primary care practitioners and mental health care workers to take depression account into the prevention and clinical treatment of osteoporotic fractures.

## Additional file

**Additional file 1: Table S1.** Characteristics of studies included in the meta-analysis. (DOCX 18 kb)

**Abbreviations**
BMD: Bone mineral density.; CI: Confidence interval; HRs: Hazard ratios; NOS: the Newcastle–Ottawa scale; RRs: Relative risks

**Funding**
Foster research fund of Hainan Medical University.

**Authors' contributions**
LQ and XXY conceived and designed the study. LQ, QY and NS searched and checked the databases according to the inclusion and exclusion criteria. YHG and XXY helped to develop search strategies. LQ and QY extracted the data and assessed their quality. LQ, NS, DDL, YXZ and XTL analyzed the data. YHG gave advice on meta-analysis methodology. LQ wrote the draft of the paper. All authors contributed toward writing, reviewing or revising the paper and read and approved the final manuscript. XXY is the guarantor of this work and had full access to all the data in the study and takes responsibility for its integrity and the accuracy of the data analysis. All authors read and approved the final manuscript.

**Consent for publication**
Not applicable.

**Competing interests**
The authors declare that they have no competing interests.

**Author details**
[1]School of Public Health, Tongji Medical College, Huazhong University of Science and Technology, 430030 Wuhan, People's Republic of China. [2]School of Management, Hainan Medical University, Haikou, People's Republic of China. [3]Department of Emergency, The Second Affiliated Hospital of Hainan Medical University, Haikou 571199, People's Republic of China. [4]Emergency and Trauma College, Hainan Medical University, Haikou 571199, People's Republic of China.

### References

1. Kendler DL, Bauer DC, Davison KS, Dian L, Hanley DA, Harris ST, McClung MR, Miller PD, Schousboe JT, Yuen CK, et al. Vertebral Fractures: Clinical Importance and Management. Am J Med. 2016;129(2):221 e221–10.
2. Singer A, Exuzides A, Spangler L, O'Malley C, Colby C, Johnston K, Agodoa I, Baker J, Kagan R. Burden of illness for osteoporotic fractures compared with other serious diseases among postmenopausal women in the United States. Mayo Clin Proc. 2015;90(1):53–62.
3. Si L, Winzenberg TM, Chen M, Jiang Q, Palmer AJ. Residual lifetime and 10 year absolute risks of osteoporotic fractures in Chinese men and women. Curr Med Res Opin. 2015;31(6):1149–56.
4. Gilbody S, Sheldon T, Wessely S. Should we screen for depression? BMJ. 2006;332(7548):1027–30.
5. Kessler RC, Berglund P, Demler O, Jin R, Koretz D, Merikangas KR, Rush AJ, Walters EE, Wang PS. The epidemiology of major depressive disorder: results from the National Comorbidity Survey Replication (NCS-R). Jama. 2003;289(23):3095–105.
6. Organization WH: Depression and other common mental disorders. 2017.
7. Gale CR, Dennison EM, Edwards M, Sayer AA, Cooper C. Symptoms of anxiety or depression and risk of fracture in older people: the Hertfordshire cohort study. Arch Osteoporos. 2012;7:59–65.
8. Cheng BH, Chen PC, Yang YH, Lee CP, Huang KE, Chen VC. Effects of depression and antidepressant medications on hip fracture: a population-based cohort study in Taiwan. Medicine (Baltimore). 2016;95(36):e4655.
9. Mussolino ME. Depression and hip fracture risk: the NHANES I epidemiologic follow-up study. Public Health Rep. 2005;120(1):71–5.
10. Wu Q, Liu J, Gallegos-Orozco JF, Hentz JG. Depression, fracture risk, and bone loss: a meta-analysis of cohort studies. Osteoporos Int. 2010;21(10):1627–35.
11. Stroup DF, Berlin JA, Morton SC, Olkin I, Williamson GD, Rennie D, Moher D, Becker BJ, Sipe TA, Thacker SB. Meta-analysis of observational studies in epidemiology: a proposal for reporting. Meta-analysis of observational studies in epidemiology (MOOSE) group. Jama. 2000;283(15):2008–12.
12. Moher D, Liberati A, Tetzlaff J, Altman DG, Grp P, Group P. The PG: Preferred reporting items for systematic reviews and meta-analyses: the PRISMA statement. PLoS Med. 2009;6(7):e1000097.
13. George W, Beverley JS, Dianne O'C, je P, Vivian W, M L, Peter T. The Newcastle–Ottawa Scale (NOS) for Assessing the Quality of Non-Randomized Studies in Meta-Analysis. Ottawa Health Res Institute. 2009.
14. Higgins JPT, Thompson SG. Quantifying heterogeneity in a meta-analysis. Stat Med. 2002;21(11):1539–58.
15. Higgins JPT. Commentary: heterogeneity in meta-analysis should be expected and appropriately quantified. Int J Epidemiol. 2008;37(5):1158–60.
16. Lau J, Ioannidis JPA, Schmid CH. Quantitative synthesis in systematic reviews. Ann Intern Med. 1997;127(9):820–6.
17. Begg CB, Mazumdar M. Operating characteristics of a rank correlation test for publication Bias. Biometrics. 1994;50(4):1088–101.
18. Egger M, Smith GD, Schneider M, Minder C. Bias in meta-analysis detected by a simple, graphical test. BMJ. 1997;315(7109):629–34.
19. S D RT. Trim and fill: a simple funnel-plot-based method of testing and adjusting for publication Bias in meta-analysis. Biometrics. 2000;56(2):455–63.
20. Williams LJ, Pasco JA, Jackson H, Kiropoulos L, Stuart AL, Jacka FN, Berk M. Depression as a risk factor for fracture in women: a 10 year longitudinal study. J Affect Disord. 2016;192:34–40.
21. Lee SC, Hu LY, Huang MW, Shen CC, Huang WL, Lu T, Hsu CL, Pan CC. Risk of vertebral fracture in patients diagnosed with a depressive disorder: a Nationwide population-based cohort study. Clinics. 2017;72(1):44–50.
22. Lewis CE, Ewing SK, Taylor BC, Shikany JM, Fink HA, Ensrud KE, Barrett-Connor E, Cummings SR, Orwoll E. Predictors of non-spine fracture in elderly men: the MrOS study. J Bone Miner Res. 2007;22(2):211–9.
23. Piirtola M, Vahlberg T, Isoaho R, Aarnio P, Kivela SL. Predictors of fractures among the aged: a population-based study with 12-year follow-up in a Finnish municipality. Aging Clin Exp Res. 2008;20(3):242–52.
24. Spangler L, Scholes D, Brunner RL, Robbins J, Reed SD, Newton KM, Melville JL, Lacroix AZ. Depressive symptoms, bone loss, and fractures in postmenopausal women. J Gen Intern Med. 2008;23(5):567–74.
25. Whooley MA, Kip KE, Cauley JA, Ensrud KE, Nevitt MC, Browner WS. Depression, falls, and risk of fracture in older women. Study of osteoporotic fractures research group. Arch Intern Med. 1999;159(5):484–90.
26. Tolea MI, Black SA, Carter-Pokras OD, Kling MA. Depressive symptoms as a risk factor for osteoporosis and fractures in older Mexican American women. Osteoporos Int. 2007;18(3):315–22.
27. Forsen L, Meyer HE, Sogaard AJ, Naess S, Schei B, Edna TH. Mental distress and risk of hip fracture. Do broken hearts lead to broken bones? J Epidemiol Community Health. 1999;53(6):343–7.
28. Bolton JM, Morin SN, Majumdar SR, Sareen J, Lix LM, Johansson H, Oden A, McCloskey EV, Kanis JA, Leslie WD. Association of Mental Disorders and Related Medication use with Risk for major osteoporotic fractures. JAMA Psychiatry. 2017;74(6):641–8.
29. Whitson HE, Sanders L, Pieper CF, Gold DT, Papaioannou A, Richards JB, Adachi JD, Lyles KW. Depressive symptomatology and fracture risk in community-dwelling older men and women. Aging Clin Exp Res. 2008;20(6):585–92.
30. Lobo E, Marcos G, Santabarbara J, Salvador-Roses H, Lobo-Escolar L, De la Camara C, Aso A, Lobo-Escolar A: Gender differences in the incidence of and risk factors for hip fracture: a 16-year longitudinal study in a southern European population. Maturitas 2017, 97:38–43.
31. Sogaard AJ, Joakimsen RM, Tverdal A, Fonnebo V, Magnus JH, Berntsen GK. Long-term mental distress, bone mineral density and non-vertebral fractures. The Tromso study. Osteoporos Int. 2005;16(8):887–97.
32. Ojo F, Al Snih S, Ray LA, Raji MA, Markides KS. History of fractures as predictor of subsequent hip and nonhip fractures among older Mexican Americans. J Natl Med Assoc. 2007;99(4):412–8.
33. Atteritano M, Lasco A, Mazzaferro S, Macri I, Catalano A, Santangelo A, Bagnato G, Bagnato G, Frisina N. Bone mineral density, quantitative ultrasound parameters and bone metabolism in postmenopausal women with depression. Intern Emerg Med. 2013;8(6):485–91.
34. Berk M, Williams LJ, Jacka FN, O'Neil A, Pasco JA, Moylan S, Allen NB, Stuart AL, Hayley AC, Byrne ML, et al. So depression is an inflammatory disease, but where does the inflammation come from? BMC Med. 2013;11:200.
35. Wu ZJ, He JL, Wei RQ, Liu B, Lin X, Guan J, Lan YB. C-reactive protein and risk of fracture: a systematic review and dose-response meta-analysis of prospective cohort studies. Osteoporos Int. 2015;26(1):49–57.
36. Moylan S, Berk M, Dean OM, Samuni Y, Williams LJ, O'Neil A, Hayley AC, Pasco JA, Anderson G, Jacka FN, et al. Oxidative & nitrosative stress in depression: why so much stress? Neurosci Biobehav Rev. 2014;45:46–62.
37. Nakamura K, Saito T, Kobayashi R, Oshiki R, Oyama M, Nishiwaki T, Nashimoto M, Tsuchiya Y. C-reactive protein predicts incident fracture in community-dwelling elderly Japanese women: the Muramatsu study. Osteoporos Int. 2011;22(7):2145–50.
38. Eriksson AL, Moverare-Skrtic S, Ljunggren O, Karlsson M, Mellstrom D, Ohlsson C. High-sensitivity CRP is an independent risk factor for all fractures and vertebral fractures in elderly men: the MrOS Sweden study. J Bone Miner Res. 2014;29(2):418–23.
39. Andreescu C, Butters MA, Begley A, Rajji T, Wu M, Meltzer CC, Reynolds CF 3rd, Aizenstein H. Gray matter changes in late life depression--a structural MRI analysis. Neuropsychopharmacology. 2008;33(11):2566–72.
40. Fossati P, Radtchenko A, Boyer P. Neuroplasticity: from MRI to depressive symptoms. Eur Neuropsychopharmacol. 2004;14(Suppl 5):S503–10.
41. Patten SB, Williams JV, Lavorato DH, Campbell NR, Eliasziw M, Campbell TS. Major depression as a risk factor for high blood pressure: epidemiologic evidence from a national longitudinal study. Psychosom Med. 2009;71(3):273–9.
42. Ojike N, Sowers JR, Seixas A, Ravenell J, Rodriguez-Figueroa G, Awadallah M, Zizi F, Jean-Louis G, Ogedegbe O, McFarlane SI. Psychological distress and hypertension: results from the National Health Interview Survey for 2004-2013. Cardiorenal medicine. 2016;6(3):198–208.
43. Pan A, Lucas M, Sun Q, van Dam RM, Franco OH, Manson JE, Willett WC, Ascherio A, Hu FB. Bidirectional association between depression and type 2 diabetes mellitus in women. Arch Intern Med. 2010;170(21):1884–91.
44. Li C, Zeng Y, Tao L, Liu S, Ni Z, Huang Q, Wang Q. Meta-analysis of hypertension and osteoporotic fracture risk in women and men. Osteoporos Int. 2017;28(8):2309–18.

45. Wang J, You W, Jing Z, Wang R, Fu Z, Wang Y. Increased risk of vertebral fracture in patients with diabetes: a meta-analysis of cohort studies. Int Orthop. 2016;40(6):1299–307.

46. Rauma PH, Honkanen RJ, Williams LJ, Tuppurainen MT, Kroger HP, Koivumaa-Honkanen H. Effects of antidepressants on postmenopausal bone loss - a 5-year longitudinal study from the OSTPRE cohort. Bone. 2016;89:25–31.

47. Eom CS, Lee HK, Ye S, Park SM, Cho KH. Use of selective serotonin reuptake inhibitors and risk of fracture: a systematic review and meta-analysis. J Bone Miner Res. 2012;27(5):1186–95.

48. Coupland C, Dhiman P, Morriss R, Arthur A, Barton G, Hippisley-Cox J. Antidepressant use and risk of adverse outcomes in older people: population based cohort study. BMJ. 2011;343:d4551.

# 13

# Obesity and depressive symptoms in mid-life: a population-based cohort study

Anwar Mulugeta[1,2]*(iD), Ang Zhou[1], Christine Power[3] and Elina Hyppönen[1,3]

## Abstract

**Background:** Obesity and depression are both highly prevalent public health disorders and evidence on their relationship is inconsistent. This study examined whether depressive symptoms are associated with current obesity, and further, whether obesity in turn is associated with an increased odds of depressive symptoms five years later after accounting for potential lifestyle confounders and depressive symptoms at baseline.

**Methods:** Data were obtained from the 1958 British birth cohort ($N = 9217$ for cross-sectional and 7340 for prospective analysis). Clinical Interview Schedule-Revised and Mental Health Inventory-5 were used for screening depressive symptoms at ages 45 and 50 years, respectively. General and central obesity were defined using measurements of body mass index (BMI) and waist circumference (WC) at 45 years, respectively.

**Results:** There was a cross-sectional association between depressive symptoms and obesity: participants with ≥2 depressive symptoms had 31% (95%CI 11% to 55%) higher odds of general and 26% higher odds of central obesity (95%CI 8% to 47%). In prospective analyses, both general and central obesity were associated with higher odds of depressive symptoms five years later among women but not in men ($P_{interaction} < 0.01$). After adjustment for depressive symptoms at baseline, sociodemographic and lifestyle factors, women with general obesity had 38% (95% CI 7% to 77%) and women with central obesity 34% (95%CI 9% to 65%) higher odds of depression compared to others.

**Conclusions:** Depressive symptoms are associated with concurrent obesity and related lifestyle factors among women and men in mid-life. Our study suggests that obesity in turn affects long-term risk of depressive symptoms in women but not in men, independently of concurrent associations, providing an important target group for the implementation of preventative strategies.

**Keywords:** General obesity, Central obesity, Depressive symptoms, Middle-age

## Background

Obesity and depression are both highly prevalent public health disorders that affect many age groups and communities [1, 2]. Globally, more than 600 million people are living with obesity while depression affects over 350 million people [1, 3]. Obesity and depression are interrelated; both are known risk factors for cardiovascular disorders and diabetes [4–6], and relate to negative health and lifestyles factors such as disturbed sleep patterns, sedentary behaviours and dysregulation in appetite and

* Correspondence: anwar.mulugeta@aau.edu.et;
gebam006@mymail.unisa.edu.au
[1]Australian Centre for Precision Health, University of South Australia Cancer Research Institute, GPO Box 2471, Adelaide, SA 5001, Australia
[2]Department of Pharmacology, School of Medicine, College of Health Science, Addis Ababa University, Addis Ababa, Ethiopia
Full list of author information is available at the end of the article

food intake [7]. These interrelations are clearly complex as use of antidepressant medication often leads to weight gain, as suggested from a review of ten clinical studies that explored the effect of antidepressants on body weight [8]. Furthermore, as evidenced by clinical trials conducted on women [9], dietary restriction targeting weight reduction in obesity may in turn exacerbate depression.

Previous observational studies on the association between obesity and depressive symptoms have provided mixed findings [10–17], with some suggesting a positive association [10], while others have reported an inverse association (obesity associated with lower risk of depression) [12], no association [13], or a u-shaped association (higher risk of depressive symptoms among underweight and obese individuals) [14]. These inconsistencies can arise from differences in population characteristics (for example, ethnicity and age) [12, 15, 18], residual confounding [19, 20], or potentially, differences in measures used to define obesity [21]. For example, a study of 3666 individuals from different ethnic groups in USA suggested an association among White but not Black or Mexican Americans [18]. A meta-analysis of 13 cross-sectional obesity-depression association studies (median $n = 1215$), indicated differences in point estimates and statistical precision based on the number of confounders included in the adjustment [20]. Furthermore, most previous studies consider "general" obesity, as measured by body mass index (BMI) [22, 23], while notably less attention has been paid to potential differences in risk based on body fat distribution. While BMI is widely used, it has well-known limitations and may reflect differences in muscle rather than adipose tissue [21]. Some studies have associated central obesity, as measured by waist circumference (WC) or waist-hip ratio (WHR), with depression risk [24]. Adipose tissue is an active endocrine organ associated with increased inflammatory response which relates to depression [25]. White adipose tissue which accumulates typically around the waist is a source of a range of inflammatory markers, which can pass the brain-blood barrier and thereby affect depression risk [26]. Another possibility is that dysregulation of the hypothalamus-pituitary-adrenal (HPA) axis could increase the accumulation of fat around the abdomen as well as leading to alterations in mood [27], possibly indicating a greater importance of central rather than general obesity with respect to depression risk.

This study used data from a large-scale population-based cohort to establish whether depressive symptoms in mid-adulthood are associated with concurrent general or central obesity and related lifestyle factors, and further, whether obesity in turn predicts the longer term risk of depressive symptoms after accounting for potential sociodemographic and lifestyle confounders and the presence of depressive symptoms at baseline.

## Methods
### Study population
This study used data from 1958 British birth cohort, which included all born in one week of 1958 in England, Scotland and Wales ($N = 17,638$) with immigrants born the same week included up to age 16 years ($N = 920$) [28]. The cohort has been followed up until adulthood, and this study primarily used data from the biomedical survey conducted at age 45 years (target sample 11,971, data collected for 9377) and from the 50 year follow-up [29].

Participants with complete information on depressive symptoms, general and central obesity at age 45 years were included for cross-sectional analysis ($N = 9217$).

Individuals from the cross-sectional analysis who also had information on depressive symptoms at 50 years ($N = 7340$) were included in the prospective analysis. The flow diagram for the selection of participants is shown in Fig. 1.

### Depressive symptoms
Depressive symptoms at 45 years were assessed using the Clinical Interview Schedule-Revised (CIS-R) [28]. CIS-R was developed for use by lay interviewers as a screening instrument for 14 common mental disorders including depression [30]. CIS-R has been reported to have an acceptable agreement with the Schedule for Clinical Assessment in Neuropsychiatry (SCAN), a clinical diagnostic tool for depression [31]. In the 1958 cohort, the CIS-R was administered by trained nurses; depressive symptoms were assessed using four questions that reflect symptom occurrence over the past week. These include "In the past week have you been able to enjoy or take an interest in things as much as usual?", "In the past week on how many days have you felt sad, miserable or depressed/unable to enjoy or taken an interest in things?", "Did you feel depressed for more than three hours in any day of the week?", and "In the

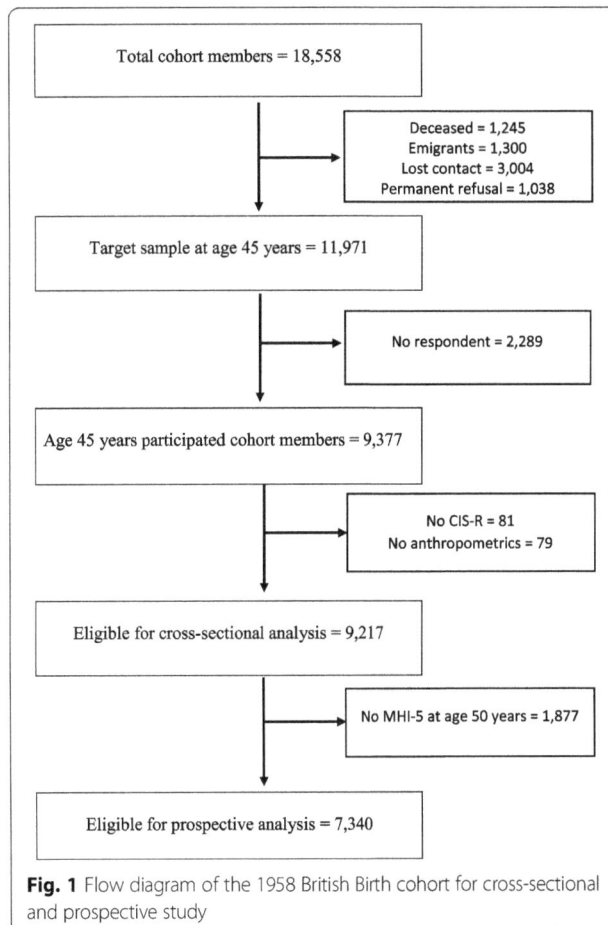

**Fig. 1** Flow diagram of the 1958 British Birth cohort for cross-sectional and prospective study

last week during depressive periods, did you feel happier when nice things happened or when you spent time with your friends?". Participants presenting with two or more depressive symptoms were considered as case in our analyses [32, 33].

Mental Health Inventory – 5 (MHI-5), a short version of MHI-38, was used to assess depressive symptoms as part of the postal survey conducted at age 50 years [29] MHI-5 shows an acceptable validity in screening for depression compared to clinical depression diagnostic tools and has an equivalent level of performance in screening depression compared to other screening tools [34, 35]. MHI-5 has five self-administered questions which assess the amount of time in the past four weeks when the participants felt [1] happy, [2] calm and cheerful [3] nervous, [4] felt down and low or [5] felt like nothing could cheer them up. Each question was rated using six Likert scale options (ranging from none to all of the time) to give a total score range of 5 to 30 [35]. Where needed, scores were converted to have lower values indicating a greater prevalence of symptoms and then scaled to 100. Scores ≤52 were used to indicate clinically significant depressive symptoms [34].

### Anthropometric measures

At age 45 years, height, weight and waist circumference were measured by trained nurses [36]. Weight (in light clothing) was measured with Tanita solar scales, and height (without shoes) with a stadiometer. Using a body tension tape, waist circumference was measured (over light clothing) between the lower ribs and iliac crest in the mid-axillary line [36]. BMI was calculated as weight (kg) over height squared ($m^2$). According to WHO classification, BMI was categorized into four groups and coded as underweight (< 18.5), normal (≥18.5 and < 25), overweight (≥25 and < 30) and obesity (≥30) [37]. Central obesity was defined as waist WC ≥102 cm for males and ≥ 88 cm for females [38].

### Covariates

Sociodemographic and lifestyle factors were taken from age 45 years or from the nearest possible age sweep where the information was provided. Region of residence at age 45 years was coded as South, Middle and Northern England, London and Scotland; highest educational level attained by 33 years was grouped as <O level (less than Secondary education), O level, A level or higher (further education) [39]; socioeconomic position at birth (based on father's occupation, or if missing, from age 7 years) and in adulthood (42 years) was categorised using the Registrar General Classification, and coded as I and II (professional/managerial), IIINM (skilled non-manual), IIIM (skilled manual) and IV and V (partially skilled and unskilled) [40, 41]. Information on smoking

(currently non-smoker, ex-smoker or smoker), and physical activity (4–7 times/week, 2–3 times/week, 1 time/week and < 2–3 times/month), fruit consumption (< 1, 1–2, and ≥ 3 days/week) were collected at 42 years. Alcohol consumption (non-drinker; light drinker, < 7 units/week; moderate drinker, 7–14 units/weeks; heavy drinker, > 14 units/week), and sedentary behaviour based on time spent viewing a TV or PC (≥ 3 h and < 3 h/day) were from the 45 year survey.

### Statistical analysis

Logistic regression was used to evaluate both the cross-sectional and prospective associations. Cross-sectional analyses of depressive symptoms and obesity (general and central) included adjustments for sex, region, and social class at birth and in adulthood. Prospective analyses of obesity at 45 years and depressive symptoms at 50 years, included adjustments for sex and baseline depressive symptoms (model 1), with further adjustment for sociodemographic factors (region, social class at birth and in adulthood; model 2), and for both sociodemographic, and lifestyle factors (full model, further including alcohol, smoking, sedentary behaviour, physical activity, and fruit consumption; model 3). Models 1 to 3 were repeated for BMI and WC as continuous variables, using linear regression, to provide trend estimates and to test for curvature (using a quadratic term) of relationships with depression. BMI and WC were analysed separately and also mutually adjusted, to assess their independent effects. Interaction by sex was tested in cross-sectional and prospective analyses, and where found, results are presented separately for men and women.

Information on one or more social or lifestyle covariates was missing for 7% of cohort members. We used multiple imputation with chained equations (ice command in Stata) and present results from pooled analyses of 15 imputed datasets. There were no notable differences in the effect sizes obtained by analyses using multiple imputation compared to complete case analyses, although associations from models with multiple imputation were typically slightly more precise. All analyses were performed using Stata/ SE 14 software.

### Results

At age 45 years, around a quarter of participants were classified as having general obesity and 35% with central obesity. The prevalence of depressive symptoms was 8.4% at 45 years and 12.4% at 50 years. Sociodemographic and lifestyle factors associated with greater prevalence of general and central obesity were mostly also associated with higher prevalence of depressive symptoms (Table 1).

Table 2 shows the cross-sectional associations of depressive symptoms with obesity and lifestyle factors at

45 years. The odds of obesity were higher for those reporting ≥2 symptoms compared to individuals with no depressive symptoms (OR 1.31, 95%CI 1.11 to 1.55 and OR 1.26, 95%CI 1.08 to 1.47, for general and central obesity, respectively). The cross-sectional associations between depressive symptoms and general or central obesity did not vary by sex (P $_{sex-interaction}$ > 0.33). Number of depressive symptoms was also related to sedentary behaviour, smoking and low fruit consumption ($P <$ 0.001 for all comparisons after adjustment for sex, region, social class at birth and in adulthood). The association of depressive symptoms with cigarette smoking and fruit consumption varied by sex (P$_{sex-interaction}$ < 0.02 for both comparisons), and both associations were observed in women but not men. Compared to women without symptoms, those with symptoms at baseline had an OR 1.82 (95% CI 1.38 to 2.19; men OR 1.05, 95% CI 0.78 to 1.40) for smoking and OR 0.51 (95% CI 0.40 to 0.67; men OR 0.76, 95% CI 0.57 to 1.00) for fruit consumption.

Both general and central obesity at 45 years were associated with higher odds of depressive symptoms at age 50 years in women but not in men (Table 3, P$_{sex-interaction}$ < 0.01 for all comparisons). In women, the observed associations between BMI and WC with depressive symptoms were somewhat attenuated by adjustment for sociodemographic and lifestyle factors, but for both obesity indicators the associations remained even after accounting for baseline symptoms, sociodemographic and lifestyle factors (BMI: OR per 10 kg/m$^2$ 1.36, 95%CI 1.15 to 1.62; WC: OR per 5 cm 1.07, 95%CI 1.03 to 1.11). In men the fully adjusted OR for BMI was 0.83 (95%CI 0.64 to 1.10, P$_{trend}$ = 0.20) and for WC 0.99 (95%CI 0.94 to 1.04, P$_{trend}$ = 0.67). In a model including all covariates and mutually adjusted for BMI and WC, the association in women for BMI was abolished (OR 0.96, 95%CI 0.77 to 1.18) while the estimate for WC remained significant (OR 1.08, 95%CI 1.02 to 1.15). Again, the corresponding mutually adjusted model among men did not suggest an association either for WC or BMI ($P$ > 0.16 for all comparisons).

To further understand the association between obesity and depressive symptoms, we explored the prospective associations between lifestyle factors and depressive symptoms. Alcohol consumption, smoking, sedentary behaviour and fruit consumption were all associated with depressive symptoms at 50 years after adjustment for depressive symptoms at 45 years, sex, sociodemographic and other lifestyle factors (Table 4). The presence of depressive symptoms at age 45 years was associated with an over four-fold greater odds of depressive symptoms at 50 years, attenuating only slightly after adjustment for obesity and lifestyle factors (OR reduced from 4.43 (95%CI 3.61 to 5.43) to 4.11 (95%CI 3.34 to

5.06)), suggesting further unmeasured influences on the tracking of depressive symptoms.

## Discussion

Tackling the current obesity epidemic both in terms of addressing its causes and consequences remains a key public health priority. Mental wellbeing has broad influences on health and as shown in our large-scale study, the presence of depressive symptoms is strongly associated both with obesity and a broad range of related lifestyle factors. However, as shown in our analyses, even after controlling for these concurrent associations, obesity several years earlier appears to affect subsequent odds of depressive symptoms among women but not in men, providing an important target group for implementation of preventative strategies. Furthermore, this study provided some support for the hypothesis that central rather than general adiposity may have a key role in contributing to the association between obesity and the risk of developing depressive symptoms, highlighting the need of further studies to establish related mechanisms and pathways.

Our work builds on an earlier analysis in the 1958 cohort, which suggested that when looking at categories of BMI from childhood to adulthood (age 7 onwards) obesity was associated with the subsequent odds of depressive symptoms in women but not in men [15]. Inclusion here of central obesity is important because BMI has known weaknesses, especially for men, due to the strong correlation with muscle mass [21]. The result from our previous work [15] is consistent with the current study, and both the analysis using BMI (or general obesity) and WC (or central obesity) suggest that obesity is affecting the likelihood of developing depressive symptoms in women only.

Our findings for higher odds of depressive symptoms by general and central obesity are consistent with several other previous studies [20, 22]. For example, a meta-analysis including eight cross-sectional studies reported the odds of depression to be 35% higher in people with obesity compared to normal weight individuals [42]. A meta-analysis reporting prospective associations also included eight studies, six of them assessed to be of poor quality by the authors, suggesting an overall 55% higher odds of depression for those with obesity compared to normal weight, with no evidence for sub-group differences by sex [22]. Another meta-analysis including 15 studies showed 38% higher odds of depression in individuals with central obesity compared to those without, with higher estimates among women than men [20]. Importantly, unlike these previous studies [20, 22], our study included an adjustment for depressive symptoms at baseline. Furthermore, the weaker effect estimate in our study compared to previous meta-analyses may be

**Table 1** Characteristics and distributions of adult obesity and depressive symptoms by sociodemographic and lifestyle factors

| Covariates | N (%) | BMI mean (SD) | General obesity N (%) | Central obesity N (%) | Depression[b] age 45y N (%) | Depression[c] age 50y N (%)[d] |
|---|---|---|---|---|---|---|
| All | 9217 | 27.4 (5.0) | 2251 (24.4) | 3208 (34.8) | 776 (8.4) | 911 (12.4) |
| Gender | | | | | | |
| Male | 4591 (49.8) | 27.8 (4.3) | 1162 (25.3) | 1503 (32.7) | 322 (7.0) | 369 (10.5) |
| Female | 4626 (50.2) | 26.9 (5.6) | 1089 (23.5) | 1705 (36.9) | 454 (9.8) | 542 (14.2) |
| P | | < 0.001 | 0.05 | < 0.001 | < 0.001 | < 0.001 |
| Social class age 42 | | | | | | |
| I & II | 3715 (40.3) | 27.2 (4.7) | 813 (21.9) | 1188 (32.0) | 231 (6.2) | 287 (9.4) |
| IIINM | 1916 (20.8) | 26.9 (5.0) | 419 (21.9) | 663 (34.6) | 172 (9.0) | 222 (14.0) |
| IIIM | 1711 (18.6) | 28.1 (4.9) | 493 (28.8) | 598 (35.0) | 127 (7.4) | 150 (11.6) |
| IV & V | 1469 (15.9) | 27.8 (5.5) | 423 (28.8) | 593 (40.4) | 167 (11.4) | 183 (16.3) |
| Others | 406 (4.4) | 27.7 (5.6) | 103 (25.4) | 166 (40.9) | 79 (19.5) | 69 (25.8) |
| P[a] | | < 0.001 | < 0.001 | < 0.001 | < 0.001 | < 0.001 |
| Alcohol (units/week) | | | | | | |
| Non-drinker | 623 (6.8) | 28.2 (6.3) | 193 (31.0) | 253 (40.6) | 108 (17.3) | 114 (24.8) |
| Light < 7 | 4476 (48.6) | 27.6 (5.3) | 1196 (26.9) | 1, 642 (36.7) | 367 (8.2) | 428 (11.9) |
| Moderate 7–14 | 2226 (24.2) | 26.8 (4.3) | 431 (19.4) | 679 (30.5) | 137 (6.1) | 185 (10.2) |
| Heavy > 14 | 1854 (20.0) | 27.3 (4.6) | 214 (21.0) | 616 (33.2) | 160 (8.6) | 182 (12.6) |
| Missing | 38 (0.4) | 27.3 (4.6) | 10 (26.3) | 18 (47.4) | 4 (10.5) | 2 (11.1) |
| P[a] | | < 0.001 | < 0.001 | < 0.001 | 0.002 | 0.008 |
| Smoking | | | | | | |
| Never | 4256 (46.1) | 27.4 (5.0) | 1024 (24.1) | 1440 (33.8) | 307 (7.2) | 386 (10.9) |
| Ex- smoker | 2497 (27.1) | 27.8 (5.0) | 645 (25.8) | 914 (36.6) | 185 (7.4) | 217 (8.7) |
| Current smoker | 2161 (23.5) | 27.0 (5.1) | 520 (24.1) | 752 (34.8) | 249 (11.5) | 282 (13.1) |
| Missing | 303 (3.3) | 27.0 (4.7) | 62 (20.5) | 102 (33.7) | 35 (11.6) | 26 (14.1) |
| P[a] | | 0.49 | 0.31 | 0.05 | < 0.001 | < 0.001 |
| Physical activity | | | | | | |
| < 2–3 times/month[e] | 3026 (32.8) | 28.0 (5.5) | 878 (29.0) | 1229 (40.6) | 317 (10.5) | 352 (14.9) |
| 1 time/week | 1670 (18.1) | 27.4 (4.8) | 415 (24.9) | 565 (33.8) | 104 (6.2) | 144 (10.4) |
| 2–3 times/week | 1932 (21.0) | 27.1 (4.5) | 413 (21.4) | 612 (31.7) | 138 (7.1) | 161 (10.3) |
| 4–7 times/week | 2295 (24.9) | 26.9 (4.9) | 484 (21.1) | 703 (30.6) | 181 (7.9) | 227 (12.2) |
| Missing | 294 (3.2) | 26.9 (4.3) | 61 (20.8) | 99 (33.7) | 36 (12.2) | 27 (15.3) |
| P[a] | | < 0.001 | < 0.001 | < 0.001 | < 0.001 | 0.003 |
| Sedentary behaviour | | | | | | |
| < 3 h/day | 5806 (63.0) | 26.9 (4.7) | 1195 (20.6) | 1751 (30.2) | 429 (7.4) | 517 (11.0) |
| ≥ 3 h/day | 2995 (32.5) | 28.4 (5.4) | 945 (31.6) | 1296 (43.3) | 293 (9.8) | 348 (14.9) |
| Missing | 416 (4.5) | 27.7 (5.4) | 111 (26.7) | 161 (38.7) | 54 (13.0) | 46 (16.7) |
| P[a] | | < 0.001 | < 0.001 | < 0.001 | < 0.001 | < 0.001 |
| Fruit consumption | | | | | | |
| < 1 day/week | 1676 (18.2) | 27.5 (5.0) | 433 (25.8) | 618 (36.9) | 195 (11.6) | 220 (17.5) |
| 1–2 days/week | 1367 (14.8) | 27.5 (5.1) | 349 (25.5) | 506 (37.0) | 113 (8.3) | 161 (15.1) |
| ≥ 3 days/week | 5879 (63.8) | 27.4 (5.0) | 1407 (23.9) | 1984 (33.8) | 432 (7.4) | 503 (10.4) |
| Missing | 295 (3.2) | 27.0 (4.3) | 62 (21.0) | 100 (33.9) | 36 (12.2) | 27 (15.3) |
| P[a] | | 0.74 | 0.13 | 0.001 | < 0.001 | < 0.001 |

[a]P-value from logistic regression adjusted for sex
[b]Depressive symptoms measured using CIS-R
[c]Depressive symptoms measured using MHI-5. [d] Cohort members who had missing data on depressive symptoms at age 50 (n = 1, 877) have been excluded. [e] include individuals who responded no for "Do you do any regular exercise?"

**Table 2** Cross-sectional association of depressive symptoms with obesity and lifestyle factors at age 45 years

| | N[c] (%) | Obesity, OR (95% CI)[a] | | Lifestyle factors[b], OR (95% CI)[a] | | | |
| --- | --- | --- | --- | --- | --- | --- | --- |
| | | General obesity | Central obesity | Sedentary behaviour | High alcohol consumption | Current smoking | Fruit consumption |
| Depressive symptoms | | | | | | | |
| None | 7683 (83.4) | Reference | Reference | Reference | Reference | Reference | Reference |
| 1 | 758 (8.2) | 1.07 (0.90, 1.27) | 1.02 (0.87, 1.19) | 1.36 (1.16, 1.59) | 1.15 (0.95, 1.40) | 1.47 (1.23, 1.74) | 0.82 (0.68, 1.00) |
| ≥ 2 | 776 (8.4) | 1.31 (1.11, 1.55) | 1.26 (1.08, 1.47) | 1.30 (1.10, 1.53) | 1.19 (0.99, 1.44) | 1.53 (1.30, 1.82) | 0.52 (0.53, 0.76) |
| $P_{unadjusted}$ | | 0.001 | < 0.001 | < 0.001 | 0.89 | < 0.001 | < 0.001 |
| $P_{adjusted}$[a] | | 0.005 | 0.01 | < 0.001 | 0.08 | < 0.001 | < 0.001 |
| $P_{sex-interaction}$[d] | | 0.33 | 0.58 | 0.52 | 0.11 | < 0.001 | 0.02 |

[a]P-value adjusted and OR (95% CI): adjustment made for sex, region, social class at birth and social class at age 42 years
[b]Sedentary behaviour, spent 3 or more hrs/day viewing a TV or PC; high alcohol consumption, > 15 units/week alcohol consumption; current smoking, smoking during age 42 sweep; fruit consumption, < 1 day/week fruit consumption vs > 1 day/week fruit consumption
[c]All the analysis done in 9217 sample population of the age 45
[d]Interaction between sex and depressive symptoms on obesity and on lifestyle factors after adjustment for sex, region, social class at birth and social class at age 42 years

due to better control for sociodemographic or other confounding factors as most previous studies included in the two meta-analyses [20, 22, 42] were either unadjusted or adjusted for limited set of confounders.

We observed a dose-dependent increase in the odds of depressive symptoms by categories of BMI, which is consistent with most previous studies [10, 13, 43]. However, in some studies, the association between general obesity and depressive symptoms has favoured the "Fat and Jolly" hypothesis, suggesting that obesity may protect against depression [44] while others show a higher

odds both for the very thin and obese individuals compared to those with normal weight [14, 16, 45]. It is possible that an increased odds of depression for those who are thin or underweight, can reflect sub-optimal health status [46]. These inconsistencies among studies could be further explained by contextual, and psychosocial influences contributing to the obesity – depression relationship. Individuals who experience stigma and discrimination due to their weight may have low self-esteem and high degree body image dissatisfaction that further aggravate psychological stress and lead to depressive

**Table 3** Prospective association between general and central obesity at age 45 years and depressive symptoms at age 50 years (n = 7340) among men and women

| | Women | | | Men | | |
| --- | --- | --- | --- | --- | --- | --- |
| | Model-1 OR (95% CI) | Model-2 OR (95% CI) | Model-3 OR (95% CI) | Model-1 OR (95% CI) | Model-2 OR (95% CI) | Model-3 OR (95% CI) |
| Body Mass Index | | | | | | |
| Underweight | 0.72 (0.21, 2.49) | 0.72 (0.20, 2.50) | 0.54 (0.15, 1.99) | 2.47 (0.45, 13.05) | 2.30 (0.41, 12.80) | 1.91 (0.33, 11.21) |
| Normal | Reference | Reference | Reference | Reference | Reference | Reference |
| Overweight | 1.11 (0.87, 1.40) | 1.08 (0.85, 1.38) | 1.10 (0.86, 1.40) | 0.87 (0.64, 1.13) | 0.87 (0.65, 1.15) | 0.86 (0.65, 1.15) |
| Obesity[a] | 1.56 (1.22, 1.98) | 1.46 (1.14, 1.86) | 1.38 (1.07, 1.77) | 0.87 (0.63, 1.21) | 0.87 (0.63, 1.21) | 0.85 (0.61, 1.18) |
| Per 10 kg/m² | 1.48 (1.26, 1.74) | 1.41 (1.20, 1.67) | 1.36 (1.15, 1.62) | 0.87 (0.66, 1.14) | 0.86 (0.65, 1.12) | 0.83 (0.64, 1.10) |
| $P_{trend}$ | < 0.001 | < 0.001 | < 0.001 | 0.31 | 0.26 | 0.20 |
| $P_{curvature}$ | 0.25 | 0.19 | 0.32 | 0.05 | 0.11 | 0.14 |
| Waist circumference | | | | | | |
| Normal | Reference | Reference | Reference | Reference | Reference | Reference |
| Central obesity[b] | 1.48 (1.21, 1.81) | 1.41 (1.15, 1.73) | 1.34 (1.09, 1.65) | 0.97 (0.75, 1.23) | 0.94 (0.73, 1.21) | 0.90 (0.70, 1.17) |
| Per 5 cm | 1.10 (1.06, 1.14) | 1.09 (1.05, 1.13) | 1.07 (1.03, 1.11) | 1.00 (0.95, 1.05) | 1.00 (0.95, 1.05) | 0.99 (0.94, 1.04) |
| $P_{trend}$ | < 0.001 | < 0.001 | < 0.001 | 0.99 | 0.88 | 0.67 |

$P_{sex-interaction}$ is the interaction between sex and obesity variables at age 45 years on depression at age 50 years (For all obesity variables, $P_{sex-interaction}$ < 0.01) Model-1, adjusted for depressive symptoms at age 45 years; Model-2, adjusted for depressive symptoms at age 45 years, and region, social class at birth and social class at adulthood; Model-3, adjusted for depressive symptoms at age 45 years, region, social class at birth, social class at adulthood, fruit consumption, physical activity, sedentary behaviour, smoking, alcohol)
[a]BMI ≥ 30 kg/m²
[b]WC ≥ 102 cm for men and WC ≥ 88 cm for women

**Table 4** Lifestyle factors and the risk of depressive symptoms at age 50 years

| | Adjusted for sex, depressive symptoms at 45y, & other factors[a] OR(95%CI) | Full adjustment[b] OR(95%CI) | $P_{sex\text{-}interaction}$ |
|---|---|---|---|
| Alcohol | | | 0.40 |
| Non-drinker | 1.98 (1.52, 2.58) | 1.88 (1.44, 2.46) | |
| Light < 7 units/week | Reference | Reference | |
| Moderate 7–14 units/week | 0.98 (0.80, 1.19) | 1.00 (0.82, 1.22) | |
| Heavy > 14 units/week | 1.23 (1.00, 1.51) | 1.17 (0.95, 1.45) | |
| P | < 0.001 | < 0.001 | |
| Smoking | | | 0.05 |
| Never | Reference | Reference | |
| Ex-Smoker | 0.96 (0.80, 1.16) | 0.93 (0.77, 1.13) | |
| Current smoker | 1.51 (1.25, 1.81) | 1.33 (1.09, 1.61) | |
| P | < 0.001 | 0.003 | |
| Physical activity | | | 0.51 |
| 2–3 times/month | Reference | Reference | |
| 1 time/week | 0.79 (0.63, 0.98) | 0.88 (0.71, 1.10) | |
| 2–3 times/week | 0.76 (0.61, 0.94) | 0.88 (0.70, 1.09) | |
| 4–7 times/week | 0.86 (0.71, 1.05) | 0.98 (0.81, 1.20) | |
| P | 0.04 | 0.52 | |
| Sedentary behaviour | | | 0.09 |
| < 3 h/day | Reference | Reference | |
| ≥ 3 h/day | 1.36 (1.16, 1.59) | 1.20 (1.02, 1.41) | |
| P | < 0.001 | 0.05 | |
| Fruit consumption | | | 0.02 |
| < 1 day/week | Reference | Reference | |
| 1–2 days/week | 0.93 (0.73, 1.18) | 0.98 (0.76, 1.25) | |
| ≥ 3 days/week | 0.60 (0.49, 0.73) | 0.67 (0.55, 0.82) | |
| P | < 0.001 | < 0.001 | |
| Depressive symptoms at age 45y | | | 0.36 |
| No | Reference | Reference | |
| Yes | 4.43 (3.61, 5.43) | 4.11 (3.34, 5.0) | |
| P | < 0.001 | < 0.001 | |

P-value based on Likelihood ratio test
[a]Sociodemographic factors included region, social class at birth and social class at age 42 years
[b]Full adjustment involved sex, depressive symptoms at age 45 years, sociodemographic factors, general and central obesity, alcohol, smoking, physical activity, sedentary behaviour, and fruit consumptions

symptoms [47]. Indeed, the possible stigma and discrimination due to excessive body weight is likely to have a greater impact on women than men which may explain the observed gender difference [47].

Mechanisms underlying the association between obesity and depression remains unclear, however, molecular and clinical studies have provided some evidence for the involvement of HPA axis, inflammatory pathways and insulin sensitivity [48], with dysregulation of HPA axis, elevation of certain inflammatory markers and insulin resistance being observed in both individuals with obesity and in individuals with depression

[49–51]. Disturbance in any of these systems may affect the secretion or metabolism of neurotransmitters, such as serotonin, norepinephrine and dopamine, in the brain and consequently influence mood [48, 52]. Findings regarding inflammatory pathways and insulin sensitivity are particularly interesting: the observed elevated inflammatory markers, including leptin, adiponectin and IL-6 and TNF-α are mainly secreted from white adipose tissue found on the abdomen [26]; abdominal obesity, in particular, places people at higher risk for developing insulin resistance [53]. All these observations resonate with our findings of an independent association for WC and highlight the particular importance of central obesity on the risk of developing depressive symptoms.

Our study also suggests that the association between obesity and depressive symptoms is in part related to socioeconomic and lifestyle factors, with obesity associations attenuating by about 30% after allowing for such factors. This attenuation was expected considering that most studies show lower socioeconomic status and unhealthy lifestyle factors to be associated with obesity and depression [54, 55] although some factors may be on the causal pathway from obesity to depressive symptoms. For example, obesity may lead to less active lifestyles as well as inactivity increasing the risk of obesity [56]. Even so, given the links shown here between lifestyle factors and depressive symptoms, our study suggests that these behaviours may be additional targets for interventions to reduce obesity and depression.

## Limitations

It is important to emphasise the following limitations of this study. Firstly, our study used the presence of depressive symptoms as the outcome rather than defining it based on the diagnosis of depressive disorder. In an earlier meta-analysis, the association between obesity and depression was found to be stronger for depressive disorder than for depressive symptoms [22]. This may explain why the associations found here are weaker than other reported estimates. Different instruments were used to assess depressive symptoms at ages 45 and 50 years, although both have been shown to be valid, with similar performance compared to standard diagnostic tools and both have been used in community-based epidemiological studies for screening of depressive symptoms [57, 58]. Another limitation relates to representativeness, as the ethnic composition of the current UK population is notably more diverse compared to the participants included here, 98% of whom were European origin [28]. Hence, the results may not be generalisable to today's more ethnically diverse population in the UK. A further limitation relates to inadequately measured or unmeasured confounding: although a broad range of lifestyle and sociodemographic factors were included, some measures (e.g. sedentary behaviour, physical activity) may have limitations, whilst in total the measures may not have captured all variation influencing the association between obesity and depressive symptoms. Finally, our study is limited in its ability to fully dissect independent effects of general and central adiposity. BMI and WC are highly correlated, and while our analyses suggest that WC may be the major influence, further studies avoiding problems with collinearity are needed to confirm this interpretation. Alternative approaches such as Mendelian randomisation may provide

further insights into the independent causal roles of central and general obesity on depression risk.

## Conclusion

Depressive symptoms are associated with obesity and related lifestyle factors in mid-life. Our study suggests that obesity affects subsequent risk of developing depressive symptoms among women independently of these concurrent associations, providing an important target group for implementation of preventative strategies. In the management of depressive symptoms, one of the alternative approaches could be targeting and managing obesity and unfavourable lifestyle factors.

## Abbreviations
BMI: Body Mass Index; CIS-R: Clinical Interview Schedule – Revised; HPA: Hypothalamus-Pituitary-Adrenal Axis; IL-6: InterLeukin-6; MHI-5: Mental Health Inventory-5; MHI-8: Mental Health Inventory-8; OR: Odds Ratio; PC: Personal Computer; SCAN: Schedule for Clinical Assessment in Neuropsychiatry; TNF-α: Tissue Necrotizing Factor—α; TV: Television; UK: United Kingdome; WC: Waist Circumference; WHO: World Health Organisation; WHR: Waist – Hip Ratio

## Acknowledgements
The authors are grateful to the Centre for Longitudinal Studies (CLS), UCL Institute of Education for the use of these data and to the UK Data Service for making them available. However, neither CLS nor the UK Data Service bear any responsibility for the analysis or interpretation of these data. The authors are thankful to Australian Research Training program Scholarship for AM's studentship support.

## Funding
The National Child Developmental study sweep 6 were funded by Economic and Social Council, and Government Departments. Medical Research Council funded the biomedical survey. Chris Power was funded by the Department of Health Policy Research Programme through the Public Health Research Consortium (PHRC) and supported by the National Institute for Health Research Biomedical Research Centre at Great Ormond Street Hospital for Children NHS Foundation Trust and University College London. The views expressed in the publication are those of the authors and not necessarily those of the Department of Health. Information about the wider programme of the PHRC is available from http://phrc.lshtm.ac.uk. Funding organisation has no role in the study design, analysis, and interpretation of results or writing of the report.

## Authors' contributions
EH conceptualised the study. AM, EH and AZ contributed to the planning, data analysis and interpretation. AM drafted the paper. EH, AZ and CP critically revised the paper and all authors approved the final manuscript.

## Consent for publication
Not applicable.

## Competing interests
The authors declare that they have no competing interests.

## Author details
[1]Australian Centre for Precision Health, University of South Australia Cancer Research Institute, GPO Box 2471, Adelaide, SA 5001, Australia. [2]Department of Pharmacology, School of Medicine, College of Health Science, Addis Ababa University, Addis Ababa, Ethiopia. [3]Population, Policy and Practice, UCL Great Ormond Street Institute of Child Health, London, UK.

## References

1. Obesity and Overweight [http://www.who.int/mediacentre/factsheets/fs311/en/]. (accessed 24.11.16)
2. Depression: A Global Public Health Concern [http://www.who.int/mental_health/management/depression/en/]. (Accessed 4 July 2016)
3. Lopez AD, Murray CJL. The global burden of disease, 1990 - 2020. Nat Med. 1998;4(11):1241–3.
4. Pan A, Lucas M, Sun Q, Van Dam RM, Franco OH, Manson JE, Willett WC, Ascherio A, Hu FB. Bidirectional association between depression and type 2 diabetes mellitus in women. Arch Intern Med. 2010;170(21):1884–91.
5. Lippi G, Montagnana M, Favaloro EJ, Franchini M. Mental depression and cardiovascular disease: a multifaceted, bidirectional association. Semin Thromb Hemost. 2009;35(3):325–36.
6. Casanueva FF, Moreno B, Rodriguez-Azeredo R, Massien C, Conthe P, Formiguera X, Barrios V, Balkau B. Relationship of abdominal obesity with cardiovascular disease, diabetes and hyperlipidaemia in Spain. Clin Endocrinol. 2010;73(1):35–40.
7. Reeves GM, Postolache TT, Snitker S. Childhood obesity and depression: connection between these growing problems in growing children. Int J Child Health Human Dev. 2008;1(2):103–14.
8. Lee SH, Paz-Filho G, Mastronardi C, Licinio J, Wong ML. Is increased antidepressant exposure a contributory factor to the obesity pandemic? Transl Psychiatry. 2016;6:e759.
9. Smith KA, Williams C, Cowen PJ. Impaired regulation of brain serotonin function during dieting in women recovered from depression. Br J Psychiatry. 2000;176:72–5.
10. Herva A, Laitinen J, Miettunen J, Veijola J, Karvonen JT, Laksy K, Joukamaa M. Obesity and depression: results from the longitudinal northern Finland 1966 birth cohort study. Int J Obes. 2006;30(3):520–7.
11. Chaiton M, Sabiston C, O'Loughlin J, McGrath JJ, Maximova K, Lambert M. A structural equation model relating adiposity, psychosocial indicators of body image and depressive symptoms among adolescents. Int J Obes. 2009;33(5):588–96.
12. Li ZB, Ho SY, Chan WM, Ho KS, Li MP, Leung GM, Lam TH. Obesity and depressive symptoms in Chinese elderly. Int J Geriatr Psychiatry. 2004; 19(1):68–74.
13. Van Gool CH, Kempen GI, Bosma H, van Boxtel MP, Jolles J, van Eijk JT. Associations between lifestyle and depressed mood: longitudinal results from the Maastricht aging study. Am J Public Health. 2007;97(5):887–94.
14. de Wit LM, van Straten A, van Herten M, Penninx BW, Cuijpers P. Depression and body mass index, a u-shaped association. BMC Public Health. 2009;9:14.
15. Geoffroy MC, Li L, Power C. Depressive symptoms and body mass index: co-morbidity and direction of association in a British birth cohort followed over 50 years. Psychol Med. 2014;44(12):2641–52.
16. Noh JW, Kwon YD, Park J, Kim J. Body mass index and depressive symptoms in middle aged and older adults. BMC Public Health. 2015;15:310.
17. Kodjebacheva G, Kruger DJ, Rybarczyk G, Cupal S. Racial/ethnic and gender differences in the association between depressive symptoms and higher body mass index. J Public Health. 2015;37(3):419–26.
18. Hicken MT, Lee H, Mezuk B, Kershaw KN, Rafferty J, Jackson JS. Racial and ethnic differences in the association between obesity and depression in women. J Womens Health. 2013;22(5):445–52.
19. Skelly AC, Dettori JR, Brodt ED. Assessing bias: the importance of considering confounding. Evid Based Spine Care J. 2012;3(1):9–12.
20. Xu Q, Anderson D, Lurie-Beck J. The relationship between abdominal obesity and depression in the general population: a systematic review and meta-analysis. Obes Res Clin Pract. 2011;5(4):e267–360.
21. Stevens J, McClain JE, Truesdale KP. Selection of measures in epidemiologic studies of the consequences of obesity. Int J Obes. 2008;32(Suppl 3): S60–6.
22. Luppino FS, de Wit LM, Bouvy PF, Stijnen T, Cuijpers P, Penninx BW, Zitman FG. Overweight, obesity, and depression: a systematic review and meta-analysis of longitudinal studies. Arch Gen Psychiatry. 2010; 67(3):220–9.
23. de Wit L, Luppino F, van Straten A, Penninx B, Zitman F, Cuijpers P. Depression and obesity: a meta-analysis of community-based studies. Psychiatry Res. 2010;178(2):230–5.
24. Janssen I, Katzmarzyk P, Ross R. Waist circumference and not body mass index explains obesity-related health risk. Am J Clin Nutr. 2004;79:6.
25. Kershaw EE, Flier JS. Adipose tissue as an endocrine organ. J Clin Endocrinol Metab. 2004;89(6):2548–56.
26. Shelton R, Miller A. Inflammation in depression: is adiposity a cause? Dialogues Clin Neurosci. 2011;13:13.
27. Thakore JH, Richards PJ, Reznek RH, Martin A, Dinan TG. Increased intra-abdominal fat deposition in patients with major depressive illness as measured by computed tomography. Biol Psychiatry. 1997;41(11):1140–2.
28. Power C, Elliott J. Cohort profile: 1958 British birth cohort (National Child Development Study). Int J Epidemiol. 2006;35(1):34–41.
29. The 1958 National Child Development Study [http://www.cls.ioe.ac.uk/page.aspx?&sitesectionid=724&sitesectiontitle=National+Child+Development+Study]. Accessed 26 July 2016.
30. Lewis G, Pelosi AJ, Araya R, Dunn G. Measuring psychiatric disorder in the community: a standardized assessment for use by lay interviewers. Psychol Med. 1992;22(2):465–86.
31. Jordanova V, Wickramesinghe C, Gerada C, Prince M. Validation of two survey diagnostic interviews among primary care attendees: a comparison of CIS-R and CIDI with SCAN ICD-10 diagnostic categories. Psychol Med. 2004;34(6):1013–24.
32. Jenkins R, Lewis G, Bebbington P, Brugha T, Farrell M, Gill B, Meltzer H. The National Psychiatric Morbidity surveys of Great Britain--initial findings from the household survey. Psychol Med. 1997;27(4):775–89.
33. Das-Munshi J, Goldberg D, Bebbington PE, Bhugra DK, Brugha TS, Dewey ME, Jenkins R, Stewart R, Prince M. Public health significance of mixed anxiety and depression: beyond current classification. Br J Psychiatry. 2008;192(3):171–7.
34. Holmes WC. A short, Psychiaatric, case-finding measure for HIV Seropossetive outpatients: performance characterstics of the 5-item mental health subscale of the SF-20 in a male, seropositive sample. Med Care. 1998;36(2):8.
35. Berwick D, Murphy J, Goldman P, Ware J, Barsky A, Weinstein M. Perfornmance of a five-item mental health screening test. Med Care. 1991;29(2):8.
36. Tehnical report on the national child development study biomedical survey 2002-2004. [www.cls.ioe.ac.uk/shared/get-file.ashx?id=369&itemtype=document]. (accessed 09.02.17)
37. BMI classification [http://www.who.int/topics/obesity/en/]. Accessed 10 Sept 2018.
38. Waist circumference and waist–hip ratio: report of a WHO expert consultation [http://whqlibdoc.who.int/publications/2011/9789241501491_eng.pdf]. (accessed 10.11.16).
39. What qualification levels mean [https://www.gov.uk/what-different-qualification-levels-mean]. Accessed 10 Aug 2018.
40. Butler NR, Bonham DG. Perinatal mortality. Edinburgh: livingstone; 1963.
41. Maddock J, Geoffroy MC, Power C, Hypponen E. 25-Hydroxyvitamin D and cognitive performance in mid-life. Br J Nutr. 2014;111(5):904–14.
42. Jokela M, Hamer M, Singh-Manoux A, Batty GD, Kivimaki M. Association of metabolically healthy obesity with depressive symptoms: pooled analysis of eight studies. Mol Psychiatry. 2014;19(8):910–4.
43. Johnston E, Johnson S, McLeod P, Johnston M. The relation of body mass index to depressive symptoms. Can J Public Health. 2004;95(3): 179–83.
44. Yu NW, Chen CY, Liu CY, Chau YL, Chang CM. Association of Body Mass Index and Depressive Symptoms in a chinese community population: Results from the Health Promotion Knowldge, Attitude, and Performance Survey in Taiwan. Chang Gung Med J. 2011;34:7.

45. Simon GE, Arterburn D, Rohde P, Ludman EJ, Linde JA, Operskalski BH, Jeffery RW. Obesity, depression, and health services costs among middle-aged women. J Gen Intern Med. 2011;26(11):1284–90.

46. Carslake D, Davey Smith G, Gunnell D, Davies N, Nilsen TIL, Romundstad P. Confounding by ill health in the observed association between BMI and mortality: evidence from the HUNT study using offspring BMI as an instrument. Int J Epidemiol. 2018;47(3):760–70.

47. Hunger JM, Major B. Weight stigma mediates the association between BMI and self-reported health. Health Psychology. 2015;34(2):172–5.

48. Bornstein SR, Schuppenies A, Wong ML, Licinio J. Approaching the shared biology of obesity and depression: the stress axis as the locus of gene-environment interactions. Mol Psychiatry. 2006;11(10):892–902.

49. Lee JH, Park SK, Ryoo JH, Oh CM, Mansur RB, Alfonsi JE, Cha DS, Lee Y, McIntyre RS, Jung JY. The association between insulin resistance and depression in the Korean general population. J Affect Disord. 2017;208:553–9.

50. Lu XY, Kim CS, Frazer A, Zhang W. Leptin: a potential novel antidepressant. Proc Natl Acad Sci U S A. 2006;103(5):1593–8.

51. Varghese FP, Brown ES. The hypothalamic-pituitary-adrenal Axis in major depressive disorder: a brief primer for primary care physicians. Prim Care Companion J Clin Psychiatry. 2001;3(4):151–5.

52. Kleinridders A, Cai W, Cappellucci L, Ghazarian A, Collins WR, Vienberg SG, Pothos EN, Kahn CR. Insulin resistance in brain alters dopamine turnover and causes behavioral disorders. Proc Natl Acad Sci U S A. 2015;112(11):3463–8.

53. Westphal SA. Obesity, abdominal obesity, and insulin resistance. Clin Cornerstone. 2008;9(1):23–9 discussion 30–21.

54. De Mello MT, Lemos Vde A, Antunes HK, Bittencourt L, Santos-Silva R, Tufik S. Relationship between physical activity and depression and anxiety symptoms: a population study. J Affect Disord. 2013;149(1–3):241–6.

55. Lee O, Lee DC, Lee S, Kim YS. Associations between physical activity and obesity defined by waist-to-height ratio and body mass index in the Korean population. PLoS One. 2016;11(7):e0158245.

56. Golubic R, Wijndaele K, Sharp SJ, Simmons RK, Griffin SJ, Wareham NJ, Ekelund U, Brage S. Physical activity, sedentary time and gain in overall and central body fat: 7-year follow-up of the ProActive trial cohort. Int J Obes. 2015;39(1):142–8.

57. Patton GC, Coffey C, Posterino M, Carlin JB, Wolfe R, Bowes G. A computerised screening instrument for adolescent depression: population-based validation and application to a two-phase case-control study. Soc Psychiatry Psychiatr Epidemiol. 1999;34(3):166–72.

58. Trainor K, Mallett J, Rushe T. Age related differences in mental health scale scores and depression diagnosis: adult responses to the CIDI-SF and MHI-5. J Affect Disord. 2013;151(2):639–45.

# 14

# Requirements for the implementation of open door policies in acute psychiatry from a mental health professionals' and patients' view: a qualitative interview study

J. Kalagi[1], I. Otte[2], J. Vollmann[2], G. Juckel[1] and J. Gather[1,2*]

## Abstract

**Background:** Treating legally committed patients on open, instead of locked wards is controversially discussed and the affected stakeholders (patients, mental health professionals) have ambiguous views on the benefits and disadvantages. The study aims to assess the opinions and values of relevant stakeholders with regard to the requirements for implementing open wards in psychiatric hospitals.

**Methods:** Semi-structured interviews were conducted with 15 psychiatrists, 15 psychiatric nurses and 15 patients, and were analyzed using qualitative content analysis.

**Results:** The interviewees identified conceptual, personnel and spatial requirements necessary for an open door policy. Observation and door watch concepts are judged to be essential for open wards, and patients appreciate the therapeutic value they hold. However, nurses find the door watch problematic. All groups suggest seclusion or small locked divisions as a possible way of handling agitated patients. All stakeholders agree that such concepts can only succeed if sufficient, qualified staff is available. They also agree that freedom of movement is a key element in the management of acutely ill patients, which can be achieved with an open door policy. Finally, the interviewees suggested removing the door from direct view to prevent absconding.

**Conclusions:** For psychiatric institutions seeking to implement (partially) open wards, the present results may have high practical relevance. The stakeholders' suggestions also illustrate that fundamental clinical changes depend on resource investments which – at least at a certain point – might not be feasible for individual psychiatric institutions but presumably require initiatives on the level of mental health care providers or policy makers.

**Keywords:** Locked wards, Coercion, Open door policy, Acute psychiatry, Implementation, Qualitative research

## Background

People suffering from severe and acute psychiatric disorders are at an increased risk of being involuntarily detained on a locked ward, especially in situations in which they pose a threat to themselves or to others. Although research by Rittmannsberger and colleagues [1], conducted in Austria, Hungary, Romania, Slovakia and Slovenia, showed more than 10 years ago that involuntarily committed patients are not necessarily referred to locked wards, it is still common practice in most European countries to treat acutely ill psychiatric patients who pose a danger to themselves or to others, at least initially on wards whose doors are permanently locked. Data from the United Kingdom even reveals that the proportion of locked wards has risen over the last decades, resulting in more than 90% locked wards out of all wards visited by the Care Quality Commission in 2015/2016 [2, 3].

In Germany, there are two legal regimes – the guardianship law (which is a federal law) and the mental health laws of each of the 16 German federal states – under which patients can be involuntarily admitted to a psychiatric

\* Correspondence: jakov.gather@rub.de
[1]Department of Psychiatry, Psychotherapy and Preventive Medicine, LWL University Hospital, Ruhr University Bochum, Alexandrinenstr. 1-3, 44791 Bochum, Germany
[2]Institute for Medical Ethics and History of Medicine, Ruhr University Bochum, Markstr. 258a, 44799 Bochum, Germany

hospital. About 10% of the admissions to a psychiatric hospital are involuntary, and the absolute number of involuntary admissions has increased significantly under both legal regimes since the 1990s [4]. Traditionally, legally committed patients are admitted to locked wards. However, in recent years, several clinicians and bodies advocated for stronger efforts to implement open door policies in psychiatry, which means to treat legally committed patients on open, rather than locked wards [5–8]. Such approaches are discussed controversially; however, some psychiatric hospitals have quite a long tradition of open door policies [9–11].

Legally, it is assumed that the treatment of legally committed patients on open, rather than locked wards, is permissible as long as hospitals take appropriate measures to guarantee that the respective patients do not abscond from the commitment [12, 13]. In North Rhine-Westphalia, which is the German federal state with the highest number of inhabitants, on 1 January 2017 a new mental health law came into force which even explicitly states that "legal commitments shall be performed in an open setting as far as possible" (Sec. 10 of the North Rhine-Westphalian PsychKG). All such demands and provisions aim to ensure the safety of the patients or others as best as possible while limiting the patients' freedom as little as possible. There is data that opening the doors might lead to less aggressive incidents [14, 15] and that absconding and suicide rates are not higher compared with closed settings [15, 16].

However, previous studies revealed that mental health professionals' and patients' attitudes towards open wards are quite ambiguous and that different stakeholders tend to not only see benefits but also certain disadvantages of open wards, such as the loss of resources due to the observation of the open door or a decrease in security and control [2, 17–20]. Open door policies challenge those who are directly involved in clinical routines and have to transform theoretical concepts into daily clinical practice. While these previous studies have primarily investigated the effects of open door policies, there is no research that we are aware of that has explored how such concepts can be newly implemented and what organizational requirements may be necessary for putting them into practice.

The present study is part of a larger mixed-methods study on clinical effects and ethical aspects of open door policies. The mixed-methods study consists (1) of a prospective cohort study, which aims to investigate – amongst others – the effects of open compared to locked doors on coercive interventions and serious incidents in a sample of all patients who were involuntarily committed to five different psychiatric hospitals during a specified 6 months period, and (2) of a qualitative interview study with mental health professionals and patients. With the interviews, we aim to explore the experiences and attitudes of different experts of psychiatric practice with the implementation of open doors in an acute psychiatric hospital. In this article, we only present results of the qualitative interview study. We intend to identify requirements for the treatment of legally committed patients on open instead of locked wards by taking into account the practical and personal knowledge of those who are needed when such fundamental changes such as an open door policy are introduced into clinical practice.

## Methods

Between February and June 2016, four members of the research team conducted 45 qualitative, open-ended, semi-structured interviews (15 interviews with patients, 15 interviews with psychiatric nurses and 15 interviews with psychiatrists). Psychiatrists and psychiatric nurses were chosen because they are directly involved in the decision making around legal commitments of psychiatric patients and in putting those into practice (amongst others by determining whether the ward's entrance door should be opened or locked). The patients were chosen because they are personally affected by the legal commitment and restricted in their freedom by the locked door.

Before starting the sampling process, the research project was presented to all psychiatrists and psychiatric nurses in their regular team meetings. The sampling process was purposive in order to obtain a diverse selection of psychiatrists and psychiatric nurses to represent a range of professional experience, hierarchical positions, ages and genders. The interviewees could get in touch or were contacted directly by the members of the research team. With regard to the patients, we contacted all patients who met the inclusion criteria and appeared in the hospital's outpatient or inpatient department during the course of the study.

The inclusion criterion for psychiatrists and psychiatric nurses was to have working experience on both open and closed acute psychiatric wards. As for the patients, the inclusion criteria were (1) having a psychiatric disorder according to ICD-10, (2) having experiences with involuntary commitments in the hospital before and/or after the implementation of the open door policy and (3) preserved mental capacity at the time of the informed consent process and the interview. In case the patient had a legal guardian, the latter also had to give informed consent.

The study was approved by the ethics committee of the Medical Faculty of the Ruhr University Bochum (Reg. No. 15-5452). Before conducting the interviews, the interviewers were trained by an experienced sociologist with the help of mock interviews.

The semi-structured interviews focused on thematic aspects, such as personal experience with the open door policy, challenges and barriers as well as suggestions for improvement. The guideline was developed based on our literature review and refined further after the first interviews, giving the interviewers the opportunity to add relevant questions to the set. The average length of an interview was 41 min (range: 21–64 min). All interviews were audio-taped, anonymized and transcribed verbatim. All transcripts were read and reread to ensure familiarity with the data. The analysis was conducted by five members of the research team, who were not involved in the treatment of the patients. The coders followed the principles of qualitative content analysis, a method that provides useful access to the large amount of data by preserving the advantages of quantitative content analysis and complementing them with qualitative-interpretative steps of analysis [21, 22]. During the analysis, using AtlasTi 6.2 software, the data was repeatedly coded, moving from concrete passages to more abstract levels of coding, from codes to categories and finally to three overarching themes. This process was both inductively deriving themes from the data and searching for repeating concepts [23], as well as deductively analyzing the data on the grounds of previously conducted literature research and the current research question. These steps were repeated as coding guidelines for each interviewee group were gradually developed. All findings were critically tested and discussed among the researchers who had different disciplinary backgrounds (sociology, psychiatry, psychology, nursing and medical ethics). Any disagreements were resolved by discussion. Since the coding system remained the same for the last interviews and the findings did not add anything significantly new to the interviews conducted previously, we concluded that we had reached theoretical saturation.

As Table 1 demonstrates, the participants varied in their age and professional background or diagnosis respectively. One psychologist was included in the group of the psychiatrists. That particular psychologist carries out many tasks of the doctors in the clinic and is therefore referred to as part of the psychiatrist group for the remainder of this article.

## Results

We identified three overarching themes in which changes are seen as necessary for the implementation of open door policy in an acute psychiatric hospital: conceptual, personnel and spatial requirements.

### Conceptual requirements

Two concepts which are often implemented in open door policies are intensive forms of observation and a door watch. The continuous or intermittent observation (e.g. 1:1 or 2:1 observation) of patients intends to ensure their safety and that of others and at the same time is a therapeutic intervention to engage the patient in a positive interaction. The door watch consists of a staff member being positioned near the door in order to prevent patients from absconding.

### Observation

Both professional groups are in favour of observation because it is less disruptive of the patients' freedom in comparison to a locked door or mechanical restraint. However, the nurses note that it is very exhausting to constantly be with a patient for lengthy periods of time. Furthermore, psychiatrists and nurses are aware that continuous observation may actually increase tension in certain patient groups. All interviewee groups acknowledge that observation is personnel intensive. Patients greatly appreciate continuous observation as it seems to achieve the right balance of feeling cared for while still remaining autonomous.

*I've had it a few times that a nurse offered me to talk a little or that I could reach out to them for a chat and I liked that very much. In general, that there are people around you and don't harass you and don't want anything but just have a look at what you're doing, how you are. [...] I've always found that pleasant. (Patient 3)*

### Door watch

While psychiatrists and patients judge the door watch as largely positive, the nurses find the concept problematic. According to the nurses, the door watch poses a big challenge for several reasons. Firstly, they find it mentally draining to watch the door. Many experience stress because so much is happening in the entrance area and they have to be continuously alert. They report it is very difficult to make sure no patient absconds when they have to interact with other patients at the same time. They also experience stress because they are afraid of being attacked and getting harmed when a patient tries to abscond. Finally, some nurses report stress due to feeling responsible when a patient absconds and even being made responsible by their superior. The role of watching the door and ensuring that patients do not abscond thus comes with a lot of emotional distress.

*For a nurse, that's not exactly a comfortable situation because you can't assume that you can make the patient, who absolutely wants to leave the clinic now, a benevolent, therapeutic offer - rather, you have to mechanically prevent him from something. That's always a negative experience to the point of quarrelling scenarios, which happen; with sounding the alarm and all that. (Nurse 9)*

Secondly, many nurses see a role conflict in being a "guard" for the door. Nurses view themselves as a caring profession whose primary concern is to support the patient. They are thus averse to the idea of having a task that puts them in a position of a guard. Moreover, they report that

**Table 1** Clinical and socio-demographic characteristics

| | Psychiatrists (N = 15) | Nurses (N = 15) | Patients (N = 15) | Total sample (N = 45) |
|---|---|---|---|---|
| Gender | | | | |
| Female | 9 (60%) | 9 (60%) | 3 (20%) | 21 (47%) |
| Male | 6 (40%) | 6 (40%) | 12 (80%) | 24 (53%) |
| Age (M ± SD) | 35.3 ± 7.0 | 35.2 ± 12.1 | 38.9 ± 14.0 | 36.5 ± 11.3 |
| Range | 28–54 | 24–63 | 20–60 | 20–63 |
| Years of professional experience (M ± SD) | 7.0 ± 7.0 | 12.0 ± 12.6 | | |
| Range | 0.5–27 | 1.25–45 | | |
| Years employed in the hospital (M ± SD) | 4.4 ± 6.0 | 6.7 ± 6.3 | | |
| Range | 0.08–23.75 | 0.75–22 | | |
| Professional background | | | | |
| Psychologist | 1 (6.7%) | | | |
| Psychiatric resident | 10 (66.7%) | | | |
| Psychiatrist (specialist) | 2 (13.3%) | | | |
| Senior psychiatrist | 2 (13.3%) | | | |
| Nursing student | | 2 (13.3%) | | |
| Nurse without academic degree | | 10 (66.7%) | | |
| Nurse with academic degree | | 3 (20%) | | |
| Diagnosis | | | | |
| Psychotic disorders (ICD-10 F2) | | | 6 (40%) | |
| Affective disorders (ICD-10 F3) | | | 6 (40%) | |
| Substance dependence (ICD-10 F1) | | | 3 (20%) | |
| Duration of the illness in years (M ± SD) | | | 17.0 ± 13.0 | |
| Number of previous hospitalizations (M ± SD) | | | 5.53 ± 6.3 | |
| With legal commitment | | | 2.00 ± 2.2 | |
| Currently legally committed | | | | |
| Yes | | | 6 (40%) | |
| No | | | 9 (60%) | |

the door watch prevents them from being able to fulfill their role as a nurse. They can no longer assist patients because they cannot leave their spot or have therapeutic conversations with them because privacy is not given in the entrance area. For this reason, the nurses judge the door watch to be too resource intensive as an entire person's capacity is taken up by a non-nursing task. Lastly, the nurses point out that repeatedly having to tell patients that they cannot leave, fosters aggression and sometimes strains the therapeutic relationship.

*You always had a bit of a bouncer feeling. You technically were rather a bouncer and not a nurse, but had to watch that he wouldn't abscond, and this one, he can leave. Well that's not really what we've studied for.* (Nurse 13)

Psychiatrists are in favour of having a nurse watch the door. They view a constant eye on the door as essential for the success of the open door concept. Psychiatrists think that when a patient leaves the ward, a fast reaction using the presence of numerous staff members is often very effective in preventing absconding. A prerequisite for this is a constant watch of the door.

*That would be, I'd say, a justifiable restriction of the respective person's freedom. He would be brought back by nurses or an alarm would be sounded and everybody comes running. That usually is sufficient in getting the patient to return to the ward, and the other patients aren't restricted one bit in their freedom of movement.* (Psychiatrist 9)

At the same time, psychiatrists acknowledge that nurses cannot be expected to verbally prevent all, especially aggressive patients, from absconding.

Patients experience a nurse paying attention to the door as largely positive. They appreciate that it gives them someone on the floor who they can talk to. Some patients feel like they are being closely monitored, which they dislike, while others mention that they do not have a feeling of being watched. Generally, patients think that by watching the door, nurses can keep a better eye on patients who are at risk of harming themselves or others which enables them to respond faster to escalating situations.

*Another one, two more would maybe be better because then maybe it would be a little more compact, right? Maybe one could leave the door open more often [...] that staff sits there and pays special attention to those who are particularly at risk.* (Patient 12)

All groups agree that the majority of the patients can be easily convinced to stay on the ward by using verbal communication but that some patients cannot be reached by these means and have a strong urge to repeatedly try to leave the ward. The challenge of an open door policy is to find a way of managing this latter group of patients. The interviewees have various ideas of how this might be accomplished. All groups agree that a successful door watch requires more staff. Psychiatrists suggest that all wards should be built in a way that the door can be viewed from the nurses' room. Another idea for managing challenging patients in an open setting involves seclusion.

### Seclusion
Patients, nurses and psychiatrists unanimously would like to have the option of seclusion in the clinic. Patients reported finding seclusion less traumatic than mechanical restraint.

*Hence the rest room, the padded room. So they can go in there and let off steam without end and when they're calm again, they can come out again; instead of being mechanically restrained. Because when you get*

*mechanically restrained, it rather causes more frustration.* (Patient 1)

Professionals view a locked door as less coercive than mechanical restraint but they critically note that it affects many patients. By having a seclusion room, nurses highlight that a situation can be effectively de-escalated without having to mechanically restrain the patient or lock the ward for many unaffected patients.

*If the locked door can result in the de-escalation of a patient, or bring the situation as a whole under control, the locked door is preferable to mechanical restraint. But I would do it on a small scale [...]. In my opinion, there should be an option to put the patient in a room, however that looks like, to lock the door and have a controlled area. I'd prefer that instead of having it affect so many patients.* (Nurse 11)

*For rather physically agitated and restless patients, if you can somehow create special options for them which lead to a reduction of this urge to move; well if you think beyond pharmacological stuff [...] possibly a sort of rage room or soft room [...] that aggression can also be released without injuries to themselves or others.* (Psychiatrist 12)

An overview of the identified conceptual requirements can be found in Table 2.

### Personnel requirements
#### More staff and strong therapeutic relationships
All interviewee groups agree that open-door policies can be implemented more successfully with more staff. Both professional groups critically note that the present staff number is insufficient when there are several acute patients on the ward or when staff members are ill. Especially continuous observation and the door watch, both of which are often carried out when the door is open, are very personnel-intensive and result in too little

**Table 2** Perceptions about conceptual requirements

|  | Psychiatrists | Nurses | Patients |
|---|---|---|---|
| Observation | + less coercive than a closed door<br>– long observation can create tension | + less coercive than a closed door<br>– long observation is exhausting | + good balance between care and autonomy |
| Door Watch | + effectively prevents most absconding<br>– not all patients can be prevented from leaving | + effectively prevents most absconding<br>– very strenuous<br>– safety risk<br>– feeling too much responsibility | + effectively prevents most absconding<br>+ conversation partner on the ward<br>+ better monitoring of dangerous patients<br>– feeling of being watched |
| Seclusion | + affects less patients than a closed ward | + affects less patients than a closed ward | + less traumatic than mechanical restraint |

+: positive; –: negative

resources for the remaining patients. The patients are also aware of this issue.

*Worst-case-scenario would be being assigned to a shift with four of us. We have 32 patients who need to be cared for, then one of us drops out because of 1:1, then the door stays open so we need to establish a door watch, then the third nurse goes out on the floor. Then we only have two people who need to support the remaining 31 patients. That's difficult. (Nurse 8)*

*The nurses are only humans, they can't keep an eye on everything. They've also got paperwork, they also have to treat other patients and so the chance to abscond is easy. No that doesn't work, it doesn't work out. (Patient 1)*

Patients and nurses critically note that having too little time to engage in activities or conversations with patients gives patients the feeling that they are not being taken seriously. As a result, tension builds up. All three groups agree that building a strong relationship between staff and patient is crucial for an open door policy.

Psychiatrists and nurses suggest that by having more staff, even students, who can engage in continuous observation or watch the door, the other nurses have more time to manage the needs of patients and form stronger therapeutic relationships. Psychiatrists and nurses highlight that a strong relationship can prevent absconding because patients have a better understanding of why they are in the clinic and that staff want to help them. Moreover, the staff have a better understanding of how exactly they need to engage and communicate with the individual patient to calm them down or prevent them from leaving the ward.

*I for one had the feeling I often had too little time to engage in adequate relationship building with the patient, that I had the feeling relationship-wise things were running smoothly, so that patients on this basis could be prevented from absconding. And speaking from my medical point of view, I think there was too little of that. I would've preferred to talk more to the patients in order to clearly and explicitly discuss with them why they are here, so that on that basis of trust, I maybe would have accomplished more, that patients don't abscond. (Psychiatrist 3)*

Patients and nurses suggest fixed opportunities for conversations with the staff. Patients report that it is important to them that they can talk to the nurses, to know that the staff regards them with benevolence and that the staff is open to make arrangements. Nurses stress that supporting patients, actively engaging and spending time with

them can be effective in preventing tension from building up, which may have otherwise resulted in absconding or aggression.

*Beneficial here is without question the communication you can have here; that you're not put off but rather that you can directly interact with the nursing staff, [...] in the locked setting it's rather that they withdraw, and with this observation there is a kind of care, you get attention and warmth and feel social proximity, and that's very conducive to your health. (Patient 2)*

### Trained staff
Nurses and psychiatrists emphasize that training staff adequately is very helpful in the implementation of open-door policies. Psychiatrists critically note that many staff members lack detailed knowledge on the legal aspects of coercive measures and legal commitments to a psychiatric hospital. Psychiatrists also admit that coercive measures, including the locked door policy, should be reviewed more regularly, because oftentimes short periods of a locked door are sufficient to de-escalate a situation. Psychiatrists suggest that there should be more standards and that the given standards regarding coercive measures should be more strictly adhered to. Nurses suggest regular supervisions or inter-professional reevaluation sessions in which the challenges and ideas for the implementation of the open door policy can be discussed.

*Technically, we are obliged to review every four hours, and also when a situation has de-escalated earlier, you should always check that you can quickly open the door again. And sometimes you become a little negligent with that. (Psychiatrist 1)*

An overview of the identified personnel requirements can be found in Table 3.

### Spatial requirements
#### Increased freedom of movement and outdoor activities
Both nurses and patients stress the importance of being surrounded by or in nature. They highlight that activities in nature have therapeutic and de-escalating effects. Patients would like to have more outside excursions with staff. Nurses express their wish to have more time to go for a walk with patients.

*That you get to do more with the group, go somewhere or go for a walk in the park, experience more nature, go for a jog or so. (Patient 11)*

Psychiatrists and nurses find a garden enclosed in the ward very valuable as patients can be outside, have a

**Table 3** Perceptions about personnel requirements

|  | Psychiatrists | Nurses | Patients |
|---|---|---|---|
| More staff | + allows for observation and door watch while still having resources for unaffected patients | + allows for observation and door watch while still having resources for unaffected patients | + allows for an open ward with resources for all patients |
| Better therapeutic relationships | + prevents absconding | + prevents build-up of tension | + assurance that staff regards them with benevolence |
| Trained staff | + can decrease length of coercive measures | + importance of re-evaluating situations | |

+: positive

smoke and more space to move around. Patients appreciate it, too, but point out that the garden should not be too small.

*The problem was that I had to walk all the time because, due to the antipsychotics I got, I had restless legs symptoms. So somehow walk all the time, and so I constantly walked in a circle in this courtyard garden and was annoyed that I couldn't get further out.* (Patient 3)

All three groups agree that it would be favourable to have a bigger space which patients can move in. However, psychiatrists note that a bigger space makes it hard to keep an overview and thus comes with safety risks.

### No visible freedom restraints

Related to an increased freedom of movement is the suggestion of moving the actual border within which patients should remain. Both nurses and psychiatrists proposed that patients should be kept on the open ward through verbal communication and that there should only be a lock system outside the ward. This system may be an alarm that automatically goes off, a door further on in the clinic which automatically locks when an alarm button is pressed or special security staff who could be called.

*If you secure the outer borders, you could have plenty of latitude to possibly let the patient abscond because then you would find him on the way to the main reception so to speak. So really a mechanical process, that you kind of move the security aspect further outside distance-wise. To present the open here so to speak, which, I find and I stand by that, holds a therapeutic quality for the patient. But the security aspect, that no one absconds who's going to run out in front of a car or who is going to kill someone or things like that.* (Nurse 9)

Another suggestion put forward by the nurses is the idea that it could be helpful to put the (open or locked) door out of line of sight for the patients. By moving the door around a corner which is not visible from the usual movement on the ward, the open door may not create

such a big temptation to abscond while the locked door may not create so much frustration. Both these ideas attempt to make the freedom restraints less visible to the patient so that they are not constantly at the top of their minds.

### Small locked divisions

Another compromise which is proposed by patients and nurses is to generally have an open setting in the clinic with an additional small locked ward or division. This locked area should have very few beds and only be for acutely dangerous patients. Furthermore, it should be highly staffed with experienced and trained personnel to ensure intensive care. Patients and nurses agree that such a ward would keep the other patients safe. The acute patients would also benefit because they could stabilize in a small, low-stimulus environment. Once they are stable again, they can return to their respective open ward.

*Maybe I would really stow them away in an extra space, well only at risk, strongly at risk [...] that you can take them out in the acute phase but then also reintegrate them back into the community because they do belong to us, we are a community after all.* (Patient 15)

An overview of the identified spatial requiremenst can be found in Table 4.

## Discussion

The interviewees identified several requirements for an implementation of open door policies which pose a challenge to the current mental health care system. These include – amongst others – door watch and special observation measures as conceptual requirements, a higher number of well trained staff as personnel requirements and more freedom of movement as well as making the door less visible as spatial requirements.

### Conceptual requirements

Special observation measures are well-established in many psychiatric institutions and an integral part of existing clinical guidelines [24]. Besides observational aspects, they entail therapeutic elements which are valuable for the

**Table 4** Perceptions about spatial requirements

|  | Psychiatrists | Nurses | Patients |
| --- | --- | --- | --- |
| Outdoor activities | + therapeutic / de-escalating effects | + therapeutic / de-escalating effects | + therapeutic / de-escalating effects |
| Increased freedom of movement | + de-escalating effects − safety risk | + de-escalating effects | + de-escalating effects |
| No visible restraints | + compromise between perceived freedom and safety | + compromise between perceived freedom and safety | |
| Small locked divisions | | + intense care for destabilized patients while maintaining an open setting | + intense care for destabilized patients while maintaining an open setting |

+: positive; −: negative

management of suicidal or aggressive patients. If one opens a locked entrance door on a psychiatric ward, one has to replace the former "mechanical" with a "human" barrier to guarantee that the staff members always know who is on the ward and who is not. This requires measures with a strong focus on observation, and such measures may contradict the professional self-conception of nurses. Moreover, such observational measures can cause emotional distress among nurses (which was described as "anxious vigilance" by Muir-Cochrane et al. [19] several years ago) and come along with a feeling of having too much responsibility. Against this background, it seems desirable to 1. clearly assign responsibilities among the multi-professional teams, especially in situations in which it comes to absconding, 2. periodically change the observing nurse to prevent emotional distress and 3. strengthen the therapeutic elements in the implementation of a door watch which means using the time of the door watch procedure to engage patients in positive contact instead of merely focusing on the observational aspect.

The psychiatrists', psychiatric nurses' and patients' call for seclusion seems to be quite contradictory at first sight, as it would merely replace one locked door (the ward's entrance door) by another (the seclusion room's door). Given that seclusion is rarely used in Germany, in comparison to other countries, and many German psychiatric hospitals do not even possess seclusion rooms (but use mechanical restraint instead [4]), this claim seems even more astonishing. Furthermore, the claim for seclusion apparently contradicts the international efforts to eliminate all coercive interventions [25–29] and seems to ignore the existing literature on negative effects of seclusion [30–32].

However, what concerns the psychiatrists and psychiatric nurses most is the management of individual agitated or aggressive patients without affecting many other patients by locking the door of the whole ward, and in this context, they regard seclusion rooms as helpful. These attitudes correspond – at least with respect to the patients' and the staff members' safety – to the results of a survey in which service users, carers and professionals to varying degrees (ranging from ca. 44 to 85%) hold the opinion that seclusion can increase the safety of service users or others [33].

The patients' claim for seclusion rooms probably can be best understood in the context of their strong disapproval of mechanical restraint [34]. Patients might see seclusion as a less restrictive alternative compared to mechanical restraint [35].

In view of our results, alongside German guidelines which already recommend the provisioning of different types of coercive measures in psychiatric institutions (to be able to take into account the patients' individual preferences [36]), psychiatric hospitals should consider providing seclusion rooms. This does not necessarily have to result in an increase of seclusion or coercive interventions in general. On the contrary, there is evidence that coercive interventions including seclusion can be significantly reduced by the introduction of an open-door policy [11, 14, 37]. Furthermore, there are less restrictive and voluntary alternatives to seclusion such as "soft rooms" which are already known from "Soteria" concepts [38]. Our interviewees suggested such facilities as helpful in the management of agitated patients.

**Personnel requirements**

All stakeholders unanimously share the view that ambitious conceptual changes, like the implementation of an open door policy, can only succeed if sufficient and well qualified staff are made available. However, most of the legal reforms and various demands for a reduction of coercion in psychiatry are not accompanied by the provision of higher financial resources. Taking the views of those who are directly involved in daily clinical routines seriously, initiatives to reduce coercion should include sufficient financial and personnel investments in order to avoid excessive demands on the part of the staff and to make such initiatives successful. At the level of mental health care providers and leaders of psychiatric institutions, strong support should be provided by internal guidelines and regular trainings which has already been identified to be a helpful and effective approach in the reduction of coercion in general [39–42].

**Spatial requirements**

Considering that legally committed patients are often tense and restless, an increased freedom of movement is presumably a key element in the management of patients in acute psychic crisis situations. Opening locked doors can both psychologically and factually increase the available space and help reduce crowding with all its negative effects on aggression and concomitant coercion [9, 15, 43–46].

With regard to the idea of moving the actual border out of sight of the patients, it is questionable whether an open door policy is still given when there is in fact a locked door further on in the building. However, the idea illustrates that professionals seek a compromise of reaping the therapeutic and ethical benefits of an open door while ensuring safety and abiding by the legal requirement of taking measures to keep the patient committed in the hospital.

Whereas such ideas would presumably require structural modifications in the hospital, this is all the more true for the idea of having small (locked) divisions for intensive care on a regular ward. The interviewees' suggestions brings the Dutch "High and Intensive Care"- model to mind which entails special "Intensive Care Units", in which patients can temporarily receive intensified care in acute crisis situations [47, 48].

All these approaches indicate that conceptual changes, at least at a certain point, often have to be accompanied by architectural changes. This is in line with the already existing evidence that modifying a hospital's architecture can contribute to a reduction of coercion [49–52].

### Strengths and limitations

To our knowledge, this study is the first qualitative interview study on open door policies in acute psychiatry which includes psychiatrists, nurses and patients, hence all stakeholders who are primarily affected by such a far-reaching change in clinical practice. A key strength of this study is its use of a qualitative method to explore a multifaceted topic, enabling mental health professionals, alongside patients, to express their attitudes towards the implementation of an open door policy. Using a qualitative method such as semi-structures interviews allows participants to expand on their responses, ideally resulting in a rich data collection that provides depth and detail which could not be achieved using a quantitative method approach. However, selection biases due to the recruitment process are possible which could result in a bias towards the participation of mental health professionals who feel generally more positively towards this topic. Nevertheless, since we have (1) strictly respected confidentiality and anonymity and also (2) obtained a variety of distinct answers that are not limited to what would be expected to be socially desirable (e.g. very critical statements), it is safe to conclude that this bias remains small.

With regard to the participating patients, one major limitation is the fact that we did not systematically assess the patients' disease severity at the time of the interviews and

that some of their viewpoints might have been influenced by their current state of disease. Furthermore, not all patients we asked agreed to participate so that we possibly missed the views of those patients who would have been more critical.

A general limitation, which applies to most qualitative studies, is the issue of generalizability. However, the aim of qualitative studies is not generalizability or statistical significance, but rather, to gain a better understanding of social phenomena such as the effects of the implementation of open door policies. Since 1) the data was gathered from a good representation of various mental health professions and 2) theoretical saturation was reached within the number of conducted interviews, we are convinced that we have achieved this aim. Nevertheless, it is unclear whether the attitudes and beliefs presented here would be shared by participants from other settings in other areas or countries.

### Conclusion

Based on their personal experiences, mental health professionals and patients point out several requirements which help to promote the process of implementing open door policies in acute psychiatric hospitals. Hence, for all psychiatric institutions which seek to (partially) open former locked wards, their insights into conceptual, personnel and spatial preconditions might have a high practical relevance. On a broader level, the suggestions also illustrate that fundamental clinical changes, such as the implementation of open door policies, depend on resource investments which, at least at a certain point, might not be realised on the level of an individual psychiatric institution but presumably require initiatives on the level of mental health care providers or policy makers.

### Abbreviations
ICD-10: International statistical classification of diseases and related health problems (10th Revision); PsychKG: Gesetz über Hilfen und Schutzmaßnahmen bei psychischen Krankheiten

### Acknowledgments
We thank Johannes Bernard, Matthias Kühne and Marco Knoll for their support in the conduction of the study and Jan Schildmann for his methodological advice. Finally, we thank all patients and mental health professionals for their participation in our interview study.

### Funding
The Medical Faculty of the Ruhr University Bochum supported this study financially by a grant for the Department of Psychiatry, Psychotherapy and Preventive Medicine (Head: Georg Juckel; Awardee: Jakov Gather; FoRUM-award Clinical Research, K093-15).

## Authors' contributions

IO, JV, GJ and JG made substantial contributions to the conception and design of the study. IO and JG recruited and interviewed the participants. JK managed the data analysis and interpretation to which IO and JG contributed. JK wrote the first draft of the manuscript, JG was a major contributor in writing the manuscript. All authors read the manuscript and were involved in revising and finalizing it. All authors read and approved the final manuscript.

## Consent for publication

Not applicable

## Competing interests

The authors declare that they have no competing interests.

## References

1. Rittmannsberger H, Sartorius N, Brad M, Burtea V, Capraru N, Cernak P, et al. Changing aspects of psychiatric inpatient treatment. A census investigation in five European countries. Eur Psychiatry. 2004;19:483–8.
2. van der Merwe M, Bowers L, Jones J, Simpson A, Haglund K. Locked doors in acute inpatient psychiatry: a literature review. J Psychiatr Ment Health Nurs. 2009;16:293–9.
3. Care Quality Commission. Monitoring the Mental Health Act in 2015/16. 2016. https://www.cqc.org.uk/sites/default/files/20161122_mhareport1516_web.pdf. Accessed 26 July 2018.
4. Steinert T, Noorthoorn EO, Mulder CL. The use of coercive interventions in mental health care in Germany and the Netherlands. A comparison of the developments in two neighbouring countries. Front Public Health. 2014;2:141.
5. Zentrale Ethikkommission bei der Bundesärztekammer (ZEKO). Zwangsbehandlung bei psychischen Erkrankungen. Dtsch Ärztebl. 2013; 110(26):A1334–8.
6. Deutsche Gesellschaft für Psychiatrie und Psychotherapie, Psychosomatik und Nervenheilkunde e.V. (DGPPN). Respect for self-determination and use of coercion in the treatment of mentally ill persons. An ethical position statement of the DGPPN. Nervenarzt. 2014;85:1419–31.
7. Juckel G. Psychiatric intensive care units – contra. Psychiatr Prax. 2015;42:238–9.
8. Beine KH. Let's open the doors.... Psychiatr Prax. 2016;43:69–70.
9. Gather J, Nyhuis PW, Juckel G. How can an open door policy be successfully implemented? Conceptual considerations on opening the doors in acute psychiatry. Recht Psychiatrie. 2017;35:80–5.
10. Zinkler M, Nyhuis PW. Open doors in psychiatric hospitals in Germany: models of care and standard procedures. Recht Psychiatrie. 2017;35:63–7.
11. Jungfer HA, Schneeberger AR, Borgwardt S, Walter M, Vogel M, Gairing SK, et al. Reduction of seclusion on a hospital-wide level: successful implementation of a less restrictive policy. J Psychiatr Res. 2014;54:94–7.
12. Henking T. Concepts of open doors in psychiatry – open, but locked anyway? Recht Psychiatrie. 2017;35:68–71.
13. Henking T. Patient rights in psychiatry – legal perspectives on beneficence and coercion. In: Gather J, Henking T, Nossek A, Vollmann J, editors. Beneficial coercion in psychiatry? Foundations and challenges. Münster: Mentis; 2017. p. 19–37.
14. Schneeberger AR, Kowalinski E, Fröhlich D, Schröder K, von Felten S, Zinkler M, et al. Aggression and violence in psychiatric hospitals with and without open door policies: a 15-year naturalistic observational study. J Psychiatr Res. 2017;95:189–95.
15. Lang UE, Hartmann S, Schulz-Hartmann S, Gudlowski Y, Ricken R, Munk I, et al. Do locked doors in psychiatric hospitals prevent patients from absconding? Eur J Psychiatry. 2010;24:199–204.
16. Huber CG, Schneeberger AR, Kowalinski E, Fröhlich D, von Felten S, Walter M, et al. Suicide risk and absconding in psychiatric hospitals with and without open door policies: a 15 year, observational study. Lancet Psychiatry. 2016;3(9):842–9.
17. Haglund K, von Essen L. Locked entrance doors at psychiatric wards – advantages and disadvantages according to voluntarily admitted patients. Nord J Psychiatry. 2005;59(6):511–5.
18. Bowers L, Haglund K, Muir-Cochrane E, Nijman H, Simpson A, van der Merwe M. Locked doors: a survey of patients, staff and visitors. J Psychiatr Ment Health Nurs. 2010;17:873–80.
19. Muir-Cochrane E, van der Merwe M, Nijman H, Haglund K, Simpson A, Bowers L. Investigation into the acceptability of door locking to staff, patients, and visitors on acute psychiatric wards. Int J Ment Health Nurs. 2012;21:41–9.
20. Ashmore R. Nurses' accounts of locked ward doors: ghosts of the asylum or acute care in the 21st century? J Psychiatr Ment Health Nurs. 2008;15:175–85.
21. Schreier M. Qualitative content analysis. In: Flick U, editor. The sage handbook of qualitative data analysis. Los Angeles: Sage; 2014. p. 170–84.
22. Forman J, Damschroder L. Qualitative analysis. In: Jacoby L, Siminoff L, editors. Empirical methods for bioethics: a primer. Bingley: Emerald Group Publishing Limited; 2007. p. 39–62.
23. Mayring P. Qualitative content analysis. Forum: qualitative social research. Volume 1, No. 2, Art. 20. 2000. http://www.qualitative-research.net/index.php/fqs/article/view/1089/2385. Accessed 26 July 2018.
24. The British Psychological Society and The Royal College of Psychiatrists. Violence and Aggression. Short-term management in mental health, health and community settings. Updated edition. Nice Guideline NG10. 2015. https://www.nice.org.uk/guidance/ng10. Accessed 26 July 2018.
25. McSherry B, Gooding P. Torture and ill-treatment in health care settings: lessons from the United Nations. J Law Med. 2013;20:712–8.
26. Juan E. Méndez. Report of the Special Rapporteur on torture and other cruel, inhuman or degrading treatment or punishment, A/HRC/22/53. 2013. https://www.ohchr.org/documents/hrbodies/hrcouncil/regularsession/session22/a.hrc.22.53_english.pdf. Accessed 26 July 2018.
27. Committee on the Rights of Persons with Disabilities. General comment no. 1. Article 12: equality before the law. CRPD/C/GC/1. 2014. https://www.ohchr.org/en/hrbodies/crpd/pages/gc.aspx. Accessed 26 July 2018.
28. Report of the Special Rapporteur on the right of everyone to the enjoyment of the highest attainable standard of physical and mental health. A/HRC/35/21. 2017. http://ap.ohchr.org/documents/dpage_e.aspx?si=A/HRC/35/21. Accessed 26 July 2018.
29. United Nations High Commissioner for Human Rights. Mental health and human rights. A/HRC/34/32. 2017. https://documents-dds-ny.un.org/doc/UNDOC/GEN/G17/021/32/PDF/G1702132.pdf?OpenElement. Accessed 26 July 2018.
30. Sailas EES, Fenton M. Seclusion and restraint for people with serious mental illnesses. Cochrane Database Syst Rev. 2000; 1: CD001163. DOI: https://doi.org/10.1002/14651858.CD001163.
31. Brophy LM, Roper CE, Hamilton BE, Tellez JJ, McSherry BM. Consumers and their supporters' perspectives on poor practice and the use of seclusion and restraint in mental health settings: results from Australian focus groups. Int J Ment Heal Syst. 2016;10:6.
32. Brophy LM, Roper CE, Hamilton BE, Tellez JJ, McSherry BM. Consumers' and their supporters' perspectives on barriers and strategies to reducing seclusion and restraint in mental health settings. Aust Health Rev. 2016;40:599–604.
33. Kinner SA, Harvey C, Hamilton B, Brophy L, Roper C, McSherry B, et al. Attitudes towards seclusion and restraint in mental health settings: findings from a large, community-based survey of consumers, carers and mental health professionals. Epidemiol Psychiatr Sci. 2017;26:535–44.
34. Whittington R, Bowers L, Nolan P, Simpson A, Neil L. Approval ratings of inpatient coercive interventions in a national sample of mental health service users and staff in England. Psychiatr Serv. 2009;60(6):792–8.
35. Steinert T, Birk M, Flammer E, Bergk J. Subjective distress after seclusion or mechanical restraint: one-year follow-up of a randomized controlled study. Psychiatr Serv. 2013;64(10):1012–7.
36. Deutsche Gesellschaft für Psychiatrie und Psychotherapie, Psychosomatik und Nervenheilkunde e.V. (DGPPN). S3-Leitlinie "Verhinderung von Zwang: Prävention und Therapie aggressiven Verhaltens bei Erwachsenen". AWMF-Register Nr. 038-022. https://www.dgppn.de/_Resources/Persistent/02645b3598e9832a01b7ba617383aaa599011369/S3%20LL%20Verhinderung%20von%20Zwang%20LANGVERSION%20FINAL%2020.7.2018.pdf. Accessed 26 July 2018.
37. Hochstrasser L, Fröhlich D, Schneeberger AR, Borgwardt S, Lang UE, Stieglitz R-D, et al. Long-term reduction of seclusion and forced medication on a hospital-wide level: implementation of an open-door policy over 6 years. Eur Psychiatry. 2018;48:51–7.

38. Ciompi L, Hoffmann H. Soteria Berne: an innovative milieu therapeutic approach to acute schizophrenia based on the concept of affect-logic. World Psychiatry. 2004;3(3):140–6.

39. Scanlan JN. Interventions to reduce the use of seclusion and restraint in inpatient psychiatric settings: what we know so far a review of the literature. Int J Soc Psychiatry. 2010;56:412–23.

40. Richter D. How to de-escalate a risk situation to avoid the use of coercion. In: Kallert T, Mezzich J, Monahan J, editors. Coercive treatment in psychiatry: clinical, legal and ethical aspects. West Sussex: Wiley-Blackwell; 2011. p. 57–80.

41. Steinert T, Lepping P. Is it possible to define a best practice standard for coercive treatment? In: Kallert T, Mezzich J, Monahan J, editors. Coercive treatment in psychiatry: clinical, legal and ethical aspects. West Sussex: Wiley-Blackwell; 2011. p. 49–56.

42. LeBel JL, Duxbury JA, Putkonen A, Sprague T, Rae C, Sharpe J. Multinational experiences in reducing and preventing the use of restraint and seclusion. J Psychosoc Nurs. 2014;52(1):22–9.

43. Palmstierna T, Huitfeldt B, Wistedt B. The relationship of crowding and aggressive behavior on a psychiatric intensive care unit. Hosp Community Psychiatry. 1991; 42(12):1237–40.

44. Nijman HLI, Rector G. Crowding and aggression on inpatient psychiatric wards. Psychiatr Serv. 1999;50:830–1.

45. Ng B, Kumar S, Ranclaud M, Robinson E. Ward crowding and incidents of violence on an acute psychiatric inpatient unit. Psychiatr Serv. 2001;52:521–5.

46. Cibis M-L, Wackerhagen C, Müller S, Lang UE, Schmidt Y, Heinz A. Comparison of aggressive behavior, compulsory medication and absconding behavior between open and closed door policy in an acute psychiatric ward. Psychiatr Prax. 2017;44:141–7.

47. Mulder NCL. Psychiatric intensive care units – pro. Psychiatr Prax. 2015;42:237–8.

48. van Melle L, Edelbroek H, Voskes Y, Widdershoven G. New developments around coercion in the Netherlands. A care ethics perspective. In: Gather J, Henking T, Nossek A, Vollmann J, editors. Beneficial coercion in psychiatry? Foundations and challenges. Münster: Mentis; 2017. p. 193–201.

49. Husum TL, Bjørngaard JH, Finset A, Ruud T. A cross-sectional prospective study of seclusion, restraint and involuntary medication in acute psychiatric wards: patient, staff and ward characteristics. BMC Health Serv Res. 2010;10:89.

50. van der Schaaf PS, Dusseldorp E, Keuning FM, Janssen WA, Noorthoorn EO. Impact of the physical environment of psychiatric wards on the use of seclusion. Br J Psychiatry. 2013;202:142–9.

51. Kalisova L, Raboch J, Nawka A, Sampogna G, Cihal L, Kallert TW, et al. Do patient and ward-related characteristics influence the use of coercive measures? Results from the EUNOMIA international study. Soc Psychiatry Psychiatr Epidemiol. 2014; 49:1619–29.

52. Dresler T, Rohe T, Weber M, Strittmatter T, Fallgatter AJ. Effects of improved hospital architecture on coercive measures. World Psychiatry. 2015;14(1):105–6.

# 15

# Attitudes of mental health clinicians toward perceived inaccuracy of a schizophrenia diagnosis in routine clinical practice

Dana Tzur Bitan[1,2], Ariella Grossman Giron[1,2], Gady Alon[2,3], Shlomo Mendlovic[2,3], Yuval Bloch[2,3] and Aviv Segev[2,3*]

## Abstract

**Background:** Mental health clinicians have previously been reported to express reservations regarding the utility and accuracy of the psychiatric classification systems. In this study we aimed to examine clinicians' experiences with instances of perceived inaccuracy of a schizophrenia diagnosis.

**Methods:** Mental health clinicians ($N = 175$) participated in an online survey assessing prevalence and perceived reasons for inaccuracies of a schizophrenia diagnosis. Respondents included psychiatric ward directors (13.1%), senior psychiatrists and psychologists (40.5%), and psychiatry and clinical psychology residents (36%).

**Results:** Fifty-three percent of respondents reported encountering instances where a schizophrenia diagnosis was assigned even though clinical presentation did not match diagnostic criteria. Seventy-three percent of senior psychiatrists in a position to determine a diagnosis declared assigning schizophrenia even when controversial among clinical staff, and 15% of them declared doing so frequently. The likelihood of frequently assigning a schizophrenia diagnosis even when clearly controversial was predicted by the perception that an inaccurate diagnosis is assigned due to the presence of negative symptoms (OR 2.20, 95% CI 1.04–4.66, $p = 0.039$) and due to patient-related factors, such as the need to facilitate rehabilitation (OR 1.77, 95% CI 1.07–2.90, $p = 0.024$).

**Conclusions:** Although a schizophrenia diagnosis is considered relatively stable and clear, our study indicates that, in clinical practice, the assignment of this diagnosis is frequently controversial. These controversies are associated with the perception that an inaccurate diagnosis is assigned due to diagnostic considerations, or due to the possibility that patients might benefit from such a diagnosis. Implications and limitations for psychiatric practice and discourse are discussed.

**Keywords:** Schizophrenia, DSM, ICD, Misdiagnosis, Rehabilitation, Negative symptoms

## Background

Surveys examining mental health clinicians' attitudes towards the classification systems indicate that mental health professionals have different views of their utility and accuracy. For example, a global survey found that psychiatrists rated the ICD diagnostic criteria to be fairly accurate and easy to use [1]. On the other hand, a World Health Organization survey found that psychologists rated several diagnostic criteria as low on goodness of fit as compared to ease of use, suggesting that they view some problems with the descriptive validity of the classification systems [2]. It was also reported that although more than 90% of psychologists use the DSM for classification purposes, most of them express serious concerns about various aspects of the diagnostic system [3].

The study of mental health clinicians' attitudes towards the accuracy of psychiatric classification is even more meaningful in the case of a schizophrenia diagnosis. Studies indicate that the label of schizophrenia in and of itself not only affects mental health and primary care providers' expectations (such as patients' adherence and ability to manage their illness), but also their actual treatment decisions [4]. Additional byproducts of schizophrenia labeling

* Correspondence: Segev_a@netvision.net.il
[2]Shalvata Mental Health Center, 13th Alyat Hanoar st, POB 94, 45100 Hod Hasharon, Israel
[3]Sackler School of Medicine, Tel Aviv University, POB 39040, 69978 Tel Aviv, Israel
Full list of author information is available at the end of the article

include self and social stigma which, regardless of illness severity, can facilitate a severe course and prognosis, and imperil chances of recovery [5–11]. Taking these implications under consideration, it is reasonable to assume that clinicians' security with assigning such a diagnosis should be relatively high.

Surprisingly, not many studies have assessed clinicians' perceptions about the accuracy and inaccuracy of a schizophrenia diagnosis as utilized in routine clinical settings. A relatively modest indication of clinicians' attitudes towards instances of schizophrenia misdiagnosis can be found in a study [12] reporting that almost 50% of surveyed psychiatrists believed that schizophrenia tends to be frequently misdiagnosed among black people. Indeed, studies addressing schizophrenia diagnosis inaccuracy have mainly concentrated on social and diagnostic factors associated with over, under, or misdiagnosis of schizophrenia, such as difficulties in differentiating schizophrenia from either axis 1 or 2 diagnoses [13–18], or misdiagnosis due to immigration or racial influences [19–22]. To the best of our knowledge, no study has systematically explored how frequently mental health clinicians encounter, or take part in, labeling patients with the diagnosis of schizophrenia, even when such a label is either controversial or subjectively perceived to be inaccurate.

In this study, we aimed to bridge this gap by examining mental health clinicians' experiences with the assignment of a schizophrenia diagnosis. Specifically, we focused on three research questions: (a) How often do mental health clinicians participate in assigning a schizophrenia diagnosis even when clinical presentation does not match diagnostic criteria? (b) How often do mental health clinicians perceive a schizophrenia diagnosis to be inaccurate even when clinical presentation matches diagnostic criteria? (c) How often do senior psychiatrists, authorized to assign a schizophrenia diagnosis, assign such a diagnosis even if controversial among clinical staff? Additionally, we aimed to explore whether the assignment of a controversial schizophrenia diagnosis is associated with specific attitudes regarding the underlying reasons for the occurrence of such instances.

## Methods
### Participants
Participants were psychiatrists, psychologists, and social workers who were on the mailing lists of any of three mental health centers in Israel: Shalvata Mental Health Center, Lev Hasharon Mental Health Center, and Geha Mental Health Center. These three centers are characterized by a diagnostic process which frequently, but not always, involves an interdisciplinary staff meeting during patient interviewing (intake) in order to establish diagnosis. Therefore, clinicians at these centers were viewed as relevant participants for the current study. During

these meetings, staff discussion is usually recorded in patients' clinical files. Information regarding the patient's diagnosis is usually shared sensitively and cautiously after the diagnosis has been assigned, and in most cases the patient does not participate in the discussion related to his/her diagnosis. The survey was also circulated in the department of psychiatry at the school of medicine of the affiliated university, as well as two classes of the psychotherapy school of the affiliated university.

### Procedure
The study was reviewed and authorized by the Institutional Review Board of the Shalvata Mental Health Center in Israel. Participants were recruited through an e-mail containing an embedded link to a Qualtrics electronic survey. The participants were informed about the subject of the study, the estimated time for its completion, and the safeguarding of anonymity, and were also informed that answering the questionnaire signified their agreement to participate in the study. Demographic and clinical characteristics were collected, and were followed by items inquiring about experiences of perceived inaccuracy of schizophrenia diagnoses in clinical settings. A 20-item questionnaire, specifically designed to assess perceptions regarding the underlying reasons for inaccuracy in schizophrenia diagnosis, followed. Participants' responses were coded using designated research codes, and their identities were completely anonymized.

### Construction of the questionnaire assessing reasons for inaccuracy in schizophrenia diagnosis
The uniquely designed questionnaire assessing reasons for inaccuracy in schizophrenia diagnosis comprised three sections (see Appendix A). The first part obtained demographic data (age, years of experience, position, exposure to patients with schizophrenia). In the second part, participants were requested to report the frequency with which they experienced instances of inaccurate diagnosis of schizophrenia. As schizophrenia is viewed to be a relatively clear diagnosis [23], we assumed that even frequent cases of inaccurate diagnosis would rarely rise above the 10% mark. Therefore, the questions and associated categories were constructed as follows: (a) How often did you participate in assigning patients a diagnosis of schizophrenia even though clinical presentation did not meet the DSM criteria (as part of a staff meeting)? Answers were *never, rarely* (less than 1% of cases), *occasionally* (1–5%), *frequently* (5–10%), and *very frequently* (more than 10%); (b) How often did you disagree with the assigned schizophrenia diagnosis despite the matched DSM criteria? (c) If you are a senior psychiatrist, and authorized to assign and document a diagnosis, how often have you given a diagnosis of schizophrenia even though other staff members opposed such a

diagnosis? The rationale for using the DSM (rather than the ICD) as common ground for diagnosis assignment was guided by the need to use a diagnostic system relatively familiar to all clinical sectors, and to serve as an archetype for any diagnostic system that is set to provide a formal diagnosis. The third section included 20 statements referring to possible reasons for inaccurate diagnosis. These statements were generated based on previous literature associating the inaccuracy of a schizophrenia diagnosis with specific diagnoses or agendas [24–27]. For example, as borderline patients are often hospitalized for prolonged periods of time due to psychotic episodes [24], which might in turn serve as a basis for inaccurate schizophrenia diagnoses, statements referring to such possible associations were constructed. For example: "A significant percentage of the patients were characterized by a tendency towards self-injury" and "A significant percentage of these patients were characterized by frequent or prolonged hospitalizations." Answers were given on a 5-point Likert-type scale (ranging from *strongly agree* to *strongly disagree*), reflecting participants' opinions regarding the reasons they felt contributed to an inaccurate diagnosis of schizophrenia. The statements pertain to symptom-based characteristics (deficit, affect, emotional dysregulation, use of drugs, etc.); management-based characteristics

(frequent admissions, drug-resistance, rehabilitation, etc.); and staff-based characteristics (experience, burnout, etc.).

## Results

Demographic and clinical characteristics of the mental health clinicians participating in the survey are presented in Table 1. A total of 175 clinicians responded to the survey. Thirteen percent of the participants were psychiatric ward directors, 71 (about 40%) were senior psychiatrists and psychologists, 32 (18%) were senior psychiatry residents (already authorized to determine psychiatric diagnoses and treat independently in a private clinic setting, though not in a hospital). The mean years of experience in the clinical field was 11.05 (*SD* = 9.80). About half of the participants were employed (either part or full-time) in psychiatric hospital wards (47.1%), and 52.9% were employed (either part of full-time) in public outpatient clinics. The vast majority of participants reported working with patients diagnosed with schizophrenia either very frequently (56%) or frequently (17.7%). A large proportion of the participants reported that they engaged, with varying frequency, in writing legal psychiatric opinions, and 35% of respondents declared that they engaged in writing legal psychiatric opinions as part of their daily work.

**Table 1** Characteristics of clinicians responding to the survey

| Main demographic and clinical characteristics | | Mean (SD) | Frequency (%) |
|---|---|---|---|
| Age | | 41.59 (8.99) | |
| Experience (in years) | | 11.05(9.80) | |
| Gender | Male | | 69 (39.4%) |
| | Female | | 106(60.6%) |
| Position | Psychiatric Ward Director | | 23 (13.1%) |
| | Senior Psychiatrist | | 37 (21.1%) |
| | Senior Psychiatry Resident | | 32 (18.3%) |
| | Junior Psychiatry Resident | | 17 (9.7%) |
| | Senior Clinical Psychologist | | 34 (19.4%) |
| | Clinical Psychology Intern | | 14 (8%) |
| | Social Worker | | 18 (10.3%) |
| Clinical work place | Hospital ward | | 82 (47.1%) |
| | Public outpatient clinic | | 92 (52.9%) |
| | Private clinic | | 68 (39.0%) |
| | Other | | 13 (7.5%) |
| Writing legal Psychiatric opinion | Frequently | | 62(35.4%) |
| | Rarely | | 42 (24%) |
| | Never | | 70 (40%) |
| Working with Schizophrenia Patients | Very Frequently | | 98 (56%) |
| | Frequently | | 31 (17.7%) |
| | Not often | | 18 (10.3%) |
| | Rarely | | 28 (16%) |

Responses of clinicians from different clinical positions to questions concerning the perceived accuracy of a schizophrenia diagnosis in daily practice are presented in Table 2.

Most respondents reported giving a diagnosis of schizophrenia even when the clinical presentation of the patient did not match DSM criteria; out of those, 42.9% reported encountering such situations rarely and 10.9% reported encountering such situations frequently. There was no significant difference between the different clinical positions. Most respondents also reported that they experienced subjective disagreement with the diagnosis even when the clinical presentation met the diagnostic criteria, either rarely (49.7%) or frequently (12.6%), with a statistically significant difference among the clinical positions. A Bonferroni correction post-hoc analysis (at alpha level of 0.005) indicated a lower frequency of psychiatrists reporting that they never had a disagreement regarding a schizophrenia diagnosis (adjusted standardized residual $Z = -3.3$, $p < 0.005$). Finally, among the senior psychiatrists (34.2% of the entire sample), 58.3% declared assigning a schizophrenia diagnosis even if controversial among clinical staff, and 15% declared encountering such situations frequently.

A principal component analysis (PCA) was next performed on the entire sample of clinicians in order to cluster the various reasons for the perceived inaccurate diagnosis. Tests for sampling adequacy included the Kaiser-Meyer-Olkin, which produced a value of 0.75, and the Bartlett test of sphericity, which was statistically significant ($p < .001$). These values are well within range [28–30] and point to the suitability of the data for factor analysis. As the factors were assumed to be interrelated, oblique

rotation was used. The PCA resulted in a six-factor solution explaining 64.73% of the variance. Four factors were retained from this analysis based on the number of highly (i.e., .40 and higher) and uniquely loaded items per factor and interpretability, resulting in one item which was excluded from analysis. These factors were found to have the following thematic organization: (A) Staff-related considerations. These included items reflecting different emotional aspects of the staff's clinical routine, such as attempting to resolve daily clinical decisions which are hard to make due to unclear diagnosis, occupational fatigue, alleviation of staff's feelings of helplessness, and conceptions of senior psychiatrists. (B) Patient-related considerations. These included items reflecting patients' therapeutic and emotional processes, such as helping patients come to terms with their severe mental states, helping patients obtain their social rights, facilitating rehabilitation programs; (C) Borderline in differential diagnosis. These included items reflecting signs and symptoms that suggest that the diagnosis should be a severe form of borderline personality disorder, such as multiple hospitalizations, tendency to self-harm, difficulties in emotional regulation, recurrent episodes of affective episodes, and treatment-resistant patients; and (D) Negative symptoms schizophrenia, which included the following items: the existence of severe and prolonged functional impairment, the existence of a significant impairment in affect, and excessive hospitalizations.

On the basis of these four factors, scale scores were then calculated by averaging the items for each scale. Means, SDs, Cronbach alpha coefficients, and Pearson correlations for the resulting four scores are presented in Table 3.

As can be seen, most scales had means slightly below the middle point of the five-point scale, and the SDs all

**Table 2** Frequency distribution of perceived accuracy of a schizophrenia diagnosis

| | Psychiatrists N = 109 N (%) | Psychologists N = 48 N (%) | Others N = 18 N (%) | Total N = 175 N (%) | Chi Square |
|---|---|---|---|---|---|
| Gave SCZ diagnosis when clinical presentation did not match DSM? | | | | | 8.56 |
| Never | 42 (38.5%) | 30 (62.5%) | 9 (50%) | 81 (46.3%) | |
| Rarely | 52 (47.7%) | 15 (31.3%) | 8 (44.4%) | 75 (42.9%) | |
| Frequently | 15 (13.8%) | 3 (6.3%) | 1 (5.6%) | 19 (10.9%) | |
| Disagreed about SCZ diagnosis despite matched DSM criteria? | | | | | 11.95* |
| Never | 30 (27.8%) | 24 (50%) | 11 (61.1%) | 65 (37.1%) | |
| Rarely | 62 (57.4%) | 19 (39.6%) | 6 (33.3%) | 87 (49.7%) | |
| Frequently | 16 (14.8%) | 5 (10.4%) | 1 (5.6%) | 22 (12.6%) | |
| Gave SCZ diagnosis when controversial? (authorized psychiatrists only) | | | | | n/a |
| Never | 16 (26.7%) | | | 16 (26.7%) | |
| Rarely | 35 (58.3%) | | | 35 (58.3%) | |
| Frequently | 9 (15.0%) | | | 9 (15.0%) | |

SCZ = Schizophrenia; DSM = Diagnostic and Statistical Manual of Mental Disorders. *$p < .05$

**Table 3** Means, standard deviations, alpha reliability coefficients, and Pearson correlations for identified four factors

|  | Mean | Standard Deviation | Alpha | A | B | C |
|---|---|---|---|---|---|---|
| A. Staff-related factors | 2.95 | 0.73 | 0.80 | | | |
| B. Patient-related factors | 2.61 | 0.72 | 0.74 | .21$^*$ | | |
| C. Borderline in differential diagnosis | 2.96 | 0.78 | 0.80 | .45$^{**}$ | .26$^{**}$ | |
| D. Presence of negative symptoms | 3.35 | 0.67 | 0.56 | .35$^{**}$ | .25$^{**}$ | .35$^{**}$ |

$* p < .05 ** p < .01$

indicate reasonable variance. The Cronbach alpha reliability coefficients ranged from 0.56 to 0.80. Correlations between the scales were all statistically significant and positive and ranged from 0.21 to 0.45.

Finally, we aimed to explore the association between the perceived reasons for inaccuracy in schizophrenia diagnosis and the assignment of a schizophrenia diagnosis by senior psychiatrists even when controversial and opposed by the clinical staff. Binary logistic regression was performed with the four factors serving as predicting variables, while the probability of frequently giving a schizophrenia diagnosis even when controversial or opposed by the clinical staff served as the dependent variable. Age and years of experience were entered as covariates. The analyses yielded a significant model, $\chi^2$ (6) = 18.82, $p < .01$, explaining between 31.9% (Cox & Snell R-squared) and 57% (Nagelkerke R-squared) of the variance of frequent assignment of a controversial diagnosis. Results of the logistic regression analysis are presented in Table 4. Results indicate that perceiving inaccuracy in a schizophrenia diagnosis as emerging from the presence of negative symptoms, or from patient-related factors, significantly predicted the probability of making a schizophrenia diagnosis even when controversial.

## Discussion

This is the first study attempting to depict clinicians' experiences with situations in which a diagnosis of schizophrenia is perceived as inaccurate. Over 50% of the mental health clinicians assessed in our study reported assigning a schizophrenia diagnosis even when DSM criteria were not met, and about 10% of them reported such events to be frequent. In addition, 49.7% reported disagreements regarding diagnosis even when patients' clinical presentation matched

DSM criteria, with 12.6% estimating that these disagreements occur frequently. Finally, the majority of senior psychiatrists authorized to assign a schizophrenia diagnosis reported assigning such a diagnosis even when controversial among the clinical staff, either rarely or frequently. It is important to note that the participants in our study were mainly experienced mental health clinicians, many of them in teaching or clinical mentoring positions while working in team-based settings. Moreover, a large proportion of the study's sample engaged in writing legal psychiatric opinions, where the assignment of a schizophrenia diagnosis can have a substantial impact.

Although the diagnosis of schizophrenia is considered stable and clear among expert clinicians [23, 31, 32], the current study suggests that among most mental health workers, the determination of such a diagnosis is not as clear as expected. Unlike general medicine, where laboratory tests or imaging procedures can corroborate or refute clinical diagnoses, psychiatric medicine still has no objective measures for diagnosis affirmation. As a result, the diagnostic system is forced to rely on phenomenological measures, which are known to be sensitive to subjective interpretation. This perspective has been previously addressed in the past, where scholars criticized the reliability-over-validity approach of the diagnostic system and the resulting "thinning out" of clinical psychiatry [33–37]. Our findings suggest that even though the revolution of the DSM-III was meant to minimize variability [33], the use of the classification system in team-based clinical settings, where interdisciplinary staff takes part in establishing a diagnosis, allows for more frequent occasions during which a diagnosis is either controversial or perceived as inaccurate. The issue of diagnostic validity can also be reflected by the

**Table 4** Logistic regression for the prediction of frequently giving a schizophrenia diagnosis even when controversial

|  | Odds Ratio | Confidence Interval | p value |
|---|---|---|---|
| Staff-related factors | 1.08 | 0.80–1.46 | > 0.1 |
| Patient-related factors | 1.77 | 1.07–2.90 | 0.039 |
| Borderline in differential diagnosis | 0.95 | 0.59–1.52 | > 0.1 |
| Presence of negative symptoms | 2.20 | 1.04–4.66 | 0.024 |

conceptual differentiation between validity and utility, where the categorical classification of mental disorders as a whole is argued to suffer from validity issues, yet remains the most frequent form of diagnosis due to its utility in predicting course, prognosis, and outcome of a specific disorder [38, 39].

An additional interesting finding that emerged from the current study is that most of the psychiatrists reported disagreeing about schizophrenia diagnosis despite matched DSM criteria, either rarely or frequently. One possible explanation is that psychiatrists have an ambivalent attitude towards the standardization of routine clinical practice, forced on them by the adoption of the DSM. Drawing from interviews with psychiatrists, it was previously suggested [40] that a trend of "sociological ambivalence" exists among psychiatrists, where professionals in this field develop "workarounds," in the form of alternative diagnostic typologies or diagnosis negotiations, in order to develop a sense of autonomy. Therefore, it is possible that the perception of inaccuracy stems from the ongoing negotiation between the need to develop a sense of autonomy in the provision of clinical diagnoses and the adherence to diagnostic standardization.

In order to assess the underlying attitudes toward inaccuracy in schizophrenia diagnosis, a measure of attitudes towards the origins of schizophrenia diagnosis inaccuracy was constructed. The results of the exploratory factor analysis indicated a four-dimension structure, which included (a) Staff-related factors: the perception that an inaccurate diagnosis is being assigned to aid the clinical staff by allowing them to strategize treatment and alleviate feelings of frustration and burnout; (b) Patient-related factors: the perception that an inaccurate diagnosis is often assigned due to the benefits that can accrue to the patient, ranging from the technical (welfare services, rehabilitation programs, etc.) to the psychological (acceptance of illness, the need for medication or supported housing, etc.); (c) Borderline in differential diagnosis: the perception that an inaccurate diagnosis of schizophrenia results from a severe form of borderline personality disorder, as expressed by impaired emotional regulation, self-harm tendencies, but also treatment-resistance and frequent or prolonged hospitalization, and (d) Presence of negative symptoms: the perception that an inaccurate diagnosis of schizophrenia results from the presence of negative symptoms, a diagnostic criterion of schizophrenia that is considered predominant in the former diagnosis of "schizophrenia simplex," which no longer exists in the DSM but is acknowledged in the ICD-10 as simple-type schizophrenia.

When we explored the association between these emerged four factors and the probability of frequently assigning a schizophrenia diagnosis even when controversial, we found such an association in two main clusters: the first is the perception that an inaccurate diagnosis stems from negative-predominant schizophrenia, whereas the second refers to patient-related factors (clusters D and B, respectively). Senior psychiatrists who reported frequently assigning a schizophrenia diagnosis, even when it was controversial to do so, tended to view these instances as resulting either from the presence of negative symptoms or for the benefit of the patients. These senior psychiatrists are experienced clinicians with much familiarity and experience with previous diagnostic systems. Negative symptoms schizophrenia, a type which no longer exists in the DSM but is acknowledged in the ICD-10 as simple-type schizophrenia, is most probably very familiar to senior psychiatrists. Our findings may therefore indicate a certain lag in the implementation of the current version of the DSM-5, which adopted a stricter stance towards a schizophrenia diagnosis by the requirement of clear positive symptoms [41].

The second association found in our study is that senior psychiatrists who report frequently assigning a schizophrenia diagnosis even when controversial view the inaccurate diagnosis as a result of a process aimed at benefiting the patients. The concept of deliberate misdiagnosis, where a certain diagnosis is given even if not accurate in order to gain benefits, has been an issue for conceptual, clinical, and ethical debate. Namely, it has been suggested that the diagnostic labeling process is constantly shaped by cultural and policy environments, in which mental health services are provided under specific diagnostic criteria [42]. Studies indicate that social workers and physicians frequently face the dilemma of altering diagnoses due to procedural aspects of clinical care, such as the attainment of reimbursement [43–45]. Although warranting further research, our findings may suggest that this phenomenon occurs not only in the diagnosis of major depression [45] but also in the diagnosis of schizophrenia, as the probability of frequently assigning a schizophrenia diagnosis was associated with the view that an inaccurate diagnosis can result from such a process. Future studies are also needed to explore whether the reasons for inaccurate diagnosis stem from clinicians' views and interpretations or, alternatively, derive from talking to service users. As the level of cooperation with service users during diagnosis assignment was not inquired about in the survey, an interesting line of research would be to explore how patients' views might affect the perceived accuracy of the diagnostic process, as well as their own views on the assigned diagnosis.

It should be noted that the association between negative symptoms and patient-related factors and frequent assignment of controversial diagnoses does not necessarily imply that clinical staff endorsing such attitudes might themselves assign controversial diagnoses on the basis of such views. Instead, our findings represent perceived attitudes that can potentially reflect the clinicians' views of the social and professional discourse towards the assignment of a schizophrenia diagnosis. The team-based approach to providing psychiatric diagnoses can be viewed as a natural ground for controversies, and can even be aimed at facilitating them. A process where a senior clinician makes a diagnosis, other members of the team question it, and a consensus then emerges, might be a valuable process, even in light of staff members' reservations. Therefore, a critical line of future research that derives from our findings would be the study of the effects of such controversies on patients' quality of care.

Several limitations should be noted. The cross-sectional design of our study does not allow for causality inferences. Future studies should assess, preferably by employing a longitudinal design, whether different views and perceptions of diagnosis inaccuracy can result in greater tolerance towards inaccurate diagnoses. As the factor structure of the scale assessing reasons for the inaccuracy of a schizophrenia diagnosis was derived from a sample of mental health clinicians, these factors can only be considered to apply to this population, and additional studies are needed to assess whether this factor structure applies across specific professional sectors. Additionally, although the study was performed in several clinical settings and across a variety of mental health professions, the sample size is considered modest. Cultural characteristics, whether social or professional, might have had an impact on study findings and may therefore affect the generalizability of our results. For example, professionals working primarily in mental health centers employing a team-based diagnostic process, such as the professionals who participated in this study, might encounter controversies more often than professionals who work in more independent settings. Additionally, the cultural and social atmosphere in Israel, and primarily the trend towards facilitating community integration of people with severe mental illness [46], might affect the level of sensitivity towards assigning a schizophrenia diagnosis, a factor which could vary across countries. Different mental health systems across the world vary in terms of professional staff, as well as of reliance on different classification systems (such as the ICD in most European countries), and can therefore present different patterns of views towards the level of accuracy of a given schizophrenia diagnosis. Further studies are needed in order to examine professionals' views of diagnostic inaccuracy of schizophrenia in different cultural and social environments, as well as towards

the different classification systems. Although the use of a survey in the current study allowed for intensive data collection and exploration of the main research questions, it should be noted that this approach is limited so as to primarily represent the explicit attitudes of participants, and therefore inferences cannot be made regarding associated potential behaviors or implicit views.

Finally, the use of volunteer sampling might have created a bias towards compliant mental health professionals; therefore, it is possible that clinicians who chose not to participate hold different views and attitudes.

## Conclusions

Despite the clear diagnostic criteria and reported stability of the schizophrenia diagnosis, our study indicates that mental health professionals' experience of inaccurate labeling occurs more frequently than expected. The probability of assigning a schizophrenia diagnosis, even when controversial among staff, is associated with a perception of inaccuracy as resulting from either diagnostic considerations (the presence of negative symptoms), or for the benefit of the patient. The indication of negative symptoms and patient-centered factors as potential rationales for diagnostic inaccuracy might point to the need for a separate function-based diagnosis. These results may suggest a lag in implementing the new strict criteria of the DSM-5 to the assignment of such a diagnosis (primarily the exclusion of schizophrenia simplex), but may also reflect a mild ambivalence towards the classification system and a need for clinical autonomy. The use of a more general diagnostic label, such as "severe mental disorder involving a decline in adaptive functions," might improve accuracy and agreement between professionals and help the clinical and research fields to improve both reliability and validity of psychiatric diagnoses, as well as improve public perception of psychiatry. Future studies are needed in order to explore these competing explanations. Finally, the association between assignment of an inaccurate diagnosis and the concept of doing so for the benefit of the patient might point to social, cultural, and policy effects on the process of diagnosis assignment. These effects should be further explored, as the current phenomenological structure of the classification system obligates professionals to rely on clinical evaluation, which is often subject to these effects. As a schizophrenia misdiagnosis can have severe clinical, social, occupational, and economic consequences, investigations into the routes leading to inaccuracy in diagnosis are highly essential. Such investigations can eventually allow for a more knowledgeable diagnostic process and reduce the prevalence of misdiagnosis in clinical settings.

# Appendix

**Table 5** The questionnaire used in this study (translated to English)

| Dimension | Item # | Description | Loading |
|---|---|---|---|
| Staff Related Factors | Q6 | It is more likely that a misdiagnosis of Schizophrenia will be made by veteran caregivers | |
| | Q9 | The diagnosis of Schizophrenia alleviated the clinical staff, in cases in which the treatment strategy was vague | |
| | Q16 | The diagnosis of Schizophrenia might or has led to deterioration or impasse in these patients' condition | |
| | Q17 | I believe that feelings of helplessness or frustration in the clinical staff are a prominent factor in the misdiagnosis of Schizophrenia | |
| | Q18 | I believe that the misdiagnosis of Schizophrenia is related, among other things, to feelings of burnout | |
| | Q19 | Eventually, assigning the diagnosis of Schizophrenia alleviated the clinical staff | |
| Patient Related Factors | Q7 | The diagnosis of Schizophrenia assisted the patient by facilitating various technical aspects (social financial aid, rehabilitation services, and medicinal re-imbursements) | |
| | Q8 | The diagnosis of Schizophrenia assisted the patient for various emotional reasons (acceptance of his referral to rehabilitation services such as assisted living, supported employment, etc.) | |
| | Q15 | Eventually, the diagnosis of Schizophrenia might or has contributed to the rehabilitation of patients in these cases | |
| | Q20 | Eventually, assigning the diagnosis of Schizophrenia alleviated the patients | |
| Borderline-Like Patient | Q5 | The patients in question were treatment resistant | |
| | Q10 | A significant part of these patients were characterized by frequent or prolonged hospitalizations | |
| | Q11 | A significant part of the patients were characterized by a tendency for self-injury | |
| | Q12 | A significant part of these patients were characterized by major impairment in their capacity for emotional regulations | |
| | Q13 | A significant part of the patients were characterized by repeating major affective episodes I | |
| Schizophrenia Simplex Type | Q1 | The patients' symptomatology did not sufficiently meet the DSM criteria of Schizophrenia | |
| | Q2 | The Schizophrenia diagnosis was given due to severe and continuous impairment in functioning | |
| | Q3 | The Schizophrenia diagnosis was given due to severe impairment in affect | |
| | Q4 | A significant part of the patients were unnecessarily or redundantly hospitalized | |

## Abbreviations
DSM: Diagnostic and Statistical manual for Mental Disorders;
ICD: International Classification of Diseases; IRB: Institutional Review Board;
PCA: Principal Component Analysis; SD: Standard Deviation

## Acknowledgements
We thank Ms. Eve Horowitz-Leibowitz for her assistance and contribution in editing and clarifying the manuscript.

## Funding
This study did not receive any specific grant from funding agencies in the public, commercial, or not-for-profit sectors.

## Availability of data and materials
The datasets used and analyzed during the current study are available from the corresponding author in the form of SPSS file upon reasonable requests.

## Authors' contributions
DTB performed the literature review, analyzed and interpreted the data and drafted the manuscript. AGG performed the literature review, analyzed the data and drafted the manuscript. GA initiated and designed the study, executed and acquired the data and critically revised the manuscript. SM initiated and designed the study, acquired the data and critically revised the manuscript. YB designed the study, interpreted the data and critically revised the manuscript. AS initiated and designed the study, executed and acquired the data, analyzed and interpreted the results, and drafted the manuscript. All authors read and approved the final manuscript.

## Ethics approval and consent to participate
The study was approved by the Shalvata Mental Health Center IRB. Informed consent was waived due to the nature of the questionnaire and the participants (clinicians), and participants were informed that answering the questionnaire signified their agreement to participate in the study.

## Consent for publication
Not applicable.

## Competing interests
The authors declare that they have no competing interests.

## Author details
[1]Department of Behavioral Sciences, Ariel University, Ramat Hagolan 65th st, 4070000 Ariel, Israel. [2]Shalvata Mental Health Center, 13th Alyat Hanoar st, POB 94, 45100 Hod Hasharon, Israel. [3]Sackler School of Medicine, Tel Aviv University, POB 39040, 69978 Tel Aviv, Israel.

Attitudes of mental health clinicians toward perceived inaccuracy of a schizophrenia diagnosis in routine...

151

## References

1. Reed GM, Mendonça Correia J, Esparza P, Saxena S, Maj M. The WPA-WHO global survey of psychiatrists' attitudes towards mental disorders classification. World Psychiatry. 2011;10:118–31.

2. Evans SC, Reed GM, Roberts MC, Esparza P, Watts AD, Correia JM, et al. Psychologists' perspectives on the diagnostic classification of mental disorders: results from the WHO-IUPsyS Global Survey. Int J Psychol [Internet]. 2013;48:177–93. Available from: http://www.pubmedcentral.nih. gov/articlerender.fcgi?artid=3725658&tool=pmcentrez&rendertype=abstract.

3. Raskin JD, Gayle MC. DSM-5: do psychologists really want an alternative? J Humanist Psychol. 2016;56:439–56 SAGE Publications Sage CA: Los Angeles, CA.

4. Sullivan G, Mittal D, Reaves CM, Haynes TF, Han X, Mukherjee S, et al. Influence of schizophrenia diagnosis on providers' practice decisions. J Clin Psychiatry. 2015;76:1068–74.

5. Link BG, Struening EL, Neese-Todd S, Asmussen S, Phelan JC. Stigma as a barrier to recovery: the consequences of stigma for the self-esteem of people with mental illnesses. Psychiatr Serv. 2001;52:1621–6.

6. Link BG, Struening EL, Rahav M, Phelan JC, Nuttbrock L. On stigma and its consequences: evidence from a longitudinal study of men with dual diagnoses of mental illness and substance abuse. J Health Soc Behav. 1997; 38:177–90.

7. Rosenfield S. Labeling mental illness: the effects of received services and perceived stigma on life satisfaction. Am Sociol Rev. 1997;62:660–72.

8. Rössler W, Joachim Salize H, Van Os J, Riecher-Rössler A. Size of burden of schizophrenia and psychotic disorders. Eur Neuropsychopharmacol. 2005:399–409.

9. Sirey JA, Bruce ML, Alexopoulos GS, Perlick DA, Friedman SJ, Meyers BS. Stigma as a barrier to recovery: perceived stigma and patient-rated severity of illness as predictors of antidepressant drug adherence. Psychiatr Serv. 2001;52:1615–20.

10. Świtaj P, Wciórka J, Smolarska-Świtaj J, Grygiel P. Extent and predictors of stigma experienced by patients with schizophrenia. Eur Psychiatry. 2009;24:513–20.

11. Sartorius N, Schulze H. Reducing the stigma of mental illness: a report from a global Programme of the world psychiatric association. Reducing stigma Ment. Illn. A Rep. From a Glob. Program. World Psychiatr. Assoc. 2005.

12. Kingdon D, Sharma T, Hart D. What attitudes do psychiatrists hold towards people with mental illness? Psychiatr Bull. 2004;28:401–6.

13. Gunderson JG, Singer MT. Defining borderline patients: an overview. Am J Psychiatry. 1975:1–10.

14. Horgan D. Change of diagnosis to manic-depressive illness. Psychol Med. 1981;11:517–23.

15. Yee L, Korner AJ, McSwiggan S, Meares RA, Stevenson J. Persistent hallucinosis in borderline personality disorder. Compr Psychiatry. 2005;46: 147–54.

16. Joyce PR. Age of onset in bipolar affective disorder and misdiagnosis as schizophrenia. Psychol Med. 1984;14:145–9.

17. Pope HG, Jonas JM, Hudson JI, Cohen BM, Tohen M. An empirical study of psychosis in borderline personality disorder. Am J Psychiatry. 1985;142: 1285–90.

18. Gonzalez-Pinto A, Gutierrez M, Mosquera F, Ballesteros J, Lopez P, Ezcurra J, et al. First episode in bipolar disorder: misdiagnosis and psychotic symptoms. J Affect Disord. 1998;50:41–4.

19. Haasen C, Yagdiran O, Mass R, Krausz M. Potential for misdiagnosis among Turkish migrants with psychotic disorders: a clinical controlled study in Germany. Acta Psychiatr Scand. 2000;101:125–9.

20. Jones BE, Gray BA. Problems in diagnosing schizophrenia and affective disorders among blacks. Hosp Community Psychiatry. 1986;37:61–5.

21. Bell CC, Mehta H. The misdiagnosis of black patients with manic depressive illness. J Natl Med Assoc [Internet]. 1980;72:141–145. Available from: https:// www.ncbi.nlm.nih.gov/pmc/articles/PMC2552475/

22. Bell CC, Mehta H. Misdiagnosis of black patients with manic depressive illness: second in a series. J Natl Med Assoc [Internet]. 1981;73:101–107. Available from: http://www.pubmedcentral.nih.gov/articlerender.fcgi?artid= 2552632&tool=pmcentrez&rendertype=abstract

23. Bromet EJ, Naz B, Fochtmann LJ, Carlson GA, Tanenberg-Karant M. Long-term diagnostic stability and outcome in recent first-episode cohort studies of schizophrenia. Schizophr. Bull. 2005;31:639–49.

24. Paris J. Is hospitalization useful for suicidal patients with borderline personality disorder? J Pers Disord [Internet]. 2004;18:240–7. Available from: https://guilfordjournals.com/doi/10.1521/pedi.18.3.240.35443. https://doi.org/10.1521/pedi.18.3.240.35443.

25. Bury JE, Bostwick JM. Iatrogenic delusional parasitosis: a case of physician-patient folie a deux. Gen Hosp Psychiatry. 2010;32:210–2.

26. Pope HG, Jonas JM, Jones B. Factitious psychosis: phenomenology, family history, and long-term outcome of nine patients. Am J Psychiatry. 1982;139:1480–3.

27. Mead MA, Hohenshil TH, Singh K. How the DSM system is used by clinical counselors: A national study. J Ment Heal Couns [Internet]. 1997;19:383. Available from: http://search.ebscohost.com/login.aspx?direct=true&db= a9h&AN=226909&site=ehost-live&scope=site.

28. Bartlett MS. A note on the multiplying factors for various X2 approximations. J R Stat Soc. 1954.

29. Kaiser HF. A second generation little jiffy. Psychometrika. 1970.

30. Kaiser HF. An index of factorial simplicity. Psychometrika. 1974.

31. Tsuang MT, Woolson RF, Winokur G, Crowe RR. Stability of psychiatric diagnosis. Schizophrenia and affective disorders followed up over a 30- to 40-year period. Arch Gen Psychiatry [Internet]. 1981;38:535–9. Available from: http://archpsyc.jamanetwork.com/data/Journals/PSYCH/12341/ archpsyc_38_5_005.pdf

32. Hollis C. Adult outcomes of child- and adolescent-onset schizophrenia: diagnostic stability and predictive validity. Am J Psychiatry. 2000;157:1652–9.

33. Frances A. The new crisis of confidence in psychiatric diagnosis. Ann Intern Med. 2013:720.

34. Kendler KS. The phenomenology of major depression and the representativeness and nature of DSM criteria. Am J Psychiatry. 2016:771–80.

35. Andreasen NC. DSM and the death of phenomenology in America: an example of unintended consequences. Schizophr Bull. 2007;33:108–12.

36. Hyman SE. The diagnosis of mental disorders: the problem of reification. Annu Rev Clin Psychol Annual Reviews. 2010;6:155–79.

37. Kendler KS. DSM issues: incorporation of biological tests, avoidance of reification, and an approach to the "box canyon problem". Am J Psychiatry. 2014;171:1248–50.

38. Kendell R, Jablensky A. Distinguishing between the validity and utility of psychiatric diagnoses. Am J Psychiatry. 2003.

39. Jablensky A. Psychiatric classifications: validity and utility. World Psychiatry. 2016.

40. Whooley O. Diagnostic ambivalence: psychiatric workarounds and the diagnostic and statistical manual of mental disorders. Sociol Heal Illn. 2010; 32:452–69.

41. American Psychiatric Association. Highlights of Changes from DSM-IV-TR to DSM-5. Am Psychiatr Assoc Washington, ... [Internet]. 2013;19. Available from: https://dsm.psychiatryonline.org/doi/abs/10.1176/appi.books. 9780890425596.changes.

42. Dobransky K. The good, the bad, and the severely mentally ill: official and informal labels as organizational resources in community mental health services. Soc Sci Med. 2009;69:722–8.

43. Wakefield JC. DSM-5 and clinical social work: mental disorder and psychological justice as goals of clinical intervention. Clin Soc Work J. 2013; 41:131–8.

44. Probst B. "Walking the tightrope:" clinical social workers' use of diagnostic and environmental perspectives. Clin Soc Work J. 2013;41:184–91.

45. Rost K, Smith R, Matthews DB, Guise B. The deliberate misdiagnosis of major depression in primary care. Arch Fam Med. 1994;3:333–7.

46. Roe D, Gross R, Kravetz S, Baloush-Kleinman V, Rudnick A. Assessing psychiatric rehabilitation service (PRS) outcomes in Israel: conceptual, professional and social issues. Isr J Psychiatry Relat Sci. 2009;46(2):103–10.

# 16

# The Prejudice towards People with Mental Illness (PPMI) scale: structure and validity

Amanda Kenny, Boris Bizumic[*] and Kathleen M. Griffiths

## Abstract

**Background:** Although there is a substantial body of research on the stigma associated with mental illness, much of the extant research has not explicitly focused on the concept of prejudice, which drives discriminatory behaviour. Further, research that has investigated prejudice towards people with mental illness has conceptual, theoretical and psychometric limitations. To address these shortcomings, we sought to develop a new measure, the Prejudice towards People with Mental Illness (PPMI) scale, based on an improved conceptualisation and integration of the stigma and prejudice areas of research.

**Methods:** In developing the new scale, we undertook a thematic analysis of existing conceptualisations and measures to identify a pool of potential items for the scale which were subsequently assessed for fidelity and content validity by expert raters. We tested the structure, reliability, and validity of the scale across three studies (Study 1 $N = 301$; Study 2 $N = 164$; Study 3 $N = 495$) using exploratory factor, confirmatory factor, correlational, multiple regression, and ordinal logistic regression analyses using both select and general community samples.

**Results:** Study 1 identified four factors underlying prejudice towards people with mental illness: fear/avoidance, malevolence, authoritarianism, and unpredictability. It also confirmed the nomological network, that is, the links of these attitudes with the proposed theoretical antecedents and consequences. Studies 2 and 3 further supported the factor structure of the measure, and provided additional evidence for the nomological network.

**Conclusions:** We argue that research into prejudice towards people with mental illness will benefit from the new measure and theoretical framework.

**Keywords:** Prejudice, Mental illness, Attitudes, Stigma, Scale development

## Background

Researchers have widely studied mental illness (MI) stigma because it has detrimental effects on people with MI, such as widespread discrimination, exacerbated symptoms, and poor treatment outcomes (e.g., [1]). The concept of stigma includes multiple components, such as stereotypes, prejudice, and discrimination [2]. Within the literature its use has been primarily confined to studies of illness. By contrast, researchers who study prejudice see it as a specific negative attitude, which has largely been studied in relation to ethnic and racial outgroups [3]. The concept of prejudice itself has rarely been the explicit focus of studies involving MI, and many scales measuring stigma do not explicitly focus on, or in some cases do not include items

* Correspondence: Boris.Bizumic@anu.edu.au
Research School of Psychology, The Australian National University, Building 39 Science Road, Canberra, ACT 2601, Australia

measuring, prejudice [1]. Recently, Phelan et al. wrote: "the strong congeniality and large degree of overlap we found between models of stigma and prejudice should encourage scholars to reach across stigma/prejudice lines when searching for theory, methods and empirical findings to guide their new endeavors" ([3], p. 365) We will follow these researchers' call, and while reviewing the broad literature on stigma, focus on the construct of prejudice towards MI and its measurement.

For the purpose of this investigation, we will use a definition of prejudice as a negative outgroup attitude [4], and an attitude as a positive or negative evaluation of an object [5]. These definitions are widely, though not universally, endorsed. According to this conceptualisation, attitudes are distinct from stereotypes, which involve generalisations about group members [6], and can be known without being endorsed. We therefore see prejudice as the central component of stigma that drives behaviour (discrimination), and the avenue with the most potential to modify the detrimental effect of these attitudes. Thus, in integrating the literature on stigma and prejudice, we will focus primarily on the concept of prejudice, its measurement, and its theoretical causes and consequences, building on both stigma and prejudice literature, and will not focus on the related concepts of stereotypes and discrimination.

**Problems in the study of prejudice towards people with MI**
Researchers have developed numerous scales to assess stigma towards people with MI, and many of these scales include items measuring prejudice [1]. The scales in this area, however, often have conceptual and psychometric problems (see [1] for a recent comprehensive summary of problems of existing stigma measures, including its psychometric properties; these researchers note that even 2/3 of all published measures of stigma have not had any psychometric evaluations, and most of those that have had such evaluations still have numerous problems.). Researchers in the field of psychological measurement have emphasised the importance of construct validity and the related nomological network, which describes the theoretical antecedents and consequences of a psychological construct [7]. Construct validity should be a central aspect of scale development, but measures in this area often do not elucidate the nomological network (e.g., [8–11]).

Many scales in the area fail to define what they measure and focus on diverse beliefs, opinions, attitudes, and stereotypes related to MI (e.g., [12–14]). This becomes important as people can be aware of stereotypes without endorsing them, and even scales designed to measure attitudes often include items presenting non-evaluative opinions (e.g., [15, 16]). Many measures do not specify the construct and their items have various targets, such as the person, MI, or treatment (e.g., [8, 14, 17–19]), which often do not contain the evaluative component central to an attitude [5] and may not be linked to behaviour and therefore influence discrimination. Construct validity is central to showing that a measure reflects the true theoretical meaning of a concept.

Although studies indicate that attitudes towards people with MI are multidimensional, and commonly found dimensions relate to avoidance, exclusion, fear, benevolence, and authoritarian control [20, 21], there is no agreement on the number and nature of dimensions. Moreover, scales often lack a replicable factor structure. For example, the factor structures of widely-used measures of attitudes towards people with MI, the Opinions about Mental Illness (OMI) scale [22], and the Community Attitudes toward the Mentally Ill scale (CAMI) [14] have not been replicated (e.g., for OMI [23, 24]; for CAMI [20, 25]). Without a clear and replicable factor structure, evaluating

any variation in attitudes over time or as a result of interventions is fraught with a lack of clarity around the mechanisms of change and influence.

On the most fundamental level, even widely-used scales, such as the OMI and CAMI, contain double-barrelled items, which are items that include two separate ideas (e.g., [13, 18, 26]). Including such items is poor psychometric practice because participants may be responding to either of two ideas. In addition, scales often fail to address acquiescent response bias (e.g., [13, 26, 27]). To reduce acquiescence, researchers construct balanced scales with equal numbers of positively-keyed and negatively-keyed items [28]. Furthermore, researchers often overlook social desirability factors when measuring negative attitudes towards people with MI [2, 29].

Researchers today are not able to specifically study prejudice, as most measures are focused on a diversity of phenomena, and therefore may miss the central attitudinal aspect of prejudice that drives discriminatory behaviours. If a diverse set of phenomena are included in a measure, then this hinders the development of our understanding of the phenomenon, including its nomological network.

It should be noted that problems that affect the study of prejudice towards people with MI could perhaps be ameliorated by including a validated measure of generalised prejudice and applying it to people with MI. There, however, does not appear to exist a well-validated and multidimensional measure of prejudice that could be applied to people with MI. We were, for example, able to find only one-item feeling thermometer measures, typically used to measure attitudes towards ethnic groups, being applied to people with MI (e.g., [30, 31]), but these measures cannot capture the multidimensional nature of prejudice against people with MI. A problem in the area of social psychological study of prejudice is that measures of prejudice are often created ad hoc, and even when they are not created ad hoc, they are often aimed at specific groups, such as specific ethnic minorities, and therefore may not be appropriate when applied to people with MI. Accordingly, a measure that specifically targets prejudice against people with MI is needed.

**Nomological network**
To inform the nomological network, we argue that prejudice towards people with a MI represents multidimensional negative attitudes towards people with MI. In addition, we argue that extensive literature from prejudice research provides a useful integration of existing fields of research into the study of negative attitudes towards people with MI. Based on the extensive research literature on prejudice, we posit the following antecedents and consequences.

*Antecedents*

Social dominance orientation (SDO) and right-wing authoritarianism (RWA) are ideological beliefs that predispose people to prejudice towards many groups [32]. SDO, as an orientation towards non-egalitarianism and preference for group-based dominance [33], predicts prejudice towards groups perceived inferior [34], and may relate to less benevolent and sympathetic attitudes towards people with MI. RWA reflects traditional, conservative, and authoritarian social attitudes, and relates to prejudice against threatening groups [30], and conceivably relates to fearfulness and authoritarian control of people with MI. RWA and SDO have been shown to be the two most important predictors of generalised prejudice, and together they explain most of its variance [35].

Research has also shown that lack of empathy predicts generalised prejudice over and above the influence of SDO and RWA [36], and may therefore relate to less benevolence towards people with MI. In addition, a meta-analysis has linked the personality traits of lower agreeableness and openness to experience to generalised prejudice and these appeared to be most important effects of personality traits on prejudice [32]. It could be expected that lower agreeableness conceivably relating to less benevolence, and lower openness to avoidance of people with MI. Finally, less contact with people with MI is associated with more negative attitudes [37], possibly predisposing people to fear and avoidance of people with MI. Contact itself has been used as a frequent cause of stigma towards people with MI, whereas RWA, SDO, empathy, and personality traits were not. Nonetheless, all these concepts have been shown to be highly important theoretical underpinnings of prejudice in general, and therefore, should be comprehensive underpinnings of prejudice against people with MI.

*Consequences*

The two main consequences of attitudes towards people with MI would be attitudes towards people with specific mental illnesses and discriminatory behaviours. Accordingly, general prejudice towards people with MI should translate into people's attitudes towards people with specific mental illnesses. Research has identified two dimensions underlying social perception: warmth and competence, which translate into disliking (low warmth) and disrespect (low competence) [38]. General prejudice towards people with MI may predispose people to dislike and/or disrespect people with a specific MI, such as schizophrenia or depression. Thus, although there may be differences in liking and respect towards people with specific mental illnesses, these attitudes are expected to be influenced by general attitudes towards people with MI. Additionally, prejudice may lead to discrimination towards

people with MI [2] because attitudes have been found to be consistently linked to behavioural outcomes [39].

**Study aims**

This project aimed to address limitations of research into prejudice towards people with MI, and develop a scale – the Prejudice towards People with a Mental Illness (PPMI) scale – to measure this prejudice. To this end, in constructing the PPMI scale we (i) limited the attitude object to *people* with MI; (ii) defined prejudice as negative attitudes, and excluded other components of stigma; (iii) aimed to develop a balanced scale; and (iv) measured social desirability to control for response biases. The items of the PPMI scale were developed to address topics identified in a thematic analysis of existing measures. The factor validity of the PPMI scale was assessed using an exploratory and confirmatory factor analyses. Based on past research we predicted that:

**Hypothesis 1:** Prejudice associated with MI is multidimensional.

Construct validity was measured by exploring relationships between the PPMI scale and antecedents and consequences. In particular, based on past research we predicted that:

**Hypothesis 2:** The prejudice towards people with MI as measured by the PPMI scale relates to antecedents of higher RWA and SDO, and lower agreeableness, openness to experience, empathy, and contact.
**Hypothesis 3:** The consequences of MI prejudice are disliking and disrespect for people with specific MI and discriminatory behaviours.

We anticipated that the precise relationships of the antecedents and consequences with the specific dimensions would depend on the nature of these dimensions. We, however, had preliminary expectations. For example, we anticipated that fearful, authoritarian, and avoidant attitudes would relate to RWA, low openness to experience, low contact with people with MI, and disliking people with specific illnesses. Similarly, we expected that possible dimensions expressing lack of benevolence or sympathy would relate to SDO, low agreeableness, low empathy, limited contact, and disrespect for people with specific illnesses. We tested the measure across three studies, two employing select samples and the third involving participants from the general community.

**Study 1**
**Method**
*Participants*
The sample consisted of 301 participants (eight were removed as multivariate outliers), comprising university

undergraduates (56.48%) and members of the general public. The mean age was 26.60 years ($SD = 11.68$), and respondents were predominantly female (78.45%) and Australian citizens (62.46%).

## Materials and procedure

We recruited participants through predominantly psychology research websites and snowball sampling on social media. Although we provided online and paper versions of the survey, containing identical items, almost all participants completed the online version (98.3%). We measured the following constructs.

**Prejudice towards people with MI** We conducted a thematic analysis [40] of the items in existing measures of attitudes and related constructs involving people with MI. Existing measures were identified based on a systematic review of the literature. The methodology employed in this review and the stages of the thematic analysis and reference measures are described in Additional file 1. We arranged items into 15 themes (see Additional file 1: Table S2). We decided to combine three themes due to content overlap, and to exclude six themes because they were not evaluations of people with MI. This left us with the seven remaining themes: dangerousness, unpredictability, authoritarianism, inferiority, social distance, interaction difficulty, and malevolence. We developed a pool of 179 items corresponding to the operational definitions of positively- and negatively-keyed items. Three experts rated items for their fidelity to the operational definitions and content validity. We selected the most highly rated items, paying attention to content overlap, to form a balanced 68-item scale with 8 or 10 items reflecting each theme. These were answered on a 9-point scale ranging from $-4$ (*very strongly disagree*) to $+4$ (*very strongly agree*).

**SDO and RWA** Social dominance orientation was measured with a 16-item SDO scale [41] ($\alpha = .93$), and RWA with the 18-item version of the Authoritarianism-Conservatism-Traditionalism (ACT) scale [42] ($\alpha = .88$). Both used the same rating scale as the measure of prejudice above.

**Empathy** We measured empathy using two 7-item subscales of the Interpersonal Reactivity Index [43]: empathic concern ($\alpha = .84$) and perspective taking ($\alpha = .78$).

**Social desirability** We used a 10-item version ($\alpha = .66$) of the Marlow-Crowne Social Desirability Scale [44].

**Big-five personality traits** Participants completed a 50-item scale of personality traits from the International Personality Item Pool [45], including 10-item measures of extraversion, conscientiousness, neuroticism, agreeableness,

and openness to experience ($\alpha$s in this study ranged from .82 to .91). These, like measures of empathy and social desirability, were answered on a 5-point Likert scale ranging from 1 (*very inaccurate*) through to 5 (*very accurate*).

**Disliking and disrespect for people with specific MI** Participants' rated disliking and disrespect on 16 feeling thermometer scales related to people with depression, specific phobia, schizophrenia, obsessive-compulsive disorder, bipolar disorder, anxiety, eating, and substance use disorders. There were eight items measuring disliking and eight measuring disrespect, and the rating scale ranged from $-50$ (*dislike* or *disrespect*) to $+50$ (*like* or *respect*). Each measure was reverse-scored to indicate negativity. Exploratory factor analysis showed that there was one factor with an eigenvalue greater than 1 in both disliking (explaining 60.8% of variance) and disrespect items (73.4% of variance). Accordingly, we averaged participants' scores and created measures of disliking ($\alpha = .91$) and disrespect ($\alpha = .94$).

**Discriminatory behaviour** We developed a measure that asked participants how often (1 = *never*, 2 = *once*, 3 = *twice*, 4 = *three or more times*) they had engaged in six behaviours relating to people with MI ($\alpha = .70$), based on a measure relating to gays/lesbians [46] (see Additional file 1).

**Contact** Participants indicated *yes* or *no* to 12 items of the Level of Contact Report [47]. This measure assessed the level of past exposure of the respondent to people with a MI.

## Results and discussion

We imputed missing data (.19%) with expectation maximisation.

### Exploratory factor analysis

We initially conducted confirmatory factor analysis (CFA),[1] but failed to support the seven-factor model. Accordingly, data analysis moved into an exploratory phase: an exploratory factor analysis (EFA) using Principal Axis Factoring with Oblimin rotation. Eigenvalues, the scree plot and parallel analysis suggested six-factor and four-component solutions (see Additional file 1: Table S3). Although we explored the six-factor solution, we could not interpret it because there was a method factor (resulting from acquiescence) and one factor with two items. The four-factor solution (see Additional file 1: Table S4) was interpretable, demonstrating a simpler structure that explained 44.05% of the variance. Factor 1 explained 18.87% of the variance, and included social distance, dangerousness, and interaction difficulty items (named "fear/avoidance"). Factor 2 comprised inferiority and malevolence items and explained 12.72% of the variance (named "malevolence" given they both reflect unsympathetic attitudes). Factors 3 and 4 reflected the proposed dimensions of "authoritarianism" (14.84%) and "unpredictability" (9.75%). This supported our expectation about multidimensionality (Hypothesis 1).

It appears that even though the thematic analysis of prejudiced attitudes suggested that certain themes could be distinguishable conceptually, participants did not make such a distinction. Factor analysis is empirical and more objective than the more subjective thematic analysis. Our thematic analysis suggested that dangerousness, interaction difficulty, avoidance, malevolence, and inferiority appeared to be different constructs. Nonetheless, participants who perceived that people with MI are dangerous would also uniformly and automatically find that it is difficult to interact with them and that people with MI should be avoided. These three facets therefore formed one latent variable. In addition, participants who had malevolent attitudes towards people with MI also uniformly and automatically perceived them as inferior. Accordingly, these two facets formed one latent variable. Thus, instead of the hypothesised complex seven dimensions, the findings suggested a more parsimonious four-dimensional solution.

Based on factor analysis and item analysis we created a 28-item balanced scale: the Prejudice towards People with Mental Illness (PPMI) scale ($\alpha = .93$), and four subscales, measuring fear/avoidance ($\alpha = .91$), malevolence ($\alpha = .80$), authoritarianism ($\alpha = .79$), and unpredictability ($\alpha = .82$). We selected items whose corrected item-to-.

subscale total correlation was above .3 and that loaded strongly onto the hypothesised factor, provided they did not load more strongly onto other factors. The scale demonstrated a readability (Flesch Reading Ease) score [48] of 60, suggesting its applicability to the general population. The dimensions were moderately to strongly intercorrelated, the strongest being between fear/avoidance and authoritarianism, $r = .64$, and the weakest between malevolence and unpredictability, $r = .31$.

### Correlational analysis

Table 1 shows that prejudice towards people with MI as measured by the 28-item PPMI related to the proposed antecedents and consequences, supporting Hypotheses 2 and 3, and supporting the nomological network and convergent validity. More specifically, prejudice towards people with MI related: positively to SDO, RWA, disliking and disrespect for people with specific MI (Additional file 1: Table S5 includes specific correlations), and past discriminatory behaviours; and negatively to empathic concern, perspective taking, agreeableness, openness to experience, and contact. The scale did not significantly correlate with social desirability, demonstrating discriminant validity and absence of response bias.

Our preliminary expectations about how the dimensions would relate to external variables appeared to be broadly supported. The semipartial correlations describing the unique associations of each subscale with external variables are shown in Table 1. First, fear/avoidance related negatively to contact, positively to disliking and disrespect for people with specific mental illnesses and, weakly, to SDO. Second, malevolence related positively to SDO and RWA, but negatively to empathic concern, perspective taking, agreeableness, and weakly positively with disliking and disrespect. Next, authoritarianism related positively to RWA and negatively to openness to experience. Finally, unpredictability related negatively to SDO, but positively to RWA, empathic concern, and agreeableness. No subscale related to social desirability. This pattern of findings and the differences in correlation sizes across subscales demonstrate convergent and discriminant validity. It should be noted that disliking and disrespect were strongly intercorrelated ($r = .64$, $p < .001$), suggesting that participants did not discriminate much between them. Interestingly, the dimensions of fear/avoidance and malevolence appeared to drive negative evaluations of people with specific MI.

As pointed out, one problem with measures in this area is the nonreplicable factor structure. In addition, in Study 1, we did not assess the relationship between the PPMI measure with an existing measure of attitudes towards people with MI and behaviours. Accordingly, we address these limitations and obtained further validity evidence in Study 2.

### Study 2

This study aimed to determine if the four-factor structure of the PPMI would be replicated in a second sample of participants. It also aimed to demonstrate concurrent validity of the PPMI scale using a widely-used measure of attitudes towards people with MI, the CAMI scale [14]. In addition, to further support the nomological network, we aimed to show that the subscales would predict behavioural intentions in situations eliciting relevant dimensions. For example, we hypothesised that fear/avoidance drives behaviours in situations where there is threat of contact with people with MI, malevolence drives behaviours related to disadvantaging people with MI, authoritarianism drives behaviours that involve controlling people with MI, and unpredictability drives unfavourable reactions to inconsistency of people with MI.

### Method
#### Participants

Participants were 164 undergraduate psychology students attending an Australian university (additional two were removed as multivariate outliers). There were 78.66% females,

**Table 1** Correlations and semipartial correlations among PPMI scale and subscales, and hypothesised criterion variables (Study 1)

| | PPMI | Fear/Avoidance | | Malevolence | | Authoritarianism | | Unpredictability | |
|---|---|---|---|---|---|---|---|---|---|
| | r | r | sr | r | sr | r | sr | r | sr |
| SDO | .55** | .50*** | .17*** | .63*** | .39*** | .44*** | .09* | .18*** | −.14** |
| RWA | .51*** | .40*** | .02 | .45*** | .22*** | .46*** | .18*** | .34*** | .10* |
| Empathic concern | −.21*** | −.19** | −.07 | −.42*** | −.37*** | −.14* | .03 | .07 | .21*** |
| Perspective taking | −.20*** | −.18** | −.06 | −.26*** | −.14* | −.16** | −.03 | −.07 | .04 |
| Extraversion | −.04 | −.10 | −.15** | −.09 | −.07 | .04 | .13* | .05 | .09 |
| Agreeableness | −.18** | −.18*** | −.01 | −.32** | −.28*** | −.10 | .05 | .05 | .16** |
| Openness to experience | −.30*** | −.22*** | .02 | −.25*** | −.10 | −.30*** | −.16** | −.21*** | −.06 |
| Conscientiousness | −.04 | −.03 | .00 | −.05 | −.03 | −.05 | −.03 | .00 | .03 |
| Neuroticism | .09 | .06 | −.01 | .11 | .09 | .06 | .00 | .05 | .02 |
| Disliking PWSMI | .42*** | .44*** | .25*** | .40*** | .16** | .34*** | .06 | .14* | −.13** |
| Disrespect PWSMI | .38*** | .39*** | .21*** | .38*** | .19*** | .28*** | .02 | .14* | −.10 |
| Contact | −.37*** | −.41*** | −.28*** | −.28*** | −.07 | −.24*** | .05 | −.22*** | −.00 |
| Social desirability | −.04 | −.07 | −.09 | .01 | .05 | −.02 | .01 | −.02 | .02 |
| Past behaviour | .13* | .12* | .04 | .20** | .15** | .11 | .02 | −.00 | −.09 |

$N = 301$. PWSMI = People with Specific Mental Illnesses
$* p < .05$. $** p < .01$. $*** p < .001$. The p values of the semipartial correlations are based on significance tests of the B coefficients obtained from the same regression analyses as the semipartial correlations

the mean age was 21.47 years ($SD = 3.31$), and most (75.61%) were Australians.

### Materials and procedure
Participants completed a paper survey in a laboratory with the following measures.

**Prejudice towards people with MI** The PPMI scale ($\alpha = .91$) was included, with subscales reflecting fear/avoidance ($\alpha = .89$), malevolence ($\alpha = .73$), authoritarianism ($\alpha = .72$), and unpredictability ($\alpha = .86$). The scale included original 27 items from Study 1, but we substituted a somewhat weaker 28th item, which was, based on factor loadings, one of the weakest items to measure fear/avoidance ("I would not be comfortable having a neighbour who is mentally ill") with a clearer item, which reflected the construct ("It is best to avoid people who have mental illness"). The original item also had the weakest factor loading and corrected item-total correlation in the final eight-item measure of all the selected items originally developed to measure dangerousness. Further, when the four factors were identified it became apparent that a clearer item reflecting the underlying construct was necessary to encapsulate the summarised construct of fear/avoidance. Following consultation with our expert panel of item raters, the decision was made to substitute a new item that more effectively reflected the fear/avoidance factor. Table 2 presents the items. The scale had an unchanged readability score (60). We also administered the CAMI scale ([14]; 40 items, $\alpha = .94$). Both measures were answered on a

9-point scale ranging from − 4 (*very strongly disagree*) to + 4 (*very strongly agree*).

**Behavioural intentions scenarios** We included a measure of behavioural intentions modelled on scenarios reflecting racial discrimination [49]. We asked participants to indicate their behaviours in five hypothetical scenarios, which reflected one of the four dimensions of prejudice towards people with MI: 1) interacting with someone who voiced the opinion that people with MI should not have children (authoritarianism would drive discriminatory behavioural intentions); 2) accepting that a coworker with MI had been passed over for promotion (malevolence should drive discrimination); 3) willingness to accept a person with MI being overlooked for a play due to possible unpredictability (unpredictability should drive discrimination); 4) willingness to live near a psychiatric institution (fear/avoidance should drive discrimination); and 5) tolerating a shopkeeper lying about a job's availability to a person with MI (malevolence should drive discrimination). The full items are in Additional file 1.

### Results and discussion
We imputed missing data (1.29%) using expectation maximisation.

### CFA
We analysed the variance-covariance matrix using maximum likelihood estimation. Given the moderate sample size, we used item parcels to reduce the number of parameter estimates [50],[2] and control for acquiescence

**Table 2** Final 28 items from the PPMI scale and their factor loadings on the respective content factors from the CFA in Study 2 (N = 164) and 3 (N = 495)

| Item | Study 2 | Study 3 |
|---|---|---|
| **Fear/Avoidance** | | |
| I would find it hard to talk to someone who has a mental illness | .62 | .63 |
| I would be less likely to become romantically involved with someone if I knew they were mentally ill | .51 | .45 |
| It is best to avoid people who have mental illness | .76 | .55 |
| I would feel unsafe being around someone who is mentally ill | .81 | .67 |
| I would be just as happy to invite a person with mental illness into my home as I would anyone else* | .76 | .77 |
| I would feel relaxed if I had to talk to someone who was mentally ill* | .70 | .75 |
| I am not scared of people with mental illness* | .74 | .68 |
| In general, it is easy to interact with someone who has mental illness* | .67 | .61 |
| **Malevolence** | | |
| People who are mentally ill are avoiding the difficulties of everyday life | .63 | .35 |
| People with mental illness should support themselves and not expect handouts | .58 | .34 |
| People who develop mental illness are genetically inferior to other people | .59 | .45 |
| People with mental illness do not deserve our sympathy | .49 | .53 |
| We, as a society, should be spending much more money on helping people with mental illness* | .48 | .61 |
| People who become mentally ill are not failures in life* | .41 | .62 |
| We need to support and care for people who become mentally ill* | .62 | .75 |
| Under certain circumstances, anyone can experience mental illness* | .42 | .67 |
| **Authoritarianism** | | |
| People who are mentally ill need to be controlled by any means necessary | .67 | .56 |
| Those who have serious mental illness should not be allowed to have children | .57 | .57 |
| People who are mentally ill should be forced to have treatment | .49 | .45 |
| People who are mentally ill should be free to make their own decisions* | .51 | .70 |
| People who are mentally ill should be allowed to live their life any way they want* | .50 | .66 |
| Society does not have a right to limit the freedom of people with mental illness* | .39 | .61 |
| **Unpredictability** | | |
| The behaviour of people with mental illness is unpredictable | .75 | .74 |
| People with mental illness often do unexpected things | .79 | .75 |
| In general, you cannot predict how people with mental illness will behave | .75 | .77 |
| The behaviour of people with mental illness is just as predictable as that of people who are mentally healthy* | .55 | .47 |
| People with mental illness behave in ways that are foreseeable* | .65 | .25 |
| I usually find people with mental illness to be consistent in their behaviour* | .67 | .37 |

\* = item was reverse-scored. All loadings were significant at $p < 001$

(we paired positively-keyed and negatively-keyed items in parcels). Guidelines [51] suggest that for acceptable model fit CFI should be larger than .95, and RMSEA and SRMR less than .08. The proposed four-factor model fit was acceptable, $\chi^2(48) = 75.99$, $p = .006$, CFI = .97, RMSEA = .06, SRMR = .04 (see Fig. 1), and better than that of alternative models: one-factor, $\chi^2(54) = 353.13$, $p < .000$, CFI = .68, RMSEA = .18, SRMR = .11, AIC = 425.13; and three-factor, which had items measuring fear/avoidance and authoritarianism loading on one factor, $\chi^2(51) = 109.12$, $p < .001$, CFI = .94, RMSEA = .08, SRMR = .06. Factor loadings of items from an

item-level CFA on their respective four content factors are in Table 2.

### Correlations

The PPMI scale and its subscales strongly correlated with the CAMI, demonstrating concurrent validity. The relationships ranged from $r = .44$ (unpredictability) to $r = .78$ (the overall scale).

### Ordinal logistic regression (OLR) analysis

We investigated the role of prejudice in behavioural intentions using OLR. As expected, fear/avoidance independently

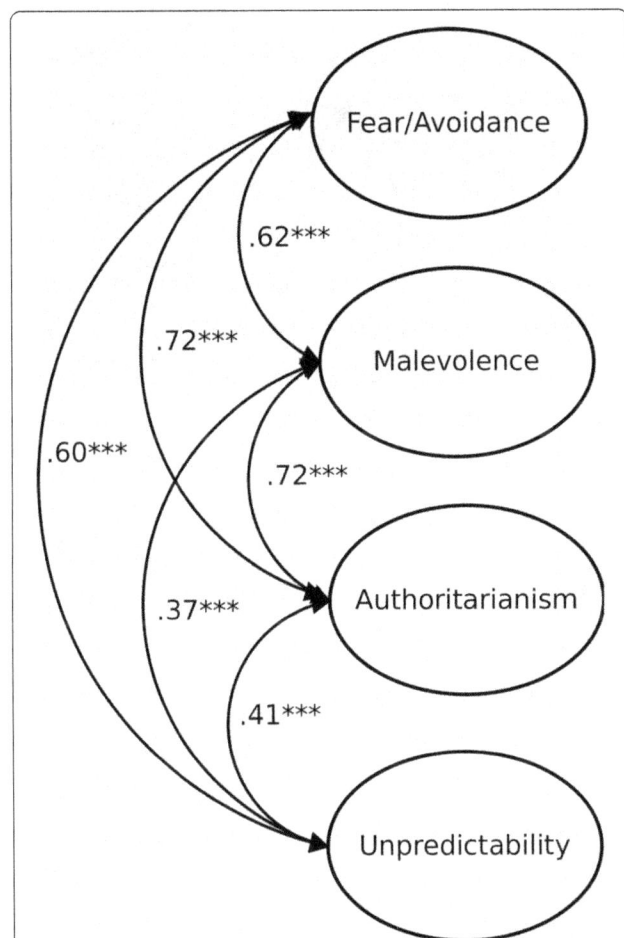

**Fig. 1** CFA of the four-factor model of Prejudice towards People with MI (Study 2). Manifest indicators are not shown. $N = 164$. *** $p < .001$

predicted unwillingness to rent an apartment near an inpatient facility, estimate = .34 [95% CI .01–.67], Wald $\chi^2(1)$ = 4.52, $p = .046$. Malevolence predicted reluctance to speak out against a shopkeeper lying about a job's availability to a person with MI, estimate = .58 [.09–1.07], Wald $\chi^2(1) = 5.30$, $p = .021$. Our expectation that authoritarianism would drive behavioural intentions in a scenario about prohibiting people with MI from having children was supported, estimate = .45 [.07–.82], Wald $\chi^2(1) = 5.32$, $p = .021$, although fear/avoidance was also a significant, though weaker, predictor, estimate = .41 [.03–.78], Wald $\chi^2(1) = 4.52$, $p = .034$. Contrary to hypotheses, malevolence, estimate = .84 [.16–1.53], Wald $\chi^2(1) = 5.81$, $p = .016$, but not unpredictability, drove discrimination in a scenario about rejecting people with MI from a role in a play, possibly because this discriminatory behaviour may disadvantage people with MI, and therefore may be elicited by malevolence. Also, contrary to predictions, malevolence did not predict lack of support for a mentally ill coworker's promotion (no dimension was a significant predictor). Full results of OLR are in Additional file 1: Table S6.

The findings, therefore, partially supported the proposed nomological network of the PPMI subscales. We did not obtain evidence for the anticipated effects in every behavioural scenario, possibly because these were originally developed to measure racial discrimination and some of them required significant adaptation to be applicable for people with MI. Moreover, general attitudes best predict discrimination across situations, and not in one situation [52]. Overall findings, nonetheless, demonstrate the utility of the PPMI scale. The sample in this study, however, was specific and not large. Accordingly, we further tested the scale and its nomological network in the general population.

## Study 3

In this study, we aimed to further investigate the stability of the four-factor solution using item-level CFA in a large community sample consisting of participants from several countries. We also investigated the proposed nomological network of prejudice in relation to RWA, SDO, agreeableness, openness to experience, contact, and specific attitudes towards people with depression and schizophrenia. Finally, we also wanted to explore whether prejudice predisposes people to positive attitudes towards people who have never had MI.

## Method
### Participants

The sample consisted of 495 participants, who were recruited through the CrowdFlower service (a website that allows researchers to access community samples for a financial compensation). Participants were all native English-speakers (58.38% females, the mean age: 38.62, $SD = 12.64$). Data from non-native English-speakers and participants who speeded, engaged in response set, or failed attention checks were removed. Participants were citizens of the US (50.71%), the UK (21.21%), Canada (17.98%), and other countries (10.10%), with 76.77% self-identifying as Anglo/White.

### Materials and procedure

Participants completed an online survey with the following measures for a small payment.

**Prejudice towards people with MI** We included the 28-item version of the PPMI scale ($\alpha = .91$) from Study 2 (Table 2), with subscales measuring fear/avoidance ($\alpha = .87$), malevolence ($\alpha = .83$), authoritarianism ($\alpha = .82$), and unpredictability ($\alpha = .79$).

**SDO and RWA** We included a newer 16-item SDO scale [33] ($\alpha = .93$), and an 18-item version of the ACT scale [42] ($\alpha = .89$). The SDO scale used a 7-point scale ranging from 1 (*strongly oppose*) to 7 (*strongly favor*). The ACT scale, like the PPMI scale, used a 9-point scale ranging from 1 (*very strongly disagree*) to 9 (*very strongly agree*).

**Big-five personality traits** Participants completed 2-item measures of agreeableness and openness to experience from the balanced Ten Item Personality Inventory [53] using a 7-point scale ranging from 1 (*disagree strongly*) to 7 (*agree strongly*). The scales' Spearman-Brown reliability coefficients were .47 for openness to experience and .57 for agreeableness.

**Contact** Participants completed the 12-item Level of Contact Report as in Study 1.

**Feeling thermometer measure** Participants indicated their level of favourability to people who have schizophrenia, depression, and those who have never had MI on a scale from − 50 (*unfavorable*) to + 50 (*favorable*).

## Results and discussion
### CFA
We analysed the items' variance-covariance matrix using maximum likelihood estimation. All tested models had content factors and two uncorrelated method factors, resulting from positively-keyed and negatively-keyed items, so that all positive items loaded on one and all negative on the other method factor; the method factors were not correlated with any other factor. This four-factor model, with additional two method factors, fitted the data well, $\chi^2(316) = 870.21$, $p < .001$, CFI = .92, RMSEA = .06, SRMR = .08. Apart from a non-significant correlation between malevolence and unpredictability, the four factors were moderately to strongly intercorrelated (see Fig. 2). A one-factor model, with two additional method factors, had a much worse fit to the data, $\chi^2(322) = 1619.27$, $p < .001$, CFI = .81, RMSEA = .09, SRMR = .14. Given the strongest intercorrelation between fear/avoidance and authoritarianism, we tested a three-factor model (also with two method factors) with items from these subscales loading on one factor. Its fit, $\chi^2(319) = 1041.00$, $p < .001$, CFI = .89, RMSEA = .07, SRMR = .12, was worse than the fit of the four-factor model. Accordingly, the analyses replicated the four-factor structure found in Studies 1 and 2. Factor loadings of items on their respective four content factors (see Table 2) tended to be similar to, though in several cases lower than, those in Study 2.

### Correlations
As in Study 1, and in support of Hypothesis 2 and 3, overall prejudice towards people with MI significantly correlated with hypothesised antecedents and consequence, supporting the nomological network (see Table 3): positively to SDO and RWA, negatively to agreeableness,

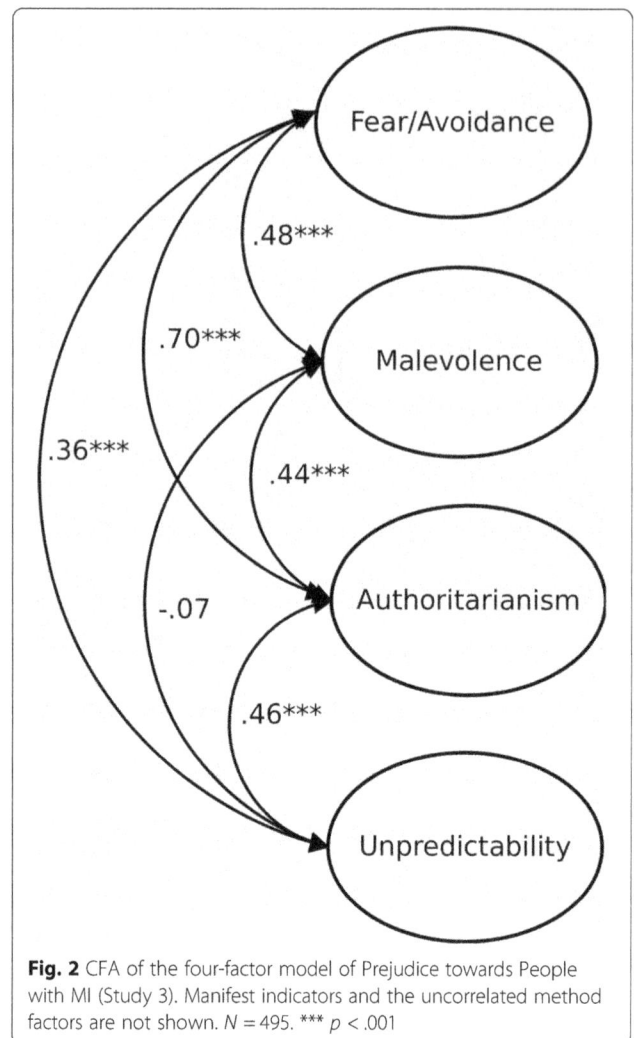

**Fig. 2** CFA of the four-factor model of Prejudice towards People with MI (Study 3). Manifest indicators and the uncorrelated method factors are not shown. $N = 495$. *** $p < .001$

openness to experience, contact, and specific attitudes towards people with schizophrenia and depression, but was unrelated to attitudes towards people who have never had MI. It should be noted that zero-order correlations of the PPMI subscales with other variables were as expected. Here, as in Study 1, we describe semipartial correlations. First, fear/avoidance related negatively to contact, agreeableness, openness to experience, and attitudes towards people with schizophrenia and depression. Second, malevolence related positively and very strongly to SDO, but more weakly to RWA; it also related negatively to agreeableness, openness to experience, attitudes towards people with schizophrenia and depression, and surprisingly to attitudes towards people who have never had MI (suggesting that malevolent prejudice may be part of a general misanthropic orientation, that is, negativity towards all humans). Next, authoritarianism related positively to RWA, and much more weakly to SDO and agreeableness. Finally, unpredictability related positively to RWA, agreeableness, and attitudes towards people who have never

**Table 3** Correlations and semipartial correlations among PPMI scale and subscales, and hypothesised criterion variables (Study 3)

| | PPMI | Fear/Avoidance | | Malevolence | | Authoritarianism | | Unpredictability | |
|---|---|---|---|---|---|---|---|---|---|
| | r | r | sr | r | sr | r | sr | r | sr |
| SDO | .52** | .38*** | −.003 | .60*** | .51*** | .41*** | .08* | .14** | .07 |
| RWA | .39*** | .24*** | −.14*** | .29*** | .17*** | .42*** | .25*** | .29*** | .16*** |
| Agreeableness | −.16** | −.20*** | −.19*** | −.23** | −.14** | −.05 | .11* | .08 | .11* |
| Openness to Experience | −.15*** | −.16*** | −.11* | −.19** | −.12** | −.08 | .05 | .01 | .04 |
| People Who Have Schizophrenia | −.43*** | −.44*** | −.25*** | −.27*** | −.08* | −.31*** | .03 | −.26*** | −.10* |
| People Who Have Depression | −.44*** | −.41*** | −.17*** | −.42*** | −.24*** | −.32*** | −.01 | −.13** | −.01 |
| People Who Have Never Had MI | −.06 | −.06 | −.03 | −.26*** | −.23*** | −.004 | .05 | .18*** | .14** |
| Contact | −.20*** | −.41*** | −.26*** | −.10* | .04 | −.13** | .06 | −.08 | .03 |

$N = 495$. * $p < .05$. ** $p < .01$. *** $p < .001$. The $p$ values of the semipartial correlations are based on significance tests of the B coefficients obtained from the same regression analyses as the semipartial correlations

had MI, but negatively to attitudes towards people with schizophrenia. The overall pattern of findings is consistent with the results from Study 1, further supporting the nomological network and conceptual distinction between the dimensions.

### National and age differences

Given that Study 3 was more diverse in participants than the previous two studies we explored group and age differences. With respect to racial/ethnic groups, 76.77% were Anglo/Whites, and the other ethnic groups had a small number of participants (of the remaining groups the largest were Chinese with only 16 participants). Accordingly, we could not meaningfully compare Anglo/Whites with any other ethnic group. We, however, had three sufficiently large national groups for comparisons. A between-groups analysis of variance (ANOVA) including participants from the US, the UK, and Canada showed that there was a significant effect of nationality on overall prejudice to people with MI, $F(2, 442) = 14.58$, $p < .001$, $\eta_p^2 = .06$, fear/avoidance, $F(2, 442) = 7.37$, $p < .001$, $\eta_p^2 = .03$, authoritarianism, $F(2, 442) = 8.71$, $p < .001$, $\eta_p^2 = .04$, malevolence, $F(2, 442) = 13.44$, $p < .001$, $\eta_p^2 = .06$, and unpredictability, $F(2, 442) = 6.04$, $p = .003$, $\eta_p^2 = .03$.

Post-hoc comparisons using the Scheffe correction were then conducted. These revealed that on prejudice towards people with MI US participants, $M = 4.30$, $SD = .97$, were significantly higher than UK participants, $M = 3.73$, $SD = 1.07$, $t(442) = 4.90$, $p < .001$, and Canadian participants, $M = 3.86$, $SD = 1.02$, $t(442) = 3.54$, $p = .002$. US participants, $M = 4.27$, $SD = 1.42$, were also significantly higher on fear/avoidance than UK participants, $M = 3.71$, $SD = 1.50$, $t(442) = 3.39$, $p = .003$, and Canadian participants, $M = 3.80$, $SD = 1.38$, $t(442) = 2.67$, $p = .029$. Further, US participants, $M = 4.39$, $SD = 1.47$, were higher on authoritarianism than UK participants, $M = 3.69$, $SD = 1.37$, $t(442) = 4.12$, $p < .001$. US participants, $M = 3.14$, $SD = 1.20$, were also higher on malevolence than UK participants, $M = 2.58$, $SD = 1.25$, $t(442) = 4.14$,

$p < .001$, and Canadian participants, $M = 2.54$, $SD = 1.01$, $t(442) = 4.15$, $p < .001$. Finally, US participants, $M = 5.50$, $SD = 1.28$, were higher on unpredictability than UK participants, $M = 5.33$, $SD = 1.23$, $t(442) = 3.29$, $p = .005$. No other national difference was significant.

There were no correlations of age with overall prejudice ($r = −.05$, $p = .23$), authoritarianism ($r = .04$, $p = .35$), and fear/avoidance ($r = −.08$, $p = .07$), but there was a significant negative correlation of age with malevolence ($r = −.26$, $p < .001$) and a significant positive correlation of age with unpredictability ($r = .21$, $p < .001$). This suggests that younger people tended to be more malevolent in their attitudes, and older perceived more unpredictability in people with MI.

### General discussion

To address limitations in the study of prejudice towards people with MI, we proposed and tested a new conceptualisation and nomological network of prejudice towards people with MI. Consistent with Hypothesis 1, prejudice was multidimensional. In contrast to our initial expectation, however, it consisted of four, and not seven, dimensions: fear/avoidance, malevolence, authoritarianism, and unpredictability. Next, supporting Hypothesis 2, prejudice related to the proposed antecedents: RWA and SDO (positively), agreeableness, openness to experience, empathy, and past contact with people with MI (negatively). This suggests that prejudice towards people with MI appears to be an outcome of ideology, personality, and past experiences. In fact, the strong associations with RWA and SDO indicated that ideology appears more important in predicting prejudice than the more widely studied contact with people with MI. Finally, supporting Hypothesis 3, prejudice predicted the proposed consequences: negative feelings for people with specific MI, past behaviours, and behavioural intentions. We demonstrated in this research that the scale measures the evaluative component of stigma, that is, prejudice, but that it is also consistently related to discrimination against people with MI. In addition, we showed that specific dimensions of prejudice lead to specific behavioural outcomes, enabling a nuanced understanding of the processes involved in stigma.

The PPMI scale demonstrated a consistent four-factor structure across three studies and in different cultural groups. This is significant as widely-used measures of attitudes towards people with MI, such as the OMI and CAMI, do not demonstrate a replicable factor structure. We demonstrated concurrent validity of the PPMI scale through correlating it with the CAMI scale [14]. This is an important finding because the PPMI scale is shorter and has improved psychometric properties.

Our findings support using both the subscales and the total scale. The model with four distinct factors was superior to the model with only one factor. Nevertheless, the four factors were intercorrelated and the overall scale was reliable, with Cronbach's alphas in each study being above .90 (Study 1 α = .93, Study 2 α = .91, Study 3 α = .91). This suggests that there was significant internal consistency present in the items to sum them up also as a scale to measure prejudice as a multidimensional construct.

Using EFA and CFA, and by consistently demonstrating unique associations between each dimension and external variables, we provided strong evidence of multidimensionality and the nomological network across samples. These findings suggest that the four dimensions have distinct antecedents and consequences. For example, malevolence appears to be a function of low empathy, low agreeableness, and high SDO, and appears to strongly drive discriminatory behaviours.

This project has emphasised the importance of using theory and research to provide a strong conceptual foundation for a new measure. Our decision to focus on prejudice, as the component of stigma that influences behaviour, was driven by theoretical and practical considerations. By reviewing measures mainly from psychiatric and general population studies, we have encapsulated the aspects of prejudice targeted by stigma reduction campaigns and interventions. Positioning prejudice within a nomological network allowed us to demonstrate construct validity in a more comprehensive way than existing conceptualisations. It should be nevertheless noted that our initial expectation for seven dimensions was not supported, but once the four dimensions were discovered, they were repeatedly shown to exist across studies.

### Limitations and suggestions for future research
Our research has several limitations. First, we inferred the antecedents and consequences from theory and research, but we did not explicitly test whether ideological beliefs, personality, and contact cause prejudice towards people with MI. Although most theoretical approaches would assume that such factors would cause social attitudes [54],

future experimental or longitudinal studies should address this issue. Next, whether it is useful to measure general attitudes towards people with MI can be questioned because there may be disparities between attitudes towards specific mental illnesses (e.g., [55, 56]). Nonetheless, Studies 1 and 3 show that general prejudice does correlate with feelings towards people with specific MI. Another limitation relates to the reliance on self-report to link prejudice with behaviour, and future research should use other methods, such as observing behaviour, to investigate the link. Finally, although we did not assess the PPMI scale for test-retest reliability, this scale was administered two weeks apart in another experiment [57], and partial correlations (controlling for the experimental condition) were satisfactory, suggesting good test-retest reliability: .73 (PPMI), .75 (fear/avoidance), .63 (malevolence), .71 (authoritarianism), and .63 (unpredictability).

By reviewing psychiatric and population research, we developed a measure that may prove useful in future research including intervention studies designed to reduce prejudice. The PPMI scale suggests that prejudice against people with MI consists of four main factors. Accordingly, anti-stigma interventions may target each of the specific attitudes separately and this may bring about more complex anti-stigma approaches. The measure could also be used to explore differences between interventions that have previously been obscured by unclear factor structures in existing measures. Indeed, our research shows that the current measure is useful in understanding nuanced changes in the four dimensions of prejudice following two interventions [57], but further investigation is needed.

### Conclusions
In this research, we clarified the structure of prejudice towards people with MI and positioned it in an empirically supported nomological network. We also presented evidence for an improved measure of prejudice, the PPMI scale. This research, therefore, provides a valuable theoretical and methodological contribution to the area, and fruitfully integrates approaches to stigma and prejudice. A novel contribution of this research is therefore the integration of stigma and prejudice literature in developing this measure, including its nomological network, and a very strong psychometric evaluation of the measure, encompassing a replicable factor structure, reliability, and validity.

Current intervention to reduce negative attitudes to people with MI are effective but the magnitude of the effects is small and there is a need to improve their effectiveness [58]. Such improvement must be informed by a better understanding of prejudice towards people with MI, including its antecedents and consequences, and by more reliable, comprehensive and precise measurement of it. The current research represents an important step towards achieving these goals.

## Endnotes

[1]The CFA for the seven-factor model did not demonstrate a clear solution, with modification indices suggesting that many items loaded strongly on two or more factors. Similarly, intercorrelations between factors were strong (up to .92, $p < .001$), indicating that several hypothesised factors measured the same construct.

[2]We also tested an item-level CFA of the four-factor model with two additional method factors (i.e., positive and negative items loading on their respective method factors). It showed acceptable fit, $\chi^2(316) = 551.32$, $p < .001$, CFI = .88, RMSEA = .07, SRMR = .08, with all items loading on their hypothesised factors. The fit was better than that of alternative models, such as one-factor and three-factor models with method factors. This analysis was somewhat affected by the moderate sample size in relation to the model's complexity.

## Additional file

**Additional file 1:** Stages of the Thematic Analysis of Items and Operational Definitions. **Table S1.** List of Measures Included in Thematic Analyses and Its Publication Reference. **Table S2.** Results of the Thematic Analysis. **Table S3.** Eigenvalues from Principal Axis Factoring and Simulated Eigenvalues from Parallel Analysis (Study 1). **Table S4.** Pattern Matrix for Principal Axis Factor Analysis with Oblimin Rotation of the PPMI Scale Items in Study 1. **Table S5.** Correlations of the PPMI Scale with Disliking or Disrespect for People with Specific Kinds of Mental Illness (Study 1). A Modified Measure of Past Behaviours Towards People with Mental Illness (Study 1). Modified Measures of Behavioural Intentions in Hypothetical Scenarios Involving People with MI (Study 2). **Table S6.** Ordinal Logistic Regression Analyses of Hypothetical Behaviour Scenarios Regressed on the PPMI Subscales (Study 2). (DOCX 42 kb)

## Abbreviations

ACT: Authoritarianism-conservatism-traditionalism; CAMI: Community attitudes toward the mentally ill; CFA: Confirmatory factor analysis; EFA: Exploratory factor analysis; MI: Mental illness; OLR: Ordinal logistic regression; OMI: Opinions about mental illness; PPMI: Prejudice towards people with mental illness; PWSMI: People with specific mental illnesses; RWA: Right-wing authoritarianism; SDO: Social dominance orientation

## Acknowledgements

We are grateful to Ross Wilkinson and John Duckitt for their feedback on this research, to Beth Gunningham for her help with data collection in Study 3 and comments on a previous version of the manuscript, and to Elizabeth Huxley, Conal Monaghan, Jaclyn Swinton, and Lachlan Smith for their comments on a previous version of the manuscript.

## Funding

This research was supported by an Australian Postgraduate Award, funded by the Australian Federal Government, to Amanda Kenny.

## Authors' contributions

AK and BB conceptualised the project. AK collected data for Study 1 and 2, whereas BB collected data for Study 3. AK and BB analysed data for Study 1 and 2, and BB analysed data for Study 3. KMG provided advice during the duration of the project and helped with methodology. AK, BB, and KMG wrote the manuscript. All authors read and approved the final manuscript.

## Consent for publication

Not applicable.

## Competing interests

The authors declare that they have no competing interests.

## References

1. Fox AB, Earnshaw VA, Taverna EC, Vogt D. Conceptualizing and measuring mental illness stigma: the mental illness stigma framework and critical review of measures. Stigma and Health.
2. Corrigan PW, Shapiro JR. Measuring the impact of programs that challenge the public stigma of mental illness. Clin Psychol Rev. 2010;30:907–22.
3. Phelan JC, Link BG, Dovidio JF. Stigma and prejudice: one animal or two? Soc Sci Med. 2008;67:358–67.
4. Stephan WG, Stephan CW. An integrated threat theory of prejudice. In: Oskamp S, editor. Reducing prejudice and discrimination. Hillsdale, NJ: Lawrence Erlbaum; 2000. p. 23–46.
5. Eagly AH, Chaiken S. The psychology of attitudes. Fort Worth, TX: Harcourt Brace Jovanovich; 1993.
6. Stigma GE. Notes on the management of spoiled identity. New Jersey. NY: Prentice-Hall; 1963.
7. Cronbach LJ, Meehl PE. Construct validity in psychological tests. Psychol Bull. 1955;52:281–302.
8. Day EN, Edgren K, Eshleman A. Measuring stigma toward mental illness: development and application of the mental illness stigma scale. J Appl Soc Psychol. 2007;37:2191–219.
9. Haghighat R. The development of an instrument to measure stigmatization: factor analysis and origin of stigmatization. Eur J Psychiatry. 2005;19:144–54.
10. Littlewood R, Jadhav S, Ryder AG. A cross-national study of the stigmatization of severe psychiatric illness: historical review, methodological considerations and development of the questionnaire. Transcult Psychiatry. 2007;44:171–202.
11. Svensson B, Markström U, Bejerholm U, Björkman T, Brunt D, Eklund M, et al. Test - retest reliability of two instruments for measuring public attitudes towards persons with mental illness. BMC Psychiatry. 2011;11:11.
12. Masuda A, Hayes SC, Lillis J, Bunting K, Herbst SA, Fletcher LB. The relation between psychological flexibility and mental health stigma in acceptance and commitment therapy: a preliminary process investigation. Behav Soc Issues. 2009;18:1–16.
13. Tanaka G, Inadomi H, Kikuchi Y, Ohta Y. Evaluating stigma against mental disorder and related factors. Psychiatry Clin Neurosci. 2004;58:558–66.
14. Taylor SM, Dear MJ. Scaling community attitudes toward the mentally ill. Schizophr Bull. 1981;7:225–40.
15. Aromaa E, Tolvanen A, Tuulari J, Wahlbeck K. Attitudes towards people with mental disorders: the psychometric characteristics of a Finnish questionnaire. Soc Psychiat Epidemiol. 2010;45:265–73.
16. Baker JA, Richards DA, Campbell M. Nursing attitudes towards acute mental health care: development of a measurement tool. J Adv Nurs. 2005;49:522–9.
17. Baker F, Schulberg HC. The development of a community mental health ideology scale. Community Ment Health J. 1967;3:216–25.
18. Kassam A, Glozier N, Leese M, Henderson C, Thornicroft G. Development and responsiveness of a scale to measure clinicians' attitudes to people with mental illness (medical student version). Acta Psychiatr Scand. 2010; 122:153–61.
19. Watson AC, Miller FE, Lyons JS. Adolescent attitudes toward serious mental illness. J Nerv Ment Dis. 2005;193:769–72.

20. Högberg T, Magnusson A, Ewertzon M, Lützén K. Attitudes towards mental illness in Sweden: adaptation and development of the community attitudes towards mental illness questionnaire. Int J Ment Health Nurs. 2008;17:302–10.

21. Morris R, Scott PA, Cocoman A, Chambers M, Guise V, Välimäki M, et al. Is the community attitudes towards the mentally ill scale valid for use in the investigation of European nurses' attitudes towards the mentally ill? A confirmatory factor analytic approach. J Adv Nurs. 2012;68:460–70.

22. Cohen J, Struening EL. Opinions about mental illness in the personnel of two large mental hospitals. J Abnorm Soc Psychol. 1962;64:349–60.

23. Anagnostopoulos F, Hantzi A. Familiarity with and social distance from people with mental illness: testing the mediating effects of prejudiced attitudes. J Community Appl Soc Psychol. 2011;21:451–60.

24. Jackson D, Heatherington L. Young Jamaicans' attitudes toward mental illness: experimental and demographic factors associated with social distance and stigmatizing opinions. J Community Psychol. 2006;34:563–76.

25. Wolff G, Pathare S, Craig T, Leff J. Community attitudes to mental illness. Br J Psychiatry. 1996;168:183–90.

26. Hirai M, Clum GA. Development, reliability, and validity of the beliefs toward mental illness scale. J Psychopathol Behav Assess. 2000;22:221–36.

27. Evans-Lacko S, Little K, Meltzer H, Rose D, Rhydderch D, Henderson C, et al. Development and psychometric properties of the mental health knowledge schedule. Can J Psychiatr. 2010;55:440–8.

28. Furr RM. Scale construction and psychometrics for social and personality psychology. London, UK: Sage; 2011.

29. Link BG, Yang LH, Phelan JC, Collins PY. Measuring mental illness stigma. Schizophr Bull. 2004;30:511–41.

30. Duckitt J, Bizumic B. Multidimensionality of right-wing authoritarian attitudes: authoritarianism-conservatism-traditionalism. Pol Psychol. 2013;34:841–62.

31. Duckitt J, Sibley C. Right wing authoritarianism, social dominance orientation and the dimensions of generalized prejudice. Eur J Personal. 2007;21:113–30.

32. Sibley CG, Duckitt J. Personality and prejudice: a meta-analysis and theoretical review. Personal Soc Psychol Rev. 2008;12:248–79.

33. Ho AK, Sidanius J, Kteily N, Sheehy-Skeffington J, Pratto F, Henkel KE, et al. The nature of social dominance orientation: theorizing and measuring preferences for intergroup inequality using the new SDO7 scale. J Pers Soc Psychol. 2015;109:1003–28.

34. Duckitt J, Sibley CG. The dual process motivational model of ideology and prejudice. In: The Cambridge handbook of the psychology of prejudice. Cambridge, UK: Cambridge University Press; 2017. p. 188–221.

35. Altemeyer B. The other "authoritarian personality". Adv Exp Soc Psychol. 1998;30:47–92.

36. McFarland S. Authoritarianism, social dominance, and other roots of generalized prejudice. Pol Psychol. 2010;31:453–77.

37. Hayward P, Bright JA. Stigma and mental illness: a review and critique. J Ment Health. 1997;6:345–54.

38. Fiske ST, Xu J, Cuddy AC, Glick P. (Dis)respecting versus (dis)liking: status and interdependence predict ambivalent stereotypes of competence and warmth. J Soc Issues. 1999;55:473–89.

39. Fazio RH, Roskos-Ewoldsen D. Acting as we feel: when and how attitudes guide behavior. In: Brock TC, Green MC, editors. The psychology of persuasion. 2nd ed. New York, NY: Allyn & Bacon; 2005.

40. Braun V, Clarke V. Using thematic analysis in psychology. Qual Res Psychol. 2006;3:77–101.

41. Pratto F, Sidanius J, Stallworth LM, Malle BF. Social dominance orientation: a personality variable predicting social and political attitudes. J Pers Soc Psychol. 1994;67:741–63.

42. Duckitt J, Bizumic B, Krauss SW. Heled E. A tripartite approach to right-wing authoritarianism: the authoritarianism-conservatism-traditionalism model. Pol Psychol. 2010;31:685–715.

43. Davis MH. A multidimensional approach to individual differences in empathy. JSAS Catalog of Selected Documents in Psychology. 1980;10:85–93.

44. Fischer DG, Fick C. Measuring social desirability: short forms of the Marlowe-Crowne social desirability scale. Educ Psychol Meas. 1993;53:417–24.

45. Goldberg LR. A broad-bandwidth, public-domain, personality inventory measuring the lower-level facets of several five-factor models. In: Mervielde I, Deary I, De Fruyt F, Ostendorf F, editors. Personality psychology in Europe. Tilburg. The Netherlands: Tilburg University Press; 1999. p. 7–28.

46. Rey AM, Gibson PR. Beyond high school: heterosexuals' self-reported anti-gay/lesbian behaviors and attitudes. Journal of Gay & Lesbian Social Services. 1998;7:65.

47. Holmes EP, Corrigan PW, Williams P, Canar J, Kubiak MA. Changing attitudes about schizophrenia. Schizophr Bull. 1999;25:447–56.

48. Kincaid JP, Fishburn RP, Rogers RL, Chissom BS. Derivation of new readability formulas (Automated Readability Index, Fog Count and Flesch Reading Ease Formula) for Navy enlisted personnel. Research Branch Report. Millington, Tennesse, Naval Air Station; 1975. http://eric.ed.gov/?id=ED108134. Accessed 27 Oct 2014.

49. Byrnes DA, Kiger G. Contemporary measures of attitudes toward blacks. Educ Psychol Meas. 1988;48:107–18.

50. Little TD, Cunningham WA, Shahar G, Widaman KF. To parcel or not to parcel: exploring the question, weighing the merits. Structural Equation Modeling: A Multidisciplinary Journal. 2002;9:151–73.

51. Schreiber JB. Core reporting practices in structural equation modeling. Res Soc Adm Pharm. 2008;4:83–97.

52. Fishbein M, Ajzen I. Attitudes towards objects as predictors of single and multiple behavioral criteria. Psychol Rev. 1974;81:59–74.

53. Gosling SD, Rentfrow PJ, WBJ S. A very brief measure of the big-five personality domains. J Res Pers. 2003;37:504–28.

54. Duckitt J. Prejudice and intergroup hostility. In: Sears DO, Huddy L, Jervis R, editors. Oxford handbook of political psychology. Oxford, UK: Oxford University Press; 2003. p. 559–600.

55. Griffiths KM, Batterham PJ, Barney L, Parsons A. The generalised anxiety stigma scale (GASS): psychometric properties in a community sample. BMC Psychiatry. 2011;11:184.

56. Reavley NJ, Jorm AF. Stigmatizing attitudes towards people with mental disorders: findings from an Australian national survey of mental health literacy and stigma. Aust N Z J Psychiatry. 2011;45:1086–93.

57. Kenny A, Bizumic B. Learn and ACT: changing prejudice towards people with mental illness using stigma reduction interventions. J Contextual Behav Sci. 2016;5:178–85.

58. Griffiths KM, Carron-Arthur B, Parsons A, Reid R. Effectiveness of programs for reducing the stigma associated with mental disorders. A meta-analysis of randomized controlled trials. World Psychiatry. 2014;13:161–75.

# 17

# Salivary cortisol in post-traumatic stress disorder: a systematic review and meta-analysis

Xiongfeng Pan[1], Zhipeng Wang[1], Xiaoli Wu[1], Shi Wu Wen[2,3] and Aizhong Liu[1*]

## Abstract

**Background:** Studies investigating salivary cortisol level as susceptibility marker for post-traumatic stress disorder (PTSD) produced inconsistent results. The aim of this study was to compare salivary cortisol concentration levels in PTSD patients with those in controls by synthesizing published data.

**Methods:** We did a systematic review, meta-analysis and meta-regression of studies comparing concentrations of salivary cortisol between patients with PTSD and controls. The electronic databases of PubMed, Embase, Web of Science and Psyc-ARTICLES were searched for relevant articles. A random-effects model with restricted maximum-likelihood estimator is used to synthesize the effect size (assessed by standardized mean difference).

**Results:** A total of 784 articles were identified of which 22 were included in the final analysis. A trend of lower salivary cortisol levels was found in PTSD patients when compared with the controls (SMD = − 0.28, 95% CI-0.53;-0.04, $p = 0.022$). Subgroup analysis showed that the salivary cortisol levels were lower in patients with PTSD than in controls in studies conducted after 2007 or in studies using saliva samples collected in the morning.

**Conclusions:** The evidence from this meta-analysis supports that salivary samples collected in the morning consistently showed a lower salivary cortisol level in patients with PTSD than in controls, although whether salivary cortisol could be used as a diagnostic tool requires further research.

**Keywords:** Post-traumatic stress disorder, Salivary cortisol, Systematic review, Meta-analysis

## Background

Post-traumatic stress disorder (PTSD) is a common psychiatric and anxiety disorder caused by traumatic events [1]. It has a negative impact on the physical and mental health of the affected patients [2], as well as their professional and social life [3, 4], which may impose a large burden on patients' families and society. Indeed, PTSD is a kind of complex disease which may also be related to genetic factors (internal factors) and environmental factors (external factors) [5, 6]. Its etiology and pathogenesis have not been fully understood [6]. However, there is plenty of evidence that PTSD might be attributed to the disorder of the Hypothalamic-Pituitary-Adrenal axis (HPA axis) [7, 8]. Cortisol is an

adrenal glucocorticoid hormones secreted by the zona fasciculata in the adrenal cortex [9, 10]. It is the end product of the HPA axis in humans. When faced with stressors the body may produce a corresponding stress response [11]. At the same time the body may secrete large amounts of cortisol to inhibit stress response by metabolic action, which in turn restores the body back to its normal functionality [12, 13]. However, if the body has been in a state of high pressure which stimulates its stress response too often, then this may lead to passivation of the HPA axis [10, 14]. Moreover, if the HPA axis is not restored to normal, then abnormal cortisol levels may arise in patients with PTSD [15]. Therefore, cortisol could be used as a biomarker for patients with PTSD [16].

Various biological specimens, including plasma, serum, saliva, cerebrospinal fluid and urine are used to measure cortisol [12, 17]. In addition, acquisition process of salivary measurement has been proposed as a noninvasive

* Correspondence: lazroy@live.cn
[1]Department of Epidemiology and Health Statistics, Xiangya School of Public Health, Central South University, Changsha, China
Full list of author information is available at the end of the article

method [18]. We focus on the salivary cortisol mainly for the consideration of practice applications. Salivary cortisol is more readily available than urine specimens, and is more convenient to collect at home for large scale epidemiological studies [19].

A much debated question is whether salivary cortisol could be used as a susceptibility marker for PTSD patients [20]. Studies investigating salivary cortisol as a susceptibility marker for PTSD patients have produced different results [12], which may be attributed to the differences in investigation time, sampling time, type of trauma, assessment tools for PTSD symptoms, and collection and analysis of salivary cortisol [21, 22].

There has been no meta-analysis specifically targeted on salivary cortisol as a susceptibility marker for PTSD patients, although some previous studies have included salivary cortisol in subgroup analyses [12].

The purpose of this study is to compare salivary cortisol levels between PTSD patients and controls using a meta-analysis of existing studies. We also used regression and subgroup analyses to explore the sources of heterogeneity among studies [23].

## Methods
### Identification and selection of studies
PRISMA guidelines were used for this systematic review and meta-analysis [24]. Online electronic databases were searched from September 1987 until September 2017 for articles published in English. These included PubMed, Embase, Web of Science and Psyc-ARTICLES. Experienced librarians designed these searches, which used the following keywords:((((((((((((cortisol in saliva [Title/Abstract]) OR saliva cortisol [Title/Abstract]) OR glucocorticoids in saliva[Title/Abstract]) OR saliva glucocorticoid[Title/Abstract])OR steroid hormones in saliva [Title/Abstract]) OR saliva steroid [Title/Abstract]) OR corticosteroids in saliva[Title/Abstract]) OR saliva corticosteroid[Title/Abstract])) OR Salivary Cortisol[Title/Abstract]))AND((PTSD[Title/Abstract]) OR Posttraumatic Stress Disorder[Title/Abstract]). These terms were adapted for the other databases and the detailed search strategies are shown in the Additional file 1. The detailed search strategies are shown in the Fig. 1.

### Eligibility criteria
Two researchers independently screened and selected the relevant articles. In case of disagreement the final decision was made after consultation with a third party [25]. Moreover, the grey literatures were not included in our study. Primary inclusion criteria for articles for this study were: the study included PTSD cases and control groups, reported PTSD diagnostic criteria, and reported the mean and standard deviation (SD) of salivary cortisol. Exclusion criteria were: studies investigating PTSD

with other comorbid disorders, or HPA axis disorder and review articles [26].

### Data extraction
This study used Note Express of Central South University in order to gain insights into analyses, and manage articles. Trauma-exposed controls (TC) and non-trauma-exposed controls (NTC) were all eligible as control groups. Since most studies reported TC for 81.8% (18/22), we chose TC as control groups when both TC and NTC were included. In addition, we analyzed the relation between PTSD and all NTC as control groups as a supplement [27]. The following characteristics were extracted from each eligible article: first author, publication year, sex, ages of participants, participant number, salivary cortisol concentration level mean ± standard deviation, country where the study was conducted (study country), trauma type [28], PTSD assessment method, saliva collection time [28], salivary cortisol collection and assay methods, inter-assay variation, intra-assay variation, sensitivity and T-frozen (temperature of frozen). Salivary cortisol unit conversion which we used was 1 g/dl = 27.59 nmol/L [29].

### Statistical analyses
All analyses were carried out using R software (version R i386 3.4.2). Meta-analysis and meta-regression analysis were performed using R software with package metafor [30]. The random-effects model with restricted maximum-likelihood estimator was used to synthesize the effect size in the studies. Standardised mean difference (SMD) was used to assess the effect size, calculated by using Cohen's d. Significance level was set at 0.05 for all statistical tests. If the SMD level was ≤0.2 then it was considered low effect; if it was 0.2–0.7 then moderate effect; if it was ≥0.8 then large effect [31, 32]. Begg's rank correlation test was used to check publication bias. The Q statistic was used to test the presence of heterogeneity and the $I^2$ statistic was used to quantify the percentage of variability. Maximal heterogeneity is indicated by an $I^2 = 100\%$ whereas no heterogeneity is indicated by an $I^2 = 0$ [33]. In addition, subgroup analyses were conducted with regard to saliva collection time and study year. We also performed meta-regression analysis to explore other sources of heterogeneity. The following 8 variables were included in this analysis: Country (USA = 1,other = 0), PTSD assessment (DSM-IV CAPS = 1, other = 0), collection time (am = 1,pm = 0), publication year (study year≥2007 = 1, < 2007 = 0), assayed methods (report = 1,Unreported = 0), inter-assay variation (report = 1,Unreported = 0), intra-assay variation (report = 1,Unreported = 0), sensitivity (report = 1,Unreported = 0) and frozen (report = 1,Unreported = 0).

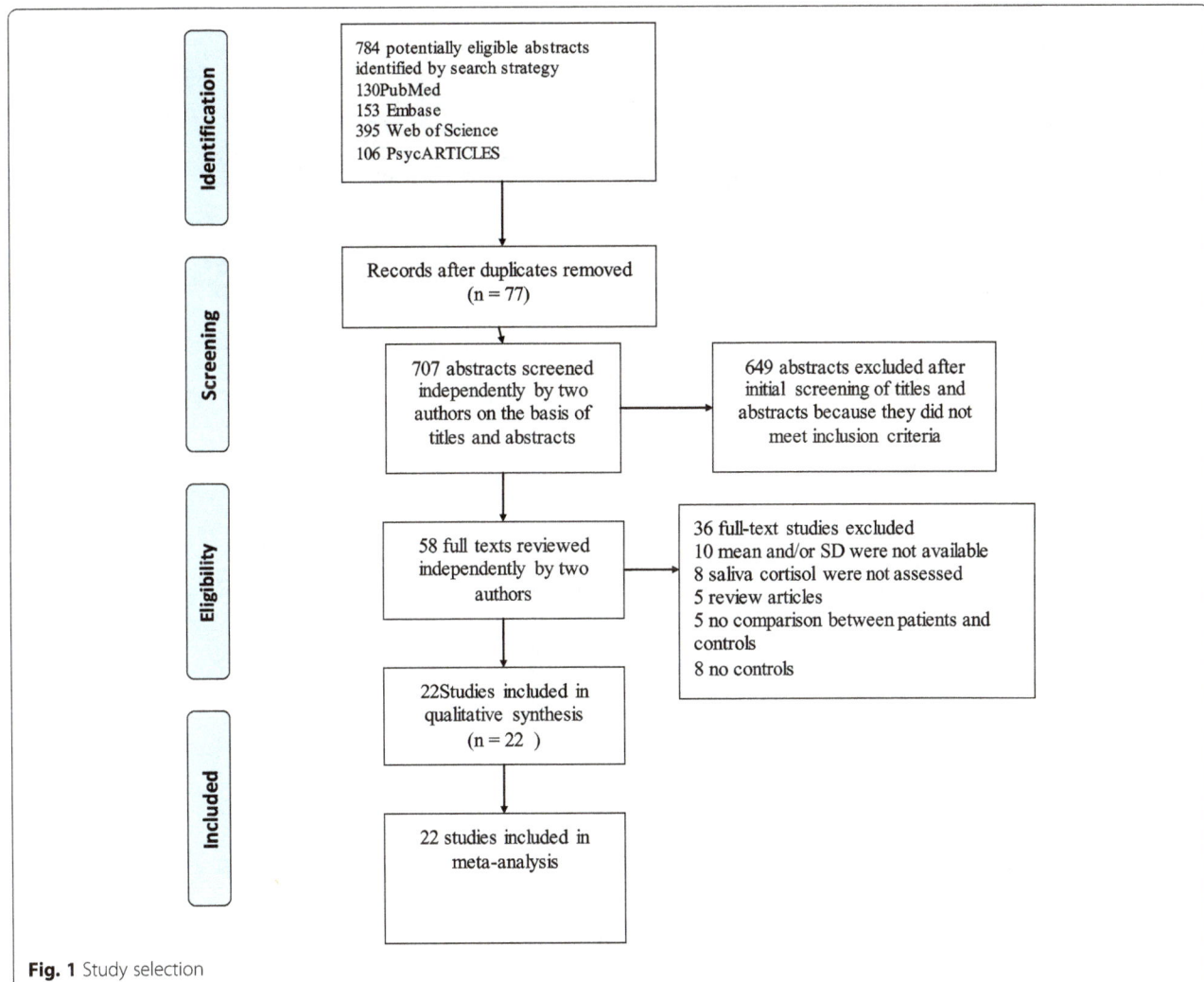

**Fig. 1** Study selection

## Results

### Literature search

Literature search produced an aggregate of 784 relevant articles of which 130 were from PubMed, 153 from Embase, 395 from Web of Science and 106 from PsycARTICLES. Of these, 77 were excluded because they were duplicates. Further assessment of abstracts of the 707 remaining articles resulted in 649 exclusions for failing to meet the inclusion criteria. The 58 full articles left were reviewed by two authors independently. Then 10 articles were excluded for not reporting means (SDs), 8 articles were excluded for not assessing saliva cortisol, 5 articles were excluded because they were review articles, 5 articles were excluded for not reporting results comparing patients and controls, and 8 articles were excluded for not reporting results in controls. In the end, 22 eligible articles were included for this study (Fig. 1).

### Characteristics of eligible articles

Table 1 presents characteristics of the 22 eligible studies. Most articles reported saliva collection time, salivary cortisol collection and assay methods, inter-assay variation, intra-assay variation, sensitivity and T-frozen.

### Salivary cortisol levels in PTSD as compared with controls

Table 2 displays the summarized salivary cortisol concentration levels between PTSD patients and the controls. A trend showing lower salivary cortisol concentration levels was observed in PTSD patients as compared to the controls (SMD = $-0.28$, 95% CI $-0.53$; $-0.04$, $p = 0.022$). There was also an overall difference in the pooled effect size between people with PTSD and NTC (SMD = $-0.33$, 95% CI $-0.63$; $-0.03$, $p = 0.032$). Figures 2 and 3 compare the salivary cortisol effect sizes (SMD) of studies using samples collected in the morning (am) with those of studies using samples collected in the afternoon (pm). The same was also compared between

**Table 1** Characteristics of studies included in the meta-analysis

| Study | N | Country | Trauma type | Controls | Female | Mean Age | PTSD Assessment | Collection time | Assayed Methods | Interassay variation | Intra-assay variation | Sensitivity | T-frozen |
|---|---|---|---|---|---|---|---|---|---|---|---|---|---|
| Carrion 2001 [43] | 51 | USA | Mixed trauma | NTC | 21 | 10.7 | DSM-IV Reaction Index | AM,PM | RIA | 12% | NR | NR | −20 °C |
| Coupland 2003 [44] | 66 | Canada | Abuse | NTC | 66 | 38 ± 11 | DSM-IV CAPS-1 | AM,PM | ELISA | 2% | 8% | 0.05 mg/dl. | −80 °C |
| Feldman 2013 [45] | 232 | Israeli | Combat | TC,NTC | 110 | 1.5–5.0 | Clinicians diagnose | AM | ELISA | 10.5% | 13.4% | NR | −20 °C |
| Gill 2008 [46] | 71 | USA | Civilian trauma | TC,NTC | 71 | 42.9 ± 7.82 | DSM-IV CAPS | PM | ELISA | 9% | 9% | NR | −80 °C |
| Kloet 2006 [47] | 83 | Netherland | Combat | TC,NTC | 0 | 34.1 ± 5.8 | DSM-IV CAPS | AM,PM | RIA | 4% | 5.5–9% | NR | −80 °C |
| Kobayashi 2014 [48] | 39 | USA | Injury | TC | 7 | 40.3 ± 10.7 | DSM-IV CAPS | AM,PM | RIA | NR | NR | NR | −20 °C |
| Lindauer 2006 [49] | 24 | Netherland | Mixed trauma | TC | 10 | 35.1 ± 11.4 | DSM-IV CAPS | AM,PM | RIA | 10% | 10% | NR | −20 °C |
| Lipschitz, DS 2003 [50] | 48 | USA | Mixed trauma | TC,NTC | 37 | 16.4 ± 2.6 | DSM-IV CTQ | AM | RIA | 8.00% | 9.00% | NR | −80 °C |
| Mcfarlane 2011 [51] | 48 | Australia | Traumatic accident | TC | 12 | 34 ± 12.7 | DSM-IV CAPS | AM,PM | RIA | NR | NR | NR | −20 °C |
| Neylan 2009 [52] | 22 | USA | Combat | TC | 0 | 51.1 ± 2.5 | DSM-IV SCID | AM | NR | NR | NR | NR | NR |
| Tucker 2010 [53] | 100 | USA | Bombing registry | TC,NTC | 54 | 47.0 ± 10.0 | DSM-IV DIS | AM | RIA | NR | NR | NR | −20 °C |
| Roth 2007 [54] | 218 | Sweden | Combat | TC | 122 | NR | DSM-IV HTQ | AM | RIA | 10% | 10% | 0.8 nmol/l | −70 °C |
| Shalev 2007 [55] | 155 | Israel | Road traffic accidents | TC | 64 | 31.2 ± 11.6 | DSM-IV CAPS | AM | NR | NR | NR | NR | −40 °C |
| Su, T 2009 [56] | 27 | China | Mixed trauma | NTC | 2 | 43.15 ± 12.8 | DSM-IV CAPS | AM | RIA | 3% | 6% | 10 pg/tube | −80 °C |
| Wahbeh 2013 [57] | 71 | USA | Combat | TC | 0 | 55.5 ± 8.9 | DSM-IV CAPS | AM,PM | ELISA | 4.74% | 3.03% | NR | NR |
| Witteveen, AB 2010 [58] | 1880 | Netherlands | Mixed trauma | TC | 141 | 47.0 ± 8.0 | DSM-IV CAPS | AM,PM | RIA | NR | NR | NR | −20 °C |
| Yehuda 2005 [59] | 63 | USA | Holocaust | TC,NTC | 36 | 69.7 ± 5.0 | DSM-IV CAPS | AM,PM | RIA | 3.90% | 12.00% | 10 ng/dl | NR |
| Yehuda, R 2005 [60] | 67 | USA | Holocaust | TC,NTC | 34 | 68.5 ± 5.9 | DSM-IV CAPS | AM,PM | RIA | 3.90% | 12.00% | 10 ng/dl | NR |
| Young, EA 2004 [61] | 516 | USA | Mixed trauma | TC,NTC | 457 | 36.8 ± 2.2 | DSM-III | AM,PM | NR | 6.50% | 5.00% | 1 ng/mL | −20 °C |
| Young 2004 [62] | 171 | USA | Mixed trauma | TC,NTC | 171 | 18–54 | DSM-III | AM,PM | NR | 10% | NR | 2 µg/dL | −20 °C |
| Steven 2004 [63] | 34 | USA | Childhood trauma | NTC | 30 | 40.3 ± 3.3 | DSM-IV CAPS | AM | ELISA | 5.70% | 6.90% | 7 µg/dL | NR |
| Neylan 2003 [64] | 32 | USA | Combat | TC | 0 | 49.4 ± 5.7 | DSM-IV CAPS | AM | NR | NR | NR | NR | NR |

*TC* Trauma-exposed controls, *NTC* Non-trauma-exposed controls, *RIA* Radioimmunoassay, *ELISA* Enzyme linked immunosorbent assay, *CAPS* Clinician-administered PTSD scale, *NR* Not report, *USA* United States of America, *T-frozen* Temperature of frozen

**Table 2** Meta-analysis of salivary cortisol markers in PTSD

| | Participants with PTSD, n | controls n | SMD (95% CI) | p value | Heterogeneity | | | Begg'S test Kendall's tau statistic (p value) |
|---|---|---|---|---|---|---|---|---|
| | | | | | Q statistic (DF; p value) | $\tau^2$ | $I^2$ | |
| all | 1064 | 2322 | −0.28 (−0.53; −0.04) | 0.022 | 236.00(33 < 0.0001) | 0.427 | 86.00% | −0.1907, p = 0.117 |
| am | 628 | 1316 | −0.39 (− 0.70; − 0.09) | 0.012 | 132.68(20 < 0.0001) | 0.412 | 84.90% | −0.2000, p = 0.219 |
| pm | 436 | 1006 | −0.11 (− 0.52; 0.30) | 0.598 | 96.40(12 < 0.0001) | 0.476 | 87.60% | −0.1795, p = 0.435 |
| <2007 | 659 | 734 | −0.13 (− 0.50; 0.23) | 0.479 | 163.59(18 < 0.0001) | 0.568 | 89.00% | −0.2281, p = 0.186 |
| ≥2007 | 405 | 1588 | −0.48 (− 0.75; − 0.20) | 0.001 | 52.71(14 < 0.0001) | 0.199 | 73.40% | −0.2952, p = 0.140 |

*PTSD* post-traumatic stress disorder, *SMD* standardised mean difference, *DF* degrees of freedom

studies conducted before 2007 and those conducted after 2007. It should be noted that a recent similar systematic review and meta-analysis on adults was published in 2007 and it performed subgroup analysis of salivary cortisol in PTSD [12]. Since then, there has been a rapid development of various salivary cortisol analyzers. Therefore, we wanted to know whether the situation had changed 10 years later after the publication of that systematic review and meta-analysis in 2007. Hence, we performed subgroup analysis related to the eligible studies published before 2007, and those published after 2007. The results of subgroup analyses showed that the differences in salivary cortisol concentration levels between PTSD patients and the controls was bigger in studies that used samples collected in the morning than in those studies that used samples collected in the afternoon. Also, higher differences were observed in studies conducted after 2007 than in those conducted before 2007. Moreover, the biggest difference in salivary cortisol concentration level was observed in studies that used

morning samples and those conducted after 2007. No differences were found for afternoon samples ($p = 0.598$), whereas in the morning people with PTSD had lower levels of cortisol than controls (SMD = − 0.39, 95% Cl − 0.70; − 0.09, $p = 0.012$). Whereas the studies conducted before 2007 did not reveal significant differences ($p = 0.479$), PTSD in studies conducted after 2007 had highly significant lower salivary cortisol levels than their comparison groups (SMD = − 0.48, 95% Cl − 0.75; − 0.20, $p = 0.001$).

### Meta-regression analyses

Table 3 presents the results of meta-regression analysis. It shows that country of study, sample collection time, study year, saliva cortisol assayed instrument reporting method, inter-assay variation reporting, intra-assay variation reporting, sensitivity reporting and frozen sample reporting were not significantly different. Recall that the meta-regression analysis was used to explore sources of heterogeneity among the eligible studies. If results indicate not

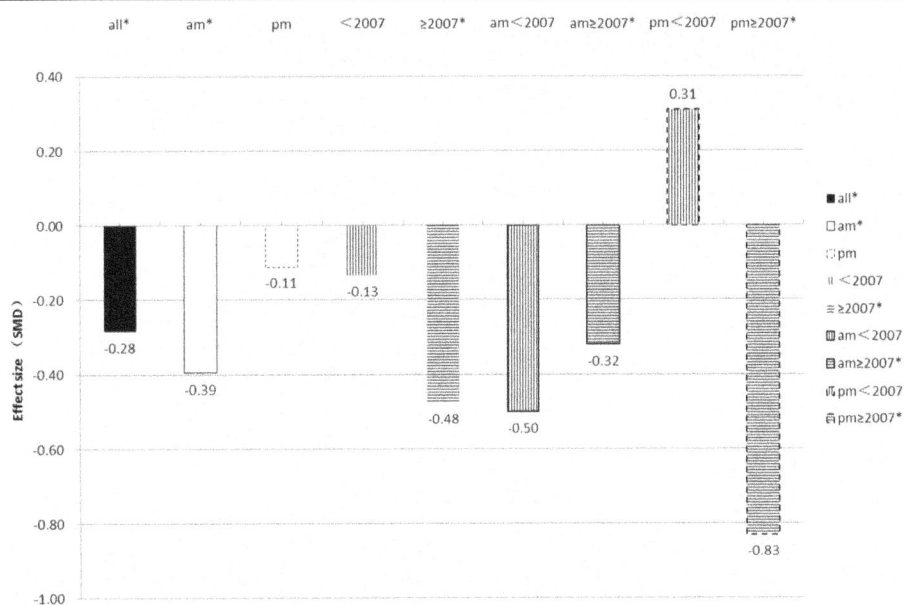

**Fig. 2** Salivary cortisol effect size. Salivary cortisol effect size (SMD) for studies examining in the morning (am), afternoon (pm), before 2007, and after 2007 levels in PTSD and control groups. PTSD,posttraumatic stress disorder; am, morning (before 12 pm); pm, afternoon (after 12 pm);<2007,before 2007;≥2007, after 2007;*p < 0.05

| Study | Total | PTSD Mean | SD | Total | Control Mean | SD | Standardised Mean Difference | SMD | 95%–CI | Weight |
|---|---|---|---|---|---|---|---|---|---|---|
| Carrion2001AM | 51 | 11.86 | 4.41 | 31 | 11.59 | 5.79 | | 0.05 | [−0.39; 0.50] | 3.2% |
| Carrion2001PM | 51 | 4.69 | 3.31 | 31 | 3.86 | 3.59 | | 0.24 | [−0.21; 0.69] | 3.2% |
| Coupland2003AM | 33 | 33.38 | 61.53 | 33 | 41.66 | 50.77 | | −0.15 | [−0.63; 0.34] | 3.2% |
| Coupland2003PM | 33 | 8.00 | 52.70 | 33 | 8.83 | 54.35 | | −0.02 | [−0.50; 0.47] | 3.2% |
| Lipschitz, D S2003 | 20 | 18.32 | 9.71 | 19 | 15.48 | 10.13 | | 0.28 | [−0.35; 0.91] | 2.9% |
| Neylan2003 | 24 | 12.50 | 5.40 | 18 | 14.20 | 6.30 | | −0.29 | [−0.90; 0.33] | 3.0% |
| Steven2004 | 17 | 22.90 | 3.59 | 17 | 29.25 | 5.24 | | −1.38 | [−2.14; −0.62] | 2.7% |
| Young, E A2004AM | 68 | 12.69 | 8.83 | 183 | 13.24 | 8.28 | | −0.07 | [−0.34; 0.21] | 3.5% |
| Young, E A2004PM | 68 | 4.69 | 4.97 | 183 | 3.86 | 4.14 | | 0.19 | [−0.09; 0.47] | 3.5% |
| Young2004AM | 70 | 13.24 | 0.83 | 16 | 11.86 | 2.21 | | 1.14 | [0.57; 1.71] | 3.0% |
| Young2004PM | 70 | 6.90 | 1.93 | 16 | 4.14 | 1.38 | | 1.48 | [0.89; 2.07] | 3.0% |
| Yehuda,R2005AM | 23 | 9.80 | 2.65 | 25 | 22.15 | 2.32 | | −4.89 | [−6.06; −3.72] | 2.0% |
| Yehuda,R2005PM | 23 | 9.94 | 2.32 | 25 | 8.08 | 2.23 | | 0.80 | [0.21; 1.40] | 3.0% |
| Yehuda2005AM | 19 | 12.19 | 6.99 | 16 | 19.70 | 9.12 | | −0.91 | [−1.62; −0.21] | 2.8% |
| Yehuda2005PM | 19 | 6.54 | 6.85 | 16 | 4.09 | 21.66 | | 0.15 | [−0.51; 0.82] | 2.9% |
| Kloet2006AM | 23 | 13.50 | 6.00 | 24 | 22.00 | 7.60 | | −1.22 | [−1.84; −0.59] | 2.9% |
| Kloet2006PM | 23 | 7.00 | 2.40 | 24 | 9.00 | 3.40 | | −0.67 | [−1.25; −0.08] | 3.0% |
| Lindauer2006AM | 12 | 28.60 | 25.70 | 12 | 9.90 | 7.00 | | 0.96 | [0.11; 1.81] | 2.5% |
| Lindauer2006PM | 12 | 8.80 | 5.50 | 12 | 7.20 | 3.40 | | 0.34 | [−0.47; 1.14] | 2.6% |
| Roth2007 | 41 | 8.69 | 2.19 | 15 | 11.51 | 9.41 | | −0.54 | [−1.14; 0.06] | 3.0% |
| Shalev2007 | 26 | 19.25 | 13.34 | 89 | 23.50 | 19.05 | | −0.24 | [−0.67; 0.20] | 3.3% |
| Gill2008 | 26 | 4.14 | 2.48 | 21 | 11.04 | 1.93 | | −3.01 | [−3.87; −2.15] | 2.5% |
| Neylan2009 | 11 | 23.89 | 8.61 | 11 | 27.23 | 11.81 | | −0.31 | [−1.15; 0.53] | 2.5% |
| Su, T2009 | 13 | 15.60 | 7.50 | 11 | 18.70 | 8.30 | | −0.38 | [−1.19; 0.43] | 2.6% |
| Tucker2010 | 11 | 9.38 | 3.31 | 50 | 6.62 | 4.41 | | 0.64 | [−0.02; 1.31] | 2.9% |
| Witteveen, A B2010AM | 39 | 13.10 | 5.90 | 588 | 14.30 | 6.50 | | −0.19 | [−0.51; 0.14] | 3.4% |
| Witteveen, A B2010PM | 40 | 8.90 | 4.50 | 575 | 10.10 | 5.40 | | −0.22 | [−0.54; 0.10] | 3.4% |
| Mcfarlane2011AM | 9 | 8.49 | 6.10 | 26 | 13.52 | 6.89 | | −0.73 | [−1.51; 0.05] | 2.6% |
| Mcfarlane2011PM | 9 | 4.46 | 4.17 | 22 | 5.49 | 3.75 | | −0.26 | [−1.04; 0.52] | 2.7% |
| Feldman2013 | 56 | 6.09 | 1.89 | 84 | 6.66 | 1.70 | | −0.32 | [−0.66; 0.02] | 3.4% |
| Wahbeh2013AM | 51 | 19.31 | 18.21 | 20 | 32.28 | 20.14 | | −0.68 | [−1.21; −0.15] | 3.1% |
| Wahbeh2013PM | 51 | 4.41 | 5.24 | 20 | 9.10 | 10.21 | | −0.67 | [−1.19; −0.14] | 3.1% |
| Kobayashi2014 | 11 | 7.70 | 3.80 | 28 | 19.30 | 18.40 | | −0.72 | [−1.43; 0.00] | 2.8% |
| Kobayashi2014 | 11 | 14.80 | 10.20 | 28 | 18.00 | 14.10 | | −0.24 | [−0.94; 0.46] | 2.8% |
| **Random effects model** | **1064** | | | **2322** | | | | **−0.28** | **[−0.53; −0.04]** | **100.0%** |
| Heterogeneity: $I^2 = 86\%$, $\tau^2 = 0.4267$, $p < 0.01$ | | | | | | | | | | |

−2 −1 0 1 2
Decreased in PTSD   Decreased in controls

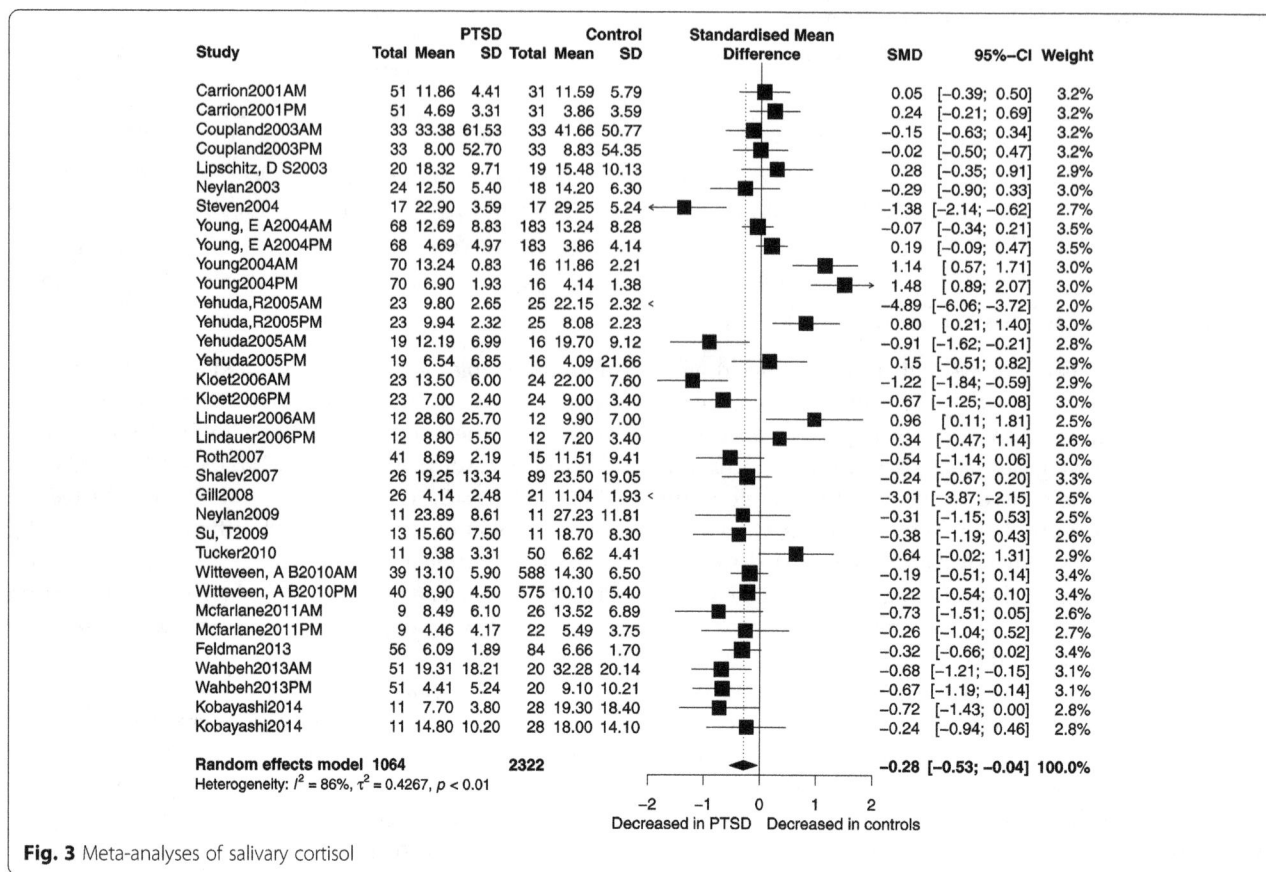

**Fig. 3** Meta-analyses of salivary cortisol

significantly different, it means the variables in question cannot explain the overall heterogeneity. However, in our case, after introducing PTSD assessment methods into the meta-regression analysis model, results showed that sources of heterogeneity can be explained by PTSD assessment methods as the difference was significant. (b = − 0.812, 95%CI -1.540;-0.084, $p = 0.0288$).

### Heterogeneity and bias analysis
Heterogeneity was reported to be high among the eligible studies ($I^2 > 75\%$). However, for the subgroup analysis stratified by study year, the combined heterogeneity

**Table 3** Separate univariate meta-regression model of salivary cortisol in PTSD, PTSD = post-traumatic stress disorder

| | Estimate | se | zval | pval | ci.lb | ci.ub |
|---|---|---|---|---|---|---|
| Collection time | − 0.306 | 0.362 | − 0.844 | 0.399 | −1.015 | 0.404 |
| Country | −0.085 | 0.362 | −0.236 | 0.814 | −0.795 | 0.624 |
| Publication year | −0.352 | 0.351 | −1.002 | 0.316 | −1.041 | 0.337 |
| PTSD assessment | −0.812 | 0.371 | −2.187 | 0.029 | −1.540 | −0.084 |
| Assayed methods | −0.344 | 0.384 | −0.896 | 0.370 | −1.097 | 0.409 |
| Inter-assay variation | −0.090 | 0.391 | −0.229 | 0.819 | −0.857 | 0.677 |
| Frozen | 0.686 | 0.390 | 1.762 | 0.078 | −0.077 | 1.450 |

of studies declined from 92 to 33%. This change in heterogeneity indicated that studies conducted after 2007 had more consistent and homogeneous results.

Begg's rank correlation test revealed no potential publication bias ($p = 0.117$), implying that there was low probability of publication bias.

### Discussion
Generally, concentrations of salivary cortisol were lower in patients with PTSD than in the controls (SMD = − 0.28, 95% CI -0.53; − 0.04, $p = 0.022$). There was also an overall difference in the pooled effect size between people with PTSD and NTC. Specifically, our findings suggest that PTSD status affects basal salivary cortisol levels; some people do not develop PTSD despite experiencing a trauma similar to that of PTSD patients [34]. The exact biological mechanisms underlying the altered long-term salivary cortisol output as a result of trauma remain largely unknown [35]. Speculatively, decreased output of salivary cortisol after developing PTSD may evolve as a compensatory anti-glucocorticoid mechanism [16, 36], to inhibit negative effects of long-term increased negative glucocorticoid feedback sensitivity of glucocorticoid receptors that have been observed in PTSD patients

irrespective of trauma-exposed status. However, this remains to be further investigated [16].

As far as we know, this is the first study to perform systematic review, meta-analysis and meta-regression on the salivary cortisol concentration levels in PTSD, particularly by considering studies reporting salivary cortisol as a susceptibility marker for PTSD. Nonetheless, there are three previous systematic reviews and meta-analyses which investigated the relationship between Cortisol and post-traumatic stress disorder. One of which included only 7 salivary cortisol studies from two databases [12], another one only used 9 PTSD salivary cortisol subgroup studies [16], and the next one used only 3 salivary cortisol studies [20]. These studies found no relationship between cortisol concentration levels and PTSD. In addition, these studies did not take into account the sample source from which cortisol concentration levels were measured. For example, they included plasma/serum, saliva or urine samples, even if it is well known that the cortisol concentration levels varied from sample to sample between sufficient samples from different sources. The use of small sample sizes might have contributed to the results of no significant relationship between cortisol concentration levels and PTSD. Noteworthy, the methods for collecting salivary cortisol, testing and analyzing cortisol concentration levels have improved in more recent years. These include immunoassay or liquid chromatography-tandem mass spectrometry (LC-MS/MS) for the measurement of salivary cortisol [37, 38]. Therefore, there is need to update literature to include these new methods when investigating the relationship between cortisol concentration levels and PTSD. Accordingly, in this study, we enlarged the scope of article searching in the online electronic databases, which eventually yielded 22 eligible studies which collectively had 1064 participants with PTSD and 2322 controls. Thus, compared with the preceding previous studies, this study used relatively larger sample size which would make conclusions more comparable and convincing. Also, unlike in the preceding studies, this study focused only on salivary cortisol concentration levels when investigating its association with PTSD because results of the same investigation, using different sample sources for cortisol concentration levels, may be problematic to interpret since cortisol concentration levels differ with different sample sources. Thus, using the 22 eligible studies, some interesting significant results were found. In the analysis according to whether saliva samples were taken in the morning or in the afternoon, it was found that PTSD patients had lower levels of salivary cortisol than controls in studies which used saliva samples taken in the morning but not in those studies which used saliva samples taken in the afternoon. With regard to methodological aspects, and due to the

pulsatile nature of adrenal steroid release, there are inherent limitations when using single-point measurements of basal salivary cortisol concentration levels [39]. More specifically, it is known that the cortisol release follows a circadian rhythm such as cortisol awakening response [40]. Additionally, specific basal morning salivary cortisol concentration levels seem to be lower in PTSD patients, while basal cortisol concentration level assessments at other times during the day do not seem to be associated with PTSD. Therefore, it could be speculated that PTSD patients' cortisol awakening response was insensitive [40], whereas that of the control groups was more nimble in the morning. Considering the preceding cortisol awakening response hypothesis, it could be suggested that the ideal time for morning saliva sampling is after awakening. We suggest that researchers control for waking when saliva samples are to be collected in the morning in practical investigation (by getting people to wake at the same time, e.g. 8.00 am).

Moreover, the indicator of publication year is selected through the group discussion and the literature review, we want to evaluate that whether the previous mixed findings on cortisol levels in PTSD could be due to time of sample collection and older assays (prior to 2007). Since the recent meta-analysis article was appear in 2007 which included subgroup analysis to distribution and function of salivary cortisol in PTSD [12]. Furthermore, in the analysis according to whether studies were conducted before 2007 or after 2007, it was observed that the difference in salivary cortisol concentration levels between PTSD patients and controls was observed only in studies which were conducted after 2007. Results of Begg's rank correlation test revealed low probability of publication bias.

In summary, this systematic review and meta-analysis found that concentrations of salivary cortisol were consistently and homogeneously lower in patients with PTSD than in the controls when the analysis included only studies conducted after 2007 and studies which used saliva samples collected in the morning. Future studies on salivary cortisol concentration levels in PTSD patients should take the following aspects into consideration:

① Saliva collection time should be unified. Considering the preceding cortisol awakening response hypothesis, it could be suggested that the ideal time for morning saliva sampling is after awakening. We suggest that researchers control for waking when saliva samples are to be collected in the morning in practical investigation (by getting people to wake at the same time, e.g. 8.00 am). Besides, the guidelines for assessment of the salivary cortisol must be strictly followed and these include: objective control of sampling adherence, participant instructions, sampling protocols and quantification strategies, as well as reporting and interpreting of salivary cortisol data [40].

② Storage methods of saliva must be unified. That is, the collected saliva sample should be stored at − 20 °C~ − 80 °C until assayed. Assay methods of saliva must be unified. We recommend using enzyme-linked im- munoassay and radioimmunoassay; and inter-assay and intra-assay coefficients of variation of lower than 10%.

③ The meta-regression analysis had 8 variables, of which only one was significant: PTSD assessment method (Table 3). It means this variable can explain the overall heterogeneity. Thus, we recommend using DSM-IVdiagnostic criteria with the clinician- administered PTSD scale (CAPS). This scale has proved to show high degree of reliability and validity, and can provide a better reference for further study of PTSD and salivary cortisol [41]. It is expected that meeting these consensus guidelines in future research could create more powerful research designs that would yield reliable and reproducible data and results. Although no biomarkers have yet demonstrated clinical applicability for PTSD [23, 41], in future, we believe that salivary cortisol could be a quick biomarker assay to assist in screening patients for PTSD hence promising a possi- bility for screening a lot of people within a short time for PTSD. After screening, clinicians can then assess symptom severity by conducting clinical interviews with those suspected of having PTSD. On the one hand, as we know from natural disasters (like earth- quake, hurricane, tsunami and flood) [42]; the affected population is generally large. Especially for developing countries such as China and India, with an enormous population density and limited psychiatrists, millions of people would be at high risk for PTSD after natural disasters. It can save a lot of clinicians and psychological guidance resources to enable the large- scale PTSD screening to become a reality.

Saliva is a specimen that is safe and easy to obtain in a large-scale epidemiological study. Therefore, develop- ment of rapid salivary cortisol test methods for PTSD screening could provide fast and cost-efficient means in large epidemiological studies, and in clinical practice, which could facilitate PTSD diagnosis, treatment, con- trol and prevention.

## Conclusions

The evidence from this meta-analysis supports that saliv- ary samples collected in the morning consistently showed a lower salivary cortisol level in patients with PTSD than in controls, although whether salivary cortisol could be used as a diagnostic tool requires further research.

## Abbreviations
<2007: Before 2007; ≥2007: After 2007; 95% CI: 95% confidence interval; Am: Morning (before 12 pm); CAPS: Clinician-administered PTSD scale; DF: Degrees of freedom; DSM-IV: Diagnostic and statistical manual of mental disorders, 4th edition; ELISA: Enzyme linked immunosorbent assay; NR: Not report; NTC: Non-trauma-exposed Controls; pm: Afternoon (after 12 pm); PRISMA: Preferred reporting items for systematic reviews and meta-analyses; PTSD: Post-traumatic stress disorder; RIA: Radioimmunoassay; SMD: Standardised mean difference; TC: Trauma-exposed controls

## Acknowledgements
We are grateful to Central South University Library for his assistance during the literature search. Besides, we are also thankful to Atipatsa C Kaminga for providing professional editing. Last but not least, we thank all the authors whose articles contributed an indispensable data for this systematic review and meta-analysis.

## Funding
This study has no funding. The corresponding author is ultimately responsible for the decision to submit it for publication and make full use of all the data in the study by Central South University Library.

## Authors' contributions
XP and AL contributed to the study design, while XP, ZW and XW contributed to the data collection. Statistical analyses and interpretation of results were performed by XP, ZW and XW. XP, AL and SW drafted the manuscript and edited the language. All the authors participated in the critical revision, and approved the final version of the manuscript.

## Consent for publication
Not applicable.

## Competing interests
The authors declare that they have no competing interests.

## Author details
[1]Department of Epidemiology and Health Statistics, Xiangya School of Public Health, Central South University, Changsha, China. [2]Department of Obstetrics and Gynaecology, University of Ottawa, Ottawa, ON, Canada. [3]Ottawa Hospital Research Institute, Ottawa, ON, Canada.

## References
1. Kornor H, Winje D, Ekeberg O, Weisaeth L, Kirkehei I, Johansen K, et al. Early trauma-focused cognitive-behavioural therapy to prevent chronic post-traumatic stress disorder and related symptoms: a systematic review and meta-analysis. BMC Psychiatry. 2008;8:81. https://doi.org/10.1186/1471-244X-8-81.
2. Feduccia AA, Mithoefer MC. MDMA-assisted psychotherapy for PTSD: are memory reconsolidation and fear extinction underlying mechanisms?

Prog Neuro-Psychoph. 2018;84(A):221–8. https://doi.org/10.1016/j.pnpbp.2018.03.003.

3. Heeke C, Stammel N, Heinrich M, Knaevelsrud C. Conflict-related trauma and bereavement: exploring differential symptom profiles of prolonged grief and posttraumatic stress disorder. BMC Psychiatry. 2017;17(1):118. https://doi.org/10.1186/s12888-017-1286-2.

4. Knezevic M, Krupic D, Sucurovic S. Emotional competence and combat-related PTSD symptoms in Croatian Howeland war veterans. Drustvena Istrazivanja. 2017;26(1):1–18. https://doi.org/10.5559/di.26.1.01.

5. Rona RJ, Burdett H, Bull S, Jones M, Jones N, Greenberg N, et al. Prevalence of PTSD and other mental disorders in UK service personnel by time since end of deployment: a meta-analysis. BMC Psychiatry. 2016;16(1):333. https://doi.org/10.1186/s12888-016-1038-8.

6. Lolk M, Byberg S, Carlsson J, Norredam M. Somatic comorbidity among migrants with posttraumatic stress disorder and depression - a prospective cohort study. BMC Psychiatry. 2016;16(1):447. https://doi.org/10.1186/s12888-016-1149-2.

7. Klaassens ER, Giltay EJ, Cuijpers P, van Veen T, Zitman FG. Adulthood trauma and HPA-axis functioning in healthy subjects and PTSD patients: a meta-analysis. Psychoneuroendocrinology. 2012;37(3):317–31. https://doi.org/10.1016/j.psyneuen.2011.07.003.

8. Savic D, Knezevic G, Damjanovic S, Spiric Z, Matic G. The role of personality and traumatic events in cortisol levels - where does PTSD fit in? Psychoneuroendocrinology. 2012;37(7):937–47. https://doi.org/10.1016/j.psyneuen.2011.11.001.

9. Lokhmatkina NV, Feder G, Blake S, Morris R, Powers V, Lightman S. Longitudinal measurement of cortisol in association with mental health and experience of domestic violence and abuse: study protocol. BMC Psychiatry. 2013;13:188. https://doi.org/10.1186/1471-244X-13-188.

10. Suliman S, Ericksen T, Labuschgne P, de Wit R, Stein DJ, Seedat S. Comparison of pain, cortisol levels, and psychological distress in women undergoing surgical termination of pregnancy under local anaesthesia versus intravenous sedation. BMC Psychiatry. 2007;7:24. https://doi.org/10.1186/1471-244X-7-24.

11. Ventura-Junca R, Symon A, Lopez P, Fiedler JL, Rojas G, Heskia C, et al. Relationship of cortisol levels and genetic polymorphisms to antidepressant response to placebo and fluoxetine in patients with major depressive disorder: a prospective study. BMC Psychiatry. 2014;14:220. https://doi.org/10.1186/s12888-014-0220-0.

12. Meewisse ML, Reitsma JB, de Vries GJ, Gersons BP, Olff M. Cortisol and post-traumatic stress disorder in adults: systematic review and meta-analysis. Br J Psychiatry. 2007;191:387–92. https://doi.org/10.1192/bjp.bp.106.024877.

13. Savic D, Knezevic G, Damjanovic S, Spiric Z, Matic G. Is there a biological difference between trauma-related depression and PTSD? DST says 'NO'. Psychoneuroendocrinology. 2012;37(9):1516–20. https://doi.org/10.1016/j.psyneuen.2012.02.005.

14. Melin EO, Thunander M, Landin-Olsson M, Hillman M, Thulesius HO. Depression differed by midnight cortisol secretion, alexithymia and anxiety between diabetes types: a cross sectional comparison. BMC Psychiatry. 2017;17(1):335. https://doi.org/10.1186/s12888-017-1495-8.

15. Fragkaki I, Thomaes K, Sijbrandij M. Posttraumatic stress disorder under ongoing threat: a review of neurobiological and neuroendocrine findings. Eur J Psychotraumatol. 2016;7:30915.

16. Morris MC, Compas BE, Garber J. Relations among posttraumatic stress disorder, comorbid major depression, and HPA function: a systematic review and meta-analysis. Clin Psychol Rev. 2012;32(4):301–15. https://doi.org/10.1016/j.cpr.2012.02.002.

17. Stalder T, Steudte-Schmiedgen S, Alexander N, Klucken T, Vater A, Wichmann S, et al. Stress-related and basic determinants of hair cortisol in humans: a meta-analysis. Psychoneuroendocrinology. 2017;77:261–74. https://doi.org/10.1016/j.psyneuen.2016.12.017.

18. Skoluda N, Linnemann A, Nater UM. The role of week(end)-day and awakening time on cortisol and alpha-amylase awakening responses. Stress. 2016;19(3):333–8. https://doi.org/10.1080/10253890.2016.1174850.

19. Olivera-Figueroa LA, Juster RP, Morin-Major JK, Marin MF, Lupien SJ. A time to be stressed? Time perspectives and cortisol dynamics among healthy adults. Biol Psychol. 2015;111:90–9. https://doi.org/10.1016/j.biopsycho.2015.09.002.

20. Morris MC, Hellman N, Abelson JL, Rao U. Cortisol, heart rate, and blood pressure as early markers of PTSD risk: a systematic review and meta-analysis. Clin Psychol Rev. 2016;49:79–91. https://doi.org/10.1016/j.cpr.2016.09.001.

21. Wild B, Stadnitski T, Wesche D, Stroe-Kunold E, Schultz JH, Rudofsky G, et al. Temporal relationships between awakening cortisol and psychosocial variables in inpatients with anorexia nervosa - a time series approach. Int J Psychophysiol. 2016;102:25–32. https://doi.org/10.1016/j.ijpsycho.2016.03.002.

22. Hankin BL, Badanes LS, Smolen A, Young JF. Cortisol reactivity to stress among youth: stability over time and genetic variants for stress sensitivity. J Abnorm Psychol. 2015;124(1):54–67. https://doi.org/10.1037/abn0000030.

23. Passos IC, Vasconcelos-Moreno MP, Costa LG, Kunz M, Brietzke E, Quevedo J, et al. Inflammatory markers in post-traumatic stress disorder: a systematic review, meta-analysis, and meta-regression. Lancet Psychiatry. 2015;2(11):1002–12. https://doi.org/10.1016/S2215-0366(15)00309-0.

24. Moher D, Liberati A, Tetzlaff J, Altman DG. Preferred reporting items for systematic reviews and meta-analyses: the PRISMA statement. Int J Surg. 2010;8(5):336–41. https://doi.org/10.1016/j.ijsu.2010.02.007.

25. Samara MT, Goldberg Y, Levine SZ, Furukawa TA, Geddes JR, Cipriani A, et al. Initial symptom severity of bipolar I disorder and the efficacy of olanzapine: a meta-analysis of individual participant data from five placebo-controlled studies. Lancet Psychiatry. 2017;4(11):859–67. https://doi.org/10.1016/S2215-0366(17)30331-0.

26. Steudte S, Kirschbaum C, Gao W, Alexander N, Schonfeld S, Hoyer J, et al. Hair cortisol as a biomarker of traumatization in healthy individuals and posttraumatic stress disorder patients. Biol Psychiatry. 2013;74(9):639–46. https://doi.org/10.1016/j.biopsych.2013.03.011.

27. Nygaard M, Sonne C, Carlsson J. Secondary psychotic features in refugees diagnosed with post-traumatic stress disorder: a retrospective cohort study. BMC Psychiatry. 2017;17(1):5. https://doi.org/10.1186/s12888-016-1166-1.

28. DeSantis AS, Adam EK, Hawkley LC, Kudielka BM, Cacioppo JT. Racial and ethnic differences in diurnal cortisol rhythms: are they consistent over time? Psychosom Med. 2015;77(1):6–15. https://doi.org/10.1097/PSY.0000000000000131.

29. Kolassa IT, Eckart C, Ruf M, Neuner F, de Quervain DJ, Elbert T. Lack of cortisol response in patients with posttraumatic stress disorder (PTSD) undergoing a diagnostic interview. BMC Psychiatry. 2007;7:54. https://doi.org/10.1186/1471-244X-7-54.

30. Barbui C, Purgato M, Ostuzzi G. Regulatory meta-analyses for the evaluation of psychotropic medicines. Lancet Psychiatry. 2017;4(9):660–1. https://doi.org/10.1016/S2215-0366(17)30161-X.

31. Bouras N, Ikkos G, Craig T. Meta-community mental health care: towards a new concept. Lancet Psychiatry. 2017;4(8):581–2. https://doi.org/10.1016/S2215-0366(17)30108-6.

32. Cohen J, Cohen P, West SG, Aiken LS. Applied multiple regression-correlation analysis. J R Stat Soc. 2010;52(4):691.

33. Tran US, Gregor B. The relative efficacy of bona fide psychotherapies for post-traumatic stress disorder: a meta-analytical evaluation of randomized controlled trials. BMC Psychiatry. 2016;16:266. https://doi.org/10.1186/s12888-016-0979-2.

34. Norrholm SD, Jovanovic T. Fear processing, psychophysiology, and PTSD. Harvard Rev Psychiat. 2018;26(3):129–41. https://doi.org/10.1097/HRP.0000000000000189.

35. Allen AP, Kennedy PJ, Cryan JF, Dinan TG, Clarke G. Biological and psychological markers of stress in humans: focus on the Trier social stress test. Neurosci Biobehav Rev. 2014;38:94–124. https://doi.org/10.1016/j.neubiorev.2013.11.005.

36. Allen AP, Curran EA, Duggan A, Cryan JF, Chorcorain AN, Dinan TG, et al. A systematic review of the psychobiological burden of informal caregiving for patients with dementia: focus on cognitive and biological markers of chronic stress. Neurosci Biobehav Rev. 2017;73:123–64. https://doi.org/10.1016/j.neubiorev.2016.12.006.

37. Jessop DS, Turner-Cobb JM. Measurement and meaning of salivary cortisol: a focus on health and disease in children. Stress. 2008;11(1):1–14. https://doi.org/10.1080/10253890701365527.

38. Bae YJ, Gaudl A, Jaeger S, Stadelmann S, Hiemisch A, Kiess W, et al. Immunoassay or LC-MS/MS for the measurement of salivary cortisol in children? Clin Chem Lab Med. 2016;54(5):811–22. https://doi.org/10.1515/cclm-2015-0412.

39. Norrholm SD, Jovanovic T, Gerardi M, Breazeale KG, Price M, Davis M, et al. Baseline psychophysiological and cortisol reactivity as a predictor of PTSD treatment outcome in virtual reality exposure therapy. Behav Res Ther. 2016;82:28–37. https://doi.org/10.1016/j.brat.2016.05.002.

40. Stalder T, Kirschbaum C, Kudielka BM, Adam EK, Pruessner JC, Wuest S, et al. Assessment of the cortisol awakening response: expert consensus

guidelines. Psychoneuroendocrinology. 2016;63:414–32. https://doi.org/10.
   1016/j.psyneuen.2015.10.010.

41. Kruger-Gottschalk A, Knaevelsrud C, Rau H, Dyer A, Schafer I, Schellong J, et
   al. The German version of the posttraumatic stress disorder checklist for
   DSM-5 (PCL-5): psychometric properties and diagnostic utility. BMC
   Psychiatry. 2017;17(1):379. https://doi.org/10.1186/s12888-017-1541-6.

42. Dai W, Kaminga AC, Tan H, Wang J, Lai Z, Wu X, et al. Long-term
   psychological outcomes of flood survivors of hard-hit areas of the 1998
   Dongting Lake flood in China: prevalence and risk factors. PLoS One. 2017;
   12(2):e171557. https://doi.org/10.1371/journal.pone.0171557.

43. Carrion VG, Weems CF, Ray RD, Glaser B, Hessl D, Reiss AL. Diurnal salivary
   cortisol in pediatric posttraumatic stress disorder. Biol Psychiatry. 2002;51(7):
   575–82.

44. Coupland NJ, Hegadoren KM, Myrholm J. Increased beclomethasone-
   induced vasoconstriction in women with posttraumatic stress disorder.
   J Psychiatr Res. 2003;37(3):221–8.

45. Feldman R, Vengrober A, Eidelman-Rothman M, Zagoory-Sharon O. Stress
   reactivity in war-exposed young children with and without posttraumatic
   stress disorder: relations to maternal stress hormones, parenting, and child
   emotionality and regulation. Dev Psychopathol. 2013;25(4pt1):943–55.
   https://doi.org/10.1017/S0954579413000291.

46. Gill J, Vythilingam M, Page GG. Low cortisol, high DHEA, and high levels of
   stimulated TNF-α, and IL-6 in women with PTSD. J Trauma Stress. 2008;
   21(6):530–9. https://doi.org/10.1002/jts.20372.

47. de Kloet CS, Vermetten E, Heijnen CJ, Geuze E, Lentjes EGWM, Westenberg
   HGM. Enhanced cortisol suppression in response to dexamethasone
   administration in traumatized veterans with and without posttraumatic
   stress disorder. Psychoneuroendocrinology. 2007;32(3):215–26. https://doi.
   org/10.1016/j.psyneuen.2006.12.009.

48. Kobayashi I, Delahanty DL. Awake/sleep cortisol levels and the development
   of posttraumatic stress disorder in injury patients with peritraumatic
   dissociation. Psychol Trauma Theory Res Pract Policy. 2014;6(5):449–56.
   https://doi.org/10.1037/a0033013.

49. Lindauer RJL, Olff M, van Meijel EPM, Carlier IVE, Gersons BPR. Cortisol,
   learning, memory, and attention in relation to smaller hippocampal volume
   in police officers with posttraumatic stress disorder. Biol Psychiatry. 2006;
   59(2):171–7. https://doi.org/10.1016/j.biopsych.2005.06.033.

50. Lipschitz DS, Rasmusson AM, Yehuda R, Wang S, Anyan W, Gueoguieva R, et
   al. Salivary cortisol responses to dexamethasone in adolescents with
   posttraumatic stress disorder. J Am Acad Child Adolesc Psychiatry. 2003;
   42(11):1310–7. https://doi.org/10.1097/01.chi.0000084832.67701.0d.

51. McFarlane AC, Barton CA, Yehuda R, Wittert G. Cortisol response to acute
   trauma and risk of posttraumatic stress disorder. Psychoneuroendocrinology.
   2011;36(5):720–7. https://doi.org/10.1016/j.psyneuen.2010.10.007.

52. Neylan TC, Schuff N, Lenoci M, Yehuda R, Weiner MW. Cortisol levels are
   positively correlated with hippocampal N-Acetylaspartate. Biol Psychiatry.
   2003;54(10):1118–21. https://doi.org/10.1016/S0006-3223(03)01974-1.

53. Tucker P, Pfefferbaum B, North CS, Kent A, Jeon-Slaughter H, Parker DE.
   Biological correlates of direct exposure to terrorism several years
   postdisaster. Ann Clin Psychiatry. 2010;22(3):186–95.

54. Roth G, Ekblad S, Ågren H. A longitudinal study of PTSD in a sample of adult
   mass-evacuated Kosovars, some of whom returned to their home country.
   Eur Psychiat. 2006;21(3):152–9. https://doi.org/10.1016/j.eurpsy.2005.11.004.

55. Shalev AY, Videlock EJ, Peleg T, Segman R, Pitman RK, Yehuda R. Stress
   hormones and post-traumatic stress disorder in civilian trauma victims: a
   longitudinal study. Part I: HPA axis responses. Int J Neuropsychopharmacol.
   2008;11(03). https://doi.org/10.1017/S1461145707008127.

56. Su T, Zhang L, Chung M, Chen Y, Bi Y, Chou Y, et al. Levels of the potential
   biomarker p11 in peripheral blood cells distinguish patients with PTSD from
   those with other major psychiatric disorders. J Psychiatr Res. 2009;43(13):
   1078–85. https://doi.org/10.1016/j.jpsychires.2009.03.010.

57. Wahbeh H, Oken BS. Salivary cortisol lower in posttraumatic stress disorder.
   J Trauma Stress. 2013;26(2):241–8. https://doi.org/10.1002/jts.21798.

58. Witteveen AB, Huizink AC, Slottje P, Bramsen I, Smid T, van der Ploeg HM.
   Associations of cortisol with posttraumatic stress symptoms and negative
   life events: a study of police officers and firefighters.
   Psychoneuroendocrinology. 2010;35(7):1113–8. https://doi.org/10.1016/j.
   psyneuen.2009.12.013.

59. Yehuda R, Golier JA, Kaufman S. Circadian rhythm of salivary cortisol in
   holocaust survivors with and without PTSD. Am J Psychiatry. 2005;162(5):
   998–1000. https://doi.org/10.1176/appi.ajp.162.5.998.

60. Yehuda R, Golier JA, Harvey PD, Stavitsky K, Kaufman S, Grossman RA, et al.
   Relationship between cortisol and age-related memory impairments in
   holocaust survivors with PTSD. Psychoneuroendocrinology. 2005;30(7):678–87.
   https://doi.org/10.1016/j.psyneuen.2005.02.007.

61. Young EA, Tolman R, Witkowski K, Kaplan G. Salivary cortisol and
   posttraumatic stress disorder in a low-income community sample of
   women. Biol Psychiatry. 2004;55(6):621–6. https://doi.org/10.1016/j.biopsych.
   2003.09.009.

62. Young EA, Breslau N. Saliva cortisol in posttraumatic stress disorder: a
   community epidemiologic study. Biol Psychiatry. 2004;56(3):205–9. https://
   doi.org/10.1016/j.biopsych.2004.05.011.

63. Lindley SE, Carlson EB, Benoit M. Basal and dexamethasone suppressed
   salivary cortisol concentrations in a community sample of patients with
   posttraumatic stress disorder. Biol Psychiatry. 2004;55(9):940–5. https://doi.
   org/10.1016/j.biopsych.2003.12.021.

64. Neylan TC, Lenoci M, Maglione ML, Rosenlicht NZ, Metzler TJ, Otte C, et al.
   Delta sleep response to metyrapone in post-traumatic stress disorder.
   Neuropsychopharmacology. 2003;28(9):1666–76. https://doi.org/10.1038/sj.
   npp.1300215.

# 18

# Direct and moderating effects of personality on stigma towards mental illness

Qi Yuan*⬛, Esmond Seow, Edimansyah Abdin, Boon Yiang Chua, Hui Lin Ong, Ellaisha Samari, Siow Ann Chong and Mythily Subramaniam

## Abstract

**Background:** While many studies have explored the concept and correlates of stigma towards individuals with mental illness, few have investigated the role of personality in this process. In the current study, we firstly examined the relationship between personality and stigma towards mental illness; and then explored the moderating effects of personality traits on the relationship between contact experience/s and stigma.

**Methods:** Participants were recruited from public medical ($N = 502$) and nursing schools ($N = 500$) from April to September 2016 in Singapore for this cross-sectional survey, and they were randomly assigned to a vignette describing one of the following mental disorders: major depressive disorder, obsessive compulsive disorder, alcohol abuse, schizophrenia, and dementia. Stigma was measured by the 'Personal and Perceived scales of the Depression Stigma Scale' and the 'Social Distance Scale'. These scales together had a 3-factor structure based on a previous national study in Singapore, namely 'weak-not-sick', 'dangerous/unpredictable' and 'social distance'. Personality was measured by the 20-item short form of the International Personality Item Pool-five factor model measure.

**Results:** Regression suggested agreeableness and openness to experience were negatively associated with all three domains of stigma. 'Weak-not-sick' and extraversion were positively associated; and 'social distance' was positively associated with higher scores on conscientiousness and neuroticism. Both close- and non-close contact were associated with more positive attitudes towards mental illness among the participants. Openness to experience moderated the relationships of close contact experience with 'weak-not-sick' and 'dangerous/unpredictable', but in different directions. The association between close contact and 'social distance' were moderated by agreeableness.

**Conclusions:** Unlike non-close contact experience, close contact with people with mental illness worked differently on stigma for individuals with different personality traits. Future studies are needed to further explore the underlying mechanisms for such differences.

**Keywords:** Personality, Stigma, Mental illness, Interpersonal contact, Moderation

## Background

The World Health Organization defined stigma as 'a distinguishing mark establishing a demarcation between the stigmatized person and others attributing negative characteristics to this person' [1]. Stigma towards mental illness is widespread, and comprises public stigma (the reaction that the general population has to people with mental illness) and self-stigma (the prejudice which people with mental illness turn against themselves) [2]. It has three components- stereotypes (negative belief about a group), prejudice (negative emotional reaction) and discrimination (behavioral response to prejudice) [2, 3]. For people with mental illness, self-stigma could affect their personal experience with others, their willingness to disclose their disease, and the subsequent help-seeking behavior [3, 4]; while for public stigma, it could affect the daily interactions between the public and the mentally ill [3, 5]. Both have the potential to lead to negative outcomes among individuals with mental disorders. Other than the general public [6, 7], health care professionals may also hold stereotypes,

* Correspondence: Qi_YUAN@imh.com.sg
Research Division, Institute of Mental Health, Singapore, Singapore

and have negative emotional reactions and behavioral responses towards people with mental illness [8, 9]. Such stigma can be detrimental with regards to the quality of health care received by the mentally ill [8]. A previous study among health care providers in the United States found that professionals who endorsed stigmatizing characteristics of patients with mental illness were more likely to view the patients as non-adherent, making them less likely to refer patients to specialists to refill medications [10]. Findings from a previous systematic review also suggested that while delivering healthcare services to patients with substance abuse disorders, healthcare professionals tended to use a more avoidant approach compared to those without such disorders, which in turn could influence the treatment outcomes [11]. Another study among family physicians in United States showed that the physicians tended to believe that the physical symptoms (e.g. headache and abdominal pain) among people with previous episodes of depression stemmed from their mental disorders and as a result they were less likely to investigate the underlying reasons [12]. To lower the negative impact on patients, it is necessary to improve the attitudes of healthcare professionals towards individuals with mental illness, especially among those with relatively high stigma. Thus, identifying factors that influence stigma could be one of the crucial steps in this endeavor.

Various studies have explored relationships between personality and prejudice, mainly from two theoretical perspectives 1) the authoritarian personality approach which proposed a direct link between personality and prejudice, and 2) a dual-process motivational approach which focused on personalities' indirect impact over prejudice [13]. For example, Ekehammar and Akrami [14, 15] tested the relationships between the Big Five personality traits and generalized prejudice (a composite measure based on scores from racial/ethnic prejudice, attitudes towards women, and attitudes towards mentally disabled people, and attitudes towards homosexuals, lesbians and gay men) among two different samples of students, and found consistent significant negative relationships of openness and agreeableness with generalized prejudice. Their findings are consistent with that from a meta-analysis exploring the relationship between personality and prejudice [13]. On the other hand, a 2008 review of 18 different models suggested that although prejudice and stigma have different emphasis and focus (i.e. subjects), their conceptual models including the cause and consequences actually have considerable overlap [16]. And the authors also suggested that this large degree of overlap should encourage scholars to reach across stigma/prejudice lines while searching for theory, methods and empirical findings [16]. As a result, findings on relationships between personality and prejudice might be extended to between personality and stigma (i.e. stigma is not always related to lack of knowledge [17],

other factors including personality might also play an important role). Preliminary evidence supports this extension - according to a study conducted by Arikan among 700 final year university students, a strong correlation between the use of narcissistic defense (i.e. narcissistic personality) and the tendency to stigmatize people was found [18]. Another study exploring the social appraisal of adults with attention deficit hyperactivity disorder (ADHD) among psychology undergraduates suggested that agreeableness, extraversion, and conscientiousness were all significantly associated with their attitudes towards people with ADHD [19]. More specifically, Brown [20] also found that after controlling for experiences of personal contact with people with mental illness, openness and agreeableness were negatively associated with stigma towards severe mental illness. However, till date studies on this topic are very limited; and none of them are among Asian populations.

Inter-group contact experience is beneficial for reducing prejudice [21]; and a similar relationship also applies for contact and attitudes to mental illness [22, 23]. One potential explanation is that contact experiences help people to understand the feelings and worldview of the stigmatized group and as a result lead to enhanced empathy towards the stigmatized groups and reduce prejudice [24]. Previous studies on personality and communication skills suggested that agreeableness and openness to experience uniquely predicted better active-empathic listening skills of individuals [25]. For those scoring higher on openness, their state of being more open-mind [26, 27] might allow them to gain more understanding on the feelings and worldview of the individuals with mental illness from the contact experience. People who score higher on agreeableness tend to be more good-natured, cooperative and tolerant [26, 27]; this in turn might enable them to have enhanced empathy towards people with mental illness. Following this rationale, we hypothesized that higher levels of these two personality traits might contribute to a more positive inter-group contact process, and ultimately lead to larger improvements on stigma towards mental illness compared to those who score lower on these traits. In other words, other than the direct relationship, personality traits including openness and agreeableness might also work as moderators which moderate the relationship between contact experience/s and stigma towards mental illness.

The current study aims to 1) examine the direct relationship between the 'Big Five' personality traits and stigma towards mental illness through a sample of health care students in Singapore; and 2) explore if agreeableness and openness to experience moderate the relationship between contact experience and stigma towards mental illness.

## Methods

### Participants and procedure

Data for the current study were extracted from a project exploring mental health literacy level of health care students using a vignette-based approach as well as factors that lead them to choose psychiatry as a career [28, 29]. This cross-sectional study used an online web survey, QuestionPro®, to collect data. The target population included medical and nursing students who were enrolled in public medical and nursing educational programmes in Singapore at the time of the study from April to September 2016. Students who were Singapore residents (Singapore Citizens or Permanent Residents) were eligible for the study.

Public medical and nursing schools in Singapore were approached by the study team members to seek their permission to recruit respondents from these institutions. Upon approval, the institutions sent a mass email on behalf of the study team to invite the students to join the study, with a pre-defined quota for each institution. The quota was based on institutions, the academic years and also the number of vignettes. This was meant to improve the representativeness of the study sample. The participation was voluntary, and an online consent form was used to obtain the informed consent from all participants. The online survey took around 20–30 min to complete; and after completion, a SG$20 voucher was given to each participant. In total, 1002 students were recruited during the recruitment period, among which 502 were medical students and 500 were nursing students.

Ethical approval of the project was granted by the National Healthcare Group Domain Specific Review Board in Singapore.

### Measurements

#### Personality traits

Personality was measured by the 20-item short form [30] of the 50-item International Personality Item Pool-Five-Factor Model measure (mini-IPIP) [31], with 4 items measuring each of the 'Big Five' personality traits (i.e. extraversion, agreeableness, conscientiousness, neuroticism, and openness to experience). Participants were required to read items such as 'I am the life of the party', 'I sympathize with others' feelings', and then rate how each item accurately describe themselves using a 5-point Likert scale, with '1 = very inaccurate' and '5 = very accurate'. An average score was calculated for each personality trait; with a higher score representing higher endorsement of the personality trait. The composite reliability statistics were 0.79 for extraversion, 0.79 for agreeableness, 0.68 for conscientiousness, 0.71 for neuroticism, and 0.76 for openness in the current study. A cut-off of 0.7 for composite reliability [32] was deemed acceptable.

### Stigma towards mental illness

Participants of the current study were randomly assigned to a vignette describing one of the following specific mental disorders: major depressive disorder, obsessive compulsive disorder (OCD), alcohol abuse, schizophrenia, and dementia; and were then asked to indicate their attitudes to the mentally ill person described in the assigned vignette using two different scales - the personal subscale of the 'Personal and Perceived scales of the Depression Stigma Scale (DSS)' [33] and the 'Social Distance Scale (SDS)' [34]. Vignettes on depression and schizophrenia were adapted from those used in previous studies [35, 36]; while those on dementia, alcohol abuse and OCD were developed by the investigators [7, 37]. All these vignettes were approved by a panel of senior clinical psychiatrists to ensure that each disorder satisfied the DSM-IV diagnostic criteria. Please refer to Additional file 1 for the details of the vignettes.

The DSS has two subscales (personal stigma and perceived stigma), and each comprises 9 different items [33]. It was originally developed to measure depression stigma. In the current study, only 8 items of the DSS-personal subscale was used (item 'I would not vote for a politician if I know they had a mental illness' was excluded) [7]. The DSS was rated based on a 5-point Likert scale, ranging from '1 = strongly disagree' to '5 = strongly agree'. The SDS has 5 different items, and it was used to measure the participants' self-reported willingness to contact the person depicted in the vignette. A 4-point Likert scale varied from '1 = definitely unwilling' to '4 = definitely willing' was used for its rating. This vignette-based approach and the measurement tools have been used in a national study on mental health literacy in Singapore before, and the factor analysis suggested a 3-factor structure – 'weak-not-sick', 'dangerous/unpredictable', and 'social distance' [7]. Following the national study, the 5 items of 'social distance' were reversed scored first; and then the scores for all three factors were calculated by summing the items included in each factor (for 'dangerous/unpredictable', item 'if I had a problem like [vignette] I would not tell anyone' was excluded from the calculation) [7]. In this case, higher scores of each factor represent more stigmatizing attitudes towards mental illness. In the current sample, we ran a confirmatory factor analysis for this 3-factor structure, and the results suggested acceptable model fit (the comparative fit index/CFI = 0.960, the Tucker-Lewis index/TLI = 0.948, the root mean square error of approximation/RMSEA = 0.084). The composite reliability statistics were 0.73, 0.73, and 0.90 for 'weak-not-sick', 'dangerous/unpredictable' and 'social distance', respectively.

### Contact experiences

Contact experiences were captured by two different questions after the participants read the assigned vignette: 1) close contact – 'has anyone in your family or close circle of friends ever had problems depicted in the vignette?'; and 2) non-close contact – 'have you ever had any experiences (e.g. volunteering, training) in dealing with a person who had problems depicted in the vignette?'. In the current study to ensure the interpretability, participants who reported 'don't know/refused' for these two contact experience questions were treated as missing in all regression analyses. The total sample included in the regression and path analyses was 870.

Other than the above-mentioned assessments, we also measured socio-demographics including age, gender, ethnicity, highest education level attained before current school, monthly household income, and type of study program (i.e. medical or nursing), vignette type and whether the participants could correctly identify the mental disorder described in the vignette assigned to them.

### Statistical analysis

Descriptive analysis was conducted for socio-demographics and other variables. Mean and standard deviation (SD) were calculated for continuous variables; while for categorical variables, their frequency and percentage were presented. To explore the direct effects of personality on stigma, linear regression analyses were conducted, with each factor of the stigma measures regressed on all 5 'Big Five' personality traits, after controlling for socio-demographics (including age, gender, ethnicity, education level, monthly income, and type of study program), contact experiences (close contact and non-close contact), and vignette-associated variables (vignette type and the status whether the participants could correctly recognize the mental disorder in the assigned vignette). The regression was done through IBM SPSS V23.0, and a two-sided $p$-value below 0.05 was considered as statistically significant.

The moderating effects of agreeableness and openness to experience were tested through path analysis following a 2-step approach. In the first step, all three domains of stigma were regressed on the two types of contacts (i.e. close contact and non-close contact) simultaneously, with the two personalities of agreeableness and openness to experience being the moderators for each of the regression paths. In step 2 based on the results from the previous step; the non-significant moderation paths were removed. Both steps controlled for socio-demographics, the vignette-associated variables, and the remaining three personality traits. Model fit was defined as 1) the comparative fit index (CFI) > 0.95; 2) the Tucker-Lewis index (TLI) > 0.95; and the root mean square error of approximation (RMSEA) < 0.06 [38]. Finally, the regression parameters from the fit model were presented. Conditional effects (both unstandardized and standardized) between contact experience and stigma based on different level of moderators and the simple slopes for the moderation analyses

were also presented. All moderation analyses were conducted using 'lavaan' package [39] in the R statistical program.

### Results

The socio-demographics of the study participants are presented in Table 1. The study sample comprised 1002 participants, among whom 500 were from nursing programs and 502 were medical students. The participants had a mean age of 21.3 years (SD = 3.3), and the majority of them were female (71.1%, $n = 712$) and Chinese (75.3%, $n = 754$). Among the participants, 75.4% ($n = 755$) correctly identified the mental disorder described in the assigned vignette. 25.1% of the participants ($n = 252$) reported that they had close friends or family members with problems similar to that depicted in the assigned vignette (i.e. close contact experience); while 33.7% ($n = 338$) mentioned that they used to deal with people had similar problems in the vignette (i.e. non-close contact experience).

Table 2 presents the descriptive statistics for personality and stigma measures. The mean scores for each of the 'Big Five' personality traits are listed below: 2.91 for extraversion, 3.93 for agreeableness, 3.40 for conscientiousness, 2.86 for neuroticism, and 3.57 for openness to experience. For the three domains of stigma towards mental illness, the mean score was 7.90, 10.09, and 11.42 for 'weak-not-sick', 'dangerous/unpredictable', and 'social distance', respectively.

The linear regression results after controlling for covariates suggested that the 'weak-not-sick' factor was significantly associated with extraversion ($B = 0.429$, $p < 0.001$), agreeableness ($B = -0.350$, $p = 0.004$), and openness to experience ($B = -0.340$, $p = 0.001$). Significant associations were also identified for 'dangerous/unpredictable' factor with agreeableness ($B = -0.467$, $p = 0.002$) and openness to experience ($B = -0.421$, $p = 0.001$); and for 'social distance' with agreeableness ($B = -0.619$, $p < 0.001$), conscientiousness ($B = 0.251$, $p = 0.028$), neuroticism ($B = 0.238$, $p = 0.040$) and openness to experience ($B = -0.419$, $p = 0.001$). Meanwhile, having close-contact and non-close contact with individuals with mental illness were both significantly correlated with more positive attitudes on the three domains of stigma towards mental illness. Details of the results are shown in Table 3.

The path analysis suggested that after removing the insignificant moderation paths, the final model (Fig. 1) showed very good fit ($\chi^2_{(df)} = 3.354_{(3)}$, CFI = 1.000, TLI = 0.990, RMSEA = 0.012). The final moderation model revealed that openness to experience moderated the relationships between close contact and 'weak-not-sick' ($B = 0.48$, z-value = 2.383, $p = 0.017$; interaction: $\Delta R^2 = 0.0040$), and between close contact and 'dangerous/unpredictable' ($B = -0.50$, z-value = -2.151, $p = 0.031$; interaction: $\Delta R^2 = 0.0038$);

**Table 1** Socio-demographic characteristics of the sample (*n* = 1002)

| Group | Frequency | Percentage |
|---|---|---|
| Age (mean, SD) | 21.3 | 3.3 |
| Gender | | |
| Male | 290 | 28.9 |
| Female | 712 | 71.1 |
| Ethnicity | | |
| Chinese | 754 | 75.3 |
| Malay | 141 | 14.1 |
| Indian or others | 107 | 10.7 |
| Highest education attained before current school | | |
| Secondary or below | 251 | 25.1 |
| Technical education | 114 | 11.4 |
| A level | 428 | 42.7 |
| Diploma | 81 | 8.1 |
| Tertiary | 128 | 12.8 |
| Monthly household income | | |
| Below 2000 | 241 | 24.1 |
| 2000-3999 | 263 | 26.3 |
| 4000-5999 | 171 | 17.1 |
| 6000-9999 | 146 | 14.6 |
| More than 10,000 | 181 | 18.1 |
| Type of study program | | |
| Medical | 502 | 50.1 |
| Nursing | 500 | 49.9 |
| Vignette type | | |
| Schizophrenia | 200 | 20.0 |
| Depression | 200 | 20.0 |
| OCD | 201 | 20.1 |
| Alcohol abuse | 200 | 20.0 |
| Dementia | 201 | 20.1 |
| Correct identification of vignette | | |
| Yes | 755 | 75.4 |
| No | 247 | 24.7 |
| Close contact | | |
| Yes | 252 | 25.1 |
| No | 648 | 64.7 |
| Don't know/refuse | 102 | 10.2 |
| Non-close contact | | |
| Yes | 338 | 33.7 |
| No | 615 | 61.4 |
| Don't know/refuse | 49 | 4.9 |

**Table 2** Descriptive statistics for 'Big Five' personality and stigma measures

| | Mean | SD | Min | Max |
|---|---|---|---|---|
| Big Five Personality | | | | |
| Extraversion | 2.91 | 0.85 | 1 | 5 |
| Agreeableness | 3.93 | 0.60 | 1 | 5 |
| Conscientiousness | 3.40 | 0.75 | 1 | 5 |
| Neuroticism | 2.86 | 0.76 | 1 | 5 |
| Openness to experience | 3.57 | 0.73 | 1 | 5 |
| Stigma | | | | |
| Weak-not-sick | 7.90 | 2.37 | 3 | 15 |
| Dangerous/unpredictable | 10.09 | 2.71 | 4 | 19 |
| Social distance | 11.42 | 2.69 | 5 | 20 |

while agreeableness moderated the relationship between close contact and 'social distance' ($B = -0.74$, z-value $= -2.631$, $p = 0.009$; interaction: $\Delta R^2 = 0.0051$).

Table 4 shows the results of the conditional effects of close contact experience on the three factors of the stigma measurements among the health care students at a specific level of openness to experience/agreeableness. Results suggest that at low openness to experience level (mean-1SD), 'weakness-not-sick' was negatively associated with close contact experience (conditional effect = $-0.625$, $p = 0.004$); however, at average (mean) or high levels of openness to experience (mean + 1SD), the relationship was not significant. For 'dangerous/unpredictable', it was negatively associated with close contact experience only among participants with average (mean) or high openness to experience level (mean + 1SD). Close contact experience predicted less 'social distance' among people with average (mean) or high level of agreeableness (mean + 1SD). The graphic demonstrations of the moderations are shown in Figs 2, 3 and 4.

## Discussion

The current study aimed to explore the direct and moderating effects of personality on stigma towards mental illness using a vignette-based approach. Similar vignettes and measurement tools had been used in a previous national study in Singapore [7]. Compared to the young adults (aged 18 to 34 years) from the study by Subramaniam et al. [7], our health care students sample (mean age 21.3 years) reported lower scores on 'weak-not-sick' (7.90 vs. 9.58) and slightly lower scores on 'dangerous/unpredictable' (10.09 vs. 10.88); however, their scores on 'social distance' did not differ too much from the young people in the general population (11.42 vs. 11.58). Moreover, the multivariate regression results showed that 'correct identification of the mental disorder depicted in the vignette' was negatively associated with 'weak-not-sick', but positively associated with higher endorsement on 'dangerous/unpredictable' and

**Table 3** Linear regression results of the direct relationships between personality and stigma (n = 870)

| | Weak-not-sick | | | | Dangerous/unpredictable | | | | Social distance | | | |
|---|---|---|---|---|---|---|---|---|---|---|---|---|
| | B | β | 95% CI | | p | B | β | 95% CI | | p | B | β | 95% CI | | p |
| Extraversion | 0.429 | 0.157 | 0.268 | 0.590 | 0.000 | 0.146 | 0.046 | −0.056 | 0.347 | 0.157 | 0.035 | 0.011 | −0.168 | 0.239 | 0.733 |
| Agreeableness | −0.350 | −0.088 | −0.587 | −0.113 | 0.004 | −0.467 | −0.102 | −0.764 | −0.170 | 0.002 | −0.619 | −0.137 | −0.918 | −0.319 | 0.000 |
| Conscientiousness | 0.081 | 0.026 | −0.096 | 0.259 | 0.370 | 0.059 | 0.016 | −0.163 | 0.282 | 0.600 | 0.251 | 0.070 | 0.026 | 0.475 | 0.028 |
| Neuroticism | −0.101 | −0.033 | −0.281 | 0.078 | 0.269 | 0.152 | 0.043 | −0.073 | 0.377 | 0.185 | 0.238 | 0.068 | 0.011 | 0.465 | 0.040 |
| Openness | −0.340 | −0.105 | −0.534 | −0.146 | 0.001 | −0.421 | −0.112 | −0.664 | −0.178 | 0.001 | −0.419 | −0.113 | −0.664 | −0.174 | 0.001 |

[a]B – unstandardized coefficient;
[b]β – standardized coefficient;
[c]Controlled for socio-demographics (i.e. age, gender, ethnicity, education level, monthly income, and type of study) + contact experiences (i.e. close contact and non-close contact) + vignette-associated variables (i.e. vignette type and the status whether the participants could correctly recognize the mental disorder in the assigned vignette);
[d]Close contact was significant in predicting 'dangerous/unpredictable' (B = − 0.439, p = 0.032), and 'social distance' (B = − 0.800, p < 0.001);
[e]Non-close contact was significant in predicting 'weak-not-sick' (B = − 0.495, p = 0.001), 'dangerous/unpredictable' (B = − 0.369, p = 0.041), and 'social distance' (B = − 0.539, p = 0.003);
[f]Correct identification of the mental disorder in the vignette was significant in predicting 'weak-not-sick' (B = − 0.372, p = 0.028), 'dangerous/unpredictable' (B = 0.460, p = 0.031), and 'social distance' (B = 0.510, p = 0.018)

'social distance' towards people with mental illness. Both findings indicate that better knowledge on mental illness does not necessarily lead to lower discrimination (i.e. social distance), similar to findings from other studies [9, 17, 40].

The consistent negative relationships of agreeableness and openness to experience with stigma towards mental illness were confirmed by the multivariate regression analyses. This finding is consistent with results from the cross-sectional study on personality and stigma to mental illness conducted by Brown [20]. Studies have suggested that increases in level of empathy and perspective taking are helpful in reducing prejudice [24, 41], which might also be applicable for stigma. People scoring higher on agreeableness are generally more good-natured, cooperative and tolerant [26, 27], and as a result more likely to have higher empathy towards others, such as towards people with mental disorders. On the other hand, those who had higher scores on openness to experience are more open-minded [26, 27] and more likely to accept new ideas; which might

ultimately contribute to a greater increase in perspective-taking towards the mentally ill among the participants. Another possible explanation could be relevant to social dominance orientation (SDO) and right-wing authoritarianism (RWA). Sibley and Duckitt [13] in their meta-analysis found that low agreeableness was associated with high SDO and low openness to experience was associated with high RWA, and both SDO and RWA were associated with more prejudice; moreover, the relationships between prejudice and agreeableness were fully mediated by SDO, while the relationships between prejudice and openness to experience were partially mediated by RWA. However, this alternative explanation assumes the similarities between prejudice and stigma [16, 42]. Since SDO and RWA were not measured in the current study, we were unable to confirm this effect in the current study.

Other than the above two personality traits, we also found significant positive associations between extraversion and 'weak-not-sick', between conscientiousness and

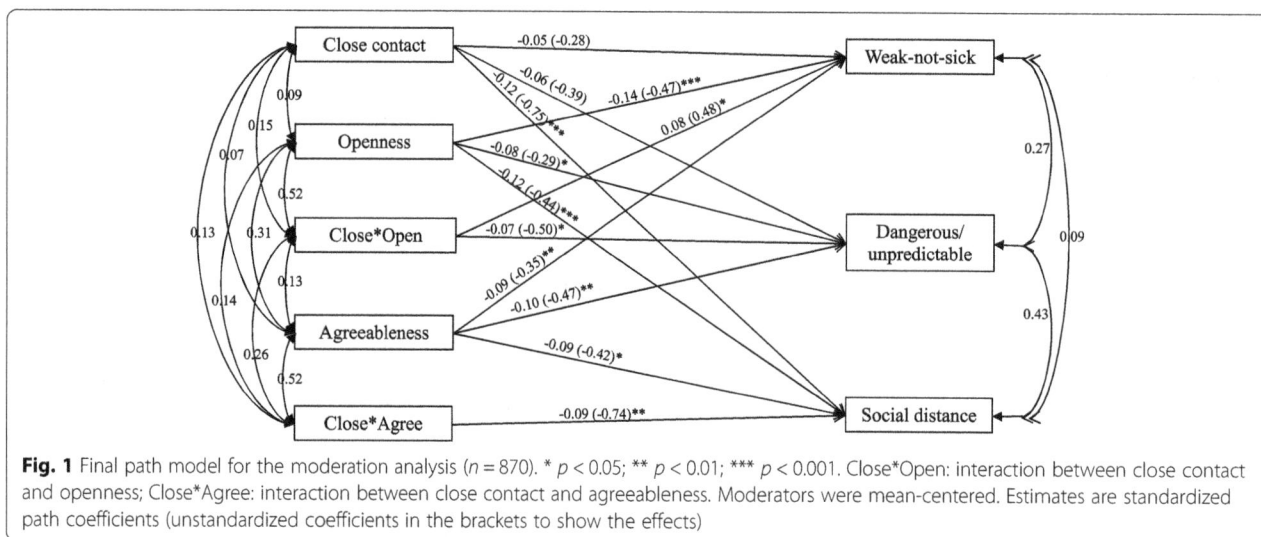

**Fig. 1** Final path model for the moderation analysis (n = 870). * p < 0.05; ** p < 0.01; *** p < 0.001. Close*Open: interaction between close contact and openness; Close*Agree: interaction between close contact and agreeableness. Moderators were mean-centered. Estimates are standardized path coefficients (unstandardized coefficients in the brackets to show the effects)

**Table 4** Conditional effects of close contact on stigma at each level of personality

| | Conditional Effect | SE | Standardized Conditional Effect | z-value | p |
|---|---|---|---|---|---|
| Weakness-not-sick | | | | | |
| Low openness (Mean-1SD) | −0.625 | 0.218 | −0.129 | −2.859 | 0.004 |
| Average openness (Mean) | −0.275 | 0.161 | −0.052 | −1.701 | 0.089 |
| High openness (Mean + 1SD) | 0.075 | 0.192 | 0.025 | 0.393 | 0.695 |
| Dangerous/unpredictable | | | | | |
| Low openness (Mean-1SD) | −0.037 | 0.263 | 0.003 | −0.139 | 0.889 |
| Average openness (Mean) | −0.398 | 0.202 | −0.066 | −1.974 | 0.048 |
| High openness (Mean + 1SD) | −0.760 | 0.234 | −0.135 | −3.247 | 0.001 |
| Social distance | | | | | |
| Low agreeableness (Mean-1SD) | −0.324 | 0.258 | −0.043 | −1.259 | 0.208 |
| Average agreeableness (Mean) | −0.768 | 0.203 | −0.129 | −3.792 | < 0.001 |
| High agreeableness (Mean + 1SD) | −1.212 | 0.242 | −0.215 | −5.009 | < 0.001 |

'social distance', and between neuroticism and 'social distance'. Extraversion refers to being sociable, energetic or outgoing; while conscientiousness is about being efficient and organized [26]. According to research on prejudice, both extraversion [43] and conscientiousness [13, 43] were positively correlated with RWA; and high RWA is strongly correlated with prejudice and negative attitudes toward outgroups [43], such as individuals with mental illness in our case. However, since RWA was not measured in this study, future studies are needed to test whether RWA mediates the relationships between extraversion and conscientiousness with stigma. Previous studies on proxemics and neuroticism suggested that people who scored higher on neuroticism had a general tendency to prefer more social distance compared to those with lower scores [44].

The moderation analyses suggested that agreeableness and openness to experience do moderate the relationship between contact experience and stigma towards mental illness. However, unlike what we had expected, the moderating effect was limited only to the relationship between close contact and stigma. For non-close contact, the moderation was non-significant. To avoid over-interpretation, a sensitivity moderation analysis

among the participants who were able to recognize the vignettes was also conducted and similar findings were identified. According to a previous literature review, contact experience of a more voluntary nature tended to be most effective in reducing negative attitudes towards people with severe mental illness [45]. Similar findings were also reported in studies on intergroup contact and prejudice, suggesting that the effect of intergroup contact experience on prejudice is not always positive; it might also lead to negative effects, especially when the contact involves involuntary contact [24, 46]. Compared to non-close contact, it is difficult for people to say 'no' to the close contact experiences, especially when the patients are family members of the participants. This difference, together with the individual differences in personality, might lead to the different results in the moderation analyses. This could be one of the potential explanations. Moreover, contact quality and valence might also contribute in this process. Barlow and colleagues [47] suggested that intergroup contacts could be positive and negative, and negative intergroup contacts could increase prejudice. In our study, since we did not gauge the differences in the quality of contact experiences, further studies are needed to explore this

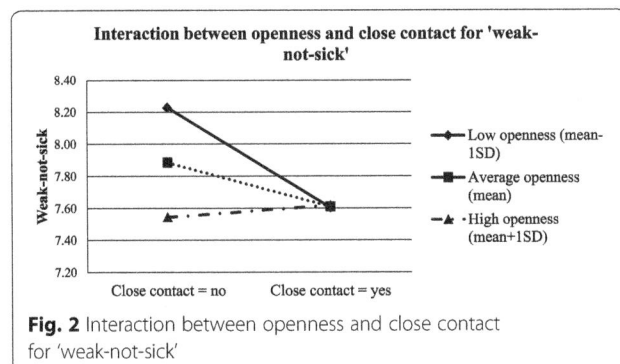

**Fig. 2** Interaction between openness and close contact for 'weak-not-sick'

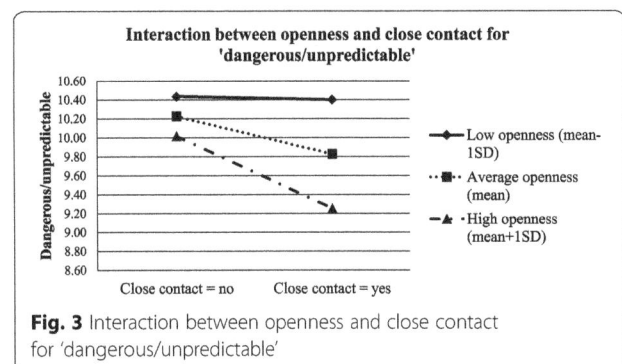

**Fig. 3** Interaction between openness and close contact for 'dangerous/unpredictable'

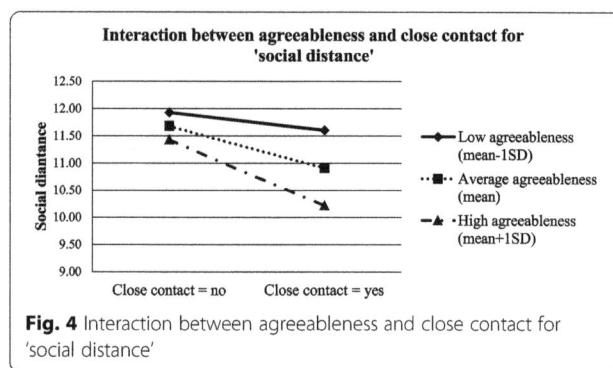

**Fig. 4** Interaction between agreeableness and close contact for 'social distance'

issue, and elucidate the exact underlying mechanism for this difference. We have also explored the potential moderation effects of the other three personality traits; however, none of them were significant.

Close contact experiences predicted significantly more positive attitudes on 'dangerous/unpredictable' among people with average or high openness to experience, and on 'social distance' among people with average or high agreeableness. However, the correlations were non-significant among those with low openness or agreeableness levels. This is in line with our hypothesis that people who scored higher on these two personality traits tend to benefit more from the contact experience. There are two possible explanations. The first relates to what we hypothesized earlier - people with higher agreeableness and openness to experiences tended to be more cooperative and perspective-taking, which could improve the quality and valence of contact experiences (i.e. positive intergroup contact experiences). The other is related to 'situational evocation and selection'. A previous study conducted by Jackson and Poulsen found that for ethnic prejudice, individuals with high agreeableness and openness tended to seek out favourable intergroup contact experiences (situational selection) and were more likely to act in a way that facilitates favourable interactions (situational evocation) [48]. In this case when contact opportunities are available, the purposive selection of favourable interactions among individuals who scored higher on agreeableness and openness ultimately lead to more positive contact experiences with the mentally ill. Although these two explanations were different, both suggest a possibility that when contact opportunities are available, individuals who scored higher on agreeableness and openness tend to have more positive contact experiences compared to their counterparts with lower scores, and such positive contacts could significantly reduce their stigma towards mental illness [47]. However, for 'weak-not-sick', close contact experience was a significant predictor only among those with low openness to experience, which is contradictory to findings from the other two stigma domains. This discrepancy might be caused by the fact that 'weak-not-sick' is more about individuals'

knowledge of mental illness which can benefit from both education and contact experiences, in contrast to the other two domains. Since the participants were all health care students who were exposed to various information on different diseases including mental illness, their knowledge depends largely on their curiosity and level of seeking and accepting new knowledge, openness to experience in other words [26, 27, 49]. Thus, health care students with higher openness would have better knowledge on mental illness and therefore lower stigmatized scores on 'weak-not-sick'. However, better knowledge also indicated there would be less room for further improvements. This could be the reason for the non-significant correlations between contact experiences and 'weak-not-sick' among participants with average or high openness. It also indicated that for individuals who are less keen in acquiring new knowledge, contact experience can be a good strategy to improve individuals' perceptions on 'weak-not-sick'.

The results of the current study have significant implications. First of all, although personality traits (as trait-like characteristics) are quite stable, there is evidence suggesting that personality traits continue to develop, especially during young adulthood [50, 51]. In this case, future studies may explore the possibility of integrating certain personality modification interventions into the attitude campaigns especially those campaigns targeting children or younger adults. Such integration could also be applied among stigma campaigns towards clinicians, especially in their earlier stages of their career such as when they are still students. This could yield better outcomes and thus might be one of the directions for future attitude campaigns. Secondly, the moderation analyses results revealed that close contact experience is beneficial for attitudes to mental illness only among specific subgroups of health care students (i.e. individuals with lower openness or agreeableness tended to benefit less from such experiences). This could be due to the possibility that health care students with higher openness or agreeableness are more likely to seek positive contact experiences with individuals with mental illness. Although further studies are still needed to determine the exact mechanism, the current study raises the importance of individual differences in the areas of stigma and indicates that it might also be necessary to also take these differences into considerations for future stigma studies or programs. Thirdly, although prejudice and stigma are different, our study suggests that theories or models of prejudice could sometimes be applied in the area of stigma, supporting that bridging the research of these two constructs could be potentially very informative [16, 42].

The current study has several strengths. To the best of our knowledge, this is the first study in Asia which has investigated the relationship between personality and stigma towards mental illness; and it is also the first study to explore the moderating effects of personality on the relationship between contact experience and stigma. Other than extending the findings from western populations into the eastern society, the current study also identified the potential individual difference on the effects of contact experience on stigma; this will be extremely helpful for us to understand the role of personality on individuals' attitudes towards mental illness in other contexts as well. Secondly, the study has a much larger sample size than the previous studies [20, 41]; which in turn makes the findings more robust. Lastly, a vignette-based approach was used in the current study. Compared to having the participants to rate their attitudes towards mental illness based on a general term 'mental illness', this approach could elicit more accurate information as 'mental illness' might indicate different diseases to different people.

The study findings should also be viewed with the following limitations in mind. First of all, the study sample comprised a group of health care students, which might limit the applicability of the findings to the general population. Second, the participants volunteered to participate in the current study; in this case, a self-selection bias might apply. Third, the vignette-based approach has its own limitations – for example, it is based on hypothetical scenarios, which might be different from real life occurrences. Fourthly, although it is common to use 1-item question to measure interpersonal contact in stigma research [45], this lacks test-retest reliability. Lastly, although we proposed that contact quality and valence might play an important role in the relationships of contact, personality and stigma, contact quality and valence were not measured in our study. Future studies are still needed to further explore this area.

## Conclusion

The current study confirmed the direct relationship between personality and stigma towards mental illness, with those who scored lower on openness to experience and agreeableness, and higher on extraversion, conscientiousness, and neuroticism tending to show more stigmatizing attitudes. Openness to experience and agreeableness moderated the relationship between close-contact and stigma, with individuals with average and higher levels of openness or agreeableness tending to benefit more from the close contact experience. Future studies should explore suitability of interventions based on personality traits; and test if the findings of this study can be extended to the general population.

## Additional file

**Additional file 1:** Vignettes used in the study (DOCX 14 kb)

## Abbreviations
ADHD: Attention deficit hyperactivity disorder; CFI: The comparative fit index; DSS: Depression stigma scale; Mini-IPIP: short form International Personality Item Pool-Five-Factor Model measure; OCD: Obsessive compulsive disorder; RMSEA: The root mean square error of approximation; RWA: Right-wing authoritarianism; SD: Standard deviation; SDO: social dominance orientation; SDS: Social distance scale; TLI: The Tucker-Lewis index

## Acknowledgements
The authors would like to thank the schools for their permissions for us to conduct the study among their students. We also want to thank the respondents for their time and efforts in the study.

## Funding
This research was supported by the Singapore Ministry of Health's National Medical Research Council under the Centre Grant Programme (Grant No.: NMRC/CG/004/2013). The funder had no role in study design, data collection and analysis, decision to publish, or preparation of the manuscript.

## Authors' contributions
QY conceived the data analysis plan and the structure of the manuscript, performed the data analysis and wrote the first draft of the manuscript. E. Seow and BYC designed the study protocol, and were in charge of the study implementation, and provided intellectual input into this article. EA provided valuable feedback on the data analysis and interpretation, and provided intellectual input into this article. MS and SAC has made substantial contribution to conception and design of the study, supervised the study implementation, and provided intellectual input into this article. HLO and E. Samari made substantial contribution to the acquisition of data, and provided intellectual input in the study and this article. All authors have read and approved the final manuscript.

## Consent for publication
Not applicable.

## Competing interests
The authors declare that they have no competing interests.

## References
1. World Health Organization. Policies and practices for mental health in Europe - meeting the challenges. Copenhagen: World Health Organization Regional Office for Europe; 2008.
2. Corrigan PW, Watson AC. Understanding the impact of stigma on people with mental illness. World Psychiatry. 2002;1(1):16–20.
3. Corrigan P. How stigma interferes with mental health care. Am Psychol. 2004;59(7):614.
4. Eisenberg D, Downs MF, Golberstein E, Zivin K. Stigma and help seeking for mental health among college students. Med Care Res Rev. 2009;66(5):522–41.
5. Centers for Disease Control and Prevention, Substance Abuse and Mental Health Services Administration, National Association of County Behavioral Health & Developmental Disability Directors, National Institute of Mental Health, Program TCCMH. Attitudes Toward Mental Illness: Results from the Behavioral Risk Factor Surveillance System. Atlanta (GA): Centers for Disease Control and Prevention, 2012.
6. Yuan Q, Abdin E, Picco L, Vaingankar JA, Shahwan S, Jeyagurunathan A, et al. Attitudes to mental illness and its demographic correlates among general population in Singapore. PloS one. 2016;11(11):e0167297.

7.  Subramaniam M, Abdin E, Picco L, Pang S, Shafie S, Vaingankar J, et al. Stigma towards people with mental disorders and its components-a perspective from multi-ethnic Singapore. Epidemiol Psychiatr Sciences. 2016:1–12.

8.  Henderson C, Noblett J, Parke H, Clement S, Caffrey A, Gale-Grant O, et al. Mental health-related stigma in health care and mental health-care settings. Lancet Psychiatry. 2014;1(6):467–82.

9.  Nordt C, Rössler W, Lauber C. Attitudes of mental health professionals toward people with schizophrenia and major depression. Schizophr Bull. 2006;32(4):709–14.

10. Corrigan PW, Mittal D, Reaves CM, Haynes TF, Han X, Morris S, et al. Mental health stigma and primary health care decisions. Psychiatry Res. 2014;218(1):35–8.

11. Van Boekel LC, Brouwers EP, Van Weeghel J, Garretsen HF. Stigma among health professionals towards patients with substance use disorders and its consequences for healthcare delivery: systematic review. Drug Alcohol Depend. 2013;131(1):23–35.

12. Graber MA, Bergus G, Dawson JD, Wood GB, Levy BT, Levin I. Effect of a patient's psychiatric history on physicians' estimation of probability of disease. J Gen Intern Med. 2000;15(3):204–6.

13. Sibley CG, Duckitt J. Personality and prejudice: a meta-analysis and theoretical review. Personal Soc Psychol Rev. 2008;12(3):248–79.

14. Ekehammar B, Akrami N. The relation between personality and prejudice: a variable-and a person-centred approach. Eur J Personal. 2003;17(6):449–64.

15. Ekehammar B, Akrami N. Personality and prejudice: from big five personality factors to facets. J Pers. 2007;75(5):899–926.

16. Phelan JC, Link BG, Dovidio JF. Stigma and prejudice: one animal or two? Social science & medicine (1982). 2008;67(3):358–67 Epub 2008/06/06. doi: https://doi.org/10.1016/j.socscimed.2008.03.022. PubMed PMID: 18524444; PubMed Central PMCID: PMCPMC4007574.

17. Thornicroft G, Rose D, Kassam A, Sartorius N. Stigma: ignorance, prejudice or discrimination? Br J Psychiatry. 2007;190(3):192–3.

18. Arikan K. A stigmatizating attitude towards psychiatric illnesses is associated with narcissistic personality traits. Isr J Psychiatry Relat Sci. 2005;42(4):248.

19. Canu WH, Newman ML, Morrow TL, Pope DL. Social appraisal of adult ADHD: stigma and influences of the beholder's big five personality traits. J Atten Disord. 2007.

20. Brown SA. The contribution of previous contact and personality traits to severe mental illness stigma. Am J Psychiatr Rehabil. 2012;15(3):274–89.

21. Pettigrew TF, Tropp LR. A meta-analytic test of intergroup contact theory. J Pers Soc Psychol. 2006;90(5):751.

22. Thornicroft G, Mehta N, Clement S, Evans-Lacko S, Doherty M, Rose D, et al. Evidence for effective interventions to reduce mental-health-related stigma and discrimination. Lancet. 2016;387(10023):1123–32.

23. Corrigan PW, Morris SB, Michaels PJ, Rafacz JD, Rüsch N. Challenging the public stigma of mental illness: a meta-analysis of outcome studies. Psychiatr Serv. 2012.

24. Pettigrew TF, Tropp LR, Wagner U, Christ O. Recent advances in intergroup contact theory. Int J Intercult Relat. 2011;35(3):271–80.

25. Sims CM. Do the big-five personality traits predict empathic listening and assertive communication? Int J Listening. 2016:1–26.

26. John OP, Srivastava S. The big five trait taxonomy: history, measurement, and theoretical perspectives. Handbook of personality: Theory and research 1999;2(1999):102–38.

27. Sibley CG, Luyten N, Purnomo M, Moberly A, Wootton LW, Hammond MD, et al. The mini-IPIP6: validation and extension of a short measure of the big-six factors of personality in New Zealand. N Z J Psychol. 2011;40(3):142–59.

28. Ong HL, Seow E, Chua BY, Xie H, Wang J, Lau YW, et al. Why is psychiatric nursing not the preferred option for nursing students: a cross-sectional study examining pre-nursing and nursing school factors. Nurse Educ Today. 2017;52:95–102.

29. Chang S, Ong HL, Seow E, Chua BY, Abdin E, Samari E, et al. Stigma towards mental illness among medical and nursing students in Singapore: a cross-sectional study. BMJ Open. 2017;7(12):e018099.

30. Donnellan MB, Oswald FL, Baird BM, Lucas RE. The mini-IPIP scales: tiny-yet-effective measures of the big five factors of personality. Psychol Assess. 2006;18(2):192.

31. Goldberg LR. A broad-bandwidth, public domain, personality inventory measuring the lower-level facets of several five-factor models. Personality psychology in Europe 1999;7(1):7–28.

32. Hair JF, Anderson RE, Tatham RL, William C. Multivariate Data Analysis. Harlow: Pearson; 2010.

33. Griffiths KM, Christensen H, Jorm AF, Evans K, Groves C. Effect of web-based depression literacy and cognitive–behavioural therapy interventions on stigmatising attitudes to depression. Br J Psychiatry. 2004;185(4):342–9.

34. Link BG, Phelan JC, Bresnahan M, Stueve A, Pescosolido BA. Public conceptions of mental illness: labels, causes, dangerousness, and social distance. Am J Public Health. 1999;89(9):1328–33.

35. Jorm AF, Korten AE, Jacomb PA, Christensen H, Rodgers B, Pollitt P. "mental health literacy": a survey of the public's ability to recognise mental disorders and their beliefs about the effectiveness of treatment. Med J Aust. 1997; 166(4):182–6 Epub 1997/02/17. PubMed PMID: 9066546.

36. Jorm AF, Wright A, Morgan AJ. Beliefs about appropriate first aid for young people with mental disorders: findings from an Australian national survey of youth and parents. Early Interv Psychiatry 2007;1(1):61–70. Epub 2007/02/01. doi: https://doi.org/10.1111/j.1751-7893.2007.00012.x. PubMed PMID: 21352109.

37. Chong SA, Abdin E, Picco L, Pang S, Jeyagurunathan A, Vaingankar JA, et al. Recognition of mental disorders among a multiracial population in Southeast Asia. BMC Psychiatry. 2016;16(1):121. Epub 2016/05/05. doi: https://doi.org/10.1186/s12888-016-0837-2. PubMed PMID: 27142577; PubMed Central PMCID: PMCPMC4855433.

38. Hu L, Bentler PM. Cutoff criteria for fit indexes in covariance structure analysis: conventional criteria versus new alternatives. Struct Equ Model Multidiscip J. 1999;6(1):1–55.

39. Rosseel Y. lavaan: An R Package for Structural Equation Modeling. 2012; 48(2):36 Epub 2012-05-24. doi: https://doi.org/10.18637/jss.v048.i02.

40. Yuan Q, Picco L, Chang S, Abdin E, Chua BY, Ong S, et al. Attitudes to mental illness among mental health professionals in Singapore and comparisons with the general population. PLoS One 2017;12(11):e0187593. Epub 2017/11/18. doi: https://doi.org/10.1371/journal.pone.0187593. PubMed PMID: 29145419.

41. Szeto AC, O'Neill TA, Dobson KS. The association between personality and individual differences and stigma toward people with mental disorders. Am J Psychiatr Rehabil. 2015;18(4):303–32.

42. Stuber J, Meyer I, Link B. Stigma, prejudice, discrimination and health. Soc Sci Med. 2008;67(3):351.

43. Ekehammar B, Akrami N, Gylje M, Zakrisson I. What matters most to prejudice: big five personality, social dominance orientation, or right-wing authoritarianism? Eur J Personal. 2004;18(6):463–82.

44. De Julio S, Duffy K. Neuroticism and proxemic behavior. Percept Mot Skills. 1977;45(1):51–5.

45. Couture S, Penn D. Interpersonal contact and the stigma of mental illness: a review of the literature. J Ment Health. 2003;12(3):291–305.

46. Pettigrew TF, Tropp LR. When groups meet: the dynamics of intergroup contact: psychology press; 2013.

47. Barlow FK, Paolini S, Pedersen A, Hornsey MJ, Radke HR, Harwood J, et al. The contact caveat: negative contact predicts increased prejudice more than positive contact predicts reduced prejudice. Personal Soc Psychol Bull. 2012;38(12):1629–43.

48. Jackson JW, Poulsen JR. Contact experiences mediate the relationship between five-factor model personality traits and ethnic prejudice. J Appl Soc Psychol. 2005;35(4):667–85.

49. Matzler K, Renzl B, Müller J, Herting S, Mooradian TA. Personality traits and knowledge sharing. J Econ Psychol. 2008;29(3):301–13.

50. Roberts BW, Mroczek D. Personality trait change in adulthood. Curr Dir Psychol Sci. 2008;17(1):31–5.

51. Roberts BW, Wood D, Smith JL. Evaluating five factor theory and social investment perspectives on personality trait development. J Res Pers. 2005; 39(1):166–84.

# 19

# Distraction towards contextual alcohol cues and craving are associated with levels of alcohol use among youth

Timo Lehmann Kvamme[1,2,3] (iD), Kristine Rømer Thomsen[1], Mette Buhl Callesen[1], Nuria Doñamayor[2,4], Mads Jensen[3], Mads Uffe Pedersen[1] and Valerie Voon[2,5,6*]

## Abstract

**Background:** Controlling drinking behaviour requires the ability to block out distracting alcohol cues in situations in which drinking is inappropriate or harmful. However, at present few studies have investigated whether distraction and response inhibition to contextual alcohol cues are related to alcohol use in adolescents and young adults. We aimed to investigate whether tendencies towards distraction and failures of response inhibition in the presence of contextual alcohol cues, and alcohol craving were associated with higher levels of alcohol consumption, beyond what could be explained by demographic variables.

**Methods:** To test this, 108 participants (Mean age = 21.7, range = 16–27), whom were both drinkers and non-drinkers performed a modified Go/NoGo task tailored to measure distraction and response inhibition in the presence of alcohol cues relative to neutral stimuli. Alcohol craving was assessed using a visual analogue scale of craving for different types of alcohol cues. Levels of alcohol use and problematic alcohol use were assessed using a self-report measure of number of drinking days in the previous month and the Alcohol Use Disorders Identification Test. Data were analysed using sequential multiple regression using a zero-inflated negative binomial distribution model.

**Results:** Drinking days correlated with distraction but not response inhibition to contextual alcohol cues. Sequential regression analyses revealed that the inclusion of distraction bias accounted for 11% additional variance (significant) in alcohol use, in addition to that explained by demographics alone (17%). Craving for alcohol explained an additional 30% variance (significant) in alcohol use.

**Conclusions:** The results reported here support the idea that both biased distraction towards alcohol cues and alcohol craving are associated with preceding drinking days, but not necessarily drinking status. Further studies are warranted that address whether cognitive distraction to alcohol-related cues cause or is an effect of alcohol use among youth.

**Keywords:** Alcohol, Distraction, Go/NoGo task, Craving, Zero-inflated negative binomial

## Background

Goal-directed behaviour can become derailed by momentary distracting stimuli such as the sight of alcohol cues [1]. Importantly, these alcohol cues are often conceptualised as acquiring their incentive value long before an individual is diagnosed with any Alcohol Use Disorder (AUD; American Psychiatric Association, 2013) [2, 3]. Initial studies on cognitive biases reported an association between attentional and approach biases to alcohol cues and indices of (problematic) alcohol consumption [4–6]. These cognitive biases have been hypothesized to be central to the aetiology and maintenance of addictive behaviours [7, 8].

Attentional biases towards alcohol cues have traditionally been measured using the Stroop task, in which participants are to report the colour of a word while ignoring its meaning (which is either substance-related or neutral). Here, heavy drinkers tend to be slower than light drinkers in reporting the colours of alcohol-related words compared to neutral words [1, 9, 10], suggesting

---

* Correspondence: vv247@cam.ac.uk
[2]Department of Psychiatry, University of Cambridge, Cambridge, UK
[5]Behavioural and Clinical Neurosciences Institute, University of Cambridge, Cambridge, UK
Full list of author information is available at the end of the article

that heavy drinkers are distracted by the presence of alcohol-related cues. In the visual-dot probe task heavy drinkers show an attentional bias indicated by reduced latencies when detecting a target that replaces an alcohol-related cue [11]. Furthermore, studies suggest that heavy drinkers display attentional biases in later stages of processing whereas abstinent alcoholics differ in initial orientation [12, 13]. Despite these findings, the purported ability of the attention bias measure to predict alcohol relapse [6] has failed replication [14, 15] and a recent review argue that the clinical relevance of attentional biases may be overstated in the literature [16].

Responses towards alcohol cues have also been investigated in the alcohol-shifting task, a variant of the Go/NoGo paradigm. In an alcohol-shifting task, the participant is asked to switch between performing two separate tasks: 1) to associate alcohol cues as Go-signals vs. neutral stimuli as NoGo-signals and 2) neutral stimuli as Go-signals and alcohol cues as NoGo-signals. Here, Noël et al. reported that both alcohol dependent and control participants were faster to respond to alcohol-related words when they were Go-signals as opposed to neutral words [17]. It was reported that alcohol dependent individuals made a higher number of false alarms (Go responses to a NoGo signal) and omission errors (NoGo responses to a Go signal) when alcohol stimuli had to be detected compared with control participants. Mixed results emerge when problem drinkers and individuals who display moderate to heavy alcohol use (but without a diagnosis of alcohol dependence) are tested. Rose and Duka report in a single sample that moderate-to-heavy drinkers have slowed responses to alcohol Go-signals [18]. In contrast, Adams et al. show faster responses to alcohol Go-signals, with no clear difference between heavy and light drinkers defined by quantity of consumption [19]. Faster responses and a higher rate of false alarm to alcohol Go-signals in general were also reported in a population of problem drinkers defined by problematic drinking severity scores [20].

The alcohol and neutral stimuli in the aforementioned variant of the Go/NoGo task can be considered task-relevant as participants are instructed to form the association between the detection of either alcohol or neutral stimuli and a motor response or inhibition. A demonstration of faster responses and a higher rate of false alarm to alcohol go-signals [20], could potentially arise from multiple cognitive processes. The alcohol stimuli could have acquired attention-grabbing properties akin to a cue-specific attention bias speeding up the detection of the target. Alternatively, the alcohol stimuli could induce enhanced motivational processes due to the associated positive affect leading to hastened motor responses as seen with approach biases [5]. In both cases the resultant overt behaviour is the same; hastened

responses and a higher rate of false alarm in the presence of alcohol.

Less explored is the option to use neutral and alcohol stimuli as task-irrelevant distractors, similar to an Emotional Stroop task [1]. In this version of the Go/NoGo task which is also modified with alcohol cues, instructions remains the same as participants are to detect a target (either the letter "P" or "F") as Go or NoGo targets, while task-irrelevant alcohol or neutral stimuli interferes with the detection of the targets [21]. Here, the task models an everyday scenario, where one is searching for a signal relevant for goal-directed behaviour while contextual salient cues interact with the cognitive process. To our knowledge, an assessment of alcohol-specific cognitive bias using this task with pictorial stimuli has not been reported in the scientific literature.

This approach is theoretically intriguing as generalized Pavlovian-instrumental-transfer theories would argue that the presence of the motivational characteristics of contextual alcohol cues might enhance the process of detection, thus hastening responses in the presence of alcohol stimuli [22, 23]. Another set of theories would argue that emotional distractors can interfere with on-going cognitive processes [24, 25]. As an example, a recent study employing distractors in a Go/NoGo task suggests that emotional cues exert distracting effects with task-irrelevant cues [26]. We propose that the repeated pairing of alcohol cues and alcohol consumption, as a rewarding outcome, might result in alcohol cues gaining emotional valence and attention-grabbing properties thus slowing responses in the presence of alcohol stimuli [27, 28].

According to the incentive-salience model, the relationship between consumption and biases towards drug-cues is not limited to the above-mentioned cognitive bias measures, but also include evaluative biases such as self-reported craving of the drug of abuse (a subjective proxy of the motivational state) [7, 8]. Studies on alcohol use are plagued by contrasting findings as some studies show higher craving scores in heavy compared to light drinkers [13] as well as a correlation between craving for alcohol and drinks/week in individuals suffering from AUDs [29]. Other studies have, in contrast, not found correlations between craving and alcohol use in social drinkers [3] and heavy drinkers [30].

As increasing levels of alcohol consumption during adolescence and young adulthood may lead to the later emergence of AUDs [2, 31], an investigation of how these cognitive and evaluative biases are associated with heightened alcohol consumption in this age-group is important.

In this study, we devised a modified Go/NoGo task in order to investigate attentional distraction and response inhibition to contextual alcohol cues and the relationship to past month drinking days in a sample of adolescents and young adults. The first aim of the study was to test for a main effect of alcohol-related distractors on response latencies and false alarms to no-go signals. On the basis of other findings [1, 26], we expected alcohol cues to act as distractors due to their elevated emotional/incentive value compared to neutral cues leading to slower reaction times and a higher percentage of false alarms. We operationalised an alcohol-specific distraction and inhibition bias as slowed responding and increased false alarms on trials with task-irrelevant alcohol cues compared with task-irrelevant neutral stimuli. Secondly, the study aimed to investigate the association between cognitive biases in the modified Go/NoGo Task and drinking days in the preceding month. We expected the retrospective alcohol consumption in the weeks leading up to cognitive testing to correlate with indices of biased distraction and inhibition towards alcohol cues. Moreover, we expected cognitive biases to explain a larger degree of variance in levels of alcohol use than what can be attributed to demographic variables of age, gender, and years of education. Finally, we explored whether craving for alcohol could explain any additional variance in levels of alcohol use.

## Methods

### Participants

The present study is part of a larger study designed to examine risk factors for problematic use of substances and non-substances among youth (for details see Rømer Thomsen et al., 2018) [36]. In order to obtain a subclinical group of youth with varying risk of developing problematic use, and with varying levels of current use, we recruited adolescents and young adults with varying degree of externalizing behavior problems. Externalizing behavioural problems have been consistently shown to increase the risk of problematic substance use and have been associated longitudinally with problematic use of alcohol and other substances [32–34].

Participants were selected from a representative national survey (*YouthMap2014 by Statistics Denmark*, $N = 3064$) based on their level of externalizing problems, measured with the EP6 [32] (EP6 consists of six items that identify externalizing behaviour problems). In total, we included 109 adolescents and young adults (aged 15–26 years) with varying levels of EP6: no externalizing problems ($N = 34$), minimal externalizing problems ($N = 19$), moderate externalizing problems ($N = 25$), and severe externalizing problems ($N = 30$).

Participants were included if they had no current major psychiatric disorder assessed with the Mini International Neuropsychiatric Inventory [35], and did not receive medication. Participants were instructed to abstain from substances (tobacco was allowed) at least 24 h prior to their participation. The study was approved by the local ethics committee and all participants received verbal and written information about the study and gave written consent prior to inclusion. Furthermore, in accordance with requirements by the local ethics committee (De Videnskabsetiske Komitéer for Region Midtjylland, case number: 1–10–72-123-15), for participants aged 15–17, parents also received written information about the study (and were offered verbal information) to ensure that the adolescent's consent was given under parental supervision.

### Self-report measures
#### Drinking days last 30 days
We measured alcohol use by asking participants to report the number of days in which they had drunk alcohol the past 30 days as part of the Addiction Severity Index [37] also used in the European Model Questionnaire, EMCDDA [38]. We regard reporting the number of days of drinking in the recent month to be less susceptible to errors of memory and other self-report response biases [39].

AUDIT scores. Problematic use of alcohol was measured using the Alcohol Use Disorder Identification Test (AUDIT) [40], which is a 10-item questionnaire developed as a screening instrument for hazardous and harmful alcohol consumption.

### Craving scores & personalization
Participants were presented with 40 alcohol pictures and instructed to rate how much they were tempted to drink this right now (In Danish; "hvor fristet er du til at drikke dette") on a computerized Visual Analog Scale from 0 to 9. It was our intention that participants would be exposed to the alcohol cues and asked to reflect on their level temptation to drink, in order to prime any attentional-distraction bias they might have to the cues.

The alcohol pictures were obtained from the internet and aimed to reflect the array of alcohol choices that are typically available to Danish youths. The alcohol pictures included bottles of beer, cider, alcopops and wine, and glasses of beer, wine, liquor and cocktails. The purpose of the picture rating was to derive a composite craving score and to select a subset of the 10 highest rated images that could be used in the subsequent Go/NoGo task.

### Go/NoGo task
Distraction and response inhibition bias to alcohol cues was measured using a modified version of the Go/NoGo Task, similar to that of Houben et al. [21]. Participants were instructed to press the space bar when Go-signals were presented and withhold responding when NoGo-signals were presented. The Go/NoGo-signals were the letters "P" and "F" (counterbalanced across participants), displayed randomly but with equal occurrence in one of the four corners of a centred image. A task-irrelevant distractor of either a neutral or an alcohol cue were presented in the centre of

the screen (Fig. 1). The alcohol cues were individualized based on participants 10 highest-rated pictures. Each alcohol picture had been matched to a neutral picture obtained from a set of standardized pictures [41], approximately matched for colour, form, and complexity. Images subtended a visual angle of $8.5° \times 13.7°$, and letters were presented at $6.7°$ of retinal eccentricity subtending $0.7° \times 0.7°$. Stimuli were presented against a white background on a 19″ monitor ($1280 \times 1024$ resolution, 60 Hz).

Participants were seated in a dimly-lit room and wore headphones for sound-attenuation. All participants completed 10 practice trials without alcohol cues. In the main task, each of the 10 different alcohol and neutral images was paired 16 times with a Go-signal (80% of trials) and 4 times with a NoGo-signal (20% of trials); totalling 400 trials taking approximately 8 min. Trials were presented in a random order.

Stimulus duration was 500 ms, the inter-trial interval was a random interval between 100 and 200 ms where a central fixation cross was displayed. If participants missed the 500 ms reaction time (RT) deadline, a 300 ms error tone of 440 Hz was delivered through the headphones accompanied by a visual feedback text "you were too slow" presented for 500 ms. False alarms (commission errors) did not lead to any feedback except in the initial practice trials where a "wrong" text was presented. The stimulation interface was custom programmed in Python using PsychoPy (Version 1.81.0) [42].

### Analysis strategy

Data analyses were performed using the statistical programming language R (Version 3.4.3). Out of the 109 participants, one participant did not complete the task. In line with prior research on cognitive biases using RT-based measures, we calculated medians to summarise participants' first level scores on the Go/NoGo task as medians minimize the effect of outliers [43, 44].

Distraction bias scores were calculated by subtracting the median RT of alcohol Go trials from neutral Go trials. To control for difference in average RT, we used the improved scoring-algorithm by Greenwald and colleagues (2003) which standardizes the bias scores by dividing the individual RT difference by a personalized standard deviation of these latencies [45]. False alarm rates were calculated for alcohol and neutral trials using signal detection theory [46]. Response inhibition bias was computed by subtracting the false alarm rate on neutral NoGo trials from the false alarm rate on alcohol cued NoGo trials. Positive bias scores indicate a tendency towards distraction or inhibition failures in the presence of alcohol cues.

Craving scores were derived from the median of the same 10 highest rated alcohol images as used in the task. We reasoned that the 10 highest rated images would likely reflect their choice of beverage if they consumed alcohol.

On the second level, the aforementioned variables were examined for outlier participants using the R package 'mvoutlier' [47], which allows for the robust evaluation of multivariate datasets. We also inspected the values that were 2.5 standard deviations (SD) from the group mean. Both approaches resulted in the detection and removal of two outliers, i.e. two participants who reported 22 and 27 days drinking in the last 30 days, reducing the final sample to 106.

### Statistical tests

One-sample t-tests were used to evaluate whether bias scores significantly deviated from zero. Pearson's correlations and sequential multiple regression analyses were used to determine the association between demographics, behavioural task measures, and alcohol use.

Despite the relative prevalence of alcohol use, many adolescents and young adults have not consumed alcohol in the last 30 days, with the underlying cause often being unknown. Consequently, a challenge in modelling

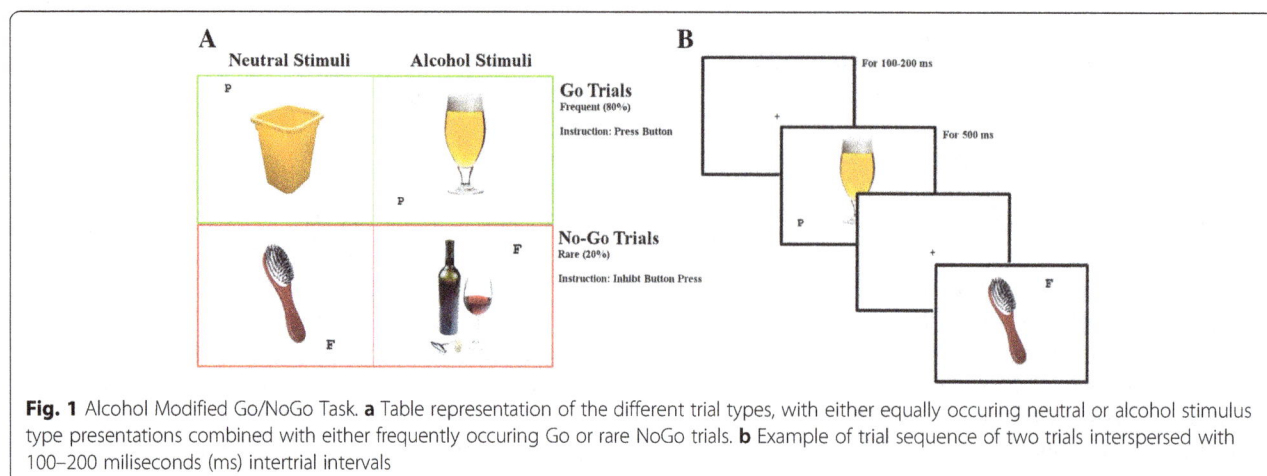

**Fig. 1** Alcohol Modified Go/NoGo Task. **a** Table representation of the different trial types, with either equally occuring neutral or alcohol stimulus type presentations combined with either frequently occuring Go or rare NoGo trials. **b** Example of trial sequence of two trials interspersed with 100–200 miliseconds (ms) intertrial intervals

alcohol consumption is to appropriately account for the large number of zeroes (potentially abstinent individuals), along with a long right tail of heavier drinkers [48]. In our analysis, the days of alcohol use within the last 30 days were not normally distributed (Shapiro-Wilk test: $p < 0.001$) and consisted of a large number of zeros (18.7%). Thus, we employed a generalized linear model (GLM). GLMs extend the ordinary least squares (OLS) regression to instances where the distribution of the response variable is non-normal and allows the magnitude of the variance to be modelled through the use of appropriate 'link' functions. Similar to other modelling approaches [49], the distribution model for alcohol use was selected after inspection of relevant histograms and QQplots, and comparison of fitted models using the Akaike information criterion (AIC).

Accordingly, the Zero-Inflated Negative Binomial (ZINB) distribution model was chosen with a logit link function consisting of a natural offset boundary at 30. The primary strength of the ZINB regression model is the explicit partitioning of the zero values into two types: "structural" zeros, i.e. those that occur because a participant has chosen to be abstinent and those zeros that occur from mere chance among eligible drinkers. The model thus simultaneously estimates a logistic component of the odds ratio of a participant being classified as a structural zero and a count component reflecting the levels of consumption along a scale from 0 to 30 days.

To assess whether distraction bias scores explained variance of alcohol use beyond what could be attributed to demographic variables, sequential multiple regression using ZINB distribution models was employed. To control for other variables, in the first step the dependent variable of alcohol use measured as drinking days within the last 30 days was regressed onto demographic variables of age, gender and years of education (Model 1), after which distraction bias was entered in a second step (Model 2). In a third step (Model 3) we explored whether the addition of craving scores significantly explained further variance in drinking days. We did not include interactions. We performed model comparisons of the difference in the log-likelihood ratio between sequential ZINB models that did or did not include additional variables of interest. This ratio approximates a $\chi^2$ distribution and can thus be compared using a likelihood ratio chi-squared test (LR $\chi^2$) to assess whether two models differ significantly, where the degrees of freedom are the difference in the free parameters of the two models. Associated $p$-values of the regression models were Bonferroni-corrected for multiple comparisons and the results were considered significant if $p < 0.05$. Regression diagnostics indicated no violation of the assumptions of multicollinearity, independence and normal distribution of errors (maximum Cook's distance = 0.036, maximum

deviance residual = 2.23). Variance inflation factors were only above 1.20 for age and years of education which were control variables, thus suggesting that multicollinearity was not a problem. The model did violate the assumption of homoscedasticity (Breusch-Pagan test: $p = 0.018$), although this is common for count models [48, 50].

To obtain effect sizes for explained variance in the regression models we compared the likelihood ratio-based $R^2$, which is a measure of fit analogous to the coefficient of determination ($R^2$) in OLS regression [51]. Although the likelihood ratio-based $R^2$ approximates an easily interpretable measure of effect size, the $R^2$ used in maximum-likelihood estimation regression is different from the $R^2$ used in OLS regression and should be interpreted with caution [52]. When estimating the total variation explained by a model, we compare the $R^2$ to a null model, which only models the dependent variable with an intercept.

## Results

We found no main stimulus differences in either distraction ($t_{105} = 0.10$, $p = 0.91$) or response inhibition ($t_{105} = 0.047$, $p = 0.96$) as bias scores did not significantly deviate from zero. Pearson's correlation coefficients are presented in Table 1 and visualized in scatter plots (Fig. 2). The distraction bias scores were moderately correlated with drinking days within the last 30 days ($r = 0.33$, $p < 0.001$), but did not correlate with AUDIT scores ($r = -0.10$, $p = 0.28$). There were no statistically significant correlations between response inhibition bias and alcohol use the last 30 days or problematic use (AUDIT). Instead, craving scores were strongly correlated with drinking days ($r = 0.51$, $p < 0.001$) and moderately correlated with problematic use (AUDIT) ($r = 0.36$, $p < 0.001$) as well as distraction bias ($r = 0.22$, $p = 0.02$).

Model 1 which was constituted by control variables explained 16.7% of the variance in drinking days which was significantly more than the null model (LR$\chi^2(2) = 19.14$, $p = 0.003$). The explained variance in Model 2, which included distraction bias, explained an additional 11.0% and was significantly higher than Model 1 (LR $\chi^2(2) = 12.25$, $p = 0.002$; see Table 2). Model 3, which included craving scores in addition to distraction bias and control variables, explained an additional 30.2% variance in drinking days, which was significantly different from Model 2 (LR $\chi^2(2) = 37.32$, p < 0.001).

Concerning the statistical significance of individual variables of the ZINB models, in Model 1, only gender was associated with drinking days, whereby expected male users tended to show more days using alcohol than expected female users. The control variables were unable to distinguish structural zeros (i.e. expected non-users) from zeroes that occurred by chance (i.e. expected users

**Table 1** Summary Statistics and Pearson's correlation coefficients

| | M [SD] | 1 | 2 | 3 | 4 | 5 | 6 | 7 | VIF |
|---|---|---|---|---|---|---|---|---|---|
| 1. Alcohol Use (Drinking Days) | 3.86 [3.44] | **1.00** | | | | | | | – |
| 2. Distraction Bias | 0.22 [22.41] | **0.33*** | **1.00** | | | | | | 1.06 |
| 3. Inhibition Bias | 0.0004 [0.10] | 0.00 | 0.04 | **1.00** | | | | | 1.03 |
| 4. AUDIT | 8.65 [5.89] | **0.23*** | − 0.10 | 0.00 | **1.00** | | | | – |
| 5. Craving | 3.16 [2.57] | **0.51*** | **0.22*** | 0.10 | **0.36*** | **1.00** | | | 1.12 |
| 6. Gender[1] | f/m 0.43% | **−0.26**** | − 0.02 | 0.07 | − 0.12 | **−0.22*** | **1.00** | | 1.14 |
| 7. Age | 21.71 [2.69] | **0.31**** | −0.01 | 0.00 | 0.08 | 0.00 | −0.08 | **1.00** | 1.85 |
| 8. Years of Education | 13.50 [1.86] | **0.20*** | −0.06 | 0.07 | 0.08 | 0.01 | 0.09 | **0.66*** | 1.87 |

[a]Gender was coded as male = 0, female = 1; M = mean; SD = standard deviation; Numbers from 1 to 7 in the top row represents each variable in the leftmost column; *VIF* Variance Inflation Factors for the sequential regression models of drinking days, *AUDIT* Alcohol Use Disorder Identification Test; Significant coefficients are in **boldface.** *$p < 0.05$, **$p < 0.01$, $p < 0.001$***

that didn't consume alcohol in the past 30 days). In Model 2, gender was still associated with drinking days while distraction bias to alcohol was positively associated with a higher number of drinking days within the last 30 days ($p = 0.004$). Higher distraction bias scores tended to relate to decreased likelihood of being a non-user but did not reach statistical significance. In Model 3, gender (being male), age, distraction bias and craving scores were all significantly positively associated with increased number of drinking days. In the third and final model, age was the only variable significantly able to discern users from non-users ($p = 0.026$), showing that as age increases the likelihood of being a non-user decreases. Results of the regression analyses are presented in Table 2.

## Discussion

Our study shows that biased distraction towards alcohol-related cues among youth is associated with number of preceding drinking days. Participants with increased proclivity for distraction in the presence of alcohol cues, as indicated by slowed responses, tended to have increased alcohol use, but not necessarily higher degree of problematic use (AUDIT score). We found no main effect of stimulus type on response latency on Go

trials or false alarms on NoGo trials, nor a statistically significant relationship between biased false alarms and drinking days or problematic alcohol use. Exploratory analyses pointed to evaluative craving scores as contributing a substantial and significant amount of explained variance in number of days drinking. The results reported here support the idea that both biased distraction towards alcohol cues and alcohol craving are associated with preceding drinking days, even when controlling for the effects of demographic variables (age, gender, and years of education). One of the primary strengths of the present study is the use of ZINB regression to separately model users and non-users as well as levels of consumption among users. Here, the results show that the variance in participants' gender, age, their distraction to contextual alcohol cues, and their alcohol craving are significantly associated with the variance in number of drinking days within expected users, but that the variance in age is the only variable able to statistically discern whether a person is a user or non-user. This is also of theoretical interest for substance use research, as it suggests that other factors than distraction to alcohol cues are more pertinent to the status of being a user or non-user.

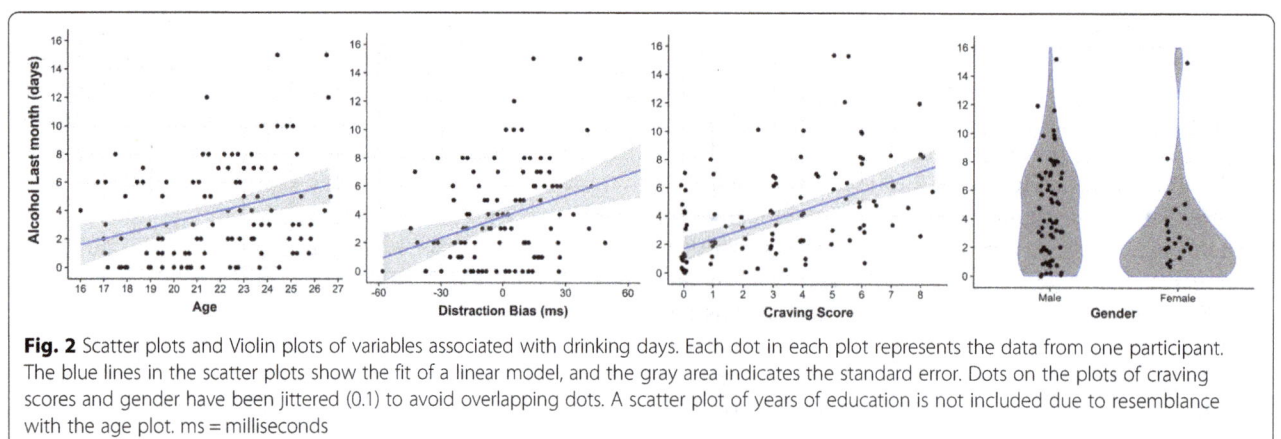

**Fig. 2** Scatter plots and Violin plots of variables associated with drinking days. Each dot in each plot represents the data from one participant. The blue lines in the scatter plots show the fit of a linear model, and the gray area indicates the standard error. Dots on the plots of craving scores and gender have been jittered (0.1) to avoid overlapping dots. A scatter plot of years of education is not included due to resemblance with the age plot. ms = milliseconds

**Table 2** Zero Inflated Negative Binominal Models of Alcohol Use

| | Logistic Component | | | | Count Component | | | |
|---|---|---|---|---|---|---|---|---|
| | β [SE] | Exp(β) | Z | P | β [SE] | Exp(β) | z | p |
| **Model 1:** Change $R^2$: 0.17 LR $\chi^2$(6) = 19.14** (AIC: 514.62) | | | | | | | | |
| Age | −0.248[0.204] | 0.780 | −1.217 | 0.224 | 0.559[0.036] | 1.057 | 1.540 | 0.124 |
| Gender | 0.652[0.792] | 1.919 | 0.823 | 0.411 | **−0.469[0.192] *** | **0.626** | **−2.434** | **0.015** |
| Years of education | −0.037[0.280] | 0.964 | −0.133 | 0.894 | 0.021[0.050] | 1.021 | 0.411 | 0.681 |
| **Model 2:** Change $R^2$: 0.11 LR $\chi^2$(2) = 12.25** (AIC: 506.36) | | | | | | | | |
| Age | −0.224[0.199] | 0.799 | −1.128 | 0.259 | 0.051[0.034] | 1.052 | 1.510 | 0.131 |
| Gender | 0.685[0.796] | 1.983 | 0.860 | 0.390 | **−0.460[0.182] *** | **0.631** | **−2.534** | **0.011** |
| Years of education | −0.079 [0.280] | 0.924 | −0.281 | 0.779 | 0.031[0.047] | 1.031 | 0.660 | 0.509 |
| Distraction Bias | −0.024[0.016] | 0.976 | −1.474 | 0.141 | **0.010[0.003] **** | **1.009** | **2.910** | **0.004** |
| **Model 3:** Change $R^2$: 0.30 LR $\chi^2$(2) = 37.32*** (AIC: 473.05) | | | | | | | | |
| Age | **−0.878[0.412] *** | **0.416** | **−2.130** | **0.032** | **0.065[0.031] *** | **1.067** | **2.086** | **0.037** |
| Gender | −1.668[1.564] | 0.188 | −1.066 | 0.286 | **−0.375[0.160] *** | **0.687** | **−2.340** | **0.019** |
| Years of education | 0.543[0.526] | 1.721 | 1.032 | 0.302 | 0.033[0.043] | 1.034 | 0.771 | 0.441 |
| Distraction Bias | −0.054[0.038] | 0.948 | −1.426 | 0.154 | **0.109[0.028] **** | **1.008** | **2.811** | **0.005** |
| Craving Scores | −4.099[2.365] | 0.017 | −1.733 | 0..083 | **0.109[0.029] ***** | **1.115** | **3.802** | **< 0.001** |

Note. $N = 106$, Gender was coded as male = 0, female = 1; Significant coefficients are in **boldface**. *$p < 0.05$, **$p < 0.01$, $p < 0.001$***. Final model $R^2$: 0.58, adjusted $R^2$: 0.48. The $R^2$ is a log-likelihood-based coefficient of determination (see method for details). LR $\chi^2$(df) Log Likelihood Ratio Chi-squared test, df degrees of freedom, β coefficients SE standard error, Exp(β) exponentiated coefficient. Exponentiated coefficient represent the odds of a structural zero score in the logistic component of the model and levels of use in the count component of the models

Our main finding is that the inclusion of distraction bias accounts for 11% additional variance, beyond what can be attributed to demographic variables, which alone accounts for 17%, and where only gender was a significant variable among these. Since both alcohol and neutral cues were task-irrelevant, slowed responding on alcohol cues compared to neutral can be interpreted as a distraction from the task-relevant ("P" versus "F") discrimination. The demonstrated association contributes to the literature linking individual cognitive biases and individual differences in substance use [1, 4, 53] by showing a robust correlation between distraction bias to alcohol cues and number of days drinking in a sample of light and moderate-to-heavy young drinkers. The results can be interpreted in the framework of Robinson and Berridge's (2001) model of drug addiction, suggesting that the alcohol cues had acquired a higher degree of emotional or incentive value for heavier drinking individuals, as a consequence of the rewarding effects of alcohol exposure [27, 28]. Our findings dovetail with recent studies reporting slower Go responses when emotional stimuli are used as distractors, which is commonly interpreted as emotional distractors drawing attention away from the cognitive task [26]. The abovementioned studies show stimulus conditions to have main effects on dependent measures, but in contrast we fail in our study to find similar effects using alcohol cues. We surmise, however, that the degree to which alcohol cues have acquired emotional valence or incentive value

depend on the relative frequency of drinking in the preceding month. We also note that we find a strong correlation between distraction bias and craving, consistent with the notion that automatic cognitive biases and evaluative craving have a mutually occurring relationship [54].

Distraction bias, as it is measured in this modified Go/NoGo task, can be understood as conceptually overlapping with attentional bias as measured with a dot-probe task [4]. Should they overlap empirically regarding alcohol use, further studies might expect distraction bias to be impacted by chronic exposure to alcohol, as it is seen in AUD [8, 15] or acute exposure to alcohol [55, 56]. Future studies employing both tasks are warranted to investigate a possible correlation between these two measures or to disentangle their potential difference.

The findings are also consistent with cognitive theories of addiction, which assert that the drinker's attention is involuntarily captured by alcohol-related cues and that this distractibility plays an important role in triggering the cognitive-behavioural processes leading to alcohol consumption. In this respect, attentional-distraction bias may serve as a novel neurocognitive biomarker that could possibly predict future alcohol use. Here, prospective studies would ideally be able to further clarify whether distraction bias can be used to predict non-problematic and problematic alcohol use, and the transition between them. It should however be noted that we did not find any correlation between distraction bias and problematic use as indicated by AUDIT.

We found no association between drinking days and inhibition bias measured as increased amount of failures to inhibit responding on trials with alcohol cues. The lack of association is consistent with a study employing the flanker task, showing increased latencies in the presence of alcohol cues, yet no effect of these cues on accuracy [57]. Similarly in a group of healthy young adults, the severity of binge drinking was not associated with inhibition on the CANTAB stop signal task [58]. One could also speculate that the degree of alcohol use correlates with specific variance in neural activity patterns as measured by functional magnetic resonance imaging (fMRI) during failed and successful response inhibition in the task without resulting in discernible overt behavioural measures, as has been demonstrated in younger age groups of drinkers [59, 60], for review see [61].

We show that, using these task parameters and this sample, a correlation between drinking days and alcohol specific lack of inhibition remains to be seen. In this regard, our results inform on recent proposals to compare bias modification effects of different variants of Go/ NoGo training paradigms, using either inhibition in the context of alcohol or general inhibition training to decrease heavy drinking days [62]. Our study also highlights a lack of correlation between drinking days and specific inhibition to contextual alcohol cues.

The results of the explorative third regression model indicated that evaluative craving scores are associated with days drinking in the preceding month, beyond distraction bias and demographic variables. Studies on the relationship between alcohol craving and alcohol use have varied findings [3, 13, 29, 30]. We stress that our craving scores are derived from a novel approach, which is different from previous studies. The noted discrepancy in the literature might relate to interindividual differences in how subjective craving may relate to drinking behaviours, to which our method of calculating craving scores is potentially more sensitive. However, unlike prior studies [3], we did not simultaneously query participant's pleasantness rating for neutral images as a way of controlling the craving scores. Thus, a limitation with our craving scores is that we cannot rule out that the relationship between craving scores and drinking days relates to a general tendency to rate images highly, although this is unlikely. One limitation with the design is that the neutral stimuli was not matched with the alcohol cues on emotional valence, and so it cannot be ruled out that the task measures general distraction to emotionally-valenced cues as opposed to specific alcohol cues. However, as a methodological strength in this study we used the craving score to individualize the stimuli for each participant, thus ensuring that participants were tested on alcohol stimuli that were salient to them.

Before concluding, the most notable limitation with the present study is that the cross-sectional nature of our design does not permit us to draw any causal inference between alcohol use and cognitive measures. Such relationships are ideally investigated in a longitudinal design, able to discern the relative predictive value of implicit and explicit cognitive biases to alcohol. In our case, despite the relatively large amount of variance explained by craving scores compared to distraction bias, it is not certain that interindividual variance in drinking behaviours across time can be explained to the same degree. Moreover, as the present study included young individuals without an AUD diagnosis, the generalization of the results to AUDs is limited. Further studies that directly assess distraction bias, craving and its relationship to traditional measures in a clinical sample is warranted to further clarify the applicability of the present findings.

## Conclusion

In conclusion, we show a novel measure of distraction bias specifically to alcohol cues and its robust association with number of drinking days within adolescents and young adults. The present study did not find evidence for a relationship between response inhibition failures to alcohol cues and drinking days. The results suggest that a beneficial avenue of research is the further investigation of distraction to alcohol cues and alcohol use behaviour across time and different AUD diagnostic populations. Identifying cognitive measures such as distraction bias and its relationship to alcohol use as it potentially leads to problematic use is crucial for the development of risk assessment and effective prevention strategies for alcohol addiction.

**Abbreviations**

AIC: Akaike information criterion; AUD: Alcohol Use Disorder; AUDIT: Alcohol Use Disorder Identification Test; fMRI: Functional magnetic resonance imaging; GLM: Generalized linear model; LR: Likelihood Ratio; OLS: Ordinary least squares; RT: Reaction Time; SD: Standard deviations; ZINB: Zero-Inflated Negative Binomial

**Acknowledgements**

We thank the participants for taking time to travel to Aarhus and take part in the study. We also wish to thank the reviewers Louise Brådvik and Robert Miranda who provided helpful comments and suggestions on the refinement of this manuscript.

## Funding
The project was supported by Aarhus University Research Foundation (AUFF), Assistant Professor Starting Grant - R46-A4016 (KRT, MBC, VV, MUP); Danish Ministry for Social Affairs and the Interior - 9173-0003 (KRT, MBC, MUP, TLK); The German Research Foundation - Research Fellowship - DO1915/1-1 (ND); The Danish Council for Independent Research - (MJ); Medical Research Council - Senior Fellowship - MR/P008747/1 (VV).

## Authors' contributions
KRT, MBC, VV & MUP were responsible for funding acquisition; KRT, MBC & VV devised the main conceptual ideas and the overall study, TLK & VV designed the task; TLK programmed the software for the task; TLK, KRT, MBC, MJ & ND collected the data; TLK analysed the data; TLK, KRT, MBC & VV interpreted the data; TLK wrote the first draft; all authors contributed to the manuscript and approved the final version of the manuscript.

## Consent for publication
Not applicable

## Competing interests
Kristine Rømer Thomsen is an Associate Editor for BMC Psychiatry. No further competing interest to declare.

## Author details
[1]Centre for Alcohol and Drug Research, School of Business and Social Sciences, University of Aarhus, Bartholins Allé 10, Building 1322, 2. Floor, Aarhus C, Denmark. [2]Department of Psychiatry, University of Cambridge, Cambridge, UK. [3]Center of Functionally Integrative Neuroscience, MINDLab, Aarhus University, Aarhus C, Denmark. [4]Department of Psychiatry and Psychotherapy, Charité – Universitätsmedizin Berlin, Berlin, Germany. [5]Behavioural and Clinical Neurosciences Institute, University of Cambridge, Cambridge, UK. [6]NIHR Biomedical Research Council, University of Cambridge, Cambridge, UK.

## References
1.  Cox WM, Blount JP, Rozak a M. Alcohol abusers' and nonabusers' distraction by alcohol and concern-related stimuli. Am J Drug Alcohol Abuse. 2000;26:489–95.
2.  American Psychiatric Association. Diagnostic and statistical manual of mental disorders (DSM-5®). In: American Psychiatric Pub; 2013.
3.  Field M, Mogg K, Bradley BP. Craving and cognitive biases for alcohol cues in social drinkers. Alcohol Alcohol. 2005;40:504–10.
4.  Field M, Cox WM. Attentional bias in addictive behaviors: a review of its development, causes, and consequences. Drug Alcohol Depend. 2008;97:1–20.
5.  Peeters M, Monshouwer K, van de Schoot RAGJ, Janssen T, Vollebergh WAM, Wiers RW. Automatic processes and the drinking behavior in early adolescence: a prospective study. Alcohol Clin Exp Res. 2013;37:1737–44.
6.  Garland EL, Franken IH, Howard MO. Cue-elicited heart rate variability and attentional bias predict alcohol relapse following treatment. Psychopharmacology. 2012;222:17–26.
7.  Franken IHA, van de Wetering BJM. Bridging the gap between the neurocognitive lab and the addiction clinic. Addict Behav. 2015;44:108–14. https://doi.org/10.1016/j.addbeh.2014.11.034.
8.  Field M, Marhe R, Franken IHA. The clinical relevance of attentional bias in substance use disorders. CNS Spectr. 2014;19:225–30. https://doi.org/10.1017/S1092852913000321.
9.  Field M, Christiansen P, Cole J, Goudie A. Delay discounting and the alcohol Stroop in heavy drinking adolescents. Addiction. 2007;102:579–86.
10. Sharma D, Albery IP, Cook C. Selective attentional bias to alcohol related stimuli in problem drinkers and non-problem drinkers. Addiction. 2001;96:285–95.
11. Townshend J, Duka T. Attentional bias associated with alcohol cues: differences between heavy and occasional social drinkers. Psychopharmacology. 2001;157:67–74.
12. Noël X, Colmant M, Van Der Linden M, Bechara A, Bullens Q, Hanak C, et al. Time course of attention for alcohol cues in abstinent alcoholic patients: the role of initial orienting. Alcohol Clin Exp Res. 2006;30:1871–7.
13. Field M, Mogg K, Zetteler J, Bradley BP. Attentional biases for alcohol cues in heavy and light social drinkers: the roles of initial orienting and maintained attention. Psychopharmacology. 2004;176:88–93.
14. Field M, Mogg K, Mann B, Bennett GA, Bradley BP. Attentional biases in abstinent alcoholics and their association with craving. Psychol Addict Behav. 2013;27:71–80. https://doi.org/10.1037/a0029626.
15. Snelleman M, Schoenmakers TM, van de Mheen D. Attentional Bias and approach/avoidance tendencies do not predict relapse or time to relapse in alcohol dependency. Alcohol Clin Exp Res. 2015;39:1734–9.
16. Christiansen P, Schoenmakers TM, Field M. Less than meets the eye: reappraising the clinical relevance of attentional bias in addiction. Addict Behav. 2015;44:43–50.
17. Noël X, Van Der Linden M, D'Acremont M, Bechara A, Dan B, Hanak C, et al. Alcohol cues increase cognitive impulsivity in individuals with alcoholism. Psychopharmacology. 2007;192:291–8.
18. Rose AK, Duka T. Effects of alcohol on inhibitory processes. Behav Pharmacol. 2008;19:284–91.
19. Adams S, Ataya AF, Attwood AS, Munafò MR. Effects of alcohol on disinhibition towards alcohol-related cues. Drug Alcohol Depend. 2013;127: 137–42. https://doi.org/10.1016/j.drugalcdep.2012.06.025.
20. Kreusch F, Vilenne A, Quertemont E. Response inhibition toward alcohol-related cues using an alcohol go/no-go task in problem and non-problem drinkers. Addict Behav. 2013;38:2520–8.
21. Houben K, Havermans RC, Nederkoorn C, Jansen A. Beer à no-go: learning to stop responding to alcohol cues reduces alcohol intake via reduced affective associations rather than increased response inhibition. Addiction. 2012;107:1280–7.
22. Cartoni E, Puglisi-Allegra S, Baldassarre G. The three principles of action: a Pavlovian-instrumental transfer hypothesis. Front Behav Neurosci. 2013. https://doi.org/10.3389/fnbeh.2013.00153.
23. Huys QJM, Cools R, Gölzer M, Friedel E, Heinz A, Dolan RJ, et al. Disentangling the roles of approach, activation and valence in instrumental and pavlovian responding. PLoS Comput Biol. 2011;7:e1002028.
24. Perlstein WM, Elbert T, Stenger VA. Dissociation in human prefrontal cortex of affective influences on working memory-related activity. Proc Natl Acad Sci. 2002;99:1736–41. https://doi.org/10.1073/pnas.241650598.
25. Dolcos F, McCarthy G. Brain systems mediating cognitive interference by emotional distraction. J Neurosci. 2006;26:2072–9. https://doi.org/10.1523/JNEUROSCI.5042-05.2006.
26. Ramos-Loyo J, Llamas-Alonso LA, González-Garrido AA, Hernández-Villalobos J. Emotional contexts exert a distracting effect on attention and inhibitory control in female and male adolescents. Sci Rep. 2017;7.
27. Everitt BJ, Dickinson A, Robbins TW. The neuropsychological basis of addictive behaviour. Brain Res Rev. 2001;36:129–38. https://doi.org/10.1016/S0165-0173(01)00088-1.
28. Robinson TE, Berridge KC. Mechanisms of action of addictive stimuli incentive-sensitization and addiction. Addiction. 2001;96:103–14. https://doi.org/10.1080/09652140020016996.
29. Murphy CM, Stojek MK, Few LR, Rothbaum AO, Mackillop J. Craving as an alcohol use disorder symptom in DSM-5: an empirical examination in a treatment-seeking sample. Exp Clin Psychopharmacol. 2014;22:43–9. https://doi.org/10.1037/a0034535.

30. MacKillop J, Miranda R, Monti PM, Ray LA, Murphy JG, Rohsenow DJ, et al. Alcohol demand, delayed reward discounting, and craving in relation to drinking and alcohol use disorders. J Abnorm Psychol. 2010;119:106–14. https://doi.org/10.1037/a0017513.

31. Ewing SWF, Sakhardande A, Blakemore S-J. The effect of alcohol consumption on the adolescent brain: a systematic review of MRI and fMRI studies of alcohol-using youth. NeuroImage Clin. 2014;5:420–37. https://doi.org/10.1016/j.nicl.2014.06.011.

32. Pedersen MU, Rømer Thomsen K, Pedersen MM, Hesse M. Mapping risk factors for substance use: introducing the YouthMap12. Addict Behav. 2017; 65:40–50. https://doi.org/10.1016/j.addbeh.2016.09.005.

33. Miettunen J, Murray GK, Jones PB, Mäki P, Ebeling H, Taanila A, et al. Longitudinal associations between childhood and adulthood externalizing and internalizing psychopathology and adolescent substance use. Psychol Med. 2014;44:1727–38. https://doi.org/10.1017/S0033291713002328.

34. Chao M, Li X, McGue M. The causal role of alcohol use in adolescent externalizing and internalizing problems: a Mendelian randomization study. Alcohol Clin Exp Res. 2017;41:1953–60.

35. Lecrubier Y, Sheehan DV, Weiller E, Amorim P, Bonora I, Sheehan KH, et al. The MINI international neuropsychiatric interview (MINI). A short diagnostic structured interview: reliability and validity according to the CIDI. Eur Psychiatry. 1997;12:224–31. https://doi.org/10.1016/S0924-9338(97)83296-8.

36. Thomsen KR, Callesen MB, Hesse M, Kvamme TL, Pedersen MM, Pedersen MU, et al. Impulsivity traits and addiction-related behaviours in youth. J Behav Addict. 2018.

37. Denis C, Fatséas M, Beltran V, Serre F, Alexandre JM, Debrabant R, et al. Usefulness and validity of the modified addiction severity index: a focus on alcohol, drugs, tobacco, and gambling. Subst Abus. 2016;37:168–75. https://doi.org/10.1080/08897077.2015.1036334.

38. EMCDDA. EMQ (European Model Questionnaire) Questions Map: Questions used in national general population survey questionnaires, 2002–12. 2013. http://www.emcdda.europa.eu/attachements.cfm/att_212814_EN_Questionnairemap.pdf.

39. Del Boca FK, Darkes J. The validity of self-reports of alcohol consumption: state of the science and challenges for research. Addiction. 2003;98:1–12. https://doi.org/10.1046/j.1359-6357.2003.00586.x.

40. Saunders JB, Aasland OG, Babor TF, de la Fuente JR, Grant M. Development of the alcohol use disorders identification test (AUDIT): WHO collaborative project on early detection of persons with harmful alcohol consumption--II. Addiction. 1993;88:791–804.

41. Blechert J, Meule A, Busch NA, Ohla K. Food-pics: an image database for experimental research on eating and appetite. Front Psychol. 2014;5.

42. Peirce JW. PsychoPy—psychophysics software in Python. J Neurosci Methods. 2007;162:8–13.

43. Wiers RW, Eberl C, Rinck M, Becker ES, Lindenmeyer J. Retraining automatic action tendencies changes alcoholic patients' approach Bias for alcohol and improves treatment outcome. Psychol Sci. 2011;22:490–7. https://doi.org/10.1177/0956797611400615.

44. Peeters M, Wiers RW, Monshouwer K, van de Schoot R, Janssen T, Vollebergh WAM. Automatic processes in at-risk adolescents: the role of alcohol-approach tendencies and response inhibition in drinking behavior. Addiction. 2012;107:1939–46.

45. Greenwald AG, Nosek BA, Banaji MR. Understanding and using the implicit association test: I. an improved scoring algorithm. J Pers Soc Psychol. 2003; 85:197–216. https://doi.org/10.1037/0022-3514.85.2.197.

46. Stanislaw H, Todorov N. Calculation of signal detection theory measures. Behav Res Methods Instrum Comput. 1999;31:137–49. https://doi.org/10.3758/BF03207704.

47. Filzmoser P, Gschwandtner M. mvoutlier: Multivariate outlier detection based on robust methods. R Packag version. 2012:1.

48. Atkins DC, Baldwin SA, Zheng C, Gallop RJ, Neighbors C. A tutorial on count regression and zero-altered count models for longitudinal substance use data. Psychol Addict Behav. 2013;27:166.

49. Tzagarakis C, Pellizzer G, Rogers RD. Impulsivity modulates performance under response uncertainty in a reaching task. Exp Brain Res. 2013;225:227–35.

50. Simons JS, Neal DJ, Gaher RM. Risk for Marijuana-Related Problems among College Students: An Application of Zero-Inflated Negative Binomial Regression. Am J Drug Alcohol Abuse. 2006;32:41–53.

51. Nagelkerke NJD. A note on a general definition of the coefficient of determination. Biometrika. 1991;78:691–2.

52. Cameron CA, Windmeijer FAG. An R-squared measure of goodness of fit for some common nonlinear regression models. J Econ. 1997;77:329–42. https://doi.org/10.1016/S0304-4076(96)01818-0.

53. Cox WM, Fadardi JS, Pothos EM. The addiction-Stroop test: theoretical considerations and procedural recommendations. Psychol Bull. 2006;132: 443–76. https://doi.org/10.1037/0033-2909.132.3.443.

54. Franken IHA. Drug craving and addiction: integrating psychological and neuropsychopharmacological approaches. Prog Neuro-Psychopharmacol Biol Psychiatry. 2003;27:563–79.

55. Duka T, Townshend JM. The priming effect of alcohol pre-load on attentional bias to alcohol-related stimuli. Psychopharmacology. 2004;176:353–62.

56. Schoenmakers T, Wiers RW, Field M. Effects of a low dose of alcohol on cognitive biases and craving in heavy drinkers. Psychopharmacology. 2008; 197:169–78.

57. Nikolaou K, Field M, Duka T. Alcohol-related cues reduce cognitive control in social drinkers. Behav Pharmacol. 2013;24:29–36. https://doi.org/10.1097/FBP.0b013e32835cf458.

58. Bø R, Aker M, Billieux J, Landrø NI. Binge drinkers are fast, able to stop - but they fail to adjust. J Int Neuropsychol Soc. 2016;22:38–46. https://doi.org/10.1017/S1355617715001204.

59. Hatchard T, Mioduszewski O, Fall C, Byron-Alhassan A, Fried P, Smith AM. Neural impact of low-level alcohol use on response inhibition: an fMRI investigation in young adults. Behav Brain Res. 2017;2016(329):12–9. https://doi.org/10.1016/j.bbr.2017.04.032.

60. Whelan R, Conrod PJ, Poline J-B, Lourdusamy A, Banaschewski T, Barker GJ, Bellgrove MA, Büchel C, Byrne M, Cummins TDR. Adolescent impulsivity phenotypes characterized by distinct brain networks. Nat Neurosci. 2012;15:920.

61. Thomsen KR, Osterland TB, Hesse M, Ewing SWF. The intersection between response inhibition and substance use among adolescents. Addict Behav. 2018;78:228–30.

62. Jones A, McGrath E, Houben K, Nederkoorn C, Robinson E, Field M. A comparison of three types of web-based inhibition training for the reduction of alcohol consumption in problem drinkers: study protocol. BMC Public Health. 2014;14:796. https://doi.org/10.1186/1471-2458-14-796.

# Barriers and facilitators of effective health education targeting people with mental illness: a theory-based ethnographic study

N. F. Hempler*, R. A. S. Pals, L. Pedersbæk and P. DeCosta⬛

## Abstract

**Background:** Health education is particularly important for people with mental illness because they are at higher risk of becoming overweight or obese and developing type 2 diabetes than are members of the general population. However, little is known about how to provide health education activities that promote engagement and motivation among people with mental illness.

**Methods:** This study used ethnographic methods to examine barriers and facilitators of effective health education targeting people with mental illness by applying the concept of flow as a theoretical framework. Flow refers to immersion in an activity and is related to motivation. Data were collected through participant observation during eight health-educating activities and were thematically analysed using the concept of flow. Fieldwork was carried out between May and July 2015 in Denmark.

**Results:** Barriers to flow included: 1) information overload, particularly of biomedical rationales for behaviour change; 2) a one-size-fits-all approach that failed to address the needs and preferences of the target group; and 3) one-way communication allowing little time for reflection. Educators promoted a state of flow when they spoke less and acted outside of a traditional expert role, thus engaging participants in the activity. Flow was facilitated when educators were attentive and responsive to people with mental illness, and when they stimulated reflection about health and health behaviour through open-ended questions, communication tools and in small group exercises.

**Conclusions:** This study suggests that more focus should be paid to training of educators in terms of skills to involve and engage people with mental illness in health education activities.

**Keywords:** Health education, Qualitative research, Patient education, Psychosocial theories

## Background

People with serious mental illness have a shorter life expectancy than do members of the general population [1–3]. Approximately 60% of this premature mortality is due to physical diseases such as cardiovascular disease and diabetes [4]. Several explanations for the excess mortality have been suggested, including unhealthy behaviours, adverse metabolic effects of antipsychotics, inadequate access to high-quality physical healthcare, and a cultural tendency to not consider physical diseases when treating mental illness [5–10].

Health behaviours are potentially modifiable. Previous research has shown that people with mental illness are as motivated as other members of the population to engage in health-promoting behaviours [11] However, eliciting behavioural change in people with mental illness has proven difficult; a review based on only 4 studies found some effect of lifestyle interventions on weight in people with psychotic disorders but no effect on blood pressure and cholesterol levels [12]. A recent study found no effect of a yearlong, intensive lifestyle coaching intervention targeting physical inactivity, unhealthy dietary habits and smoking, in people with schizophrenia [13]. This calls for rethinking and developing health education interventions focusing on

* Correspondence: nana.folmann.hempler@regionh.dk
Diabetes Management Research, Steno Diabetes Center Copenhagen, Niels Steensens Vej 6, 2820 Gentofte, Denmark

educator behaviour to improve the treatment of people with mental illness. It has been suggested that lifestyle interventions within mental healthcare require tailoring to address the needs of people with mental illness and that further research is needed to explore barriers and facilitators for participation in health education activities from the perspective of people with mental illness [14–16].

People with mental illness report that the level of engagement and attitudes of educators play an important role in their motivation to engage in health behaviour change [14, 17–20]. For example, educators' lack of motivation for physical activity can negatively affect the motivation of people with mental illness [20]. Another study supports incorporating the beliefs and perspectives on physical activity of people with mental illness into treatment for depression [17]. Educators report that patients' poor state of health as well as a lack of cooperation with other groups of educators pose significant barriers to lifestyle changes [21]. Although existing literature addresses barriers and facilitators of health behaviour change among people with mental illness, little is known about how to facilitate health education activities that promote motivation for behaviour changes in this population. As traditional health education appears unsuccessful, it is relevant to explore alternative approaches, drawing on methods and models from behavioural science, using the experiences of the target group to inform and direct health education activities in practice. This study aims to identify barriers and facilitators of engaging health education across health education activities targeting people with mental illness, through multisided ethnographic fieldwork.

## Methods
### Theoretical framework
Flow refers to an inherently rewarding experiential state that can encourage a person to persist in and return to an activity, such as health behaviours; the theory of flow also focuses on interactionism, which highlights the importance of context [22, 23]. The concept of flow emerged from qualitative interviews about the nature of the experience when a particular activity goes well and is rooted in positive psychology [22, 24]. Flow research originates from examinations of intrinsic motivation, which is a key aspect in the self-determination theory. Intrinsic motivation occurs when an activity or behaviour is driven by an internal reward such as enjoyment, rather than being a means to obtain an external goal or a reward. [23]. According to Nakamura and Csikszentmihalyi, flow is a powerful motivating force [23]. When individuals are fully involved in an activity, they tend to find it enjoyable and intrinsically rewarding. Attention plays a key role in entering into and staying in a flow state.

The theory of flow focuses on the dynamic system composed of person and environment, thereby acknowledging the importance of context [23]. Motivation emerges in the interaction rather than being dictated by a pre-existing structure located within the individual or the environment [23]. Flow is associated with highly engaging activities and situations [22]. In a state of flow, thoughts, feelings and intentions are in harmony, and the activity itself is perceived as meaningful and associated with positive emotions. Activities that create flow tend to be remembered because they are associated with positive emotions and evaluated very positively by participants. Flow has also been associated with perceived competence: People with low perceived competence are likely to experience anxiety or boredom, depending on whether they value performing well at an activity. People with high perceived competence and efficacy are likely to report higher intrinsic motivation to perform an activity [25, 26].

Facilitators of flow include clear goals of activities, immediate feedback from educators and a challenge level that is just manageable for participants. An example of a barrier to flow is activity goals that focus on the needs of staff, e.g. reducing clinical risk and symptoms and improving medication adherence, rather than needs of individual participants [27]. In addition, long-term goals that are too easy or difficult for participants to manage may result in apathy, boredom, and anxiety [27]. Conditions in which flow is stimulated include:

- A balance between perceived skills and perceived challenges. When skills match challenges, participants' attention is completely absorbed. If challenges exceed perceived skills, individuals typically become anxious; if perceived skills exceed challenges, they relax and may become bored.
- A clear set of goals that provides direction and purpose. The value of goals lies in channelling attention to structure the experience, rather than being ends in themselves.
- Clear and immediate feedback on progress. Immediate feedback allows individuals to make changes that improve activity-related performance [23, 24].

Flow was chosen as the theoretical framework in this study as it 1) addresses motivation and learning which is focus points in health education and 2) focuses on context; the interaction between educators and PMI as well as environment of importance for the delivery of health education.

### Data collection
Data collection was part of a larger study to develop a framework for a health education program targeting

people with mental illness (PMI), based on a user-driven approach involving PMI, educators, and family members of PMI. The findings presented here represent the study's initial phase, which focused on the identification of barriers and facilitators of effective health education among PMI. Insights from the fieldwork informed content and focus of workshops with PMI, educators, and family members which is reported elsewhere [28]. The larger study also involved professional development of 152 educators and testing of new methods in practice based on the developed framework (unpublished data).

We conducted multisided ethnographic fieldwork between May and July 2015 in Denmark. Ethnographic fieldwork studies groups and individuals in context, including interactions between people and their physical, material and institutional surroundings [29]. The fieldwork comprised participant observation of health-promoting activities in different care settings, including informal conversations with educators and PMI involved in the activities. Observations included 16 educators and 27 PMI in total. Health educating activities included individual lifestyle/health education consultations and group-based health education e.g. cooking classes, and physical activity.

Settings were identified in collaboration with health educators involved in the project. Educators at the identified municipal and regional care settings were contacted by e-mail or phone with a request to participate in the study. Inclusion of observation settings was based on geographical distribution, availability of individual and group-based activities, and municipal and regional outpatient care settings (Table 1). Inpatient clinics were excluded because the study excluded PMI who were hospitalised during the

observation period. All activities targeted PMI in general, rather than individuals with specific diagnoses. One or two educators, such as social workers, nurses, and physiotherapists, facilitated each activity. Informed consent was obtained from participants before observations.

In Denmark, health activities targeting PMI, can be embedded in ambulatory psychiatry services and in the municipalities. However, format, approach and methods vary substantially from setting to setting. Also, general practitioners can play a role in terms of health behaviour and act as gatekeepers for PMI access to health activities.

### Observation

The aim of observations was to explore the activities, including the physical characteristics of social situations, and participation, dialogue and engagement among PMI, informed by the theoretical framework of flow. The themes were specified in an observation guide, and observations were documented in extensive field notes taken during activities. Themes comprised e.g. the role of the educator (facilitator, teacher or participant) and the role of PMI (proactive, active or passive) and were elaborated in the field notes. The observer participated in activities while maintaining the analytical and intellectual distance needed to interpret the social setting and record field notes [30]. The observers had a background in communication and public health science and were experienced with fieldwork in various health settings. No observers had work experience from psychiatry services. The participation of the observers was passive to moderate, depending on the activity [30].

**Table 1** Characteristics of fieldwork settings

| Setting | Activity | Participants | Data collection |
|---|---|---|---|
| Outpatient clinic | Individual lifestyle consultation | 1 professional 3 PMI | Observations of 3 consultations. |
| Community health center | Group-based cooking class | 3 professionals 5 PMI | Observation. Informal interview |
| Community health center | Individual cooking class followed by a communal meal | 3 professionals 4 PMI (1 PMI and 1 professional participated in the cooking class) | Observation. Informal interview |
| Community health center | Group-based exercise/physical activity | 2 professionals (students) 4 PMI | Observation. Informal interview. |
| Community health center | Group-based education including a walk in the forest | 3 professionals 5 PMI | Observation. Informal interview. |
| Day care center | Individual lifestyle consultation | 1 professional 1 PMI | Observation. |
| Social home | No specific activity | 2 professionals 4 PMI | Observation. Informal interview. |
| Outpatient clinic | Lifestyle consultation/screening | 1 professional 1 PMI | Observation. |

## Data analysis

In order to explore the conditions in which health education activities were meaningful for the participants, the theory of flow was applied to the data analysis. We identified observable markers of flow including balance between challenges and skills, concentration, involvement and enjoyment. For example, a situation involved a dialogue between a PMI and an educator regarding daily life and food preferences; flow was noted as the PMI was engaged verbally (active participation by expressing and sharing needs and preferences with the educator) and non-verbally (concentrating and looking at the educator). Absence of flow included signs of apathy, boredom and anxiety. The analysis of barriers and facilitators of flow was concerned with forms of participation and the content of health-promoting activities. The analysis followed several steps: 1) extracting issues related to facilitators and barriers to flow by reading and re-reading observation notes; 2) analysis of the extracted data and identification of themes by writing down possible themes and categories, additional research questions, and ideas; and 3) interpretation of the data within each theme by identifying recurrent common and contrasting themes across observations. The categorization of themes was informed by the three conditions for flow as defined by Nakamura and Csikszentmihalyi; a balance between perceived skills and perceived challenges, a clear set of goals that provides direction and purpose, and clear and immediate feedback on progress [23].

Two of the authors, NFH and PD, independently coded the data and compared their interpretations, discussing any discrepancies until final agreement was reached. All authors participated in interpreting and discussing themes and categorizations of empirical material.

## Results

### Barriers to flow

#### Lack of balance between skills and challenges due to information overload

In many activities, communication was one-way; the educator did most of the talking and PMI were passive recipients of knowledge. Information overload often inhibited flow. This pattern occurred in both individual health education and group-based activities, such as cooking classes and walks. Educators dominated conversations with closed-ended questions about lifestyles and a strong focus on biomedical reasons for engaging in health behaviour. Educators offered solutions quickly and supported them with biomedical information about 'cause and effect'. This is illustrated in the following excerpt from observation notes:

*At one point, the conversation turns to the fact that the PMI lacks vitamin D. The educator rationalises*

*that this is linked to the fact that he 'barricades' himself indoors and thus does not get any daylight. The educator informs the PMI that there is something called a pineal gland, which produces melatonin. It needs sunlight. If he does not get it, he gets symptoms similar to depression. Therefore, he must at least go for a walk daily.* (Observation, individual lifestyle consultation)

PMI often had difficulty grasping educators' specialised knowledge about triglycerides, hormones, carbohydrates and the like. Communicating knowledge was a central objective for educators, as articulated by one educator after a consultation:

*'I think that I managed to communicate what I wanted to.'* (Observation, individual lifestyle consultation)

While some PMI displayed signs of boredom or apathy in response to information overload, some tried to interrupt the educator. One instance of this occurred during a nature-based education session that included a walk in the forest. The participants were not encouraged to share or reflect on their experiences with nature. At one point, in response to the educator showing a PowerPoint presentation on nature's positive effect on mental health, a PMI interrupted to state:

*'I cannot use all this theory. You are giving us too much information'. Another person adds: 'We get the point. Getting out in nature is good for us. What you have just shown us is more appropriate for educators.'* (Observation, group education followed by a walk)

As exemplified here, the educator's goal seemed to be communicating information, rather than allowing PMI to have and reflect on personal experiences of nature. Information overload was a reoccurring theme across activities and settings. Although the nature-based education session involved both classroom activities and a nature walk, the change of setting did not affect the educator's approach. The educator dominated throughout the session.

### Educator-defined goals

Many health education activities were organized under a comprehensive, structured plan. Although structure could provide direction for activities, a 'one size fits all' focus created a barrier to flow by channelling attention towards the plan rather than the needs of participants. In individual activities, programs, questionnaires, information and organisation of activities failed to take account of PMI individual characteristics or social backgrounds. Group-based activities demonstrated little focus on individual prerequisites, e.g. physical fitness.

Advice was often embedded in logical arguments, and educators told participants what they thought was good for them, a pattern that is antithetical to the experience of flow. A recurrent theme reflected the belief that increased knowledge about cause and effect of healthy lifestyle choices would elicit predetermined behavioural changes in PMI. One example was observed during a group education session in nature. Throughout the session, the educator focused squarely on communicating the positive effects of nature on health:

*'Walking is good for the brain' and 'exercise will promote reflection.'* (Observation, group education followed by a walk)

Another example from observation of an individual lifestyle consultation:

*The educator is talking quite a lot, since there is an agenda to get through (the entire health form must be completed). The educator interrupts [the participant] once in a while to continue with the questions* (Observation, individual screening and lifestyle consultation)

The goal of most activities seemed predefined and static, with little room to adjust to participants' current needs, feedback or personal interests.

### One-way communication and little feedback
The focus of health education activities tended to be on the predefined agenda rather than on responses from PMI. Most educators did not encourage reflection or feedback from participants. This was evident in observations of both group-based and individual settings:

*When the educator integrates some stones into the teaching and passes them around, some participants start to share [personal stories] and show some interest. None of the educators ask questions or follow up on participants' stories.* (Observation, group education followed by a walk)

Educators failed to acknowledge or address cues from participants and continued with the original agenda. Sometimes the educator addressed the concern with a rational solution, instead of exploring the issue further:

*The educator asks if PMI are familiar with the logo 'nøglehulsmærket' (a nutrition label stating that a food fulfils certain requirements for dietary fibre, saturated fat, sugar and salt). The PMI explains that he is familiar with it, but he does not know if he finds it trustworthy. The educator replies: 'But it is [trustworthy].' At the end of the session, the PMI again voices his concerns about 'nøglehulsmærket', to which the educator responds: 'You can trust it'.* (Observation, individual health education and screening)

During one observation, a PMI explained that he experienced persistent stomach pain, nausea and vomiting. He raised this concern several times during the observation. The observer noted:

*It seems like his stomach problems weigh heavily on his mind and that this problem needs to be addressed before he will be able to work on any lifestyle changes.* (Observation, individual lifestyle consultation)

The cues from the PMI about his pain and nausea were not addressed. The educator continued the session as planned, assessed the PMI's risk of diabetes, and gave advice on diet and lifestyle. Another example of participant engagement being overlooked by educators in favour of following a predefined plan is evident in the following observation:

*At one point the group stops at a bench. For the first time during the nature walk, everyone in the group is actively engaging in conversation and seems to be enjoying themselves. The educator interrupts: 'We've got to get going, sorry'. A PMI responds: 'I thought that the point [of the walk] was to talk to one another'.* (Observation, group education followed by a walk)

The need of educators to follow a pre-defined schedule rather than responding to cues and providing constructive feedback is illustrated in the following excerpt from observation notes:

*The educator asks if the patient would like to know his risk of diabetes. He says that he doesn't believe that he has diabetes. The educator doesn't respond to this but starts a screening test for diabetes. She [the educator] asks him a lot of questions. He scores 9 points, which indicates that he is at increased risk of type 2 diabetes. The educator then asks: 'What are your thoughts about that?' He answers: 'It doesn't concern me'. She continues: 'Would you like to know what you can do?' The patient doesn't reply. She continues by telling him what to be aware of, e.g. a potbelly.* (Observation, individual lifestyle consultation)

The educator's attention was often not directed at the PMI. The primary purpose of feedback from the PMI could be interpreted as enabling the educator to complete required forms, rather than engaging the PMI in a dialogue about health practices:

*The educator is looking at her screen a lot and at the paper schedule lying on her desk. Several times she talks to the PMI while she is looking at the screen, so they do not always have eye contact* (Observation, individual lifestyle consultation).

### Facilitators of flow
#### Active involvement channelled attention in activities
Flow was observed when PMI were actively included in an activity and when the educator dominated less. During these times, less information was conveyed, and PMI were given an opportunity to focus on specific tasks. This created an opportunity for PMI-perceived skills to match with the challenge at hand, stimulating flow:

*The PMI is using her body actively during the cooking session. The PMI appears to concentrate and initiates many tasks on her own.* (Observation, individual cooking session)

Competition stimulated flow among some participants during a badminton session. However, the element of competition was not motivating for a woman who was unable to follow the counting of points:

*All participants are engaged [playing badminton], educators as well as PMI. A young male participant is especially committed during the competition where you can gain points. This has the opposite effect on a female participant who cannot keep up with the points.* (Observation, sports café)

As illustrated in this observation, maintaining a balance between challenges and skills was integral to sustaining flow in an activity.

#### Goals related to everyday life of participants
Flow was facilitated most frequently when PMI were actively involved in determining the direction of the activity. Health education activities that actively included PMI, such as cooking sessions and sports cafes, facilitated flow on occasion by engaging participants. Flow was also stimulated when educators engaged actively as equals in health-promoting activities. During individual sessions, flow was observed primarily in response to the educator asking open-ended questions concerning the PMI's background and everyday life:

*At the end of the session, diet, smoking, alcohol and exercise are discussed in relation to the PMI's work.*

*This leads the PMI to open up and share details about his everyday life and what he likes. The PMI becomes more engaged.* (Observation, individual screening and lifestyle consultation)

#### Collective feedback from educators and participants
In the observed health-promoting activities, flow seemed to be stimulated when educators and participants were attentive and responded to other participants' goals and related concerns. In a cooking session, educators asked open-ended questions about diet and weight loss, which encouraged dialogue among participants and educators:

*One of the educators contributes to this [dialogue] by asking open-ended questions of the participants. A participant talks about losing 13 kg. Another educator asks how, and the participant says that she has counted calories and been physically active. Another participant tells that she lost 15 kg without doing much. The educators praise the participants for having lost weight. A third participant expresses that she cannot accept that the medicine [she is taking] means that she does not feel full. This leads to a dialogue among the participants about medication, including how different medicines affect them.* (Observation, group-based cooking session)

Another example of collective feedback from participants occurred at the badminton session. The participants encouraged each other during the game, creating a positive and supportive environment:

*The dialogue is praising, acknowledging, and positive. This is also the case among participants. They encourage each other; especially [name of PMI] encourages [name of PMI] who has difficulties hitting the ball.* (Observation, sports café)

During the badminton session, the educators paid close attention to the participants, which also contributed to a supportive and positive environment. This is illustrated in the following excerpt from observation notes:

*A participant hurts his arm after 15 minutes. One of the educators leaves the session with him to do stretching exercises while the others continue to play.* (Observation, sports café)

### Discussion
Flow refers to an inherently rewarding experiential state that can encourage a person to persist in and return to

an activity, such as health behaviours; the theory of flow also focuses on context. By using the concept of flow as a theoretical framework, this study sought to explore barriers and facilitators of effective health education targeting PMI, through multisided ethnographic fieldwork.

Information overload was a recurrent barrier to flow throughout the observations; the quantity and detailed nature of the information provided by educators indicated an imbalance between expected behavioural changes and the individual skills and resources of PMI. Educators often provided similar information based on a predefined goal that did not consider participants' individual goals. The one-way communication approach and highly structured agenda did not allow time for reflection or understanding of PMI's current motivation for health behaviour change. Educators continually overlooked cues from participants. Flow was observed more often when PMI were actively involved in the health-promoting activity. Active involvement was facilitated through open-ended questions related to PMIs' skills and resources, dialogue, and constructive feedback. When PMIs were more engaged, educators provided less information overall, and the information provided was more likely to match the skills and resources of the PMI.

### Information overload is counterproductive

Behaviour change is more complex than merely providing advice on healthy lifestyles [31, 32]. The findings of this study indicate that advice on healthy lifestyles can be counterproductive if it is generalised or fails to take individuals' motivations and resources into account. There is a risk that health education activities may become demotivating to PMI. In accordance with this finding, studies have shown that healthcare professionals may lack confidence in the ability of PMI to complete tasks and reach goals, which they find very discouraging [21, 33, 34].

The self-determination theory provides a useful framework for understanding the relationship between the provision of healthy lifestyle advice and individuals' motivation for engaging in health behaviour change. Self-determination refers to an individual's capacity to make choices that are the primary determinants of action [35]. This implies an experience of choice and decision-making directed at meeting self-selected goals. In contrast, an individual can experience choices as pressure to perform, e.g. to act in accordance with healthy lifestyle advice. The individual may not experience a sense of choice, leading to non-autonomous motivation for action. Health-promoting activities facilitated without consideration of individuals' resources, skills and goals can be associated with feelings of guilt and shame if the recipients feel that they cannot comply with the recommended practices [36]. To address these

negative consequences of non-autonomous motivation, Ryan and Deci [35] suggest that healthcare professionals help individuals explore their sense of choice and reflect on their reasons for action.

### One size does not fit all

Educators relied on a 'one size fits all' approach that undermined a focus on participants' skills and resources and belied the complexity of health education. The 'one size fits all' approach can also be referred to as a biomedical 'top-down' approach in which educators are viewed as experts [37]. This approach contrasts with the 'bottom-up' approach, in which participants' individual experiences and needs are considered. According to Jormfeldt [38], these paradigms co-exist and contradict each other within mental health care; a tendency exists to focus on measuring absence of symptoms (remission criteria), which is regarded as appropriate for evidence-based practice. However, remission criteria largely overlook patients' subjective experiences that appear to be crucial to stimulating experiences of flow. In this study, the focus of educators on providing biomedical information prevented them from being curious about the individual needs and cues of the target group. Being sensitive and responsive to cues from PMI about their needs could have guided educators in directing the health education activity towards the concerns of PMI. This would have represented a bottom-up approach, acknowledging and attending to positive dimensions of health such as self-esteem, quality of life, and social relations [18, 27, 39, 40]. Bruun Jensen points to the same issue of contradictory paradigms in health education interventions. He posits a need to focus on a broad concept of health, embracing dimensions of a good life and social relations, rather than defining health as merely the opposite of disease [40].

### How can flow be promoted?

The experience of flow increases motivation to engage in a given activity [25, 26]. In this study, flow was observed in situations in which educators spoke less and operated outside the role of an expert. By tailoring advice or a specific health education activity to individuals' interests and motivations, educators can encourage a state of flow to promote positive health behaviour among PMI. To do so, educators must move towards a more person-centred approach to health education. As health behaviour change necessitates active engagement with individuals' values, goals and knowledge, a need arises for professionals to be more attentive and responsive to these issues [31]. Consistent with our findings, studies have shown that the facilitator style of educators is critical to engaging PMI [15, 31, 33]. This style includes educators' behaviour during discussions, including showing openness and honesty and the choice of communication techniques and materials [33]. For example, interactive tools such as quizzes, small group tasks and the use of flipcharts/whiteboards can encourage attendance and stimulate reflection.

However, for health education activities to be truly democratic, PMI must have the opportunity to influence both the content and process of health education activities. Simovska refers to this as genuine participation and posits that it encourages development of personal meaning and allows PMI ownership of their learning processes [41]. Feedback from educators and other participants in a group activity can also facilitate flow and create a supportive environment. Group activities are an important social forum, allowing PMI to interact, feel a sense of belonging and gain support from other individuals in a similar situation [33]. However, our study showed that joining group activities can be a barrier to participating in health education activities for some PMI. The process of joining a new group can be eased if participants know each other and are organized into small groups. Another aspect concerns cognitive impairment and negative symptoms such as hallucinations, which may limit the benefit of the health intervention in PMI.

### Implications for health education practice

Many professionals agree with the philosophy of person-centred approaches to health education, but implementing these approaches in practice remains a challenge. On a structural level, a need exists to consider how health is defined and operationalised in the given context; e.g. are positive dimensions of health taken into account? Does the context allow for a broad definition of health, which is important in hardly-reached group such as PMI? Training and supervision of healthcare professionals' communication skills could enhance the likelihood of stimulating intrinsic motivation of PMI in practice. Educator approaches and attitudes towards PMI are important to consider. Focus should be on the collaboration about health in a broad sense that incorporates PMI's needs and views on their health and what is important to them. Techniques from motivational interviewing and recovery approaches such as personal goals may enable educators to better understand and support individual's personal reasons for behaviour change and facilitate discussions [27, 42, 43]. The setting is also likely to play a role in supporting PMI. Lavie-Ajayi et al. point to general practitioners as key persons in relation to health behaviour change, due to a long-term and trusting relationship with PMI [44]. Although this study focused on PMI, the findings may be transferable to other hardly-reached groups and PMI populations in other domains of rehabilitation and community integration not focusing on health.

### Strengths and limitations

A key strength of this study is its qualitative approach. The application of the theoretical framework of flow and ethnographic methods provided an in-depth understanding of the issues that facilitate and impede flow for PMI in health education activities. The framework sheds light on the interaction. Additionally, the large number and geographical dispersion of study sites are strengths. A limitation of the study is that we were able to conduct observations in only a limited number of sessions at each site. It would be beneficial to follow health education activities over a longer time period. Including the perspectives of PMI regarding facilitators and barriers to the experience of flow would also strengthen the findings. However, it was not possible to conduct formal interviews.

It is also possible that PMI are attentive but not in a state of flow, which observations might not be able to uncover. Also, it is not certain that observers always were able to detect flow when it occurred. To reach saturation for the identified themes, we documented observations in extensive field notes and analysed data using a validated approach relying on continuous monitoring and conceptualisation of data [45].

### Conclusion

This study sought to identify barriers and facilitators of flow in health education settings. A focus on flow could act as a starting point to improve health education targeting PMI. Instead of focusing on a specific activity more attention should be paid to the way activities are shaped and conducted that allow a sense of flow e.g. how to create a balance between goals and challenges, how to deliver feedback and how to create a playful environment. Creating flow is in line with an individualised approach, person-centeredness and a bottom-up approach. Promoters of flow in our study included attentiveness and responsiveness to individuals' values, goals, knowledge and everyday life. Several barriers were also identified suggesting that more focus should be paid to training of educators to promote flow in the educational setting.

**Abbreviation**
PMI: People with mental illness

## Acknowledgements
We would like to express our sincere thanks to the participating PMI and professionals for allowing observations of health education activities and providing valuable contributions. We thank our partners involved in this project including the Region of Southern Denmark, University College South Denmark and the 22 municipalities in Southern Denmark. In addition, we acknowledge Jennifer Green, Caduceus Strategies, for editorial assistance.

## Funding
The work was supported by a grant from the Danish Ministry of Health [grant number 1403120]. The funding body had no involvement in any aspect of the research or publication of this article.

## Authors' contributions
NFH designed and conceptualised the study with support from RASP. NFH, RASP and LP collected and analysed the data with support from PD. NFH drafted the manuscript with support from RASP, LP and PD. All authors revised the manuscript critically for important intellectual content and approved the final version of the manuscript.

## Consent for publication
Not applicable.

## Competing interests
The authors declare that they have no competing interests.

## References
1. Wahlbeck K, Westman J, Nordentoft M, Gisler M, Laursen T. Outcomes of Nordic mental health systems: life expectancy of patients with mental disorders. Br J Psychiatry. 2011;199:453–8.
2. Saha S, Chant D, McGrath J. A systematic review of mortality in schizophrenia: is the differential mortality gap worsening over time? Arch Gen Psychiatry. 2007;64:1123–31.
3. Harris EC, Barraclough B. Excess mortality of mental disorder. Br J Psychiatry. 1998;173:11–53.
4. Nordentoft M, Wahlbeck K, Hallgren J, Westman J, Osby U, Alinaghizadeh H, et al. Excess mortality, causes of death and life expectancy in 270,770 patients with recent onset of mental disorders in Denmark, Finland and Sweden. PLoS One. 2013;8(1):e55176.
5. Correll CU, Detraux J, De Lepeleire J, De Hert M. Effects of antipsychotics, antidepressants and mood stabilizers on risk for physical diseases in people with schizophrenia, depression and bipolar disorder. World Psychiatry. 2015;14(2):119–36.
6. Laursen TM, Munk-Olsen T, Agerbo E, Gasse C, Mortensen PB. Somatic hospital contacts, invasive cardiac procedures, and mortality from heart disease in patients with severe mental disorder. Arch Gen Psychiatry. 2009;66(7):713–20.
7. Brown S, Birtwistle J, Roe L, Thompson C. The unhealthy lifestyle of people with schizophrenia. Psychol Med. 1999;29(3):697–701.
8. Laursen T, Nordentoft M. Heart disease treatment and mortality in schizophrenia and bipolar disorder - changes in the danish population between 1994 and 2006. J Psychiatr Res. 2011;45:29–35.
9. McCreadie RG. Diet, smoking and cardiovascular risk in people with schizophrenia: descriptive study. Br J Psychiatry. 2003;183:534–9.
10. Archie SM, Goldberg JO, Akhtar-Danesh N, Landeen J, McColl L, McNiven J. Psychotic disorders, eating habits, and physical activity: who is ready for lifestyle changes? Psychiatr Serv. 2007;58(2):233–9.
11. Nordentoft M, Krogh J, Lange P, Moltke A. Psykisk sygdom og ændringer i livsstil. København: Vidensråd for forebyggelse; 2015.
12. Bruins J, Jorg F, Bruggeman R, Slooff C, Corpeleijn E, Pijnenborg M. The effects of lifestyle interventions on (long-term) weight management, cardiometabolic risk and depressive symptoms in people with psychotic disorders: a meta-analysis. PLoS One. 2014;9(12):e112276.
13. Speyer H, Christian Brix Nørgaard H, Birk M, Karlsen M, Storch Jakobsen A, Pedersen K, et al. The CHANGE trial: no superiority of lifestyle coaching plus care coordination plus treatment as usual compared to treatment as usual alone in reducing risk of cardiovascular disease in adults with schizophrenia spectrum disorders and abdominal obesity. World Psychiatry. 2016;15(2):155–65.
14. Roberts SH, Bailey JE. Incentives and barriers to lifestyle interventions for people with severe mental illness: a narrative synthesis of quantitative, qualitative and mixed methods studies. J Adv Nurs. 2011;67(4):690–708.
15. Small N, Brooks H, Grundy A, Pedley R, Gibbons C, Lovell K, et al. Understanding experiences of and preferences for service user and carer involvement in physical health care discussions within mental health care planning. BMC psychiatry. 2017;17(1):138.
16. Ward MC, White D, Druss BG. A meta-review of lifestyle interventions for cardiovascular risk factors in the general medical population: lessons for individuals with serious mental illness. J Clin Psychiatry. 2015;76(4):e477–86.
17. Searle A, Calnan M, Lewis G, Campbell J, Taylor A, Turner K. Patients' views of physical activity as treatment for depression: a qualitative study. Br J Gen Pract. 2011;61(585):149–56.
18. Hultsjö S, Hjelm K. Organizing care for persons with psychotic disorders and risk of or existing diabetes mellitus type 2. J Psychiatr Ment Health Nurs. 2012;19:891–902.
19. Shiner B, Whitley R, Van Citters A, Pratt S, Bartels S. Learning what matters for patients: qualitative evaluation of a health promotion program for those with serious mental illness. Health Promot Int. 2008;23(3):275–82.
20. McDevitt J, Snyder M, Miller A, Wilbur J. Perceptions of barriers and benefits to physical activity among outpatients in psychiatric rehabilitation. J Nurs Scholarsh. 2006;38:50–5.
21. Xiong G, Ziegahn L, Schuyler B, Rowlett A, Cassady D. Improving dietary and physical activity practices in group homes serving residents with severe mental illness. Prog Community Health Partnersh. 2010;4(4):279–88.
22. Csikszentmihalyi M. Flow og engagement i hverdagen. 1st ed. Virum: Dansk Psykologisk Forlag; 2007.
23. Nakamura J, Csikszentmihalyi M. The concept of flow. In: Snyder C, Lopez S, editors. Handbook of positive psychology. New York: Oxford University Press; 2002. p. 89–105.
24. Csikszentmihalyi M. Beyond boredom and anxiety. San Francisco: Jossey-Bass Publishers; 2000; 1975.
25. Ryan R. Control and information in the intrapersonal sphere: an extension of cognitive evaluation theory. J Pers Soc Psychol. 1982;43:450–61.
26. Vallerand R, Reid G. On the causal effects of perceived competence on intrinsic motivation: a test of cognitive evaluation theory. J Sport Psychol. 1984;6:94–102.
27. Slade M. Mental illness and well-being: the central importance of positive psychology and recovery approaches. BMC Health Serv Res. 2010;10(1):26.
28. Pals RAS, Hempler NF. How to achieve a collaborative approach in health promotion: preferences and ideas of users of mental health services. Scand J Caring Sci. 2018;32:1188–96.
29. Spradley J. Participant observation. Fort Worth: Harcourt Brace Johanovich College Publishers; 1980.
30. Pedersen M, Klitmøller J, Nielsen K. Deltagerobservation: en metode til undersøgelse af psykologiske fænomener. Copenhagen: Hans Reitzels Forlag; 2012.
31. Frates EP, Bonnet J. Collaboration and negotiation: the key to therapeutic lifestyle change. Am J Lifestyle Med. 2016;10(5):302–12.
32. Morris HL, Carlyle KE, Elston Lafata J. Adding the patient's voice to our understanding of collaborative goal setting: how do patients with diabetes define collaborative goal setting? Chronic Ill. 2016;12(4):261–71.
33. Roberts SH, Bailey JE. An ethnographic study of the incentives and barriers to lifestyle interventions for people with severe mental illness. J Adv Nurs. 2013;69(11):2514–24.
34. Mahony G, Haracz K, Williams LT. How mental health occupational therapists address issues of diet with their clients: a qualitative study. Aust Occup Ther J. 2012;59(4):294–301.
35. Ryan R, Deci E. Self-determination theory and the facilitation of intrinsic motivation, social development and well-being. Am Psychol. 2000;55(1):68–78.
36. Guttman N, Salmon CT. Guilt, fear, stigma and knowledge gaps: ethical issues in public health communication interventions. Bioethics. 2004;18(6):531–52.

37.  Lindsey E, Hartrick G. Health-promoting nursing practice: the demise of the nursing process? J Adv Nurs. 1996;23(1):106–12.

38.  Jormfeldt H. Supporting positive dimensions of health, challenges in mental health care. Int J Qual Stud Health Well Being. 2011;6(2). https://doi.org/10.3402/qhw.v6i2.7126.

39.  Jensen BB. A case of two paradigms within health education. Health Educ Res. 1997;12(4):419–28.

40.  Grabowski D, Aagaard-Hansen J, Willaing I, Jensen BB. Principled promotion of health: implementing five guiding health promotion principles for research-based prevention and management of diabetes. Societies. 2017;7:10.

41.  Simovska V. The changing meanings of participation in school-based health education and health promotion: the participants' voices. Health Educ Res. 2007;22(6):864–78.

42.  Moran GS, et al. Perceived assistance in pursuing personal goals and personal recovery among mental health consumers across housing services. Psychiatry Res. 2017;249:94–101.

43.  Wagner CC, Ingersoll KS. Motivational interviewing in groups. New York: The guilford Press; 2013.

44.  Lavie-Ajayi M, Moran GS, Levav I, Porat R, Reches T, Goldfracht M, et al. Using the capabilities approach to understand inequality in primary health-care services for people with severe mental illness. Isr J Health Policy Res. 2018;7(1):49.

45.  Bowen GA. Naturalistic inquiry and the saturation concept: a research note. Qual Res. 2008;8(1):137–52.

# 21

# Dementia severity at death: a register-based cohort study

Jesutofunmi Aworinde[1], Nomi Werbeloff[1,2], Gemma Lewis[1], Gill Livingston[1,2] and Andrew Sommerlad[1,2*] (iD)

## Abstract

**Background:** One third of older people are estimated to die with dementia, which is a principal cause of death in developed countries. While it is assumed that people die with severe dementia this is not based on evidence.

**Methods:** Cohort study using a large secondary mental healthcare database in North London, UK. We included people aged over 65 years, diagnosed with dementia between 2008 and 2016, who subsequently died. We estimated dementia severity using mini-mental state examination (MMSE) scores, adjusting for the time between last score and death using the average annual MMSE decline in the cohort (1.5 points/year). We explored the association of sociodemographic and clinical factors, including medication use, with estimated MMSE score at death using linear regression.

**Results:** In 1400 people dying with dementia, mean estimated MMSE at death was 15.3 (standard deviation 7.0). Of the cohort, 22.2% (95% confidence interval 20.1, 24.5) died with mild dementia; 50.4% (47.8, 53.0) moderate; and 27.4% (25.1, 29.8) with severe dementia.
In fully adjusted models, more severe dementia at death was observed in women, Black, Asian and other ethnic minorities, agitated individuals, and those taking antipsychotic medication.

**Conclusions:** Only one quarter of people who die with dementia are at the severe stage of the illness. This finding informs clinical and public understanding of dementia prognosis. Provision of end-of-life services should account for this and healthcare professionals should be aware of high rates of mild and moderate dementia at end of life and consider how this affects clinical decision-making.

**Keywords:** Dementia, Prognosis, Epidemiology, Health records, Mortality, Death

## Background

Dementia is a principal cause of death in England and Wales [1] and the United States [2], and it is estimated that a third of people over the age of 60 die with the condition [3]. Estimates of survival after disease onset have varied between 3.3 and 11.7 years [4] – and the uncertainty over prognosis creates difficulties for patients and their family carers about planning their life and how to prepare for end of life care [5]. The variability in survival time in dementia is most likely a consequence of other illnesses affecting survival. Some studies report a trend in recent years towards compression of morbidity, where the onset of the first chronic illness occurs at a later age, thus compressing the time living with chronic illnesses [6].

There is increasing emphasis on providing good end of life care in dementia, which tends to focus on the challenges of delivering it to people with severe dementia [7]. The proportion of people who have mild, moderate, and severe dementia at end of life has important implications for clinician- and public-awareness of prognosis, how healthcare services plan and implement treatment, and how clinicians provide evidence-based end of life care. Severe dementia is associated with lack of insight and capacity [8] to make decisions about healthcare, requiring others to make decisions on behalf of patients [9]. Someone with mild dementia is more likely to be able to make these decisions, but may require support to do so and to implement them. If many people who have dementia die with a mild form of the condition, this would have implications for palliative settings and may suggest a greater need for support for decision

* Correspondence: a.sommerlad@ucl.ac.uk
[1]Division of Psychiatry, University College London, 6th Floor, Maple House, 149 Tottenham Court Road, London W1T 7NF, UK
[2]Camden and Islington NHS Foundation Trust, London, UK

making and management strategies. One study reported that 31/68 (46%) people with dementia being managed at end of life by a general practitioner were described by the clinician as having mild dementia, [10] however there has been, to our knowledge, no study examining the distribution of dementia severity in a large cohort of people with dementia at time of death.

In this study, we therefore aim to investigate the severity of dementia at death, in a secondary mental healthcare service cohort of older people with a diagnosis of dementia and explore the association between demographic and clinical factors, including medication use (antidepressant, sedative and antipsychotic drugs, and those for cognition in dementia), and dementia severity at death.

## Methods

### Study setting and data source

We conducted a retrospective cohort study using routinely collected data from clinical dementia services in Camden and Islington NHS Foundation Trust (CIFT), a large mental health trust providing mental healthcare services including dementia assessment and treatment to a catchment area of 470,000 people in two London boroughs. We obtained our data using the Clinical Record Interactive Search (CRIS) system, a platform designed to facilitate the use of routinely collected electronic health records for research, which has been used to address a number of research hypotheses in mental health and dementia research [11]. CRIS allows the extraction of data from electronic health records' structured and unstructured (e.g. progress notes, clinic letters) fields using the General Architecture for Text Engineering (GATE) program, which uses natural language processing (NLP) algorithms [12], to identify text relating to diagnosis, treatment or other clinical information. The Camden and Islington CRIS database holds pseudo-anonymised electronic mental health records dating from 1st January 2008 for over 116,000 people who have had contact with CIFT services [13]. Individual patient consent is not required for inclusion in the database.

### Study patients

We retrieved records from eligible patients who had clinical contact with CIFT services during the study window (1st January 2008 to 30th September 2016).

Individuals were included if they:

- were aged 65 years or over at dementia diagnosis, ascertained either using a structured field diagnosis of International Classification of Diseases (ICD) 10 codes F00–03 [14], or an unstructured diagnosis (derived though NLP application)

- had their cognitive function assessed and recorded using the Mini-Mental State Examination (MMSE) [15]
- died before 30th September 2016

We excluded patients who received a diagnosis of Mild Cognitive Impairment (MCI) after dementia diagnosis ($n = 15$); this was judged to be an active clinical decision to replace dementia diagnosis with MCI, as it is not possible to have MCI and dementia simultaneously.

### Study data

#### Outcome

Dementia severity at death was assessed using the last recorded MMSE score before death. The MMSE scale is commonly used by healthcare professionals to assess cognitive impairment and monitor progression of decline in people with dementia. It is scored out of 30, and has been found to have acceptable psychometric properties to rate dementia severity [16]. We extracted all recorded MMSE scores from the unstructured fields of patient records, using the NLP application. Each MMSE score was accompanied by a post processing rule (PPR) code which provided information about the quality of the score recording and extraction [17]. A PPR code of 0 indicates that the MMSE has been optimally recorded and codes from 1 to 12 indicated a range of possible problems, such as that the numerator was higher than the denominator, or that more than one record with different scores were recorded on the same date. For all eligible patients, we used the PPR codes to select the valid MMSE records.

We validated the application for extracting and coding MMSE score. We calculated the positive predictive value (PPV) by randomly selecting MMSE scores and dates ($n = 100$) and determining if these were accurate by manually searching through the source documents in which they had been recorded. To obtain sensitivity, we extracted and read through a random set of documents ($n = 100$) which contained the word 'MMSE' to ascertain whether there was mention of MMSE score, then determining if this agreed with the coding performed by the NLP. The PPV for MMSE scores was 98%, though the accuracy of dates was substantially lower (67% overall) due to a technical problem which meant that a large proportion were marked with the date of migration to a new electronic clinical record system; so we manually corrected these dates. The sensitivity of the MMSE application was 94%.

#### Covariates

We obtained information on age at diagnosis, sex, ethnicity (White, Black, Asian, and other), marital status and the last recorded dementia subtype (categorised into 5 groups; Alzheimer's disease, vascular dementia, dementia with Lewy bodies, other, and unspecified). We estimated socio-economic status using the area-level of socio-economic deprivation by matching lower super output area (LSOA) score to the 2010 Index of Multiple Deprivation (IMD) [18]. We obtained information on clinical presentation using patient's Health of The Nations Outcome Scales (HoNOS) score within a year of diagnosis. HoNOS is a 12 subscale assessment tool with acceptable psychometric properties [19] which is routinely administered at 6 monthly intervals after initial assessment. We used the domains covering the neuropsychiatric symptoms of clinical interest- agitation, hallucination and depressed mood. Because only scores ≥2 are considered clinically significant, we categorised each domain as binary, with 0–1 categorised as 'no problem' and 2–4 as evidence of 'problem'.

Data on recorded medication use (derived from a GATE text extraction) [20] any time after dementia diagnosis, including drugs for cognition (acetyl-cholinesterase inhibitors and memantine), antipsychotics, antidepressants and sedatives (benzodiazepine or 'z-drug' hypnotics), were also extracted using NLP application.

## Statistical analysis

We first described the sociodemographic and clinical characteristics of our sample.

### Estimating dementia severity at death

We assumed that cognition would decline during the time between the last MMSE assessment and death. We therefore estimated MMSE at death by calculating the mean annual MMSE decline using individuals' last two MMSE scores and, for each patient, multiplying the duration between their last MMSE and death by the cohort's annual MMSE decline. We report this, as well as the distribution of dementia severity at death, rating MMSE ≥20 points as mild dementia, < 20 and ≥ 10 as moderate, and < 10 as severe dementia, with 95% confidence intervals for these proportions. As we judged that variable interval between last recorded MMSE and death might reduce the accuracy of our adjustment procedure, we conducted a sensitivity analysis using a subgroup of patients who had been assessed close to death (last recorded MMSE score within one year of their death), with the same adjustment procedure.

### Exploring predictors of dementia severity at death

We examined associations between estimated MMSE scores (continuous outcome variable) and each covariate (predictor variables), using linear regression. We first conducted univariable analyses of the association between each covariate and severity of dementia at death and then our planned primary mutually-adjusted multivariable analysis of the association between these factors and dementia severity at death. Due to a large amount

of missing data, with slight differences in sex, ethnicity and socio-economic status between those with complete data and those with missing data, we also conducted an analysis without the HoNOS variables. We also conducted a sensitivity analysis using the same regression analysis on the subgroup whose last MMSE was within a year of their death. In all multivariable analyses, we adjusted for time between diagnosis and death as we considered that this would be a strong confounding factor.

### Exploring the influence of medication use after dementia diagnosis on dementia severity at death

We conducted univariate and multivariable analyses for associations between our outcome and use of drugs for cognition, antipsychotics, antidepressants and sedatives after dementia diagnosis, adjusting for all the covariates and each medication individually.

All data analysis was completed using STATA (version 11).

### Ethics approval and access to the data

Ethical approval for the analysis of the CIFT CRIS database was obtained from the National Research Ethics Service Committee East of England—Cambridge Central (14/EE/0177).

## Results

The clinical and demographic characteristics of the cohort are displayed in Table 1. Our final cohort consisted of 1400 people. The median age at diagnosis was 84.6 years, and the mean time between diagnosis and death was 1.9 years (standard deviation (s.d.) = 1.7) and maximum time from diagnosis to death was 11.9 years. For those who died with mild dementia, mean time between diagnosis and death was 1.6 (1.4) years; for moderate dementia 1.9 (1.7) and for severe dementia 2.2 (1.9). The majority of individuals were White, and Black people formed the largest minority group. Of those with a recorded diagnosis, Alzheimer's disease was the most common subtype, followed by vascular dementia. Mean MMSE closest to time of diagnosis was 18.2 (6.6). Around one quarter of patients had clinically significant agitation at diagnosis and one fifth had depressive symptoms. Just under half were recorded as taking medication for cognition in dementia after their diagnosis and 30% took antidepressants.

### Severity of dementia at death

The mean last MMSE score was 17.0. The mean annual MMSE decline between penultimate and last MMSE assessment was 1.5 points and the mean time from last MMSE score to death was 1.4 years (s.d. = 1.64). The mean estimated MMSE score at death was 15.3 (s.d. = 7.0) (Table 2). We found that 27.4% (95% confidence interval 25.1, 29.8) had severe dementia, 50.4% (47.8,

**Table 1** Clinical and demographic characteristics of patients (*n* = 1400)

| Characteristic | | All people with dementia |
|---|---|---|
| | | n (%) |
| Age at diagnosis (*years*) | Median (IQR p25, p75) | 84.6 (79.4, 88.8) |
| | Range | 65.1–104.3 |
| | *65–69* | 44 (3.1) |
| | 70–74 | 104 (7.4) |
| | 75–79 | 234 (16.7) |
| | 80–84 | 349 (24.9) |
| | 85–89 | 412 (29.4) |
| | 90+ | 257 (18.4) |
| Sex | Female | 758 (54.1) |
| Ethnicity | White | 1073 (85.0) |
| | Black | 111 (8.8) |
| | Asian | 41 (3.2) |
| | Other | 38 (3.0) |
| | *Missing* | 137 |
| Marital status | Married | 388 (33.2) |
| | Widowed | 412 (35.3) |
| | Divorced | 133 (11.4) |
| | Single | 235 (20.1) |
| | *Missing* | 232 |
| Last recorded dementia type | Alzheimer's disease | 645 (46.1) |
| | Vascular dementia | 258 (21.1) |
| | Dementia with Lewy bodies | 32 (2.3) |
| | Other | 135 (9.6) |
| | Unspecified | 330 (23.6) |
| IMD | Mean (SD) | 31.0 (12.6) |
| | *Missing* | 115 |
| HoNOS at diagnosis – problems with*: | Agitation | 149 (25.3) |
| | Hallucinations | 95 (16.2) |
| | Depressed mood | 123 (21.0) |
| | *Missing*** | 810 |
| Any recorded use of medication, after diagnosis of dementia | Anti-dementia drugs | 662 (47.3) |
| | Antidepressants | 422 (30.1) |
| | Antipsychotics | 264 (18.9) |
| | Sedatives | 277 (19.8) |
| MMSE score at diagnosis | Mean (SD) | 18.2 (6.6) |
| Time between diagnosis and death – (*years*) | Mean (SD) | 1.9 (1.7) |

KEY: SD = standard deviation; IQR = interquartile range; IMD = Index of Multiple Deprivation; HoNOS = Health of the Nation Outcome Scales; MMSE = Minimental state examination
Notes: *HoNOS categories dichotomised to 0–1 (no or minor problem) and 2–4 (problem behaviour); ** The number of missing data varies according to HoNOS items (between 808 and 810)

53.0) had moderate dementia at death, and 22.2% (20.1, 24.5) died with mild dementia (Table 2). The estimated MMSE scores at death were normally distributed except that 46 people had a floor MMSE score estimated as 0 (Fig. 1).

In our sensitivity analysis, which included only the 782 people who had their last MMSE within one year of death (Table 2), we found a similar proportion of people had moderate dementia but that a higher proportion (32.1%) had severe dementia at death. The mean MMSE was however, slightly higher (16.3 (s.d. = 6.8)).

### Clinical and demographic predictors of dementia severity at death

In the fully adjusted linear regression model (Table 3), we included 452 people with all the covariates recorded. This showed that women, those of minority ethnicity background, those from more socio-economically deprived backgrounds, and those with agitation died with more severe dementia. Women were estimated to score 1.4 MMSE points lower at death (0.1, 2.8, *p* = 0.04). Similarly, those from a Black, Asian and other ethnic origin scored 3.5 (1.5, 5.5, *p* = 0.001) points, 4.7 (0.5, 9.0, *p* = 0.03) and 5.2 (0.8, 9.7, *p* = 0.02) points lower respectively on the estimated MMSE, compared to White people. Worse score on the IMD was associated with dying with more severe dementia, with each 10 point increase in deprivation score associated with 0.4 points lower on the MMSE (0.0, 0.8, p = 0.04). Having problems with agitation was associated with estimated MMSE 2.5 points (1.0, 4.0, p = 0.001) lower. Conversely, those who were divorced scored 2.2 points (0.0, 4.3, *p* = 0.05) higher on the MMSE. In the regression analysis without the HoNOS variables, which included 1131 people, the results were similar to that of our primary analysis, with the exception that those who were single died with less severe dementia (1.3 points higher on the MMSE (0.1, 2.5, *p* = 0.03) and no association for 'other' ethnic origin with dementia severity at death was found. In our sensitivity analysis assessing factors associated with estimated MMSE in the 291 people who had been assessed within one year of death and had complete covariate data (Additional file 1), similar results were obtained, except that ethnicity was no longer associated with dementia severity at death.

### Association between use of medication and dementia severity at death

Multivariable analysis of the association between different medication use after dementia diagnosis and severity of dementia at death (Table 4), showed that use of antipsychotics was associated with scoring 2.7 points lower on the MMSE at death than individuals who had not taken antipsychotics (0.9, 4.6, *p* = 0.004). Use of other

## Dementia severity at death

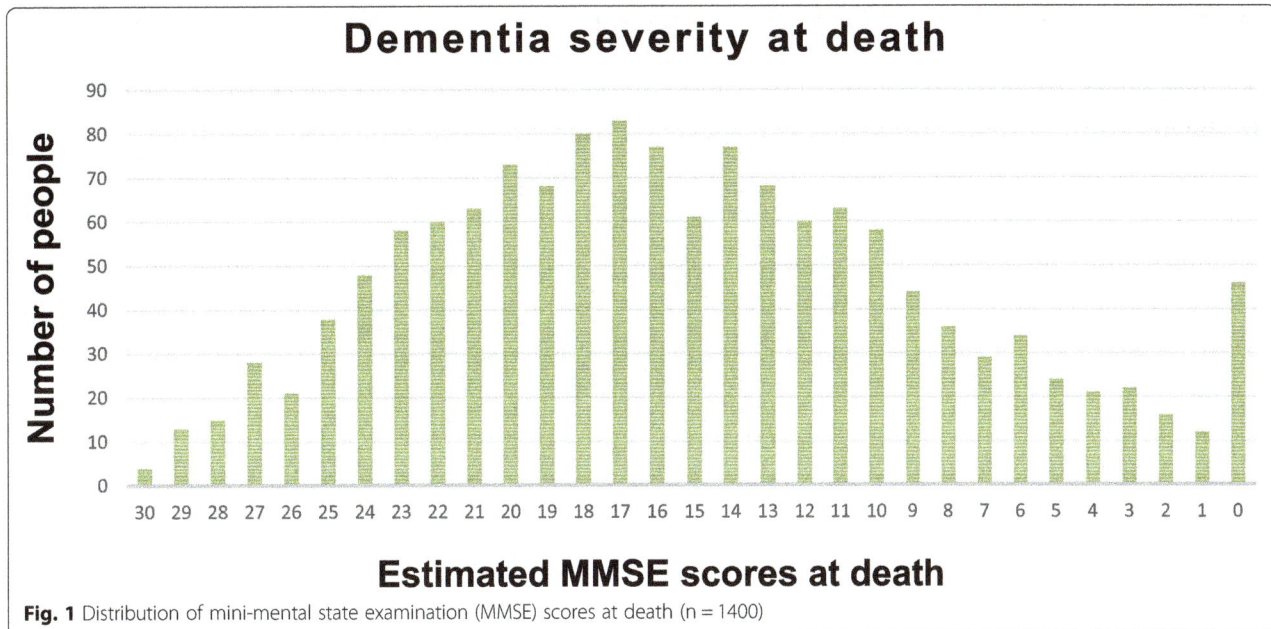

**Fig. 1** Distribution of mini-mental state examination (MMSE) scores at death (n = 1400)

psychotropic medication was not associated with dementia severity at death.

## Discussion

This is the first study, to our knowledge to report the severity of dementia at death of a cohort of people with dementia. Importantly we find that only one quarter had severe dementia, half had moderate dementia and the rest had mild dementia at death. The mean MMSE at death was 15.3 and we found a normal distribution of estimated MMSE scores at death except for those with estimated MMSE score of 0, a consequence of the floor effect of the MMSE assessment.

This result was unexpected as we had anticipated that most people in the cohort would die with severe dementia. It suggests that most of our cohort died from other illnesses rather than solely from the consequences of advanced dementia, although the presence of dementia may have led to a worse prognosis than others with the same illness [21]. The age-specific incidence of dementia has decreased in the UK over the past 20 years [22], meaning that the condition occurs later now than in previous generations, and is therefore more likely to

coexist with other illnesses. Around 70% of people with dementia have at least two comorbid chronic diseases and these increase the risk of hospitalisation and mortality [23]. This elevated mortality may have contributed to a large proportion of our cohort dying with milder forms of the disease. Furthermore, a major drive in dementia policy in the UK and other countries has been early diagnosis of dementia [24] and the services whose data we used have been successful at increasing dementia diagnosis [25], so our naturalistic cohort includes many who had dementia diagnosed at very mild stages, who may have died from other conditions, with less severe dementia.

The mean MMSE was slightly lower in the whole sample than in our sensitivity sub-group of people assessed within one year of their death, as the whole cohort included a higher number of people (46 v 24 people) whose estimated MMSE was 0, due to a long interval between their last MMSE and death. In the sensitivity analysis, a higher proportion of people had severe dementia than in the main analysis, which may be because our method underestimated the decline, which may be more precipitous before death, or because people with more

**Table 2** Distribution of dementia severity at death, using estimated mini-mental state examination scores

| | | Estimated MMSE scores (n = 1400) | Estimated MMSE scores within 1 year of death (n = 782) |
|---|---|---|---|
| *Mean (SD)* | | 15.3 (7.0) | 16.3 (6.8) |
| Dementia severity n (% (95% CI)) | Mild | 311 (22.2 (20.1, 24.5)) | 142 (18.2 (15.6, 21.0)) |
| | Moderate | 706 (50.4 (47.8, 53.0)) | 389 (49.7 (46.3, 53.2)) |
| | Severe | 383 (27.4 (25.1, 29.8)) | 251 (32.1 (28.9, 35.5)) |

KEY: MMSE = mini-mental state examination
Notes: Mild dementia = estimated MMSE 20–30; moderate dementia = 10–19; Severe dementia = 0–9

**Table 3** Association between clinical and demographic characteristics and mini-mental state examination scores at death

| Characteristic | | Univariable analysis | | | Multivariable analysis (n = 452) | | |
|---|---|---|---|---|---|---|---|
| | | Coefficient | 95% CI | P-value | Coefficient | 95% CI | P-value |
| Age at diagnosis (per 1 year increase) | | 0.0 | −0.0 to 0.1 | 0.20 | −0.0 | −0.1 to 0.1 | 0.75 |
| Sex | Reference category: Male | | | | | | |
| | Female | −0.8 | −1.5 to −0.1 | 0.04 | −1.4 | −2.8 to −0.1 | 0.04 |
| Ethnicity | Reference category: White | | | 0.001* | | | 0.001* |
| | Black | −3.4 | −4.8 to −2.0 | 0.001 | −3.5 | −5.5 to −1.5 | 0.001 |
| | Asian | −2.7 | −4.9 to −0.5 | 0.02 | −4.7 | −9.0 to −0.5 | 0.03 |
| | Other | −0.3 | −2.6 to 2.0 | 0.80 | −5.2 | −9.7 to −0.8 | 0.02 |
| Marital status | Reference category: Married | | | 0.001* | | | 0.26* |
| | Widowed | 0.7 | −0.3 to 1.7 | 0.18 | 0.8 | −0.9 to 2.4 | 0.36 |
| | Divorced | 1.3 | −0.1 to 2.7 | 0.07 | 2.2 | 0.0 to 4.3 | 0.047 |
| | Single | 1.8 | 0.7 to 2.9 | 0.002 | 0.7 | −1.1 to 2.5 | 0.45 |
| Dementia type | Reference category: Alzheimer's disease | | | 0.004* | | | 0.43* |
| | Vascular dementia | −0.2 | −1.2 to 0.8 | 0.71 | −1.1 | −2.9 to 0.9 | 0.28 |
| | Dementia with Lewy bodies | 0.5 | −1.9 to 3.0 | 0.68 | 1.8 | −3.0 to 6.6 | 0.46 |
| | Other | 1.8 | 0.5 to 3.0 | 0.008 | 1.0 | −1.0 to 3.0 | 0.33 |
| | Unspecified | 1.4 | 0.4 to 2.3 | 0.004 | 0.3 | −1.2 to 1.9 | 0.69 |
| IMD (per 10-unit increase in deprivation) | | −0.3 | −0.5 to −0.0 | 0.04 | −0.4 | −0.8 to −0.0 | 0.04 |
| HoNOS at diagnosis – problems with**: | Agitation | −2.3 | −3.6 to −1.1 | 0.001 | −2.5 | −4.0 to −1.0 | 0.001 |
| | Hallucinations | −1.8 | −3.3 to −0.4 | 0.02 | −0.7 | −2.4 to 1.0 | 0.43 |
| | Depressed mood | −0.3 | −1.6 to 1.1 | 0.70 | 0.7 | −0.8 to 2.3 | 0.37 |
| Time between diagnosis and death (per 1 year later) | | −0.7 | −0.9 to −0.5 | 0.001 | −0.5 | −1.1 to 0.0 | 0.06 |

KEY: IMD = Index of Multiple deprivation; HoNOS = Health of the Nation Outcome Scales; clinical symptoms were derived from HoNOS scale
Notes: * overall class effect for categorical variables; ** HoNOS categories dichotomised to 0–1 (no or minor problem) and 2–4 (problem behaviour))

advanced dementia were more likely to have been seen and cognitively assessed by the clinical service close to death.

More severe dementia at death was associated with being female, from ethnic minority background, more socioeconomically deprived, showing symptoms of agitation and taking antipsychotic medication. Divorced people died with less severe dementia. Our observational analyses of the association between sociodemographic and clinical factors and dementia severity cannot establish a causal relationship. The identified factors may cause dementia to progress more rapidly; they may indicate people with lower cognitive reserve [26] and therefore more severe cognitive impairment at the same pathological stage of the disease; or they may indicate those with better physical health who therefore live longer with dementia and have the condition more severely when they die.

**Table 4** Association between medication use and mini-mental state examination score at death

| Any recorded use of medication after dementia diagnosis | Univariable analysis | | | Multivariable analysis [a] (n = 452) | | |
|---|---|---|---|---|---|---|
| | Coefficient | 95% CI | P-value | Coefficient | 95% CI | P-value |
| Acetylcholinesterase inhibitors / memantine | −0.6 | −1.3 to 0.2 | 0.12 | −0.0 | −1.6 to 1.6 | 0.97 |
| Antidepressants | 0.2 | −0.7 to 0.9 | 0.72 | 0.1 | −1.4 to 1.6 | 0.94 |
| Sedatives | −1.6 | −2.5 to −0.7 | 0.001 | −1.1 | −2.8 to 0.7 | 0.24 |
| Antipsychotics | −2.7 | −3.6 to −1.8 | < 0.001 | −2.7 | −4.6 to −0.9 | 0.004 |

Notes: [a] adjusted for age, sex, ethnicity, marital status, IMD, dementia type, problems with agitation, hallucinations and depression (from HoNOS scale) and time between diagnosis and death

We found that women died with more severe dementia than men, which may result from this cohort of women having received less education [27] and therefore having less cognitive reserve so showing more severe cognitive symptoms for the same level of pathology, or be a consequence of their greater life-expectancy, allowing more dementia progression before death. Our finding that people from minority ethnic background died with more severe dementia than their white counterparts may also reflect lower cognitive reserve related to less education [28]. In addition, people from ethnic minority backgrounds develop dementia at a younger age [29] and may therefore live longer with the disease. A final explanation is that people from minority groups present later [30], so those who die with less severe illness may never have presented to memory services. Alternatively, people from ethnic minority origins may engage less with management of their condition [31], thus experience a more precipitous cognitive decline. Higher neighbourhood level socioeconomic deprivation being associated with more severe dementia at death is also likely to result from lower cognitive reserve and younger development of dementia [32]. Our finding that divorced individuals died with less severe dementia compared to married people may be due to the mortality risks associated with being divorced [33] meaning divorced individuals died earlier and with milder dementia than married people.

Our results showed agitation to be associated with more severe dementia at death and this is likely to be because agitation at diagnosis is a consequence of more severe dementia, which increases in severity as dementia progresses [34]. An alternative is that agitation caused more rapid dementia progression, supported by studies suggesting that neuropsychiatric symptoms increase neuropathological burden [35]. Antipsychotics are used for psychosis or sometimes agitation, which are markers of more severe dementia, although the potential contribution of antipsychotic use to cognitive decline [36] needs further exploration.

### Strengths and limitations

This is the first study, to our knowledge, to evaluate dementia severity at death and examine demographic and clinical predictors. Our database allowed analysis of all routinely collected clinical data, with no requirement for explicit consent to involvement in the database, meaning that we had a large naturalistic cohort of people who had been clinically-diagnosed with dementia before dying. Our results are likely to be representative of people with clinically-diagnosed dementia living in similar areas, as memory services are the mainstay of UK dementia diagnosis and assessment [24] and CIFT has a high estimated diagnosis rate – 84% of people in the catchment area estimated to have dementia from

epidemiological studies, have a formal diagnosis [25] – but our findings may not generalise to people with dementia who have not been diagnosed, who may have been more likely to die with milder dementia.

Our study has limitations; the use of electronic health records which were not collected for research purposes meant that we could only adjust for routinely recorded factors. We would have liked to adjust for education, which would be a more sensitive marker of cognitive reserve than socioeconomic deprivation, and would have ideally had more sensitive measures of physical-ill health, enabling us to examine in detail the potential confounding effect of physical illness on dementia severity at death. Our analysis assumed a linear decline in MMSE at end of life, and applied the average MMSE decline to the whole sample, whereas this may not be the case. Rate of decline likely depends on a number of factors including initial severity, type of dementia, age, neuropsychiatric symptoms, medication, sex and education and we did not have data on all these domains to allow us to predict decline for each patient individually, so we used the mean rate of decline in the sample. The mean annual rate of decline in our sample was 1.5 MMSE points. One study reported 6 month MMSE decline of 0.9 points [37], whilst others have reported an annual decline of 2.2–2.3 points [38, 39], although these studies only examined people with Alzheimer's disease, whereas we included people with all dementia types and the rate of decline differs according to dementia type [40]. Finally, for some patients, it is possible that MMSE testing was abandoned when they had more severe dementia as the patient may struggle to complete testing and/or the clinician may deem that it does not add significant information, although clinicians would often record the MMSE score at the point of abandoning the test; however, reduced recording of MMSE in severe dementia may mean that dementia severity is underestimated in this study.

### Conclusions

We found the majority of people in the sample died with moderate dementia and only one quarter had severe dementia at death. This study provides important information for clinicians and the public about the prognosis of people with dementia and should inform the development of end-of-life services tailored to the condition. Dying with severe dementia is a major concern for people with early disease [41], but we found that this occurs less frequently than expected. People with dementia, their family carers, and healthcare professionals involved in their care may delay decisions related to end-of-life, assuming this may not be relevant, and research suggests that take-up of advance care plans has been low; [42] however, our research supports the need for professionals to encourage early discussions about who may help with decisions and end-of-life preferences. All palliative care in older people should consider if the individual has dementia and how this affects their decision-making ability, the possible treatments and their ability to carry out a plan without help. People with mild to moderate dementia often appear unimpaired in social contexts to people who do not know them and it is easy to miss the disability that their cognitive impairment may cause. Clinicians involved in end of life care should consider the presence of dementia in people with less obvious signs of the condition and take this into account when explaining clinical information and making treatment decisions.

## Additional file

**Additional file 1: Appendix 1.** Association between clinical and demographic characteristics and the mini-mental state examination at death, using only scores recorded within one year of death. **Appendix 2.** Flow diagram of study patient inclusion/exclusion. (DOCX 41 kb)

## Abbreviations

CIFT: Camden and Islington NHS Foundation Trust; CRIS: Clinical Record Interactive Search; GATE: General Architecture for Text Engineering; HoNOS: Health of The Nation Outcome Scales; ICD: International Classification of Diseases; IMD: Index of multiple deprivation; LSOA: Lower super output area; MCI: Mild Cognitive Impairment; MMSE: Mini-Mental State Examination; NLP: Natural language processing; PPR: Post processing rule; PPV: Positive predictive value

## Acknowledgements
Not applicable.

## Funding
During the conduct of this study, AS was funded by a Wellcome Trust fellowship (200163/Z/15/Z). The data resource is funded by a grant from the Department of Health. NW, GL1, GL2 and AS were supported by the University College London Hospitals National Institute of Health Research Biomedical Research Centre.

## Authors' contributions
JA was involved in the conception and design of the study, analysis and interpretation of data, and drafting of the manuscript. NW was involved in the acquisition, analysis and interpretation of all data. GL1 was involved in the interpretation of all data. GL2 was involved in the conception and design of the study and interpretation of data. AS was involved in the conception and design of the study, analysis, interpretation of data and drafting of the manuscript. All authors read critically and approved the final manuscript.

## Consent for publication
Not applicable.

## Competing interests
All authors have completed the ICMJE uniform disclosure form at www.icmje.org and declare: GL2 was funded by a grant from the UK Department of Health, AS was funded by a fellowship from the Wellcome trust (200,163/Z/15/Z), and NW, GL1, GL2 and AS were supported by the University College London Hospitals National Institute of Health Research Biomedical Research Centre during the conduct of the submitted work. All authors declare no financial relationships with any organisations that might have an interest in the submitted work in the previous three years; no other relationships or activities that could appear to have influenced the submitted work.

## References
1. Statistics O. Deaths registered in England and Wales (series DR), 2011. Newport: Office for National Statistics; 2012.
2. Heron MP. Deaths: leading causes for 2011. 2015.
3. Sampson EL, Burns A, Richards M. Improving end-of-life care for people with dementia. Br J Psychiatry. 2011;199(5):357–9
4. Todd S, Barr S, Roberts M, Passmore AP. Survival in dementia and predictors of mortality: a review. Int J Geriatr Psychiatry. 2013;28(11):1109–24.
5. Thuné-Boyle IC, Sampson EL, Jones L, King M, Lee DR, Blanchard MR. Challenges to improving end of life care of people with advanced dementia in the UK. Dementia. 2010;9(2):259–84.
6. Chatterji S, Byles J, Cutler D, Seeman T, Verdes E. Health, functioning, and disability in older adults—present status and future implications. Lancet. 2015;385(9967):563–75.
7. Rexach L. Palliative care in dementia. European Geriatric Medicine. 2012;3(2): 131–40.
8. Livingston G, Leavey G, Manela M, Livingston D, Rait G, Sampson E, et al. Making decisions for people with dementia who lack capacity: qualitative study of family carers in UK. BMJ. 2010;341:c4184.
9. Johnston C, Liddle J. The mental capacity act 2005: a new framework for healthcare decision making. J Med Ethics. 2007;33(2):94–7.
10. Evans N, Pasman HRW, Donker GA, Deliens L, Van den Block L, Onwuteaka-Philipsen B, et al. End-of-life care in general practice: a cross-sectional, retrospective survey of 'cancer','organ failure'and 'old-age/dementia'patients. Palliat Med. 2014;28(7):965–75.
11. Perera G, Broadbent M, Callard F, Chang C-K, Downs J, Dutta R, et al. Cohort profile of the South London and Maudsley NHS Foundation Trust biomedical research Centre (SLaM BRC) case register: current status and recent enhancement of an electronic mental health record-derived data resource. BMJ Open. 2016;6(3):e008721.
12. Cunningham H. GATE, a general architecture for text engineering. Comput Humanities. 2002;36:223–54.
13. Werbeloff N, Osborn DPJ, Patel R, Taylor M, Stewart R, Broadbent M, et al. The Camden & Islington Research Database: using electronic mental health Records for Research. PLoS One. 2018; [In Press].
14. World Health Organization. International Statistical Classification of Diseases and Health Related Problems (The) ICD-10 2004. Geneva: World Health Organization; 2004.
15. Folstein MF, Folstein SE, McHugh PR. "Mini-mental state": a practical method for grading the cognitive state of patients for the clinician. J Psychiatr Res. 1975;12(3):189–98.
16. Perneczky R, Wagenpfeil S, Komossa K, Grimmer T, Diehl J, Kurz A. Mapping scores onto stages: mini-mental state examination and clinical dementia rating. Am J Geriatr Psychiatry. 2006;14(2):139–44.
17. Stewart R, Soremekun M, Perera G, Broadbent M, Callard F, Denis M, et al. The South London and Maudsley NHS foundation trust biomedical research Centre (SLAM BRC) case register: development and descriptive data. BMC Psychiatry. 2009;9(1):51.

18. Gill B. The English indices of deprivation 2015-statistical release. London: England Office for National Statistics; 2015.
19. Pirkis JE, Burgess PM, Kirk PK, Dodson S, Coombs TJ, Williamson MK. A review of the psychometric properties of the health of the nation outcome scales (HoNOS) family of measures. Health Qual Life Outcomes. 2005;3(1):76.
20. Kadra G, Stewart R, Shetty H, Jackson RG, Greenwood MA, Roberts A, et al. Extracting antipsychotic polypharmacy data from electronic health records: developing and evaluating a novel process. BMC Psychiatry. 2015;15(1):166.
21. Kingston A, Wohland P, Wittenberg R, Robinson L, Brayne C, Matthews FE, et al. Is late-life dependency increasing or not? A comparison of the cognitive function and ageing studies (CFAS). Lancet. 2017;390(10103):1676–84.
22. Matthews F, Stephan B, Robinson L, Jagger C, Barnes LE, Arthur A, et al. A two decade dementia incidence comparison from the cognitive function and ageing studies I and II. Nat Commun. 2016;7:11398.
23. Poblador-Plou B, Calderón-Larrañaga A, Marta-Moreno J, Hancco-Saavedra J, Sicras-Mainar A, Soljak M, et al. Comorbidity of dementia: a cross-sectional study of primary care older patients. BMC psychiatry. 2014;14(1):84.
24. Department of Health. Living well with dementia: A National Dementia Strategy 2009. London: Department of Health; 2009.
25. NHS England. Dementia diagnosis rate workbook – March 2017. 2017.
26. Stern Y. Cognitive reserve in ageing and Alzheimer's disease. Lancet Neurol. 2012;11(11):1006–12.
27. Vincent-Lancrin S. The reversal of gender inequalities in higher education: An on-going trend. Higher education to. 2008;2030(1):265–98.
28. Meng X, D'Arcy C. Education and dementia in the context of the cognitive reserve hypothesis: a systematic review with meta-analyses and qualitative analyses. PLoS One. 2012;7(6):e38268.
29. Adelman S, Blanchard M, Rait G, Leavey G, Livingston G. Prevalence of dementia in African–Caribbean compared with UK-born white older people: two-stage cross-sectional study. Br J Psychiatry. 2011;199(2):119–25.
30. Cooper C, Tandy AR, Balamurali TB, Livingston G. A systematic review and meta-analysis of ethnic differences in use of dementia treatment, care, and research. Am J Geriatr Psychiatry. 2010;18(3):193–203.
31. Moriarty J, Sharif N, Robinson J. SCIE Research briefing 35: Black and minority ethnic people with dementia and their access to support and services. (Research Briefings). Social Care Instutute for Excellence; 2011.
32. Karp A, Kåreholt I, Qiu C, Bellander T, Winblad B, Fratiglioni L. Relation of education and occupation-based socioeconomic status to incident Alzheimer's disease. Am J Epidemiol. 2004;159(2):175–83.
33. Dupre ME, Beck AN, Meadows SO. Marital trajectories and mortality among US adults. Am J Epidemiol. 2009;170(5):546–55.
34. Peters ME, Schwartz S, Han D, Rabins PV, Steinberg M, Tschanz JT, et al. Neuropsychiatric symptoms as predictors of progression to severe Alzheimer's dementia and death: the Cache County dementia progression study. Am J Psychiatr. 2015;172(5):460–5.
35. Zahodne LB, Gongvatana A, Cohen RA, Ott BR, Tremont G. Are apathy and depression independently associated with longitudinal trajectories of cortical atrophy in mild cognitive impairment? Am J Geriatr Psychiatry. 2013;21(11):1098–106.
36. Vigen CL, Mack WJ, Keefe RS, Sano M, Sultzer DL, Stroup TS, et al. Cognitive effects of atypical antipsychotic medications in patients with Alzheimer's disease: outcomes from CATIE-AD. Am J Psychiatr. 2011;168(8):831–9.
37. Livingston G, Walker AE, Katona CL, Cooper C. Antipsychotics and cognitive decline in Alzheimer's disease: the LASER-Alzheimer's disease longitudinal study. J Neurol Neurosurg Psychiatry. 2007;78(1):25–9.
38. Zhao Q, Zhou B, Ding D, Teramukai S, Guo Q, Fukushima M, et al. Cognitive decline in patients with Alzheimer's disease and its related factors in a memory clinic setting, Shanghai, China. PLoS One. 2014;9(4):e95755.
39. Xie SX, Ewbank DC, Chittams J, Karlawish JH, Arnold SE, Clark CM. Rate of decline in Alzheimer's disease measured by a dementia severity rating scale. Alzheimer Dis Assoc Disord. 2009;23(3):268.
40. Smits LL, van Harten AC, Pijnenburg YA, Koedam EL, Bouwman FH, Sistermans N, et al. Trajectories of cognitive decline in different types of dementia. Psychol Med. 2015;45(5):1051–9.
41. Steeman E, Casterlé D, Dierckx B, Godderis J, Grypdonck M. Living with early-stage dementia: a review of qualitative studies. J Adv Nurs. 2006;54(6):722–38.
42. Dening KH, Jones L, Sampson EL. Preferences for end-of-life care: a nominal group study of people with dementia and their family carers. Palliat Med. 2013;27(5):409–17.

# 22

# The burden of depressive disorders in South Asia, 1990–2016: findings from the global burden of disease study

Felix Akpojene Ogbo*⑩, Sruthi Mathsyaraja[†], Rajeendra Kashyap Koti[†], Janette Perz and Andrew Page

## Abstract

**Background:** Globally, depressive disorders are one of the most common forms of mental illness. Using data from the most recent Global Burden of Disease, Injury, and Risk Factor Study 2016 (GBD 2016), we aimed to describe the burden of disease attributable to depressive disorders in terms of prevalence and disability-adjusted life years (DALYs) in South Asia countries (namely India, Pakistan, Bangladesh, Nepal and Bhutan).

**Methods:** GBD 2016 used epidemiological data on depressive disorders (major depression and dysthymia) from South Asia and a Bayesian meta-regression tool (DisMod-MR 2.1) to model prevalence and DALYs of depressive disorders by age, sex, country and year. DALYs were calculated from the years lived with disability (YLDs), derived from the prevalence of depressive disorders and disability weights, obtained from a community and internet-based surveys. The analyses adjusted for comorbidity, data sources and multiple modelling, and estimates were presented with 95% uncertainty intervals (UI).

**Results:** In 2016, the age-standardised prevalence of depressive disorders in South Asia was 3.9% (95% UI: 3.6–4.2%), 4.4% (95% UI: 4.4–4.8%) in Bangladesh, 3.9% (95% UI: 3.6–4.2%) in India, 3.0% (95% UI: 2.8–3.3%) in Pakistan, 4.0% (95% UI: 3.7–4.3%) in Nepal and 3.7% (95% UI: 3.4–4.1%) in Bhutan. In South Asia, depressive disorders accounted for 9.8 million DALYs (95% UI: 6.8–13.2 million) or 577.8 (95% UI: 399.9–778.9) per 100,000 population in 2016. Of these, major depressive disorders (MDD) accounted for 7.8 million DALYs (95% UI: 5.3–10.5 million). India generated the largest numbers of DALYs due to depressive disorders and MDD, followed by Bangladesh and Pakistan. DALYs due to depressive disorders were highest in females and older adults (75–79 years) across all countries.

**Conclusion:** Our findings show the substantial public health burden of depressive disorders in South Asian populations and healthcare systems. Given the scale of depressive disorders, improvement in overall population health is possible if South Asian countries prioritise the prevention and treatment of depressive disorders.

**Keywords:** Depressive disorders, Depression, Global Burden of Disease, South Asia

## Background

Depressive disorders are one of the most common mental health illnesses worldwide, affecting approximately 121 million people and accounting for 5% of disability-adjusted life years (DALYs) globally [1, 2]. A previous global study suggested that major depressive disorder (MDD) would become the second leading cause of disease burden by 2020, after heart disease [3]. South Asia represents approximately 23% of the global population and one-fifth of the world's mental health cases [4]. In the past five decades, significant advances have been made in the management of depressive disorders, including the development of various pharmacological and non-pharmacological interventions that have improved patients outcomes [5, 6]. However, the higher cost of drugs, prolonged use of medications and regular clinician appointments have been shown to be impediments to pharmacological and psychotherapeutic treatments of depressive disorders in many communities in South Asia

* Correspondence: felgbo@yahoo.co.uk
[†]Sruthi Mathsyaraja and Rajeendra Kashyap Koti contributed equally to this work.
Translational Health Research Institute (THRI), School of Medicine, Western Sydney University, Locked Bag 1797, Penrith, NSW 2571, Australia

and may have led people with depressive disorders to seek alternative therapies [7, 8].

Previous studies of MDD based on the diagnostic criteria reported that the proportion of people with MDD in South Asian countries was among the highest globally [4, 9]. A recent population-based mental health survey based on case definitions of mental disorders from India indicated that the prevalence of MDD was approximately 3.0% [10], substantially lower than estimates (21–83%) from other small-scale studies which assessed MDD with symptom scales [11–13]. Past studies which also used symptom scales in other South Asian countries also reported higher figures, 46% in urban Pakistan [14], 29% in regional Bhutan [15] and rural Bangladesh [16], respectively. In many developing countries (including South Asia), there is an increasing societal awareness and better acknowledgement of mental illness [10, 17, 18]. This increasing recognition of mental disorders in many communities has led to global, regional and national efforts to address the burden of mental illness, including depressive disorders [19, 20].

Depressive disorders are associated with adverse health outcomes and reduced life-expectancy, including chronic diseases such as diabetes, arthritis, coronary heart disease and cancers [6], and may lead to poor maternal and perinatal health outcomes, disruptions of family relationships [21, 22], poor work performance, physical inactivity, increased risk of self-injury, substance abuse and adverse life events (such as suicide) [23, 24]. To scale up and prioritise interventions to promote positive mental health requires an understanding of how mental illness differs across population groups and geographies [25]. Specifically, detailed knowledge of the burden of depressive disorders is essential to inform policy decision-making and health advocacy to ensure the development and/or revision of mental health programmes to improve population health outcomes.

The Global Burden of Disease, Injury and Risk Factor (GBD) study provides comprehensive and comparable health data for 195 countries and territories to facilitate timely and policy decision-making processes. In many instances, detailed expositions of the GBD findings for various health focus areas and geographies are further highlighted in additional publications to better characterise the results for researchers, clinicians and/or policy decision-makers to identify high-priority populations, as well as assess where resources could be best allocated [9, 26–29]. Therefore, an up-to-date assessment of the burden of depressive disorders focused in South Asian countries is essential for decision-makers and health professionals in the region to inform strategic mental health actions. The present study aimed to describe the prevalence and disability-adjusted life years (DALYs) associated with depressive disorders by country, sex and age in the South Asian countries of India, Pakistan, Bangladesh, Nepal and

Bhutan, using data from the most recent GBD 2016 study. DALYs are a population health measure of overall disease burden, defined as the number of years lost due to ill-health, disability or premature death. DALYs have been used previously for priority-setting and resource allocation in health care delivery [30, 31].

## Method

The GBD study provides estimates of incidence, prevalence, cause of morbidity and mortality, and health loss, by age, sex, year, location, income group and overtime for diseases, injuries and key risk factors. The GBD study is a signatory to the Guidelines for Accurate and Transparent Health Estimates Reporting (GATHER) protocol. GATHER promotes good practice and transparency in reporting health estimates and permits researchers and decision-makers to assess the quality of the estimates [32]. The overall conceptual and analytical framework for the calculation of prevalence and DALYs for depressive disorders have been described in detail elsewhere [2, 33.]. In this study, we provide an overview of the methodology used to acquire relevant epidemiologic data and the estimation process of depressive disorders in South Asia.

### Case definition

In GBD 2016, depressive disorders included MDD and dysthymia. Depressive disorders were defined based on the criteria proposed in the Diagnostic and Statistical Manual of Mental Disorders-IV (DSM-IV) and the International Classification of Diseases 10 (ICD-10) [33]. The DSM-IV and ICD-10 definitions of the depressive disorders as described in this study are published in GBD 2015 and 2016 nonfatal health outcome papers [33, 34] and supplement [35]. The DSM-IV (296.21–24, 296.31–34) describes MDD as an episodic disorder with a prolonged outcome and an increased risk of death [36], comparable to ICD-10's description of recurrent depressive disorder (F32.0–9, F33.0–9) [37]. MDD is the presence of at least one major depressive episode (i.e., an experience of depressed mood almost all day, every day, for at least 2 weeks). Dysthymia is a less severe depressed mood compared to MDD, lasting several years, with low rates of remission and no increased risk of death (DSM-IV: 300.4 [36]; ICD-10: F34.1 [37]).

### Data sources

The GBD 2016 study used prevalence, incidence, remission or duration, and excess mortality data from a systematic review employed for GBD 2010 [38], and additional reviews conducted between January 2013 and September 2016 to generate current estimates [2]. The reviews involved electronic searches of the peer-reviewed literature (PsycINFO, Embase and PubMed), the grey literature, expert consultations, as well as institutional collaborations, including the partnership between the GBD study team and the Indian Council of Medical Research and the Public Health Foundation of India [33]. The search yielded twenty-seven sources of epidemiological data for South Asian countries which were used for the estimation of prevalence and DALYs in those countries (Additional file 1: Table S1) [2, 33].

The inclusion criteria for the reviews included: (i) studies which reported prevalence, incidence, duration and/or excess mortality data from 1980 onward; (ii) "caseness" based on clinical threshold, consistent with the DSM or ICD criteria; (iii) detailed information must be provided on the study method and sample characteristics to assess the study quality; and (iv) study samples must be representative of the general population. Studies which reported information on an inpatient or pharmacological treatment, case studies, veterans or refugee samples were excluded [2].

Data sources used for the estimation of depressive disorders in GBD 2016 for South Asian countries can be accessed in the Global Health Data Exchange website (http://ghdx.healthdata.org/gbd-2016/data-input-sources). GBD 2016 provides up-to-date prevalence and DALYs data of depressive disorders based on country-specific epidemiologic data in the global health data exchange repository (GHDx) and improvements in methodological approaches to GBD 2010 [39], 2013 [40] and 2015 [34] studies. The GHDx provides researchers, clinicians and policy-makers access to GBD 2016 input sources, results and creates opportunities for discussing population health based on the best available data. GHDx also raises awareness about different groups collecting data globally and provides standardised citations to encourage appropriate acknowledgement of data owners' contributions [41].

### Data analysis

In the estimation of each depressive disorder, epidemiological data were generated using DisMod-MR 2.1 – a Bayesian meta-regression tool. DisMod-MR 2.1 was the primary method used in GBD 2016 to combined all data sources, and adjust for variability and study quality to estimate the epidemiology of depressive disorders. Country-specific epidemiological data on depressive disorders from the systematic reviews were modelled in DisMod-MR 2.1 to estimate prevalence and DALYs by age and year, which also propagated uncertainty around the raw data through to the final estimates [2, 33]. Additionally, study- and location-level covariates were used to accommodate between-study variability and to indicate a positive association between conflict status and the proportion of depressive disorders, respectively [2].

In the GBD, DALYs are calculated by summing years lived with disability (YLDs) and years of life lost (YLLs) for each country, sex, age and year, wherein they measure the gap between the health of a population and the maximum lifespan spent in full health [33]. YLLs are calculated by multiplying the number of deaths attributable to the particular disorder at a specific age by the standard life expectancy for that age. [33]. In the present analysis, however, the YLL component was not calculated given that depression is not a cause of death in GBD study, consistent with the ICD-10 criteria for categorical designation of the cause of death to a single underlying cause [2]. Thus, DALYs were estimated for depressive disorders from the YLD component. YLDs were defined as the years of life lived with any short-term or long-term health loss, and were calculated by multiplying depression-specific prevalence data by disability weights [33]. Disability weights are population assessment of severity of health loss from a specific cause. GBD 2016 used disability weights, obtained from multi-country population-based surveys, where individuals were asked to indicate which person they perceived to be in good health, ranging from 'perfect health,' coded as '0' to death, coded as '1' [2].

YLDs were adjusted for comorbidity given that individuals can have more than one disease at a particular time. Microsimulations were performed to assess individual comorbidity, and a multiplicative method was employed to estimate the combined disability experience among individuals with multiple diseases [2]. The rationale for comorbidity adjustment is that it estimates the difference between the mean disability weight in people with one disease and combined disability weight in those with more than one disease. This analytical strategy was similar to the approaches used in GBD 2013 [9] and 2015 [34].

To determine the proportion of people within each levels of severity for a depressive disorder, data from the US National Epidemiological Survey on Alcohol and Related Conditions (NESARC, conducted between 2001 and 2005) and the Australian National Survey of Mental Health and Wellbeing of Adults (NSMHWB, conducted in 1997) were used to estimate the proportions of MDD and dysthymic cases, categorised as asymptomatic and symptomatic (mild, moderate and severe) [2]. This approach captures the main features of MDD and dysthymia based on the DSM-IV and ICD-10 criteria, consistent with methodologies employed in the previous GBD studies [9, 34].

Corresponding 95% uncertainty intervals (UIs) for prevalence and DALYs estimates were generated from 1000 draws from the posterior distribution of each estimation process [33]. Unlike confidence intervals, UIs do not only adjust for sampling error but also capture uncertainty from several analytical modelling stages and adjust for type and quality of data sources [33].

## Results

### Prevalence of depressive disorders

In 2016, the age-standardised prevalence of depressive disorders was 3.9% (95% UI: 3.6–4.2%) in South Asia. In

Bangladesh, age-standardised prevalence was 4.4% (95% UI: 4.4–4.8%), 3.9% (95% UI: 3.6–4.2%) in India, 3.0% (95% UI: 2.8–3.3%) in Pakistan, 4.0% (95% UI: 3.7–4.3%) in Nepal and 3.7% (95% UI: 3.4–4.1%) in Bhutan in the same year (Table 1).

### YLDs and DALYs due to depressive disorders

In 2016, depressive disorders contributed 577.8 (95% UI: 399.9–778.9) per 100,000 population in South Asian countries, an increase of 9% (Table 1) or a total of 9.8 million DALYs (95% UI: 6.8–13.2 million) in 2016 (Table 2). The majority of DALYs (7.8 million, 95% UI: 5.3–10.5 million) were due to MDD. In South Asia, MDD accounted for 2% (95% UI: 1–3%) of the total cause of DALYs in 2016 for both sexes and all age groups and was ranked the 19th leading cause of disease burden – an increase from a ranking of 30th leading cause of disease burden in 1990, data not shown.

India had the most substantial numbers of DALYs for all depressive disorders in 2016 at 7.7 million DALYs (95% UI: 5.3–10.3 million), accounting for more than two-thirds of the DALYs in South Asia. Bangladesh followed with 1.1 million DALYs (95% UI: 756,521–1.5 million) and Pakistan at 907,016 DALYs (95% UI: 625,699–1.2 million). Similarly, India had the highest numbers of DALYs for MDD at 6.1 million DALYs (95% UI: 4.2–8.2 million), followed by Bangladesh at approximately 1 million DALYs (95% UI: 619,061–1.2 million) (Table 2).

Figure 1 shows the age-standardised rate of depressive disorders by sex and country. Between 1990 and 2016, higher rates of DALYs were evident in all South Asian countries. Over the same period, DALYs rates were relatively higher in females compared to their male counterparts in South Asia, but this was not statistically significant. A stratified analysis of the rate of DALYs by age groups showed that the burden of depressive disorders was highest among older age groups (75–79 years) in all countries (Figs. 2 and 3). Between 1990 and 2016, age-standardised YLDs were highest in Bangladesh for both sexes, with higher levels seen among females compared to males but this was not statistically significant (Additional file 2: Figure S1).

### Discussion

The global prevalence of depressive disorders in 2016 was 3.7% [2], which is comparable to the reported age-standardised prevalence of 3.9% in South Asia. MDD was the largest contributor to the total burden of depressive disorders in all South Asian countries. Similarly, MDD ranks first among other mental and substance use disorders, and sixth in all diseases and injuries in the GBD 2016 study [1]. Age-standardised rate of DALYs was largest in Bangladesh, with a higher burden in females and older adults but this was not statistically significant.

The current study showed that MDD accounted for the largest proportion and numbers of DALYs due to

**Table 1** Age-standardised prevalence and absolute rate of DALYs for depressive disorders in South Asia, 1990–2016

|  |  | % (95% UI) | 1990 rate* (95% UI) | 2016 rate* (95% UI) | % change of DALYs rate 1990–2016 |
|---|---|---|---|---|---|
| Depressive disorders | South Asia | 3.9 (3.6–4.2) | 529.5 (366.4–718.7) | 577.8 (399.9–778.9) | 9.1 |
|  | India | 3.9 (3.6–4.2) | 536.3 (370.8–729.4) | 581.1 (403.6–785.2) | 8.3 |
|  | Pakistan | 3.0 (2.8–3.3) | 434.3 (298.1–592.6) | 475.0 (327.7–643.6) | 9.4 |
|  | Bangladesh | 4.4 (4.4–4.8) | 583.0 (405.6–787.4) | 680.6 (467.3–925.6) | 16.7 |
|  | Nepal | 4.0 (3.7–4.3) | 466.3 (321.4–633.8) | 534.7 (366.9–725.7) | 14.7 |
|  | Bhutan | 3.7 (3.4–4.1) | 453.6 (314.9–619.3) | 530.3 (361.6–716.3) | 16.9 |
| Major depressive disorder | South Asia | 2.6 (2.4–2.8) | 430.7 (297.5–585.1) | 457.4 (314.5–617.5) | 6.2 |
|  | India | 2.5 (2.3–2.8) | 436.2 (300.6–592.3) | 458.5 (315.8–620.9) | 5.1 |
|  | Pakistan | 2.3 (2.1–2.6) | 341.7 (233.5–470.9) | 367.0 (251.3–502.7) | 7.4 |
|  | Bangladesh | 3.1 (2.8–3.5) | 488.9 (335.3–664.5) | 561.7 (382.4–763.5) | 14.9 |
|  | Nepal | 2.6 (2.1–2.9) | 371.5 (254.8–508.7) | 424.4 (288.0–573.4) | 14.3 |
|  | Bhutan | 2.4 (2.2–2.7) | 361.3 (248.7–495.4) | 412.6 (281.0–557.6) | 14.2 |
| Dysthymia | South Asia | 1.4 (1.2–1.6) | 98.8 (66.6–143.8) | 120.4 (81.2–174.1) | 21.9 |
|  | India | 1.4 (1.2–1.6) | 100.2 (67.6–145.2) | 122.6 (82.5–177.2) | 22.4 |
|  | Pakistan | 1.4 (1.2–1.6) | 92.7 (62.6–135.6) | 108.0 (72.7–156.5) | 16.5 |
|  | Bangladesh | 1.4 (1.2–1.6) | 94.2 (63.2–138.0) | 118.9 (79.9–174.4) | 26.3 |
|  | Nepal | 1.4 (1.2–1.6) | 94.9 (64.1–139.6) | 110.3 (74.4–159.6) | 16.3 |
|  | Bhutan | 1.4 (1.2–1.6) | 92.2 (62.4–133.7) | 117.8 (78.9–171.8) | 27.7 |

%: prevalence; *rate is per 100,000 population; *UI* uncertainty interval, *DALYs* disability-adjusted life years

**Table 2** Numbers of disability-adjusted life years by depressive disorders in South Asia, 1990–2016

| | | 1990<br>DALYs (95% UI) | 2016<br>DALYs (95% UI) | % change of DALYs<br>numbers 1990–2016 |
|---|---|---|---|---|
| Depressive disorders | South Asia | 5,800,499 (4,014,423-7,873,652) | 9,821,063 (6,797,636-1323,9210) | 69.3 |
| | India | 4,632,923 (3,202,901-6,300,340) | 7,647,086 (5,311,795-10,332,886) | 65.1 |
| | Pakistan | 470,327 (322,832-641,750) | 907,016 (625,699-1,228,954) | 92.8 |
| | Bangladesh | 607,410 (422,605-820,278) | 1,101,909 (756,521-1,498,522) | 81.4 |
| | Nepal | 87,429 (60,251-118,821) | 160,820 (110,353-218,278) | 83.9 |
| | Bhutan | 2410 (1673-3291) | 4232 (2885-5716) | 75.6 |
| Major depressive disorder | South Asia | 4,718,648 (3,259,338-6,410,444) | 7,774,678 (5,345,086-1,0496,504) | 64.8 |
| | India | 3,767,801 (2,596,567-5,116,562) | 6033,551 (4,155,478-8,171,522) | 60.1 |
| | Pakistan | 369,982 (252885–509,986) | 700,813 (479,865-959,981) | 89.4 |
| | Bangladesh | 509,304 (349,326-692,269) | 909,375 (619,061-1,236,065) | 78.6 |
| | Nepal | 69,641 (47,763-95,369) | 127,647 (86,607-172,470) | 83.3 |
| | Bhutan | 1920 (1321-2632) | 3292 (2242-4449) | 71.5 |
| Dysthymia | South Asia | 1,081,851 (729,209-1,575,227) | 2,046,386 (1,380,766-2,958,677) | 89.2 |
| | India | 865,123 (584,292-1,254,327) | 1,613,535 (1,086,278-2,332,034) | 86.5 |
| | Pakistan | 100,345 (67,839-146,800) | 206,203 (138,778-298,937) | 105.5 |
| | Bangladesh | 98,106 (65,798-143,768) | 192,534 (129,339-282,364) | 96.3 |
| | Nepal | 17,787 (12,016-26,176) | 33,173 (22,367-48,012) | 86.5 |
| | Bhutan | 490 (331–711) | 940 (629–1371) | 91.7 |

*DALYs* disability-adjusted life years, *UI* uncertainty interval

depressive disorders in South Asia. This finding is consistent with a previous study which found that the majority of depressive disorders worldwide related to MDD [9]. The previous study also suggested that the burden of depressive disorders was higher among high-income North American and European countries compared to Asian countries [9]. Possible reasons for this finding may be due to the under-reporting of mental illness or a lack of high-quality epidemiological data on mental health disorders in many developing countries [9, 42]. Under-reporting of depressive disorders in the South Asian region may also be partly due to a high level of stigma and discrimination associated with mental health disorders in South Asian countries [43–47].

A study conducted in Nepal indicated that stigma and discrimination were the most common factors associated with a lack of uptake of mental health treatment, where self-disclosure of traumatic events is socially stigmatised. Additionally, people believe that disclosing one's traumatic experience may affect the reputation of a person and their family [48]. Since 2006, the Government of Nepal introduced the Mental Health Act to improve the mental health outcomes of the population [49], including the involvement of medical colleges to strengthen collaboration between researchers and community stakeholders [50]. However, mental health initiatives in Nepal remain under-resourced as only 0.1% of the national health budget is allocated to mental health interventions [49]. To

promote the mental health of the Nepalese population, government at all levels in Nepal would have to increase funding for mental health programmes and be committed to supporting evidence-based and culturally-appropriate interventions.

The study showed that Bangladesh had the highest age-standardised prevalence of MDD, and it was one of the leading contributors to the burden of depressive disorders in the South Asian region, consistent with previous studies [9, 17] and a World Health Organisation (WHO) report [51]. In Bangladesh, there are efforts to reduce the burden of mental health disorders. For example, between 2005 and 2006, the Government of Bangladesh in collaboration with the WHO and primary health sector introduced programmes to create awareness and educate people on mental illness, increased the number of mental health professionals, as well as developed research capacities [51]. However, improvement in mental health funding will be required given that Bangladesh – where over 65% of health expenditures is out-of-pocket – recently allocated only 0.5% of the total health budget to mental health initiatives [52].

In South Asian countries, depressive disorders are more common among people from lower socio-economic background, those with no or lower education, those unemployed, divorced or widowed (especially women), and the elderly [10, 53–56]. Consistent with previous reports [9, 57, 58], the present study showed that the burden of

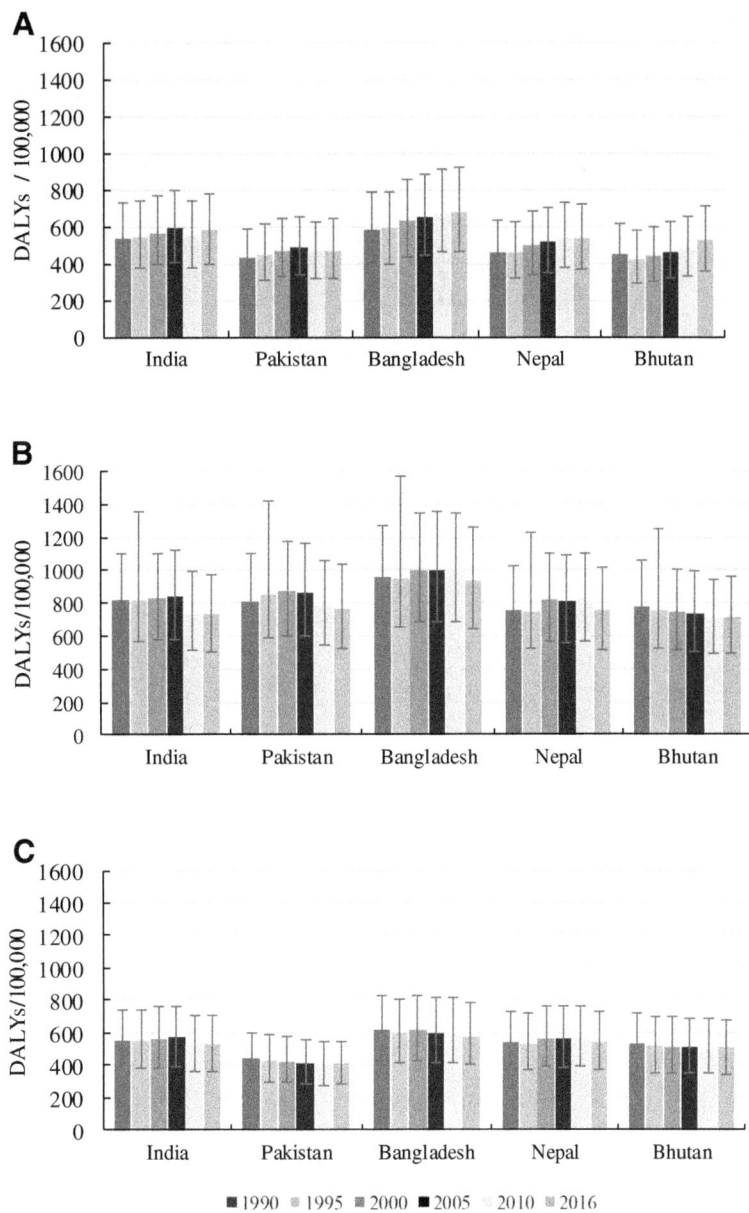

**Fig. 1** Age-standardised rate of DALYs due to depressive disorders by sex in South Asia, 1990–2016. **a** Both sexes; (**b**) Females; (**c**) Males

depressive disorders was higher among females and older adults compared to males and young people, respectively, in all South Asian countries. Past studies have reported that compared to males, females are more likely to experience adverse life events that are strongly associated with the onset of depressive episodes, including gender discrimination, physical and sexual abuse, relationship breakdown, intimate partner violence, antenatal and postnatal stress, and adverse cultural norms [59–61]. There is limited evidence to attribute a hormonal or biological mechanism as a potential explanation for the higher burden of depressive episodes among women than men [62]. To improve mental health outcomes in South Asia, mental health interventions should target the general population, particularly females and those in vulnerable environments.

The present study showed that the age-standardised prevalence of MDD and dysthymia was 2.5% and 1.4%, respectively in India, in line with previous reports [9, 10]. However, studies from regional areas of India have indicated that the prevalence of MDD ranged from 21 to 83% [11–13]. This variation is due to differences in case definitions and the measurement of depressive episodes, wherein those small-scale studies assessed MDD with symptom scales. Since the 1970s [63, 64], India has taken

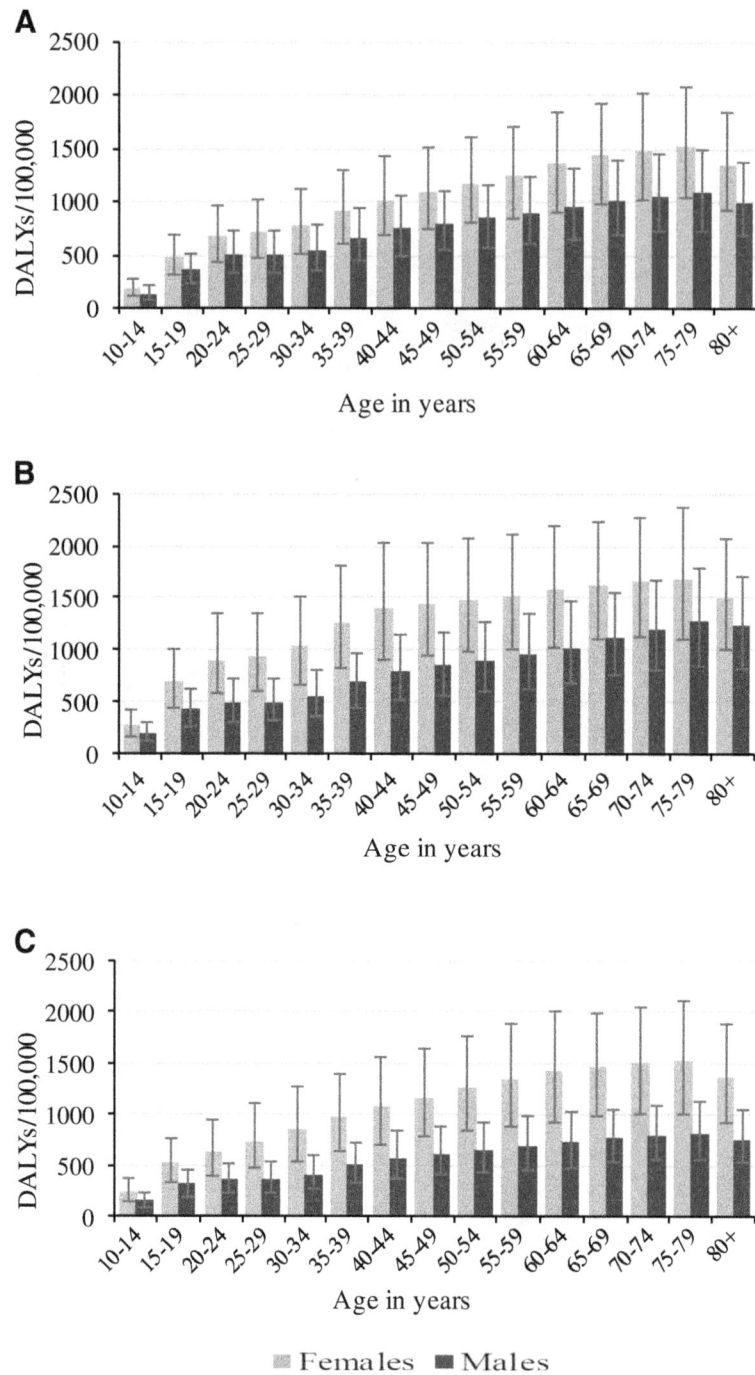

**Fig. 2** Rate of DALYs due to depressive disorders by age in India, Bangladesh and Pakistan, 2016. **a** India; (**b**) Bangladesh; (**c**) Pakistan

necessary steps to address mental health issues, including increasing funding for mental health programmes, improving institutional care and research, and motivating relevant stakeholders to implement mental health laws at all levels of government [65, 66]. However, the shortages of healthcare professionals and stigma associated with mental health illness remain an obstacle to the uptake of relevant health care measures in the country [67–69].

Task-sharing (such as training of non-physicians) to provide focused and relevant health services in addition to health care workers in communities, designing and promoting life skills and family education programmes have been advocated to improve mental health outcomes in India [65, 67].

Among the South Asian countries studied, Pakistan had a lower prevalence of depressive disorders at 3.0%,

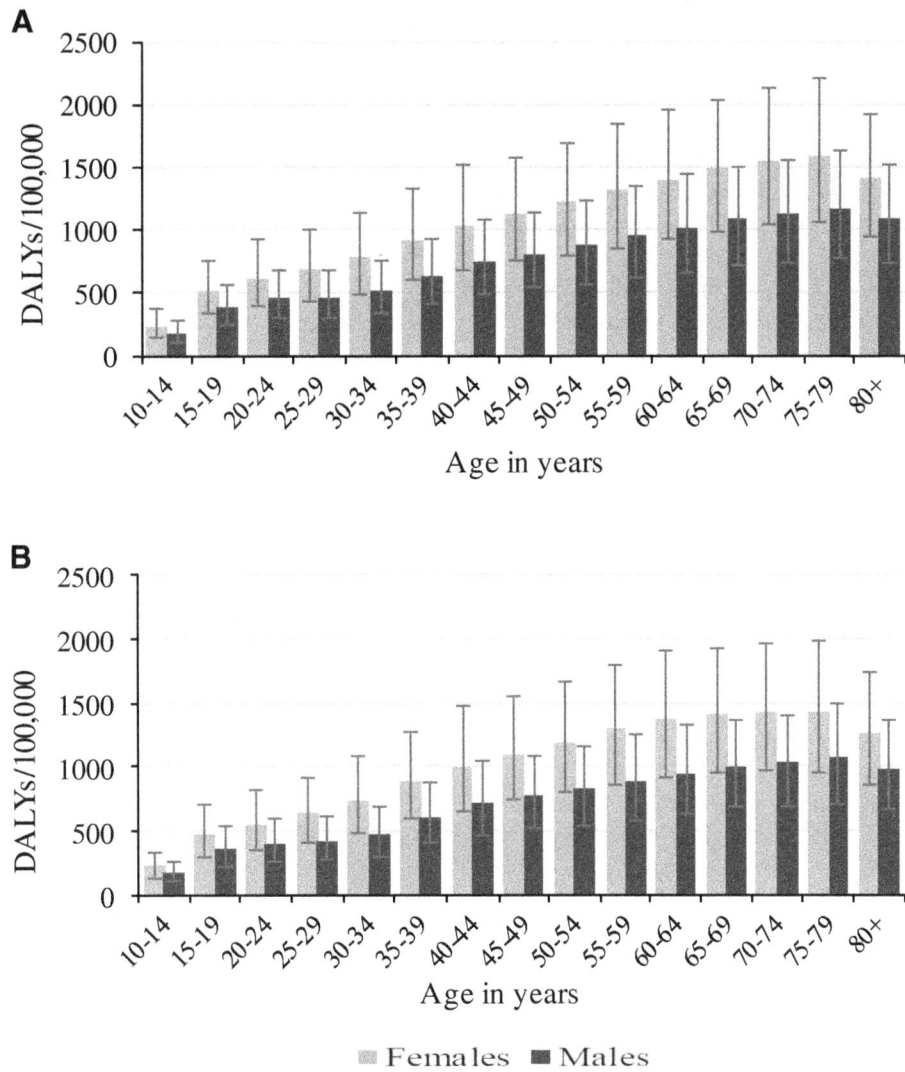

**Fig. 3** Rate of DALYs due to depressive disorders by age in Nepal and Bhutan in 2016. **a** Nepal; (**b**) Bhutan

which may be attributable to under-reporting and a lack of high-quality epidemiologic data. Previous reports suggested that weakening of traditional values and family systems due to urbanisation, fear of wars and natural disasters may be associated with an increasing burden of depressive disorders in Pakistan [47, 70]. The prevalence of depressive disorders in Bhutan was 3.7%, with an associated higher rate of DALYs attributable to depressive disorders. Like the Pakistanis [47], Bhutanese people often believe that 'Karma' (previous life) and attitudes strongly influence a person's propensity to experience mental illness. Consequently, more than 99% of Bhutanese with mental illness seek alternative therapies such as faith and religious healing [71].

In the last decade, Bhutan has introduced a number of mental health initiatives to increase accessibility and availability of primary mental health services, with a

subsequent increase in mental health awareness [71, 72]. These efforts have been revised to incorporate other key measures (such as 'National Happiness Index') to promote the well-being of individuals and inform policy decision-making [25]. Nevertheless, improvements are still needed in Bhutan as the country has no trained psychiatrists in community-based mental health programmes [71]. For Pakistan, the mental health strategy has multiple weaknesses, including inadequate funding and a lack of service integration [14, 73]. Training of health workers, development of research capacity and epidemiological data collection, and refinement of current mental health programmes, as well as an increase in mental health financing, galvanised with strong political will at all levels, are warranted in those countries [15, 72].

The study has a number of limitations, which have been described in detail in the Lancet Series for the

GBD and supplement [2, 9, 33]. Briefly, we describe specific limitations. First, DSM-IV and ICD-10 criteria for depressive disorders may not be applicable across all cultural sub-population groups in South Asia as people prefer not to disclose mental health issues as a result of stigma and discrimination. Second, GBD study used disability weights to capture health loss while not accounting for the impact of depressive disorders on economic productivity and family socio-emotional interaction. Third, the lack of assessment of YLLs for depressive disorders presents challenges in the full estimation of health loss due to depressive disorders as they are not coded as causes of death in the GBD study based on the ICD-10 criteria for listing causes of death. Fourth, it is possible that the study may have underestimated the 'full burden' of depressive disorders given data availability and a time lag between the in-country release of data and their subsequent incorporation into the GBD study. The lack of high-quality epidemiological data for all countries is possibly reflected in the wide uncertainty intervals. However, underestimation of data may be less likely in India given gbd 2016 access to recent epidemiological data and improvements in methodological and modelling strategies.

## Conclusion

The study indicates that the prevalence of depressive disorders in South Asia is comparable to the global estimate, and Bangladesh and India has higher proportions of people with depressive disorders in South Asia. Additionally, females and older adults (75–79 years) have the highest burden of depressive disorders across all countries in the region. The findings suggest that mental health services and programmes should be prioritised and scaled up across South Asian countries, with significant contributions and involvement of national and subnational governments to improve population health and well-being.

## Additional file

> **Additional file 1: Table S1.** Data sources used for estimating the burden of depressive disorders in South Asian countries. (DOCX 18 kb)
>
> **Additional file 2: Figure S1.** Age-standardised rate of YLDs due to depressive disorders by sex in South Asia, 1990–2016. (A) Both sexes; (B) Females; (C) Males. (DOCX 30 kb)

## Abbreviations

DALYs: Disability-adjusted life years; GBD: Global Burden of Disease; YLDs: Years lived with disability; YLLs: Years of life lost

## Acknowledgements

The authors are grateful to the Institute for Health Metrics and Evaluation, Seattle, USA for providing the data.

## Funding

Bill & Melinda Gates Foundation funded GBD 2016. The authors receive no specific funding from a private/public organisation for the study.

## Authors' contributions

FAO conceived and designed the study, obtained the data, interpreted the data, drafted the manuscript and critically revised the final manuscript as submitted. SM and RKK contributed to the study conceptualisation, interpreted data and contributed to the drafting of the manuscript, as well as critically revised the manuscript draft as submitted. JP and AP provided advise on the manuscript structure, interpreted data and critically revised the manuscript as submitted. All authors read and approved the final manuscript.

## Consent for publication

Not applicable.

## Competing interests

The authors declare that they have no competing interests.

## References

1. Institute for Health Metrics and Evaluation. GBD Compare Seattle, WA, USA: IHME, University of Washington; 2017 [November 22 2017]. Available from: http://vizhub.healthdata.org/gbd-compare.
2. Vos T, Abajobir AA, Abbafati C, Abbas MK, Abate KH, Abd-Allah F, et al. Global, regional, and national incidence, prevalence, and years lived with disability for 328 diseases and injuries for 195 countries, 1990–2016: a systematic analysis for the Global Burden of Disease Study 2016. Lancet. 2017;390:1211–59.
3. Murray CJ, Lopez AD, World Health Organization. The global burden of disease: a comprehensive assessment of mortality and disability from diseases, injuries, and risk factors in 1990 and projected to 2020: Summary. 1996.
4. Bishwajit G, O'Leary DP, Ghosh S, Yaya S, Shangfeng T, Feng Z. Physical inactivity and self-reported depression among middle-and older-aged population in South Asia: world health survey. BMC Geriatr. 2017;17(1):100.
5. Goesling J, Clauw DJ, Hassett AL. Pain and depression: an integrative review of neurobiological and psychological factors. Current Psychiatry Rep. 2013; 15(12):421.
6. Moussavi S, Chatterji S, Verdes E, Tandon A, Patel V, Ustun B. Depression, chronic diseases, and decrements in health: results from the world health surveys. Lancet. 2007;370(9590):851–8.
7. Louie L. The effectiveness of yoga for depression: a critical literature review. Issues Ment Health Nurs. 2014;35(4):265–76.
8. Amin F, Islam N, Gilani A. Traditional and complementary/alternative medicine use in a south-Asian population. Asian Pacific J Health Sci. 2015;2:36–42.
9. Ferrari AJ, Charlson FJ, Norman RE, Patten SB, Freedman G, Murray CJ, et al. Burden of depressive disorders by country, sex, age, and year: findings from the global burden of disease study 2010. PLoS Med. 2013;10(11):e1001547.
10. Gururaj G, Varghese M, Benegal V, Rao GN, Pathak K, Singh LK, et al. National Mental Health Survey of India, 2015–16. Bengaluru, India: National Institute of Mental Health and Neuro Sciences, 2016.
11. Poongothai S, Pradeepa R, Ganesan A, Mohan V. Prevalence of depression in a large urban south Indian population—the Chennai urban rural epidemiology study (CURES–70). PLoS One. 2009;4(9):e7185.
12. Pothen M, Kuruvilla A, Philip K, Joseph A, Jacob K. Common mental disorders among primary care attenders in Vellore, South India: nature, prevalence and risk factors. Int J Soc Psychiatry. 2003;49(2):119–25.
13. Nambi S, Prasad J, Singh D, Abraham V, Kuruvilla A, Jacob K. Explanatory models and common mental disorders among patients with unexplained somatic symptoms attending a primary care facility in Tamil Nadu. Natl Med J India. 2002;15(6):331–5.

14. Gadit AAM, Mugford G. Prevalence of depression among households in three capital cities of Pakistan: need to revise the mental health policy. PLoS One. 2007;2(2):e209.

15. Pelzang R. Mental health care in Bhutan: policy and issues. WHO South-East Asia J Public Health. 2012;1(3):339–46.

16. Asghar S, Hussain A, Ali S, Khan A, Magnusson A. Prevalence of depression and diabetes: a population-based study from rural Bangladesh. Diabet Med. 2007;24(8):872–7.

17. Hossain MD, Ahmed HU, Chowdhury WA, Niessen LW, Alam DS. Mental disorders in Bangladesh: a systematic review. BMC Psychiatry. 2014;14(1):216.

18. Gilbert BJ, Patel V, Farmer PE, Lu C. Assessing development assistance for mental health in developing countries: 2007–2013. PLoS Med. 2015;12(6):e1001834.

19. World Health Organization. Social determinants of mental health. Geneva: World Health Organization; 2014.

20. Saxena S, Funk M, Chisholm D. World health assembly adopts comprehensive mental health action plan 2013–2020. Lancet. 2013;381(9882):1970–1.

21. Eastwood J, Ogbo FA, Hendry A, Noble J, Page A, Early Years Research Group. The impact of antenatal depression on perinatal outcomes in Australian women. Plos One. 2017;12(1):e0169907. https://doi.org/10.1371/journal.pone.0169907.

22. Ogbo FA, Eastwood J, Hendry A, Jalaludin B, Agho KE, Barnett B, et al. Determinants of antenatal depression and postnatal depression in Australia. BMC Psychiatry. 2018;18(1):49.

23. Mackenzie S, Wiegel JR, Mundt M, Brown D, Saewyc E, Heiligenstein E, et al. Depression and suicide ideation among students accessing campus health care. Am J Orthopsychiatry. 2011;81(1):101–7.

24. Holmstrand C, Bogren M, Mattisson C, Brådvik L. Long-term suicide risk in no, one or more mental disorders: the Lundby study 1947–1997. Acta Psychiatr Scand. 2015;132(6):459–69.

25. Barry MM. Addressing the determinants of positive mental health: concepts, evidence and practice. Int J Ment Health Promot. 2009;11(3):4–17.

26. Fitzmaurice C, Allen C, Barber RM, Barregard L, Bhutta ZA, Brenner H, Fleming T. Global, regional, and national cancer incidence, mortality, years of life lost, years lived with disability, and disability-adjusted life-years for 32 cancer groups, 1990 to 2015: a systematic analysis for the global burden of disease study. JAMA oncology. 2017;3(4):524–48.

27. Melaku YA, Appleton SL, Gill TK, Ogbo FA, Buckley E, Shi Z, et al. Incidence, prevalence, mortality, disability-adjusted life years and risk factors of cancer in Australia and comparison with OECD countries, 1990–2015: findings from the global burden of disease study 2015. Cancer Epidemiol. 2018;52:43–54.

28. Mokdad AH. Diabetes mellitus and chronic kidney disease in the Eastern Mediterranean Region: findings from the Global Burden of Disease 2015 study. International Journal of Public Health. 2017;63(Supplement 1):177–86.

29. Akinyemiju T, Abera S, Ahmed M, Alam N, Alemayohu MA, Allen C, et al. The burden of primary liver Cancer and underlying etiologies from 1990 to 2015 at the global, regional, and National Level: results from the global burden of disease study 2015. JAMA oncology. 2017;3(12):1683–91.

30. Robberstad B. QALYs vs DALYs vs LYs gained: What are the differences, and what difference do they make for health care priority setting? Norsk epidemiologi. 2009;15:2.

31. Oostvogels A, De Wit G, Jahn B, Cassini A, Colzani E, De Waure C, et al. Use of DALYs in economic analyses on interventions for infectious diseases: a systematic review. Epidemiol Infect. 2015;143(9):1791–802.

32. Stevens GA, Alkema L, Black RE, Boerma JT, Collins GS, Ezzati M, et al. Guidelines for accurate and transparent health estimates reporting: the GATHER statement. PLoS Med. 2016;13(6):e1002056.

33. Hay IS, Abajobir AA, Abate KH, Abbafati C, Abbas KM, Abd-Allah F, et al. Global, regional, and national disability-adjusted life-years (DALYs) for 333 diseases and injuries and healthy life expectancy (HALE) for 195 countries and territories, 1990–2016: a systematic analysis for the global burden of disease study 2016. Lancet. 2017;390(10100):1260–344.

34. Vos T, Allen C, Arora M, Barber RM, Bhutta ZA, Brown A, et al. Global, regional, and national incidence, prevalence, and years lived with disability for 310 diseases and injuries, 1990-2015: a systematic analysis for the global burden of disease study 2015. Lancet. 2016;388(10053):1545.

35. Charara R, Bcheraoui EC, Mokdad HA, Khalil I, Moradi-Lakeh M, Afshin A, et al. The burden of mental disorders in the Eastern Mediterranean region, 1990–2015: Findings from the global burden of disease 2015 study. International journal of public health 2017:1–13.

36. American Psychiatric Association. Diagnostic and statistical manual of mental disorders (DSM-IV-TR). Washington, DC: American Psychiatric Association; 2000.

37. World Health Organization. The ICD-10 classification of mental and behavioural disorders: clinical descriptions and diagnostic guidelines: World Health Organization; 1992.

38. Ferrari A, Somerville A, Baxter A, Norman R, Patten S, Vos T, et al. Global variation in the prevalence and incidence of major depressive disorder: a systematic review of the epidemiological literature. Psychol Med. 2013;43(3):471–81.

39. Vos T, Flaxman AD, Naghavi M, Lozano R, Michaud C, Ezzati M, et al. Years lived with disability (YLDs) for 1160 sequelae of 289 diseases and injuries 1990- 2010: a systematic analysis for the global burden of disease study 2010. Lancet. 2013;380(9859):2163–96.

40. Vos T, Barber RM, Bell B, Bertozzi-Villa A, Biryukov S, Bolliger I, et al. Global, regional, and national incidence, prevalence, and years lived with disability for 301 acute and chronic diseases and injuries in 188 countries, 1990-2013: a systematic analysis for the global burden of disease study 2013. Lancet. 2015;386(9995):743.

41. Institute for Health Metrics and Evaluation (IHME). Global Burden of Disease Study 2016 (GBD 2016) Data Input Sources Tool Online: IHME; 2018 [cited 2018 29 March]. Available from: http://ghdx.healthdata.org/gbd-2016/data-input-sources.

42. Bromet E, Andrade LH, Hwang I, Sampson NA, Alonso J, De Girolamo G, et al. Cross-national epidemiology of DSM-IV major depressive episode. BMC Med. 2011;9(1):90.

43. Bilkhu RK. Why do many South Asians regard mental illness as taboo? Online: BBC; 2016 [cited 2017 October 7]. Available from: http://www.bbc.com/news/uk-england-36489893.

44. Niaz U, Hassan S. Culture and mental health of women in South-East Asia. World Psychiatry. 2006;5(2):118.

45. Chaudhry T. The Stigma of Mental Illness in South Asian Cultures. Online: Wellesley College, 2016 Contract No.: Honors Thesis Collection. 390.

46. Kallivayalil RA, Chadda RK. Culture, ethics and medicine in South Asia. Int J Person Cent Med. 2011;1(1):56–61.

47. Afridi MI. Mental health: priorities in Pakistan. JPMA J Pak Med Assoc. 2008; 58(5):225.

48. Luitel NP, Jordans MJ, Sapkota RP, Tol WA, Kohrt BA, Thapa SB, et al. Conflict and mental health: a cross-sectional epidemiological study in Nepal. Soc Psychiatry Psychiatr Epidemiol. 2013;48(2):183–93.

49. Nicholas B. Report on Initial Planning Work in Nepal: The Australia-Nepal Mental Health Network; 2015 [cited 2017 September 20]. Available from: https://www.nepalmentalhealth.org.au/downloads.

50. World Health Organization, Ministry of Health and Population. WHO-AIMS Report on Mental Health System in Nepal: A report of the assessment of the mental health system in Nepal using the World Health Organization – Assessment Instrument for Mental Health Systems (WHO-AIMS). Nepal: 2006.

51. World Health Organization & Ministry of Health & Family Welfare. WHO-AIMS Report on Mental Health System in Bangladesh: A report of the assessment of the mental health system in Bangladesh using the World Health Organization – Assessment Instrument for Mental Health Systems (WHO-AIMS). Dhaka, Bangladesh: 2007.

52. Islam A, Biswas T. Mental health and the health system in Bangladesh: situation analysis of a neglected domain. Am J Psychiatry Neurosci. 2015;3(4):57–62.

53. Grover S, Dutt A, Avasthi A. An overview of Indian research in depression. Indian J Psychiatry. 2010;52(Suppl1):S178.

54. Mirza I, Jenkins R. Risk factors, prevalence, and treatment of anxiety and depressive disorders in Pakistan: systematic review. BMJ. 2004;328(7443):794.

55. Patel V, Kirkwood BR, Pednekar S, Pereira B, Barros P, Fernandes J, et al. Gender disadvantage and reproductive health risk factors for common mental disorders in women: a community survey in India. Arch Gen Psychiatry. 2006;63(4):404–13.

56. Trivedi J, Mishra M, Kendurkar A. Depression among women in the south-Asian region: the underlying issues. J Affect Disord. 2007;102(1):219–25.

57. Abate KH. Gender disparity in prevalence of depression among patient population: a systematic review. Ethiopian Journal Of Health Sciences. 2013; 23(3):283–8 PubMed PMID: 24307828.

58. McLean CP, Asnaani A, Litz BT, Hofmann SG. Gender differences in anxiety disorders: prevalence, course of illness, comorbidity and burden of illness. J Psychiatr Res. 2011;45(8):1027–35. https://doi.org/10.1016/j.jpsychires.2011.03.006 PubMed PMID: 21439576.

59. Keita GP. Psychosocial and cultural contributions to depression in women: considerations for women midlife and beyond. J Manag Care Pharm. 2007; 13(9 Supp A):12–5.

60. Patel V, Rodrigues M, DeSouza N. Gender, poverty, and postnatal depression: a study of mothers in Goa, India. Am J Psychiatr. 2002;159(1):43–7.

61. Trivedi JK, Sareen H, Dhyani M. Rapid urbanization-its impact on mental health: a south Asian perspective. Indian J Psychiatry. 2008;50(3):161.
62. Patel V, Kirkwood BR, Pednekar S, Weiss H, Mabey D. Risk factors for common mental disorders in women. Br J Psychiatry. 2006;189(6):547–55.
63. Wig NN, Murthy SR. The birth of national mental health program for India. Indian J Psychiatry. 2015;57(3):315.
64. Murthy RS. Mental health initiatives in India (1947–2010). 2011.
65. Government of India. National Mental Health policy of India. In: India Department of Health and Family welfare, editor. Department of Health and Family welfare; 2014.
66. Sharma DC. India's new policy aims to close gaps in mental health care. Lancet. 2014;384(9954):1564.
67. Sharma DC. India still struggles with rural doctor shortages. Lancet. 2015; 386(10011):2381–2.
68. Hazarika I. Health workforce in India: assessment of availability, production and distribution. WHO South-East Asia J Public Health. 2013;2(2):106.
69. Bagcchi S. Rethinking India's psychiatric care. Lancet Psychiatry. 2014;1(7): 503–4.
70. Khalily MT. Mental health problems in Pakistani society as a consequence of violence and trauma: a case for better integration of care. Int J Integrated Care. 2011;11:e128-e.
71. Pelzang, R. Mental health care in Bhutan: policy and issues. WHO South-East Asia journal of public health. 2012;1(3):339.
72. Trivedi JK, Goel D, Kallivayalil RA, Isaac M, Shrestha DM, Gambheera HC. Regional cooperation in South Asia in the field of mental health. World Psychiatry. 2007;6(1):57.
73. Hussain S. Mental Health in Pakistan: Myths and Facts Online: Journal of pioneering medical sciences blog; 2014 [updated june 17; cited 2017 September 18]. Available from: http://blogs.jpmsonline.com/2014/06/17/mental-health-in-pakistan-myths-and-facts/.

# 23

# Illness beliefs about depression among patients seeking depression care and patients seeking cardiac care: an exploratory analysis using a mixed method design

Julia Luise Magaard[1*] (iD), Bernd Löwe[2], Anna Levke Brütt[1,3†] (iD) and Sebastian Kohlmann[2†]

## Abstract

**Background:** Treatment of depression in cardiac patients is difficult. Patients' illness beliefs regarding depression are associated with outcomes. The aim of the mixed-methods study was to test whether patients in routine care for depression differ from patients with depression in routine care for cardiac diseases regarding illness beliefs about depression.

**Methods:** A consecutive sample of $n = 217$ patients with depressive disorder was recruited from routine care for depression ($N = 148$) and routine care for cardiac diseases ($N = 69$). Beliefs about depression were measured by the Brief-Illness Perception Questionnaire. Causal beliefs were categorized using qualitative methods. To investigate differences regarding other illness beliefs, we performed an ANCOVA controlling for sociodemographic and clinical differences by propensity score matching.

**Results:** Patients in routine care for cardiac diseases attributed their depression more often to physical illnesses (48% vs. 16%) and less often to their self (30% vs. 47%), problems at work (25% vs. 35%), childhood (25% vs. 30%), and negative life events (19% vs. 25%) in contrast to patients in routine care for depression. Patients in routine care for cardiac diseases reported beliefs of lower disability, burden, and treatment-control and of higher self-control in contrast to patients in routine care for depression.

**Conclusions:** Illness beliefs especially causal beliefs differ between patients in routine care for cardiac diseases and routine care for depression. Future research should investigate effects of these illness beliefs. We recommend exploring patients' illness beliefs about depression in routine care for cardiac diseases and routine care for depression.

**Keywords:** Causal beliefs, Coronary heart disease, Depression, Illness representations

## Background

Major depression is one of the most significant clinical disorders with a lifetime prevalence of 11.6% [1]. Depression is among the leading causes of premature death [2], suicide, and the progression of chronic physical conditions such as coronary heart disease [2].

Effective psychotherapeutic and psychopharmacological treatment options are available. In contrast to patients with depression without somatic comorbidity, psychotherapeutic and psychopharmacological treatments have only modest effects on depression severity among patients with depression and cardiac diseases [3–6]. To target and individualize psychological treatments, research is required to investigate the effects of individual factors on treatment [4]. Besides potential biological influences of cardiac risk markers (e.g. thyroid hormones and inflammatory blood markers) on response to depression treatment [7], patients'

* Correspondence: j.magaard@uke.de

†Anna Levke Brütt and Sebastian Kohlmann contributed equally to this work.

[1]Department of Medical Psychology, University Medical Center Hamburg-Eppendorf, Hamburg, Germany

Full list of author information is available at the end of the article

illness beliefs have been identified as possible antagonists for effective depression treatment [8, 9]. However, illness beliefs might differ between patients seeking help for depression and depressed patients seeking help for cardiac diseases. Thus, illness beliefs, irrespective of being correct or false, might be dysfunctional and inhibit effective treatment.

Individuals who experience symptoms or are faced with a new diagnosis will develop an organized pattern of beliefs about their health threat including cognitive and emotional representations [10, 11]. In order to build these so-called illness beliefs, individuals use their own knowledge as well as experiences of others with similar symptoms or diagnoses [10, 11]. Leventhal's common sense model of illness representations states that illness beliefs affect patients' coping behavior and their appraisal of the outcome of their efforts [11]. According to the model, patients' illness beliefs are grouped into five dimensions, namely identity, timeline, cause, consequences, and cure/control [10, 11]: The first includes beliefs about the label as well as about symptoms associate with the condition. The second includes beliefs about the duration of an illness ranging from acute to chronic. Causal beliefs are individual conceptions about what had caused an illness. Beliefs about consequences comprise effects of the illness on daily life, whereas cure/control beliefs contain perceived possibilities to cure or to control the condition through treatment or personal behavior [10, 11]. The common sense model is widely used and empirically confirmed among patients with somatic diseases [12, 13] and among patients with depression [14–19]. In patients with heart diseases, it has been shown that illness beliefs about heart failure are associated with psychological well-being [13]. In patients with major depression, illness beliefs affect illness-related behaviors [15, 20] and treatment outcomes like psychological health [8] and quality of life [9]. Illness beliefs may affect depression treatment outcomes in many ways: For example, a considerable number of patients believes that antidepressant use leads to addiction [21], which in turn may explain non-adherent medication intake. A longitudinal study among patients with depression in primary care reported that illness beliefs at baseline influenced the depression severity 6 months later [8]. For instance, beliefs that physical exercise and psychotherapy are helpful to control depression predicted improved depression scores [8]. In terms of help-seeking behavior, a study showed that patients who did not believe in effectiveness of treatment and believed in short-term depression not affecting their everyday lives, did not sought depression treatment [20]. Focusing on patients' causal beliefs, studies showed that patients' causal beliefs about depression are associated with severity of depression [22, 23], coping [15, 16], and outcome

[18, 23]. Cornwall et al. [22] concluded that biological reasons for patients' depression are associated with severity of depression. Brown et al. [15] reported that individuals believing stress or interpersonal problems caused their depression, are more likely to vent or blame themselves and exhibit poorer psychosocial functioning. Bann and colleagues [23] have shown that strong beliefs in external causes, i.e. biological abnormality are associated with less improvement. Additionally, the belief in bio-genetic causes is associated with reduced perceived positive outcomes in a sample of patients taking antidepressants [18]. Taken together, the investigation of depression related illness beliefs provides insights how depression treatment can be optimized.

Major depression often occurs comorbid with chronic somatic diseases [24]. Especially in patients with heart diseases, the rate of depression is heightened, and constitutes an independent risk factor for morbidity and mortality [25]. Regarding illness beliefs of depressed patients with comorbid somatic diseases, qualitative studies show that the beliefs regarding different illnesses often interact: Patients experience their conditions as either independent or related in terms of causing each other [26–28], forming far more complex illness representations. A qualitative interview study conducted among primary care patients with depression and a chronic disease (i.e. coronary heart disease or diabetes) showed that they not necessarily considered their depressive symptoms as depression and felt responsible for resisting depression [29]. In line with these findings, patients with depression and chronic heart failure experienced lower levels of cognitive-emotional depression symptoms like depressed mood, worthlessness, or guilt compared to depressed patients without chronic heart failure [30]. Identifying dysfunctional illness beliefs among patients with comorbid heart disease could facilitate an increased awareness of patients' perspectives and help to establish a more patient-centered care. In addition, understanding these complex depression related illness representations in patients with chronic physical diseases is important, because they appear to impact self-management [27], could have implications for engagement with depression screening [31] and, thus, for the provision of care [27]. With respect to modest effects of depression treatment among patients with heart diseases [3–6], the investigation of depression related illness beliefs appears to be promising.

Taken together, investigating depression related illness beliefs in patients with cardiac disease could unveil new insights into how to optimize care. However, a deeper understanding about how depression related illness beliefs in patients seeking help for cardiac care might differ from patients seeking help for primarily depression care is currently lacking. Accordingly, the aim of this study is to contrast patients with depression in routine care for cardiac disease (RCC) to patients in routine care for depression (RCD) with regard to their depression related illness beliefs.

## Methods

### Study participants and study design

A consecutive sample of $n = 217$ patients was recruited from routine care for depression ($N = 148$) and routine care for cardiac disease ($N = 69$). Patients were included if they had at least moderate depression severity (Patient Health Questionnaire: PHQ-9 ≥ 10) and indicating that they were diagnosed with major depression. Data from patients in RCD is based on a study about help-seeking behavior among patients with depression. Participants in RCD were recruited between August 2015 and May 2016 from three primary care practices ($N = 25$), two psychotherapeutic practices ($N = 5$), a psychiatric outpatient clinic ($N = 14$), and three inpatient clinics ($N = 104$) in Hamburg and in the surrounding area. 218 participants agreed to participate, 156 fulfilled the criteria of PHQ-9 Score ≥ 10 and 8 were excluded because of missing data. Patients in RCC were consecutively recruited between October 2011 and October 2013 from three cardiology centers in Hamburg, Germany. This cross-sectional data is from the DEPSCREEN-INFO trial (ClinicalTrials.gov, Identifier: NCT01879111). DEPSCREEN-INFO is a randomized controlled trial, which examines depression-screening strategies in patients with coronary heart disease or hypertension. Out of 355 cardiac patients with PHQ-9 ≥ 10, 69 patients indicated that they were diagnosed with major depression and filled in a questionnaire about illness beliefs, and thus, were included in the analysis. All patients filled in a questionnaire about patients' illness beliefs, about sociodemographic characteristics, depression treatment as well as depression severity. Guideline recommended depression treatment was defined as receiving psychotherapy, pharmacotherapy or a combination of both.

### Study variables

Illness beliefs were measured by the Brief-Illness Perception Questionnaire (Brief-IPQ, [32, 33]). Items assess cognitive illness beliefs like consequences, timeline, personal control, treatment control, and identity as well as illness comprehensibility. All of these items are rated using a 0-to-10 response scale. Causal representations are assessed by an open-ended response item, which asks patients to list the three most important causal factors in their illness. Depression severity was measured by the Patient Health Questionnaire-9 (PHQ-9, [34, 35]), ranging from 0 to 27. The following categories regarding severity were used: 10–14 (moderate), 15–19 (moderately severe), and 20–27 (severe) [35]. In addition, age, gender, educational level, and marital status were

documented. Among the participants recruited from RCC, severity of cardiac illness was measured by structured self-report measures reflecting the New York Heart Association (NYHA) Functional Classification system as well as the Canadian Cardiovascular Society (CCS) Angina Grading Scale.

### Data analyses

#### Qualitative analyses

A previously developed category system of causal beliefs about mental disorders [36] was used and all statements were deductively assigned to the category system to analyze the qualitative data. The category system describes twelve content-related categories with subcategories, namely "problems at work", "problems in social environment", "self/internal states", "unspecific stress and overload", "negative life events", "childhood, youth, parental home", "physical complaints and illnesses", "predisposition", "social situation", "insufficient treatment", "fate", and "lack of causal beliefs" [36]. Three researchers (ALB, SK, JLM) assigned all statements to the category system. An inter-rater reliability of Fleiss Kappa = .76 was accomplished on the level of categories in the categorization process [37, 38], which can be interpreted as a substantial agreement [39]. Mismatching categorizations were discussed until consensus was reached and categorizations were checked to improve coherence. Frequencies of patients stating at least one causal belief referring to a category were calculated. We contrasted these frequencies in patients in RCC to patients in RCD.

#### Quantitative analyses

Before comparing the differences in illness beliefs between the samples, we conducted a propensity score matching (PSM) procedure to minimize the effect of other covariates. Individual propensity scores were calculated through logistic regression modeling based on age, gender, years of formal school education, living situation, and depression severity. PSM was performed according to statistical recommendation [40] using exact matching standard caliper size of 0.2 × log [SD of the propensity score]. Standardized differences were estimated before and after matching to evaluate the balance of covariates. To investigate whether patients in RCD differ from patients in RCC with regard to their illness beliefs, we performed an ANCOVA using the scores of the Brief-IPQ subscales as dependent variable. The PSM score was used as a covariate. Given that multiple tests were performed, a false discovery rate approach (Benjamini-Hochberg procedure) was applied when judging the significance of each test to reduce the risk of alpha inflation [41].

Missing data was less than 2% on every PHQ-9 item and Brief-IPQ item. Thus, missing data were not imputed and all available information was used (pairwise deletion). Analyses were performed using SPSS Version 22.0 (Chicago Inc).

## Results

### Sample description

Sample characteristics are shown in Table 1. On average, participants from RCD had higher educational levels, were younger, to a higher percentage female (73% vs. 55%, $\chi^2$ (2, $N = 217$) = 6.85, $p = .009$)), and unmarried (76% vs. 52%, $\chi^2$ (2, $N = 217$) = 11.99, $p = .001$)) compared to participants from RCC. There was no difference between participants from RCC and RCD with regard to depression severity. On average, both groups were moderately severe depressed (Table 1) and 33% (RCC) vs. 39% (RCD), 45% (RCC) vs. 33% (RCD), and 22% (RCC) vs. 28% (RCD) were classified as moderate, moderately severe, and severe depressed, respectively ($\chi^2$ (2, $N = 217$) = 2.86, $p = .239$)). Using propensity scores as covariates, samples no longer differed regarding age, gender ($\chi^2$ (2, $N = 69$) = 0.26, $p = .614$), formal education, and marital status ($\chi^2$ (2, N = 69) = 2.65, $p = .104$). During study period 48% ($N = 33$) of the patients in RCC and 93% ($N = 135$, N = 2 Missing) of the patients in RCD received guideline recommended depression treatment. Depression severity was positively associated with consequences ($r = .385$, $p < .001$), timeline ($r = .337$, $p < .001$), and identity ($r = .406$, $p < .001$), negatively associated with personal control ($r = -.213$, $p = .002$) and treatment control ($r = -.156$, $p = .022$) and not associated with comprehensibility ($r = -.058$, $p = .399$), irrespective of controlling for RCD and RCC or not.

Among patients in RCC, 59% suffered from coronary heart disease and 41% from hypertension. According to NYHA classification, 20%, 26%, 26%, and 28% of the RCC participants were classified to class I (asymptomatic), class II (mild), class III (moderate), and class IV (severe), respectively. Among patients in RCC, NYHA classification was not significantly associated with depression severity ($r_s$ (Spearman's rank correlation) = 0.126 ($p = .302$)) or with five of the six illness beliefs measured by Brief-IPQ items. An exception is a negative association between the Brief-IPQ item treatment control and NYHA classification ($r_s = - 0.271$ ($p = .024$)).

Regarding angina pectoris, 32% of the participants reported experiencing no symptoms, 39% reported experiencing symptoms without physical activity, 15% reported experiencing symptoms when under light and 15% reported experiencing symptoms when under intense physical activity.

### Causal beliefs of patients in RCD and patients in RCC

Figure 1 shows the percentages of patients stating at least one causal belief in a category ordered by frequency in the sample. Stated causal beliefs could be assigned to all causal beliefs categories, apart from insufficient treatment.

Most frequently, stated causal beliefs were assigned to the categories problems in social environment, the self, problems at work, experiences from childhood and youth, physical complaints and illnesses, and negative life events. Patients' beliefs referring to the category problems in social environment subsumed actual family problems, relationship problems, illnesses of close relatives and their consequences, isolation and lack of appreciation, and private problems. For instance, "drinking problem of my partner" was assigned to illnesses of close relatives. The category self/internal states subsumed statements regarding anxiety, depressive symptoms, and high self-demands whereas the category negative life events consists of statements related to experience of abuse, accidents, and bereavement. Statements about interpersonal problems at work, financial problems as well as problems with working conditions were stated as causal beliefs relating to work. Independently from the care setting, every second patient stated causal beliefs concerning the social environment. Nearly half of the patients with depression in RCC attributed their depression to physical complaints (e.g. pain) and illnesses, whereas only 16% of the patients in RCD stated such causal beliefs. Contrasted to patients in RCC, patients in RCD attributed their depression more often to their self (47% vs. 30%), problems at work (35% vs. 25%), circumstances during childhood and youth (30% vs. 25%), and negative life events (25% vs. 19%).

### Illness beliefs of patients in RCD and patients in RCC

Using propensity score matching (PSM) to adjust for age, gender, years of formal school education, living

**Table 1** Sample characteristics

|  | Not adjusted | | | Adjusted | | |
|---|---|---|---|---|---|---|
|  | RCD ($N = 148$) | RCC ($N = 69$) | P-value | RCD ($N = 148$) | RCC ($N = 69$) | P-value |
| Age in years, M (SE) | 42.47 (1.06) | 59.59 (1.56) | < 0.001 | 47.88 (0.69) | 47.97 (1.10) | .95 |
| ≥ 10 years of formal education, M (SE) | 0.87 (0.03) | 0.55 (0.05) | < 0.001 | 0.77 (0.03) | 0.77 (0.05) | .98 |
| PHQ-9, M (SE) | 16.29 (0.34) | 16.45 (0.50) | .80 | 16.34 (0.37) | 16.34 (0.59) | .99 |

Legend: *RCD* routine care for depression, *RCC* routine care for cardiac diseases, *M* mean, *SE* Standard error, *PHQ-9* Patient Health Quesionnaire-9. Dummy coding: years of education, 1 ≥ 10 years of formal education, 0 < 10 years of formal education. Sample characteristics were adjusted using Propensity Score Matching

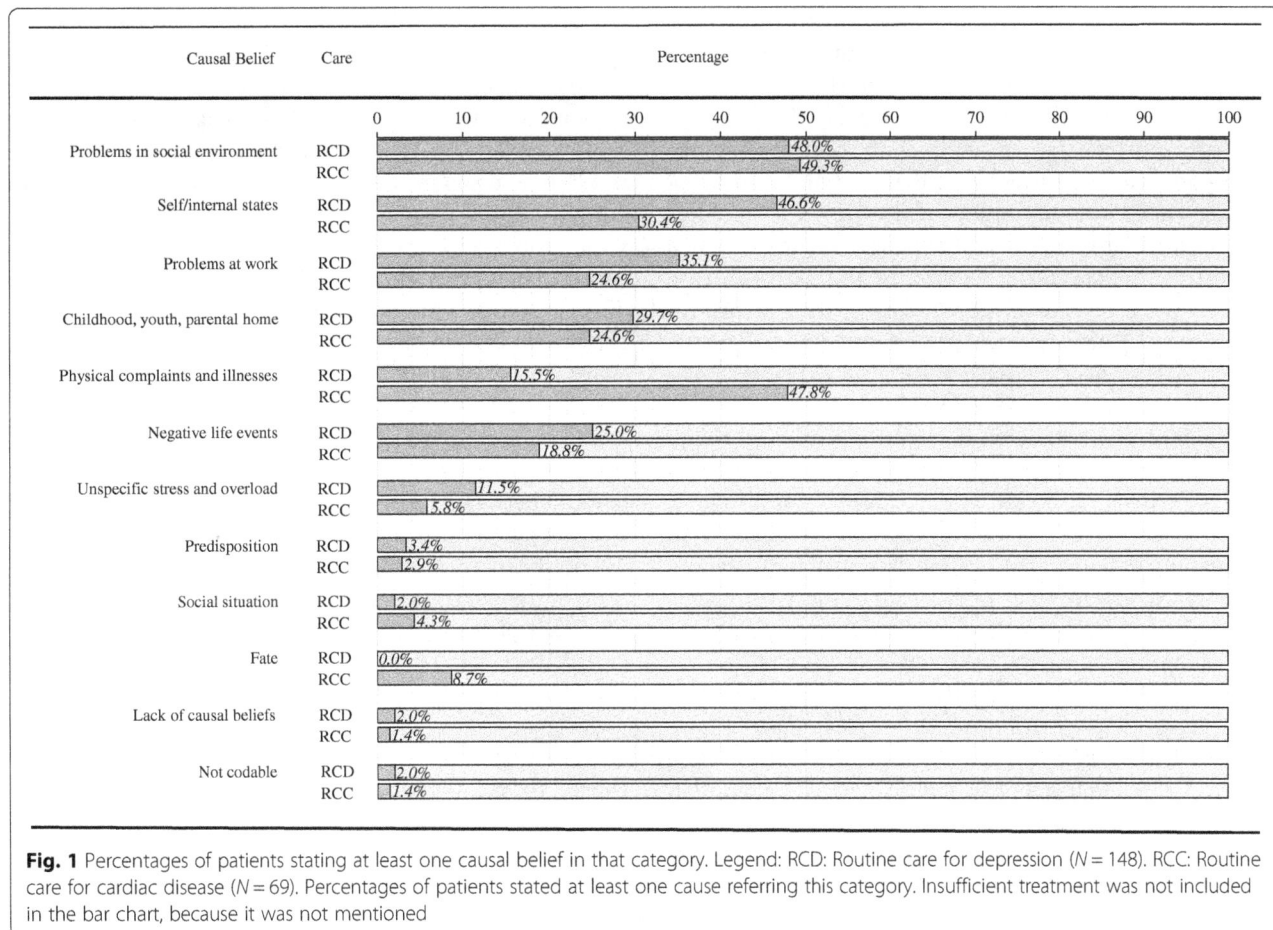

**Fig. 1** Percentages of patients stating at least one causal belief in that category. Legend: RCD: Routine care for depression (N = 148). RCC: Routine care for cardiac disease (N = 69). Percentages of patients stated at least one cause referring this category. Insufficient treatment was not included in the bar chart, because it was not mentioned

situation, and depression severity, patients in RCD rated their depression as more disabling in contrast to patients in RCC (Mean (M) Standard error (SE), 7.93(0.19) vs. 6.42(.30), $F = 15.36$, $p < .001$). Patients in RCD had lower beliefs regarding self-control in contrast to patients in RCC (M(SE), 3.93 (0.21) vs. 5.26(.33), $F = 9.89$, $p = .002$). In contrast, patients in RCD had a stronger beliefs that depression treatment would help compared to patients with RCC (M(SE), 6.96(0.22) vs. 5.90(.35), $F = 5.55$, $p = .02$). Patients in RCD also reported higher subjective symptom burden in contrast to patients in RCC (M(SE), 7.49 (0.19) vs. 6.68(.30), $F = 4.34$, $p = .038$). No differences between groups were indicated for timeline and coherence beliefs.

## Discussion

The aim of the study was to contrast patients in RCD to patients with depression in RCC regarding causal beliefs and other illness beliefs using a mixed method approach.

We found that patients with depression in RCC reported physical causal beliefs more frequently in contrast to patients in RCD. Whereas nearly half of the patients in RCC attributed their depression to physical complaints, only 16% of the patients in RCD referred their

depression to physical causes. In contrast to patients with depression in RCC, patients in RCD more frequently stated causal beliefs referring to problems at work, self and internal states, circumstances during childhood and youth, and negative life events. Despite the fact that patients were comparable regarding the level of depression severity, patients in RCD differed also from patients in RCC concerning other illness beliefs: Patients in RCD reported higher beliefs about disability, symptom burden, and treatment control compared to patients in RCC. In contrast, patients in RCC reported beliefs of higher self-control compared to patients in RCD.

The patients in both care settings held a variety of different causal beliefs referring to psychosocial problems and physical illnesses predominantly. The content of causal beliefs of patients in the current sample were similar compared to causal beliefs of patients with depression in primary care [42] and in inpatient mental health care [36]. In line with previous qualitative research (e.g. [36, 42]), only a few patients in both settings emphasized the relevance of genetic influences.

Half of the patients in RCC did and half of the patients did not emphasize chronic illness like e.g. coronary heart disease as a cause for their depression. This is in line with mainly qualitative research about causal beliefs among patients with depression and chronic somatic diseases [26, 29], diabetes [27], and heart disease [28]. Studies reported that patients with both conditions experience their illnesses as either related in terms of causing each other or independent [26–28]. Findings from a qualitative study among elderly primary care patients with depressive symptoms and heart disease can provide a deeper insight into patients' perspective about heart disease causing depression: Patients explained that heart disease can cause depression because of medication side effects, being frightened by the diagnosis, limitations in daily activities through heart disease, and loss of control as a consequence of navigating the health care system [28].

Besides causal beliefs about depression referring to chronic illnesses, our findings indicate that causal beliefs referring to private and work related social problems and internal states are also important among patients with comorbid coronary heart diseases. Similar to patients in RCD, half of the patients in RCC believed in problems in social environment as a major cause of their depression. This is in line with results from SL Alderson, R Foy, L Glidewell and AO House [29], who reported that comorbid primary care patients' causal beliefs about depression were complex, preferentially referring to external events like bereavement and relationship breakdowns besides chronic illnesses.

Causal beliefs, irrespective of being correct or false, have been associated with impairment [22, 23], coping [15, 16], and outcome [18, 23]. With our design, we were not able to provide evidence for the impact of illness beliefs on coping and outcome. Thus, future research is needed especially among patients with depression in RCD and RCC.

In our study patients in RCC perceived a lower symptom burden, less disability, believed in higher levels of self-control and lower levels of treatment control compared to patients in RCD. These differences cannot be explained by variations between samples regarding depression severity, age, gender, education, and marital status. These differences regarding appraisal and perception of symptoms is in line with results from N Holzapfel, T Müller-Tasch, B Wild, J Jünger, C Zugck, A Remppis, W Herzog and B Löwe [30]. They found that patients with depression and chronic heart failure experience less cognitive-emotional symptoms compared to patients without chronic heart failure. Both groups experience somatic symptoms of depression to a comparable extent [30]. Findings from a systematic review about illness beliefs about depression in primary care patients with chronic physical diseases indicated that some patients believe that depression is a normal part of life [31]. Similarly,

a qualitative study about beliefs about depression among GP patients with coronary heart disease or diabetes found out that patients do not necessarily understand their distress as depression, which makes recognition of depression difficult [29]. These findings are in line with our result that patients in RCC believed in lower symptom burden and less disability compared to patients in RCD although both patient groups do not differ with respect to depression severity. In line with our result of higher levels of self-control among patients in RCC, patients with depression and coronary heart disease or diabetes feel responsible to take control of the situation and make the changes needed to work towards cure of depression [29]. Comparing our findings to the results of a study among primary care patients [20], interesting parallels can be discovered between illness beliefs of patients in RCC and GP patients not seeking treatment for depression: GP patients did not belief in effectiveness of treatment and believed in short-term depression not affecting their everyday lives [20]. Compared to patients in RCD, patients in RCC perceived their depression also as less burdening with lower effects on their everyday lives and reported lower beliefs regarding effectiveness of depression treatment. Taken together, in spite of comparable depression severity, illness beliefs among patients in RCC differ from patients in RCD. At the present point of view, we do not know if these illness beliefs among patients in RCC are adaptive (e.g. through less experiences of impairment) or mal-adaptive (e.g. through impeding help-seeking behavior). Further research is needed to investigate if certain illness beliefs impede help-seeking, recognition of depression, and treatment or are even protective regarding subjective impairment. To test whether the different illness beliefs and causal attributions predict depression treatment and health outcomes in RCC, longitudinal study designs are needed.

Our results also provide initial information for tailoring depression treatment regarding the illness beliefs in patients seeking cardiac care. A focus on changing illness beliefs likely to be dysfunctional could help improve depression treatment in cardiac patients. For instance, E Broadbent, CJ Ellis, J Thomas, G Gamble and KJ Petrie [43] demonstrated that an illness perception intervention can change illness beliefs and improve rates of returning to work in myocardial infarction patients. Future research is needed to first identify dysfunctional beliefs and then prove appropriate interventions.

We believe this is the first study to specifically contrast patients in RCC to patients in RCD regarding beliefs about depression. By using a mixed-methods design, results from the qualitative analysis of causal beliefs were enriched by quantitative comparisons of other illness beliefs. Different frequencies of causal beliefs between the samples cannot be attributed to differences regarding depression severity, because both samples do not differ with respect to depression severity. In order to minimize the effects of age, gender, education, marital status and depression severity on the quantitative comparison of illness beliefs between the samples, we conducted a PSM procedure.

As a major limitation of the study, we need to discuss the implications of the differences of the groups besides the health care setting. The fact that patients in the RCC group have cardiac diseases, are older, and thus have a higher chance of having other somatic diseases may have an influence on patients' causal beliefs in this group. We have no information about prior episodes of depression among both groups and sequence of onset of depression and cardiac disease among the RCC group. We did not assess whether patients seeking depression care were also diagnosed with a somatic disease like cardiac disease, thus, we could not control this factor. In addition, it is possible that patients in the RCD group have sought help for their depression, because they have thought psychosocial reasons could be involved. This is also true for the 35% of RCC patients, currently receiving mental health treatment. Thus, our findings focus on causal beliefs common among patients in a certain health care setting and we cannot draw conclusions about the influence of having or not having cardiac diseases on illness beliefs about depression. Future studies may further investigate whether a diagnosis of a cardiac disease is associated with certain depression-related illness beliefs. Additionally, patients were included based on their self-reported diagnoses of major depression and a depression cut-off, as opposed to having a formal and confirmed diagnosis. Although the PHQ-9 is an established, reliable, and valid screening instrument for screening and severity of depression and a PHQ-9 score of $\geq 10$ has a sensitivity of 88% and a specificity of 88% for major depression [34, 35], it does not replace a thorough evaluation of psychiatric disorders. Including patients who reported the diagnoses of major depression was necessary, as illness beliefs regarding depression can only be asked for, when people are aware of their disease. Nevertheless, this inclusion criterion limits our results to this certain sample. Future research may find ways to assess illness beliefs independently from patients' awareness of diagnoses. The difference between RCD and RCC sample sizes might be a source of bias. As we analyzed written material about casual beliefs, it was not possible to clarify the statements of participants.

## Conclusions

The results of this study suggest that patients in RCD differ regarding depression related illness beliefs from patients in RCC although patient groups do not differ with respect to depression severity. These results could be used to facilitate an increased awareness of patients' perspective and to help to establish a more patient-centered care in these settings. Future research among patients with depression and comorbid heart disease should investigate progressions of illness beliefs about depression as well as relationships between illness beliefs about depression and help-seeking and outcomes to develop interventions for patients at risk.

We suggest health service providers examining patients with depression in different care settings to explore the patients' beliefs about depression in detail. Moreover, mismatching causal beliefs between patient and treatment provider should be uncovered and discussed in order to enhance concordance between patient and treatment provider regarding illness perception and to develop shared treatment plans. Among patients in RCC, psychosocial as well as physical causal beliefs should be considered in order to plan depression interventions.

**Abbreviations**

ALB: Anna Levke Brütt; BL: Bernd Löwe; BMBF: German Federal Ministry of Education and Research; Brief-IPQ: Brief Illness Perception Questionnaire; CCS: Canadian Cardiovascular Society; DFG: German Research Foundation; JLM: Julia Luise Magaard; M: Mean; NYHA: New York Heart Association; PHQ-9: Patient Health Questionnaire - 9; PSM: Propensity score matching; RCC: Routine care for cardiac disease; RCD: Routine care for depression; SE: Standard error; SK: Sebastian Kohlmann

**Acknowledgements**

We would like to thank all participants, the cooperating institutions and providers of depression care. We would also like to thank the cooperating institutions and providers of cardiac care: University Heart Center (Prof. Dr. Blankenberg), Cardiologicum Hamburg (Dr. Noak, Dr. Walter).

**Funding**

This work was funded by the German Research Foundation (DFG) for a pilot study about help-seeking behavior among patients with depression [grant number: BR4859/3–1], the German Federal Ministry of Education and Research (BMBF), Germany [grant number: 01GX1004] and internal funds by the Department of Psychosomatic Medicine and by the Department of Medical Psychology, University Medical Center Hamburg-Eppendorf. No funding body had a role in the development, design, data collection, analysis, interpretation and in the decision to submit the article for publication.

**Authors' contributions**

JLM, ALB & SK had full access to all data in the study and take responsibility for the integrity of the data and the accuracy of the data analysis. Study concept and design: JLM, ALB & SK. Acquisition of data: all authors. Analysis and interpretation of data: JLM, BL, ALB & SK. Drafting of the manuscript: JLM, ALB & SK. Critical revision of the manuscript for important intellectual content: all authors. Administrative, technical, or material support: all authors. Study supervision: all authors. Approving the final article: all authors.

**Consent for publication**

Not applicable.

**Competing interests**

The authors declare that they have no competing interests.

**Author details**

[1]Department of Medical Psychology, University Medical Center Hamburg-Eppendorf, Hamburg, Germany. [2]Department of Psychosomatic Medicine and Psychotherapy, University Medical Center Hamburg-Eppendorf, Hamburg, Germany. [3]Department of Health Services Research, School of Medicine and Health Sciences, Carl von Ossietzky University Oldenburg, Oldenburg, Germany.

**References**

1. Busch M, Maske U, Ryl L, Schlack R, Hapke U. Prevalence of depressive symptoms and diagnosed depression among adults in Germany. Bundesgesundheitsblatt. 2013;56:733–9.
2. Murray CJ, Lopez AD. Measuring the global burden of disease. N Engl J Med. 2013;369(5):448–57.
3. Baumeister H, Hutter N, Bengel J. Psychological and pharmacological interventions for depression in patients with coronary artery disease. Cochrane Database Syst Rev. 2011;9:1-75.
4. Dickens C, Cherrington A, Adeyemi I, Roughley K, Bower P, Garrett C, Bundy C, Coventry P. Characteristics of psychological interventions that improve depression in people with coronary heart disease: a systematic review and meta-regression. Psychosom Med. 2013;75(2):211–21.
5. Thombs BD, Roseman M, Coyne JC, de Jonge P, Delisle VC, Arthurs E, Levis B, Ziegelstein RC. Does evidence support the American Heart Association's recommendation to screen patients for depression in cardiovascular care? An updated systematic review. PLoS One. 2013;8(1):e52654.
6. Nieuwsma JA, Williams JW Jr, Namdari N, Washam JB, Raitz G, Blumenthal JA, Jiang W, Yapa R, McBroom AJ, Lallinger K, et al. Diagnostic accuracy of screening tests and treatment for post–acute coronary syndrome depression: a systematic review. Ann Intern Med. 2017;167(10):725–35.
7. Carney RM, Freedland KE, Steinmeyer B, Rubin EH, Mann DL, Rich MW. Cardiac risk markers and response to depression treatment in patients with coronary heart disease. Psychosom Med. 2016;78(1):49–59.
8. Lynch J, Moore M, Moss-Morris R, Kendrick T. Do patients' illness beliefs predict depression measures at six months in primary care; a longitudinal study. J Affect Disord. 2015;174:665–71.
9. Glattacker M, Heyduck K, Meffert C. Illness beliefs and treatment beliefs as predictors of short and middle term outcome in depression. J Health Psychol. 2013;18(1):139–52.
10. Petrie K, Weinman J. Why illness perceptions matter. Clin Med. 2006;6(6):536–9.
11. Leventhal H, Nerenz DR, Steele DJ. Illness representations and coping with health threats. In: Baum A, Taylor SE, Singer JE, editors. Handbook of Psychology and Health, Volume IV: Social Psychological Aspects of Health. Hillsdale, NJ: Erlbaum; 1984. p. 219–52.
12. Hagger MS, Orbell S. A meta-analytic review of the common-sense model of illness representations. Psychol Health. 2003;18(2):141–84.
13. Morgan K, Villiers-Tuthill A, Barker M, McGee H. The contribution of illness perception to psychological distress in heart failure patients. BMC Psychology. 2014;2(1):50.
14. Balck F, Preuss M, Hendrischke A, Lippmann M. Change of illness representations and quality of life during the course of a psychotherapeutic-psychosomatic treatment [German]. Z Psychosom Med Psychother. 2012;58(4):357–73.

15. Brown C, Battista DR, Sereika SM, Bruehlman RD, Dunbar-Jacob J, Thase ME. Primary care patients' personal illness models for depression: relationship to coping behavior and functional disability. Gen Hosp Psychiatry. 2007;29(6):492–500.
16. Brown C, Dunbar-Jacob J, Palenchar DR, Kelleher KJ, Bruehlman RD, Sereika S, Thase ME. Primary care patients' personal illness models for depression: a preliminary investigation. Fam Pract. 2001;18(3):314–20.
17. Fortune G, Barrowclough C, Lobban F. Illness representations in depression. Br J Clin Psychol. 2004;43(4):347–64.
18. Read J, Cartwright C, Gibson K, Shiels C, Haslam N. Beliefs of people taking antidepressants about causes of depression and reasons for increased prescribing rates. J Affect Disord. 2014;168:236–42.
19. Witteman C, Bolks L, Hutschemaekers G. Development of the illness perception questionnaire mental health. J Ment Health. 2011;20(2):115–25.
20. Elwy AR, Yeh J, Worcester J, Eisen SV. An illness perception model of primary care patients' help seeking for depression. Qual Health Res. 2011;21(11):1495–507.
21. Prins MA, Verhaak PF, Bensing JM, van der Meer K. Health beliefs and perceived need for mental health care of anxiety and depression-the patients' perspective explored. Clin Psychol Rev. 2008;28(6):1038–58.
22. Cornwall PL, Scott J, Garland A, Pollinger BR. Beliefs about depression in patients and their partners. Behav Cogn Psychother. 2005;33(2):131–8.
23. Bann CM, Parker CB, Bradwejn J, Davidson JR, Vitiello B, Gadde KM. Assessing patient beliefs in a clinical trial of Hypericum perforatum in major depression. Depress Anxiety. 2004;20(3):114–22.
24. Scott KM, Lim C, Al-Hamzawi A, Alonso J, Bruffaerts R, Caldas-de-Almeida JM, Florescu S, De Girolamo G, Hu C, De Jonge P. Association of mental disorders with Subsequent Chronic Physical Conditions: world mental health surveys from 17 countries. JAMA Psychiatry. 2016;73(2):150–8.
25. Lichtman JH, Froelicher ES, Blumenthal JA, Carney RM, Doering LV, Frasure-Smith N, Freedland KE, Jaffe AS, Leifheit-Limson EC, Sheps DS, et al. Depression as a risk factor for poor prognosis among patients with acute coronary syndrome: systematic review and recommendations a scientific statement from the American Heart Association. Circulation. 2014;129:1350–69.
26. DeJean D, Giacomini M, Vanstone M, Brundisini F. Patient experiences of depression and anxiety with chronic disease: a systematic review and qualitative meta-synthesis. Ont Health Technol Assess Ser. 2013;13(16):1–33.
27. Mc Sharry J, Bishop FL, Moss-Morris R, Kendrick T. 'The chicken and egg thing': cognitive representations and self-management of multimorbidity in people with diabetes and depression. Psychol Health. 2013;28(1):103–19.
28. Bogner HR, Dahlberg B, de Vries HF, Cahill E, Barg FK. Older patients' views on the relationship between depression and heart disease. Fam Med. 2008;40(9):652.
29. Alderson SL, Foy R, Glidewell L, House AO. Patients understanding of depression associated with chronic physical illness: a qualitative study. BMC Fam Pract. 2014;15(1):37.
30. Holzapfel N, Müller-Tasch T, Wild B, Jünger J, Zugck C, Remppis A, Herzog W, Löwe B. Depression profile in patients with and without chronic heart failure. J Affect Disord. 2008;105(1):53–62.
31. Alderson SL, Foy R, Glidewell L, McLintock K, House A. How patients understand depression associated with chronic physical disease–a systematic review. BMC Fam Pract. 2012;13(1):41.
32. Broadbent E, Petrie KJ, Main J, Weinman J. The brief illness perception questionnaire. J Psychosom Res. 2006;60(6):631–7.
33. Rief W. Die deutsche Version des B-IPQ. [The German Version of the B-IPQ.] In: Illness Perception Questionnaire. 2018. www.uib.no/ipq/pdf/B-IPQ-German.pdf. Accessed 01 Nov 2018.
34. Löwe B, Kroenke K, Herzog W, Gräfe K. Measuring depression outcome with a brief self-report instrument: sensitivity to change of the patient health questionnaire (PHQ-9). J Affect Disord. 2004;81(1):61–6.
35. Kroenke K, Spitzer RL, Williams JB. The Phq-9. J Gen Intern Med. 2001;16(9):606–13.
36. Magaard JL, Schulz H, Brütt AL. What do patients think about the cause of their mental disorder? A qualitative and quantitative analysis of causal beliefs of mental disorder in inpatients in psychosomatic rehabilitation. PLoS One. 2017;12(1):e0169387.
37. Inter-Rater Agreement with multiple raters and variables. [https://nlp-ml.io/jg/software/ira/]. Accessed 01 Nov 2018.
38. Fleiss JL. Measuring nominal scale agreement among many raters. Psychol Bull. 1971;76(5):378–82.
39. Landis JR, Koch GG. The measurement of observer agreement for categorical data. Biometrics. 1977;33(1):159–74.

40. Austin PC. Statistical criteria for selecting the optimal number of untreated subjects matched to each treated subject when using many-to-one matching on the propensity score. Am J Epidemiol. 2010;172(9):1092–7.

41. Glickman ME, Rao SR, Schultz MR. False discovery rate control is a recommended alternative to Bonferroni-type adjustments in health studies. J Clin Epidemiol. 2014;67(8):850–7.

42. Hansson M, Chotai J, Bodlund O. Patients' beliefs about the cause of their depression. J Affect Disord. 2010;124(1–2):54–9.

43. Broadbent E, Ellis CJ, Thomas J, Gamble G, Petrie KJ. Further development of an illness perception intervention for myocardial infarction patients: a randomized controlled trial. J Psychosom Res. 2009;67(1):17–23.

# Permissions

The contributors of this book come from diverse backgrounds, making this book a truly international effort. This book will bring forth new frontiers with its revolutionizing research information and detailed analysis of the nascent developments around the world.

We would like to thank all the contributing authors for lending their expertise to make the book truly unique. They have played a crucial role in the development of this book. Without their invaluable contributions this book wouldn't have been possible. They have made vital efforts to compile up to date information on the varied aspects of this subject to make this book a valuable addition to the collection of many professionals and students.

This book was conceptualized with the vision of imparting up-to-date information and advanced data in this field. To ensure the same, a matchless editorial board was set up. Every individual on the board went through rigorous rounds of assessment to prove their worth. After which they invested a large part of their time researching and compiling the most relevant data for our readers.

The editorial board has been involved in producing this book since its inception. They have spent rigorous hours researching and exploring the diverse topics which have resulted in the successful publishing of this book. They have passed on their knowledge of decades through this book. To expedite this challenging task, the publisher supported the team at every step. A small team of assistant editors was also appointed to further simplify the editing procedure and attain best results for the readers.

Apart from the editorial board, the designing team has also invested a significant amount of their time in understanding the subject and creating the most relevant covers. They scrutinized every image to scout for the most suitable representation of the subject and create an appropriate cover for the book.

The publishing team has been an ardent support to the editorial, designing and production team. Their endless efforts to recruit the best for this project, has resulted in the accomplishment of this book. They are a veteran in the field of academics and their pool of knowledge is as vast as their experience in printing. Their expertise and guidance has proved useful at every step. Their uncompromising quality standards have made this book an exceptional effort. Their encouragement from time to time has been an inspiration for everyone.

The publisher and the editorial board hope that this book will prove to be a valuable piece of knowledge for researchers, students, practitioners and scholars across the globe.

# List of Contributors

**Stephan Doering, Victor Blüml, Karin Feichtinger and Antonia Wininger**
Department of Psychoanalysis and Psychotherapy, Medical University of Vienna, Währinger Gürtel 18-20, A-1090 Wien, Austria

**Karoline Parth**
Department of Psychoanalysis and Psychotherapy, Medical University of Vienna, Währinger Gürtel 18-20, A-1090 Wien, Austria
Department of Psychology, Webster Vienna Private University, Wien, Austria

**Maria Gruber and Marion Freidl**
Department of Social Psychiatry, Medical University of Vienna, Wien, Austria

**Martin Aigner**
Department of Psychiatry, University Hospital Tulln, Tulln, Austria

**Hemma Rössler-Schülein**
Vienna Psychoanalytic Society, Wien, Austria

**Chika Tanaka and Hiroya Matsuo**
Graduate School of Health Sciences, Kobe University, 701, 2-6-2, Yamamoto-dori, Chuo-ku, Kobe, Hyogo 650-0003, Japan

**Maria Teresa Reyes Tuliao**
City Health Office, City Government of Muntinlupa, Muntinlupa, Philippines

**Eizaburo Tanaka**
Hyogo Institute for Traumatic Stress, Kobe, Japan

**Tadashi Yamashita**
Kobe City College of Nursing, Kobe, Japan

**Robert Ferdinand**
Department of Child and Adolescent Psychiatry, GGZ Delfland, 2600, GA, Delft, The Netherlands

**Richard Vijverberg**
Department of Child and Adolescent Psychiatry, GGZ Delfland, 2600, GA, Delft, The Netherlands
Amsterdam UMC, location VUmc and GGZ inGeest, Department of psychiatry, Amsterdam, The Netherlands
Amsterdam Public Health Research Institute, Amsterdam, The Netherlands

**Aartjan Beekman**
Amsterdam UMC, location VUmc and GGZ in Geest, Department of psychiatry, Amsterdam, The Netherlands
Amsterdam Public Health Research Institute, Amsterdam, The Netherlands

**Berno van Meijel**
Amsterdam UMC, location VUmc and GGZ in Geest, Department of psychiatry, Amsterdam, The Netherlands
Amsterdam Public Health Research Institute, Amsterdam, The Netherlands
Inholland University of Applied Sciences, Amsterdam, The Netherlands
GGZ-VS, Academy for Masters in Advanced Nursing Practice, Utrecht, The Netherlands
Parnassia Psychiatric Institute, The Hague, The Netherlands

**Sarah E. Romans**
Department of Psychological Medicine, University of Otago Wellington, Wellington 6242, New Zealand

**Susanna Every-Palmer and Mark A. Huthwaite**
Department of Psychological Medicine, University of Otago Wellington, Wellington 6242, New Zealand
Capital and Coast District Health Board, Wellington, New Zealand

**Eve Grant**
Capital and Coast District Health Board, Wellington, New Zealand

**Jane L. Elmslie**
University of Otago Christchurch, Christchurch, New Zealand

**Nathan Wilson and Bei Bei**
Monash Institute of Cognitive and Clinical Neurosciences, School of Psychological Sciences, Monash University, 18 Innovation Walk, Clayton Campus, VIC 3800, Australia

**Karen Wynter**
Global Public Health Unit, School of Public Health and Preventative Medicine, Monash University, Clayton, Victoria, Australia
Centre for Quality and Patient Safety Research – Western Health Partnership, School of Nursing and Midwifery, Faculty of Health, Deakin University, Burwood, VIC, Australia

**Jane Fisher**
Global Public Health Unit, School of Public Health and Preventative Medicine, Monash University, Clayton, Victoria, Australia
Masada Early Parenting Centre, Masada Private Hospital, East St Kilda, VIC, Australia

**Xi Xia, Mei Ding, Jin-feng Xuan, Jia-xin Xing, Hao Pang, Bao-jie Wang and Jun Yao**
School of Forensic Medicine, China Medical University, No. 77 Puhe Road, Shenbei New District, Shenyang 110122, China

**Linnet Ongeri, Phelgona Otieno, Jane Mbui and Elizabeth Juma**
Kenya Medical Research Institute, 00200, Mbagathi Road, Nairobi, Kenya

**Valentine Wanga and Ann Vander Stoep**
University of Washington, Jefferson St. Seattle WA 98104, Nairobi 908, Kenya

**Muthoni Mathai**
University of Nairobi, Off Ngong Road, Nairobi, Kenya

**Tore Børtveit**
Haukeland University Hospital, OCD-team, 5021 Bergen, Norway

**Gerd Kvale and Bjarne Hansen**
Haukeland University Hospital, OCD-team, 5021 Bergen, Norway
Department of Clinical Psychology, University of Bergen, Bergen, Norway

**Kristen Hagen**
Haukeland University Hospital, OCD-team, 5021 Bergen, Norway
Molde Hospital, Molde, Norway

**Stian Solem**
Haukeland University Hospital, OCD-team, 5021 Bergen, Norway
Department of Psychology, Norwegian University of Science and Technology, Trondheim, Norway

**Odile A. van den Heuvel**
Haukeland University Hospital, OCD-team, 5021 Bergen, Norway
Department of Psychiatry and Department of Anatomy and Neurosciences, VU university medical center (VUmc), Amsterdam, The Netherlands

**Lars-Göran Öst**
Haukeland University Hospital, OCD-team, 5021 Bergen, Norway

Department of Psychology, Stockholm University, Stockholm, Sweden

**Thröstur Björgvinsson and Kerry J. Ressler**
McLean Hospital, Belmont, MA, USA
Harvard Medical School, Boston, MA, USA

**Svein Haseth**
Nidaros DPS, Division of Psychiatry, St. Olav University Hospital, Trondheim, Norway

**Unn Beate Kristensen**
Oslo University Hospital, Oslo, Norway

**Gunvor Launes**
Sørlandet Sykehus, Kristiansand, Norway

**Arne Strand**
Norwegian OCD-foundation, Ananke, Oslo, Norway

**Bo Bach**
Center of Excellence on Personality Disorder, Psychiatric Research Unit, Region Zealand, Slagelse Psychiatric Hospital, Fælledvej 6, Bygning 3, 4200 Slagelse, Denmark

**Michael B First**
Department of Psychiatry, New York State Psychiatric Institute, Columbia University, New York, NY, USA

**Lu Yuan and Cun-Xian Jia**
Department of Epidemiology, School of Public Health, Shandong University and Shandong University Center for Suicide Prevention Research, Jinan, Shandong, China

**Dong-Fang Wang**
Department of Preventive Medicine, School of Basic Medical Sciences, Shandong University of Traditional Chinese Medicine, Changqing, Jinan, Shandong, China

**Bob Lew**
Department of Social Psychology, Faculty of Human Ecology, Putra University of Malaysia, Serdang, Selangor, Malaysia

**Augustine Osman**
Department of Psychology, One UTSA Circle, The University of Texas at San Antonio, San Antonio, TX, USA

**Lynn McCleary**
Department of Nursing, Brock University, St. Catharines, Canada

**Genevieve N Thompson**
College of Nursing, University of Manitoba, Winnipeg, Canada

**Lorraine Venturato**
Faculty of Nursing, University of Calgary, Calgary, Canada

**Abigail Wickson-Griffiths**
Faculty of Nursing, University of Regina, Regina, Canada

**Paulette Hunter**
Department of Psychology, St. Thomas More College, University of Saskatchewan, Saskatoon, Canada

**Tamara Sussman**
School of Social Work, McGill University, Montreal, Canada

**Sharon Kaasalainen**
School of Nursing, McMaster University, Hamilton, Canada

**Qin Yang, Na Sun, Dandan Li, Yuxin Zhao, Xiaotong Li, Yanhong Gong and Xiaoxv Yin**
School of Public Health, Tongji Medical College, Huazhong University of Science and Technology, 430030 Wuhan, People's Republic of China

**Lei Qiu**
School of Public Health, Tongji Medical College, Huazhong University of Science and Technology, 430030 Wuhan, People's Republic of China
School of Management, Hainan Medical University, Haikou, People's Republic of China

**Chuanzhu Lv**
Department of Emergency, The Second Affiliated Hospital of Hainan Medical University, Haikou 571199, People's Republic of China
Emergency and Trauma College, Hainan Medical University, Haikou 571199, People's Republic of China

**Ang Zhou**
Australian Centre for Precision Health, University of South Australia Cancer Research Institute, Adelaide, SA 5001, Australia

**Anwar Mulugeta**
Australian Centre for Precision Health, University of South Australia Cancer Research Institute, Adelaide, SA 5001, Australia
Department of Pharmacology, School of Medicine, College of Health Science, Addis Ababa University, Addis Ababa, Ethiopia

**Elina Hyppönen**
Australian Centre for Precision Health, University of South Australia Cancer Research Institute, Adelaide, SA 5001, Australia

Population, Policy and Practice, UCL Great Ormond Street Institute of Child Health, London, UK

**Christine Power**
Population, Policy and Practice, UCL Great Ormond Street Institute of Child Health, London, UK

**J. Kalagi and G. Juckel**
Department of Psychiatry, Psychotherapy and Preventive Medicine, LWL University Hospital, Ruhr University Bochum, Alexandrinenstr. 1-3, 44791 Bochum, Germany

**J. Gather**
Department of Psychiatry, Psychotherapy and Preventive Medicine, LWL University Hospital, Ruhr University Bochum, Alexandrinenstr. 1-3, 44791 Bochum, Germany
Institute for Medical Ethics and History of Medicine, Ruhr University Bochum, Markstr. 258a, 44799 Bochum, Germany

**I. Otte and J. Vollmann**
Institute for Medical Ethics and History of Medicine, Ruhr University Bochum, Markstr. 258a, 44799 Bochum, Germany

**Dana Tzur Bitan and Ariella Grossman Giron**
Department of Behavioral Sciences, Ariel University, Ramat Hagolan 65th st, 4070000 Ariel, Israel
Shalvata Mental Health Center, 13th Alyat Hanoar st, 45100 Hod Hasharon, Israel

**Gady Alon, Shlomo Mendlovic, Yuval Bloch and Aviv Segev**
Shalvata Mental Health Center, 13th Alyat Hanoar st, Hod Hasharon, Israel
Sackler School of Medicine, Tel Aviv University, 69978 Tel Aviv, Israel

**Amanda Kenny, Boris Bizumic and Kathleen M. Griffiths**
Research School of Psychology, The Australian National University, Building 39 Science Road, Canberra, ACT 2601, Australia

**Xiongfeng Pan, Zhipeng Wang, Xiaoli Wu and Aizhong Liu**
Department of Epidemiology and Health Statistics, Xiangya School of Public Health, Central South University, Changsha, China

**Shi Wu Wen**
Department of Obstetrics and Gynaecology, University of Ottawa, Ottawa, ON, Canada
Ottawa Hospital Research Institute, Ottawa, ON, Canada

**Qi Yuan, Esmond Seow, Edimansyah Abdin, Boon Yiang Chua, Hui Lin Ong, Ellaisha Samari, Siow Ann Chong and Mythily Subramaniam**
Research Division, Institute of Mental Health, Singapore, Singapore

**Kristine Rømer Thomsen, Mette Buhl Callesen and Mads Uffe Pedersen**
Centre for Alcohol and Drug Research, School of Business and Social Sciences, University of Aarhus, Bartholins Allé 10, Building 1322, 2. Floor, Aarhus C, Denmark

**Timo Lehmann Kvamme**
Centre for Alcohol and Drug Research, School of Business and Social Sciences, University of Aarhus, Bartholins Allé 10, Building 1322, 2. Floor, Aarhus C, Denmark
Department of Psychiatry, University of Cambridge, Cambridge, UK
Center of Functionally Integrative Neuroscience, MINDLab, Aarhus University, Aarhus C, Denmark

**Nuria Doñamayor**
Department of Psychiatry, University of Cambridge, Cambridge, UK
Department of Psychiatry and Psychotherapy, Charité – Universitätsmedizin Berlin, Berlin, Germany

**Valerie Voon**
Department of Psychiatry, University of Cambridge, Cambridge, UK
Behavioural and Clinical Neurosciences Institute, University of Cambridge, Cambridge, UK
NIHR Biomedical Research Council, University of Cambridge, Cambridge, UK

**Mads Jensen**
Center of Functionally Integrative Neuroscience, MINDLab, Aarhus University, Aarhus C, Denmark

**N. F. Hempler, R. A. S. Pals, L. Pedersbæk and P. DeCosta**
Diabetes Management Research, Steno Diabetes Center Copenhagen, Niels Steensens Vej 6, 2820 Gentofte, Denmark

**Jesutofunmi Aworinde and Gemma Lewis**
Division of Psychiatry, University College London, 6th Floor, Maple House, 149 Tottenham Court Road, London W1T 7NF, UK

**Nomi Werbeloff, Gill Livingston and Andrew Sommerlad**
Division of Psychiatry, University College London, 6th Floor, Maple House, 149 Tottenham Court Road, London W1T 7NF, UK
Camden and Islington NHS Foundation Trust, London, UK

**Felix Akpojene Ogbo, Sruthi Mathsyaraja, Rajeendra Kashyap Koti, Janette Perz and Andrew Page**
Translational Health Research Institute (THRI), School of Medicine, Western Sydney University, Locked Bag 1797, Penrith, NSW 2571, Australia

**Julia Luise Magaard**
Department of Medical Psychology, University Medical Center Hamburg-Eppendorf, Hamburg, Germany

**Anna Levke Brütt**
Department of Medical Psychology, University Medical Center Hamburg-Eppendorf, Hamburg, Germany
Department of Health Services Research, School of Medicine and Health Sciences, Carl von Ossietzky University Oldenburg, Oldenburg, Germany

**Bernd Löwe and Sebastian Kohlmann**
Department of Psychosomatic Medicine and Psychotherapy, University Medical Center Hamburg-Eppendorf, Hamburg, Germany

# Index

www.ingramcontent.com/pod-product-compliance
Lightning Source LLC
Chambersburg PA
CBHW080513200326

41458CB00012B/4188